Physiotherapy in Obstetrics and Gynaecology

SECOND EDITION

Edited by

Jill Mantle BA FCSP DipTP
Senior Visiting Fellow, University of East London, London, England, UK

Jeanette Haslam MPhil GradDipPhys MCSP SRP
Senior Visiting Fellow, University of East London, London, England, UK

Sue Barton MSc DipEd MCSP DipTP DipRG&RT DipTHRF SRP
Health Senior Lecturer, School of Health Studies, University of Bradford, England, UK

Foreword by

Professor Linda Cardozo MD FRCOG
Private Practitioner, London, UK

D1581866

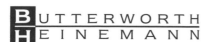
BUTTERWORTH
HEINEMANN

EDINBURGH LONDON NEW YORK OXFORD PHILADELPHIA ST LOUIS SYDNEY TORONTO 2004

BUTTERWORTH-HEINEMANN
An imprint of Elsevier Limited

First edition 1990
Second edition 2004
    Reprinted 2005

ISBN 0 7506 2265 2

British Library Cataloguing in Publication Data
A catalogue record for this book is available from the British Library

Library of Congress Cataloguing in Publication Data
A catalogue record for this book is available from the Library of Congress

Note
Medical knowledge is constantly changing. Standard safety precautions must be followed, but as new research and clinical experience broaden our knowledge, changes in treatment and drug therapy may become necessary or appropriate. Readers are advised to check the most current product information provided by the manufacturer of each drug to be administered to verify the recommended dose, the method and duration of administration, and contraindications. It is the responsibility of the practitioner, relying on experience and knowledge of the patient, to determine dosages and the best treatment for each individual patient. Neither the Publisher nor the author assumes any liability for any injury and/or damage to persons or property arising from this publication.

                                                        The Publisher

The publisher's policy is to use **paper manufactured from sustainable forests**

Printed and bound in China

Contents

Contributors   vii

Foreword to the second edition   ix
Professor Linda Cardozo

Foreword to the first edition   xi
Dame Josephine Barnes

Preface to the second edition   xiii
Jill Mantle

Preface to the first edition   xv
Margaret Polden, Jill Mantle

Introduction   xvii
Jill Mantle

1. Anatomy   1
   Jeanette Haslam

2. Physiology of pregnancy   27
   Jeanette Haslam

3. Physical and physiological changes of labour
   and the puerperium   53
   Jeanette Haslam

4. The antenatal period   93
   Jo Fordyce

5. Relieving the discomforts of pregnancy   141
   Sue Barton

6. Preparation for labour   165
   Sue Barton

7. The postnatal period   205
   Sue Barton

8. The climacteric   249
   Pauline Walsh

9. Common gynaecological conditions   269
   Jeanette Haslam

10. Gynaecological surgery   309
    Teresa Cook

11. Urinary function and dysfunction   333
    Jill Mantle

12. Bowel and anorectal function and
    dysfunction   383
    Jeanette Haslam and Jill Mantle

Appendix 1: Standardisation of terminology of lower
urinary tract function   427

Appendix 2: Standardisation of terminology of lower
urinary tract function   449

Index   473

Contributors

Sue Barton MSc DipEd MCSP DipTP DipRG&RT DipTHRF SRP
Health Senior Lecturer, School of Health Studies, University of Bradford, England, UK

Teresa Cook GradDipPhys MCSP SRP
Clinical Specialist, Physiotherapist in Women's Health, James Paget Hospital, Great Yarmouth, Norfolk, England, UK

Jo Fordyce GradDipPhys MCSP SRP
Clinical Specialist, Physiotherapist in Women's Health, St George's Hospital, London, England, UK

Jeanette Haslam MPhil GradDipPhys MCSP SRP
Senior Visiting Fellow, University of East London, London, England, UK

Jill Mantle BA FCSP DipTP
Senior Visiting Fellow, University of East London, London, England, UK

Pauline Walsh MCSP SRP
Clinical Specialist Physiotherapist in Obstetrics and Gynaecology, Mount Alvernia Hospital, Guildford, Surrey, England, UK; Royal Surrey County Hospital NHS Trust, Guildford, Surrey, England, UK

Foreword to the second edition

Since 1995 it has been a great pleasure, privilege and honour to serve as the President of the Association of Chartered Physiotherapists in Women's Health (ACPWH). This has enabled me to attend council meetings as well as the Annual Meeting of the Association on several occasions. The ACPWH is an active, enthusiastic group of specialist physiotherapists who promote the importance of physiotherapy in all aspects of obstetrics and gynaecology.

It is well recognised that antenatal education facilitates easier childbirth and a faster return to 'normal' in the post partum period. However many under estimate the value of physiotherapy throughout a woman's life in the promotion of good health by preventing or ameliorating a wide range of physical problems. For example urinary incontinence and pelvic organ prolapse are exceedingly common with a life-time risk of approximately 11% requiring surgery for one or other of these conditions, a third of whom will require re-operation. Thus a huge proportion of the adult female population suffer from symptoms which, although not life threatening, undoubtedly significantly impair quality of life and lead to embarrassment and inability to perform routine activities of daily living. Approximately two thirds of women with urinary incontinence will benefit from physiotherapy and, whilst this may not provide a complete cure, it is likely to avoid or defer the need for surgery until a suitable time e.g. when a woman's family is complete and she is fit and willing to undergo surgical intervention.

All women with lower urinary tract problems and pelvic organ prolapse benefit from the advice of a physiotherapist who can not only provide the appropriate exercises to strengthen the pelvic floor but can advise on life style interventions in order to improve symptoms and help individual women to lead a normal lifestyle. Unfortunately, at present, there are not enough physiotherapists trained in women's health to take care of the needs of all those women who would benefit from such advice and treatment.

The second edition of *Physiotherapy in Obstetrics and Gynaecology* is an excellent book written by dedicated women's health physiotherapists specifically for physiotherapists. However it will also be of use to all midwives, health visitors, obstetricians and gynaecologists and others who are involved in the care of women before, during and after pregnancy and who share the management of women with the common sequelae of childbearing. The text has been written in an 'easy to read' style and is well referenced and will, I am sure, be used as a reference book for many of us dealing with problems related to women's health. I am sure that this book will continue to be the authoritative work on the subject until the third edition of *Physiotherapy in Obstetrics and Gynaecology* is published!

Linda Cardozo, 2004

Foreword to the first edition

The physiotherapist has been an important member of the maternity team for years, in fact since at least 1912. Then, the physiotherapist Minnie Randall together with the obstetrician J. S. Fairbairn at St. Thomas' Hospital developed special interests in the management of pregnancy, labour and the puerperium. Later the scope was extended to gynaecological cases.

Out of this has grown the Association of Chartered Physiotherapists in Obstetrics and Gynaecology. Its special contribution was recognised in the joint statement by the Royal College of Midwives, the Health Visitors' Association and the Chartered Society of Physiotherapy.

This recognition makes this new book especially timely. The training of a physiotherapist does not necessarily include the role in obstetrics and gynaecology. The book is a definitive statement. It therefore includes chapters on all aspects of the physiotherapist's role in obstetrics and gynaecology, from the basic sciences through to incontinence, a symptom which causes great distress and restriction of life to so many women and one which can so often be helped by the skills of the physiotherapist.

On a personal note I am happy to say that throughout my professional life in obstetrics and gynaecology I was always conscious of the contribution physiotherapists could bring to our work. I was privileged to know and to work with Helen Heardman who did so much to promote preparation for childbirth and the relief of discomfort. The obstetric physiotherapist was always a valued member of the team attending teaching rounds and of course conducting antenatal classes for mothers, and fathers. They have a special role which cannot be properly undertaken by others not trained in their methods.

I am therefore very glad to welcome this book with all the care and effort that has gone into its production, not least in the excellent illustrations and the bibliography which follows each chapter and which makes it an excellent work of reference.

The book has a scope and interest far beyond its authors' intention.

Dame Josephine Barnes, 1990

Preface to the second edition

It gave Margie and me great pleasure to receive many assurances from colleagues that our 'off-spring' was proving useful. As we travelled the world we were encouraged by the sight of well-thumbed copies in departments and libraries, and we heard our book referred to as 'the bible' more than once.

When in 1994 the publishers first mooted the desirability of a second edition, we were exercised as to what to recommend and advise, especially with respect to physiotherapy in obstetrics. The publication in 1993 by the Department of Health (DoH) of the report of the Expert Maternity Group, entitled *Changing childbirth*, was followed by a very unsettled period within the UK Maternity Services as a variety of new service models were tried. We were dismayed by the absence of any mention within the report of the obstetric physiotherapist and, in the light of an acute shortage of midwives, we considered the emphasis upon each pregnant woman having a named midwife to support her throughout each entire childbearing episode to be unrealistic.

By 1997, publisher pressure mounted, the book was still selling well but Butterworth Heinemann wanted an upgrade and we were increasingly aware of progressions in knowledge, so once again we set to work in Margie's kitchen. Receiving the news of Margie's tragic and untimely death on Monday the 16th March 1998 is etched into the memory bank of many. All writing ceased and the second edition went on hold. It has been gradually resurrected with encouragement from Margie's husband, Martin and the family, and from colleagues. It has only been actually realised with an enormous amount of help from colleagues, in particular Jeanette Haslam, Sue Barton, Jo Fordyce, Pauline Walsh, Teresa Cook, Elizabeth Crothers, Morag Thow, Margaret Brownlee, and Deborah Fry, but also there are many others who responded to our queries. To all these people I offer my heartfelt thanks. May this edition enable the memory of Margie to continue to inspire colleagues to holistic, up-to-date best practice in this specialty.

Jill Mantle   London, 2004

Reference

DoH 1993 Changing childbirth, Part 1 Report of the Expert Maternity Group. HMSO, London.

Preface to the first edition

This book was conceived in a coach travelling between Bristol and Bath, and the first cell divisions occurred in the humid atmosphere of the Roman Baths and the Regency Pump Room. Implantation of the developing morula took place in the offices of Heinemann Medical Books, then in London, and the pregnancy was subsequently confirmed.

The gestation proved to be much longer than originally anticipated. About the length of two elephant's pregnancies, and a period we will certainly never forget! The physical stresses – writer's cramp, aching bottoms and backs – have been great, but in no way did they approach the psychological and emotional traumas to ourselves and our nearest and dearest. We have used every known coping strategy and invented several more to cope with the labour necessary to give birth.

Now in the postpartum period, we are, like all new mothers, relieved but apprehensive as to how our offspring will be received. We very much hope that it will prove to be a useful and valued contribution to society.

We would like to thank all those who gave their time so freely to answer the numerous queries that arose in our efforts to make sure that information in the book is accurate and up to date; our thanks also to Shona Grant, our illustrator, for her patience, Ricky Hoole, Margaret Nokes and Sarah Polden, our long-suffering typists, and most particularly, our dear husbands who have endured our raised catecholamine levels over an extended period. They have suffered, like many pregnant fathers, and are undoubtedly hoping that life will now 'get back to normal' – whatever that might mean.

Margaret Polden, Jill Mantle   London, 1990

Introduction

Jill Mantle

At the start of a new edition, it is inspiring to review briefly the history of physiotherapists' involvement in obstetrics and gynaecology. It is also prudent to take stock of relevant changes in policy and practice within society and the National Health Service since the publication of the first edition, and to reconsider the purpose of this book and the important issues for physiotherapists in the specialty now.

In the late nineteenth century the physiotherapy, nursing and midwifery professions shared a common rootstock. In the UK, educating more than just a few privileged women was a new philosophy, and formal and accredited training for occupations thought suitable for women, such as nursing and midwifery, was at best elementary. In addition, professional bodies were only just being formed. Women who wanted to work outside the home and were inclined to care for people took whatever training was offered, first in one aspect of caring, then in another.

In 1886, Dame Rosalind Paget, a nursing sister at the London Hospital who was also a midwife, joined the Midwives Institute, which later became the Royal College of Midwives (RCM). In 1902 she was involved in the formation of the Central Midwives Board and appears as number two on their list of members. Also in 1886 Dame Rosalind became interested in a new therapy – Swedish massage. She, and others like her, underwent training and then returned to their hospitals to teach the techniques to their colleagues. However, through her insistence on high standards and her anxiety that properly trained, reputable masseuses

should not be confused with those of 'ill repute', she became one of the founding members of the Society of Masseuses and in 1895 became its first Chairman of Council. Over the years the group prospered, extended its focus to include remedial exercise and electrotherapy, and developed into the Chartered Society of Physiotherapy (CSP). Dame Rosalind held membership number one.

Early in the twentieth century, Miss Minnie Randell OBE, a sister at St Thomas's Hospital London, had also trained both as a nurse and a midwife. She became interested in both the massage and the remedial exercises being propounded by the Swede, Per Henrik Ling. She was appointed as Sister-in-Charge and then Principal of the School of Massage and Medical Gymnastics at St Thomas' Hospital. In 1912, J. S. Fairbairn, a leading consultant obstetrician at St Thomas' who believed in 'preventive obstetrics', asked Miss Randell to devise a system of 'bed exercises' for his postnatal mothers. Because newly delivered women remained in bed for about 3 weeks at that time, many problems that are rarely seen today were rife. The exercises were designed to aid postnatal physical recovery and to train women to rest through relaxation. Thus Miss Randell was one of the first to bring the principles of physiotherapy to obstetrics. Later, Miss Randell turned her attention to antenatal instruction, once again urged on by Mr Fairbairn, who thought that more should be done preventatively to help pregnant women (Fairbairn 1923). She was greatly influenced by Dr Kathleen Vaughan who had noticed, while working in Kashmir, that women who had a sedentary, confined and inactive lifestyle frequently had more difficult labours and deliveries than the boat-women and peasants who led much more active lives. Dr Vaughan believed that heredity was not the only factor that determined the shape of the pelvis and the mobility of its joints and those of the lower spine – the way women used their bodies in their everyday lives was also an important influence. Apart from incorporating squatting into her antenatal programme as a preparation for labour, Miss Randell introduced many of the pelvic- and lumbar-spine-mobilising exercises which were based on the movements made by Kashmiri boat-women, and encouraged women to adopt different positions of comfort in labour.

In 1936 Heinemann published a book entitled *Maternity and Postoperative Exercises*; written by Margaret Morris, an ex-ballet dancer, who had been one of Miss Rendell's students. It is of interest that, in it, women in the puerperium were encouraged to practise repeated 'pelvic floor tensing', trying 'to invert the sphincters … until it becomes habitual'; it was recommended that this be performed to the strains of Schubert's waltzes 16, no. 2 (Morris 1936). In her book, *Fearless Childbirth* published by Churchill in 1948, Minnie Randell explained that the purpose of the tensing was to prevent and treat symptoms of urine leakage and prolapse (Randell 1948). It is important to appreciate that in the early part of the twentieth century far fewer books were published than today and women authors were rare. Yet these pioneers started a tradition that has continued, and has promoted and enriched the specialty down the years.

In the 1930s Dr Grantly Dick-Read was a further notable source of influence on Miss Randell with his theory of the fear–tension–pain cycle in labour. Fearful women who expected to feel pain became tense as labour began. This led to tension in their minds and, according to Grantly Dick-Read, in their cervices too. This, he claimed, gave rise to more pain, which in turn increased their fear. He encouraged his labouring mothers to relax and breathe deeply through their contractions, a system which Miss Randell built into her antenatal classes. In the late 1930s, Margaret Morris, suggested to Miss Randell that women should actually rehearse labour antenatally in the same way that dancers rehearse for a performance.

It was another physiotherapist, Helen Heardman, who in the 1940s drew together the threads of relaxation, breathing and education for childbirth into antenatal preparatory courses for labour and parenthood (Heardman 1948). Before her tragic death in 1949, she was instrumental in gathering together the group of like-minded physiotherapists from around the UK who formed the Obstetric Physiotherapist's Association in 1948. It was one of the first special interest groups of the CSP, and in 1961 became the Obstetric Association of Chartered Physiotherapists. Antenatal classes mushroomed through the 1950s, often taken entirely by so called 'obstetric physiotherapists', and women were routinely offered postnatal exercise sessions and advice postnatally during their 5–7-day hospital stay. Midwives were invited to contribute and gradually have become the dominant profession in this aspect of care.

In the 50 and more years since then, much has changed in obstetric physiotherapy, midwifery and obstetrics, and many dedicated physiotherapists have added their expertise to the specialty. In 1963 Laura Mitchell introduced her method of relaxation, which has been used extensively ever since. In 1977 Dorothy Mandelstam was invited to be the first non-medical member of the International Continence Society and her name will always be associated with the ending of the taboo on incontinence. Together with Shelia Harrison, she worked tirelessly through the 1970s to encourage OACP members to expand the field to include gynaecology and the treatment of incontinence. In 1978 the Association adopted the title of the Association of Chartered Physiotherapists in Obstetrics and Gynaecology (ACPOG). In the late 1980s there was further international pressure to think holistically of women's health issues, which led to another change of title in 1994 to the Association of Chartered Physiotherapists in Women's Health (ACPWH) and to physiotherapists employed in the field being called 'women's health physiotherapists'.

The Association is one of the largest clinical interest groups in the CSP and, down the years, it has played the lead role in developing postregistration courses for physiotherapists wishing to specialise in the field. It is regrettable that, despite the fact that half the UK population is female and childbearing is the norm for the majority, the basic physiotherapy training contains very little specific material to prepare physiotherapists to assist women in pregnancy and the puerperium. Neither does it enable them to take informed account of the effects of childbearing when treating patients with pathologies. There is also a deficit in basic training regarding the promotion of continence and the treatment of incontinence. This is largely due to the fact that obstetric, gynaecological and urogynaecological placements for students are optional and there are very few university staff with expert knowledge of these areas. It is also true that few physiotherapy managers have in-depth specialist knowledge or experience of the specialty. Consequently it has fallen to the specific interest group to provide appropriate training and this responsibility it has faithfully discharged for more than half a century, often with tutors giving their time gratis. Today there are courses accredited and run by universities and shorter courses organised by ACPWH and by individuals – see contact details at the end of the chapter. Fortunately it is now more widely recognised by other health professionals that specialist physiotherapists are to be preferred throughout obstetrics, gynaecology and urogynaecology.

This book was designed to assist the following categories:

- physiotherapy students making their first contact with this field or whose training has failed to include needed information
- newly qualified physiotherapists on obstetric and gynaecological rotations
- physiotherapists embarking on relevant specialist postregistration training
- physiotherapists who are actively involved in the specialty (as a resource book).

The Association is fortunate to count among its members, both past and present, many women who have reached the top of their profession as specialist clinicians, educators, authors and researchers. They have gained the respect, not only of their colleagues, but also of the members of the midwifery, health visitor and medical professions. This mutual respect among individuals led ACPOG into increasing dialogue and collaboration with the RCM and the Health Visitors' Association (HVA). The result was the publication of the following statement, negotiated by ACPOG with the RCM and the HVA, and endorsed by the CSP in March 1987, and further confirmed in 1994, entitled *Working Together in Psychophysical Preparation for Childbirth*. This statement was endorsed by the CSP at its Council meeting on 11 March 1987. It was revised in 1994 and is published by CSP as Information paper no. PA13:

> Midwives, Health Visitors and Obstetric Physiotherapists all have important specialist contributions to make in preparation for childbirth and parenthood. This contact with parents also provides a valuable opportunity for more general health promotion, health education and preventative medicine. In the delivery of such a service in a locality, it is important that the professional team demonstrates a flexible approach and takes account of the views and needs of all parents.

The midwife
The role of the midwife is that of the practitioner of normal midwifery, caring for the woman within the hospital and community throughout the continuum of pregnancy, childbirth and the puerperium. She has an important contribution to make in health education, counselling and support. In this context her aim is to facilitate the realization of the woman's needs, discuss expectations and air anxieties. She has the responsibility of monitoring the woman's physical, psychological and social wellbeing and is in a unique position to be able to correlate parent education with midwifery care.

The health visitor
The role of the Health Visitor in this field is to offer advice to the parents-to-be on the many health, psychological and social implications of becoming parents and the development of the child. She is in a very special position in the family scene to inform them of the services available and encourage them to use them. The health visitor should always have a participatory role within the team to provide continuity of care to the family.

The obstetric physiotherapist
The role of the Obstetric Physiotherapist is to promote health throughout the childbearing

period and to help the woman adjust advantageously to the physical and psychological changes of pregnancy and the post-natal period so that the stresses of childbearing are minimised. Antenatally and post-natally she advises on physical activity associated with both work and leisure and is a specialist in selecting and teaching appropriate exercises to gain and/or maintain fitness including pelvic floor education. Where necessary she gives specialised treatment e.g. therapeutic ultrasound post-natally to alleviate perineal discomfort. She also assesses and treats musclo-skeletal problems such as backache and pelvic floor muscle weakness. In addition she is a skilled teacher of effective relaxation, breathing awareness and positioning and thus helps the woman to prepare for labour.

Liaison

In order for the services of the team to be of maximum benefit to parents there should be a close liaison between members. Liaison, planning and shared learning sessions help to ensure that techniques and advice are consistent, up to date, related to current practice and meet the needs of parents. This is particularly important when there is no available member of one of the specialist professions. Where this is the case, advice should be sought from the relevant professional body. To enhance continuity of care, new members of the team must always have a period of inter-disciplinary induction. The Midwife, Health Visitor and Obstetric Physiotherapist should be in regular contact and operate an effective referral system.

The aims of parenthood education

- To enable parents to develop a confident and relaxed approach to pregnancy, childbirth and parenthood.
- To enable parents to be aware of the choices in care based on accurate and up to date information.
- To provide continuity of high quality care as previously defined to parents by means of team collaboration and co-operation between professionals including specialised treatments where needed.

- To ensure that appropriate, consistent and clear advice is given with full cognisance of safety factors.
- To promote health and preventative medicine.

Frequently new methods of education in parenthood are introduced e.g. aqua-natal and fitness classes. In such instances it is necessary for guidance to be sought on appropriate exercises from the local obstetric physiotherapist or alternately the Chartered Society of Physiotherapy, and further training may be required.

Since the publication of the first edition of this book in 1990 there have been several government-funded developments of relevance to the specialty and the demand, particularly within the continence services, for specialist physiotherapists has risen steeply. In 1992, the Continence Foundation was established as an umbrella organisation that has provided a focus for all those individuals and organisations concerned to improve the quality and availability of services for sufferers with continence problems. The Foundation, initially government funded but now a charity, seeks to raise awareness, foster education and research, provide information, advice and expertise and influence policy makers and providers.

As the result of much collaboration and lobbying at all levels of government, a great deal has been achieved in 10 years. Conferences and literature, for example, *Guidelines for Continence Care* (ACA 1993), *Incontinence: Causes, Management and Provision of Services* (RCP 1995), raised awareness. This culminated in 1998 in the formation of a multidisciplinary expert working group (including a physiotherapist), by the Parliamentary Under Secretary of State for the Department of Health (DoH). The brief of the working group was to look at continence services and advise on how they might be improved. Their report *Good Practice in Continence Services* was published in 2000, highlighting the problems and making strong recommendations. Although not mandatory, it clearly maps out the envisaged service, the professionals needed to provide the service and the priority groups to be served. The Continence Foundation speedily published two supporting publications *Incontinence: a Challenge and an Opportunity for Primary Care* (CF 2000a) and

Making the Case for Investment in an Integrated Continence Service (CF 2000b) designed to raise awareness of the government guidelines and of the need for better services. In 2001/2 research, jointly funded by the Continence Foundation and the Royal College of Nursing, took place to survey continence service commissioning and provision across England. A further aim of this research was to encourage those engaged in the management of people with incontinence to work towards providing the best possible services (CF 2002).

In 1997 the report of the Pennell Initiative for Women's Health, funded jointly by the government and by the pharmaceutical company Wyeth and chaired by Dame Rennie Fritchie, was published. The objective was to gain an overview of what was known about women's health in later life (45–105+) and to explore the positive steps that could be taken to improve every woman's prospects of living well into a healthy old age. Recommendations were made for policy makers, for health-care professionals, and for women and representative organisations. The recommendations prioritised education, better early preventative care and prompt assessment and treatment of problems as they arose.

The National Service Framework for Older People (DoH 2001) reflects thinking from the Pennell report (1998) and *Good Practice in Continence Services* (DoH 2000) requiring identification of those with osteoporosis and those at risk of falls, and setting the target for an integrated continence service by 2004. In addition, the requirement for evidence-based practice throughout the National Health Service (NHS) has produced a plethora of research, especially related to continence care. 'Quality of life' has become a valued outcome measure. Conservative treatment has returned to favour as the first line of treatment for many with continence problems and consequently specialist physiotherapists have been in greater demand.

Progress in the maternity services has been less positive. In 1993 the DoH published the report of an expert committee entitled *Changing Childbirth*. The committee, which did not include a physiotherapist, was chaired by Julia Cumberlege, Under-Secretary of State for Health. In essence, the recommendations were that the service should ensure that the woman and her partner felt supported and fully informed throughout pregnancy

and were prepared for the birth and the care of the baby. The committee recommended that women should be able to book with a midwife for the entire episode of care, including delivery. There followed a very unsettled period, particularly for midwives, as a variety of service provision models were tested. There was much talk of 'informed choice' for and 'empowerment' of mothers-to-be. The combination of an acute shortage of midwives, most pregnant women also being employed, and the need to hold down NHS costs, made these recommendations virtually impossible to achieve. As two leaders in the midwifery field wrote:

> It is almost impossible for women to have a decent discussion on options ... in a one off visit, with a stranger they may never see again, in a busy maternity clinic ... While we espouse the right of informed choice, we are giving the women of Britain a clear message; it is alright for you to have informed choice so long as you choose hospital birth, caesarean section, epidural anaesthesia and active management.
>
> (Page & Penn 2000)

The concern with the rising caesarean section rate continues with the 2000/1 figure for England and Wales at 21.3% (DoH 2002), and questions are now being asked as to whether women are made aware of the risks and disadvantages of caesarean section. Statistics are now being collected of the number of 'normal births', that is, spontaneous onset, and without regional anaesthesia, augmentation of labour or episiotomy. Data prepared by BirthChoiceUK.com (Dodwell 2002) from DoH statistics for England suggest a patchy picture and a fall in 'normal births' from 60% in 1999 to 41.5% in 2001. The debate regarding home delivery as an option for mothers-to-be is being clouded by the unaffordable insurance premiums being demanded of independent midwives.

Changing Childbirth failed to mention physiotherapists, and did not address the health needs of mothers in the puerperium and beyond. These needs were powerfully exposed by MacArthur et al (1991). Many of the problems highlighted could possibly be prevented by early intervention by a physiotherapist specialising in women's health and, if problems arise, would probably benefit from assessment and treatment by one. To cut costs and to reduce the risk of hospital-based infections being passed to mother or infant, women now are discharged within 1–4 days of delivery into the hands of community midwives. Shortages of midwives, holidays, sickness and urban road congestion make this service problematical. More recently the fact that postnatal women are not happy with their care has been raised (Singhe & Newburn 2000). Women now work through pregnancy, often right up to delivery. Antenatal class attendance is poor, and early discharge after delivery leaves physiotherapists struggling to deliver an effective service, even to those at risk.

Support from research and expert opinion for providing routine input to modern maternity care by women's health physiotherapists is weak; that for prevention, assessment and treatment of conditions like symphysis pubis dysfunction and incontinence is stronger (Fry 1992, Morkved 2001, Reilly et al 2002). Attempts to show benefit from antenatal class attendance has been disappointing. To deal with this uncertainty, a well-constructed body of research is needed. This is unlikely to be of interest to obstetricians and midwives. Women's health physiotherapists are the affected group and those in post must take up the challenge. The collaborative multicentre approach and carefully planned auditing would provide first stage evidence on which to base more detailed studies.

When preparations for the first edition of this book were under way, physiotherapists in urogynaecology felt they were struggling and were undervalued. What a dramatic change has occurred! Now it is those in obstetrics who are constantly being required to argue their case for existence. Hopefully this book will offer support, information and ideas. The motivation of those who have collaborated to produce this second edition is a deep conviction that thorough and effective physiotherapy is essential in this field, and that physiotherapists are the most appropriate professionals to carry it out. There is no better forum for health education, in its widest sense, than is offered by the contact between the whole obstetrical health-care team and women experiencing pregnancy, labour and the puerperium; and the benefits go on and on, into later years. The knowledge so gained radiates out, like the ripples from a stone tossed into a pool, and influences whole families and the wider community. The physiotherapist has a great deal to offer in this field, particularly in terms of fitness, coping with stress, wise back care and the promotion of continence.

We have tried not to perpetuate information that has been stated and restated in other textbooks without proper testing, and have been very careful not to dictate prescriptions for treatment, as careful educated assessment is the key to appropriate therapy. In a book of this size we have had to set limits on what is included and the depth at which it is covered; some knowledge is assumed. We have tried to write clearly and simply, with a minimum of jargon, explaining underlying physiology and the reasoning behind certain approaches. We include references for further reading in each aspect of the subject. Cross-references have been used extensively, but, in places, material has been repeated to avoid an irritating break in the reader's train of thought caused by having to turn to another page. We hope that other physiotherapists will be infected by our enthusiasm for the specialty, and will enjoy, as we do, working with our midwifery, health visitor and medical colleagues, for the benefit of women of all ages.

References

ACA (Association for Continence Advice) 1993 Guidelines for continence care. ACA, London.

CF (Continence Foundation) 2000a Incontinence: a challenge and an opportunity for primary care. Continence Foundation, London.

CF (Continence Foundation) 2000b Making the case for investment in an integrated continence service. Continence Foundation, London.

CF (Continence Foundation) 2002 Good, better and best Practice. Continence Foundation, London.

CSP (Chartered Society of Physiotherapy) 1994 Working together in psychophysical preparation for childbirth. Information paper no. PA13. CSP, London.

Dodwell M 2002 BirthChoiceUK.com: introduction to birth statistics. New Digest, August, p 8–9.

DoH (Department of Health) 1993 Changing childbirth, part 1 and 2. HMSO, London.
DoH (Department of Health) 2000 Good practice in continence services. DoH, London.
DoH (Department of Health) 2001 The national service framework for older people. DoH, London.
DoH (Department of Health) 2002 NHS maternity statistics, England and Wales. 1998–99 to 2000–01. Stationery Office, London.
Fairbairn J S 1923 Introduction. In: Liddiard M The mothercraft manual, Churchill, London.
Fry D 1992 Diastasis symphysis pubis. Journal of the Association of Chartered Physiotherapists in Obstetrics and Gynaecology 71:10–13.
Heardman H 1948 A way to natural childbirth. Livingstone, London.
MacArthur C, Lewis M, Knox E 1991 Health after childbirth. HMSO, London.
Morkved S, Salvesen K A, Scheil B et al 2001 Prevention of urinary incontinence during pregnancy – a randomised controlled trial of primiparous women. International Urogynecology Journal 12:S1.
Morris M 1936 Maternity and postoperative exercises. Heinemann, London, p 109–111.
Page L, Penn Z 2000 Informed choice has become a hollow phrase. New Generation, June: 12.
Pennell Initiative 1998 The Pennell Report on Women's Health 1998. Health Service Management, University of Manchester, Manchester, p 64–65.
Randall M 1948 Fearless childbirth. Churchill, London.
RCP (Royal College of Physicians) 1995 Incontinence: causes, management and provision of services. RCP, London.
Reilly E T C, Freeman R M, Waterfield A E et al 2002 Prevention of post partum stress incontinence in primigravidae with increased bladder neck mobility; a randomised controlled trial of antenatal pelvic floor exercises. British Journal of Obstetrics and Gynaecology 109:68–76.
Singhe D, Newburn M. 2000 Women's experiences of postnatal care. National Childbirth Trust, London.

Further reading

Continence Foundation 2000a Incontinence: a challenge and an opportunity for primary care. Continence Foundation, London.
Continence Foundation 2000b Making the case for investment in an integrated continence service. Continence Foundation, London.
Continence Foundation 2001 Good, better and best practice. Continence Foundation, London.
DoH (Department of Health) 1993 Changing childbirth, part 1 and 2. HMSO, London.
DoH (Department of Health) 2000 Good practice in continence services. DoH, London.
DoH (Department of Health) 2001 The national service framework for older people. DoH, London.
NCT 2002 Evidence based briefing. Caesarean section – Part 1. New Digest Edition 19, National Childbirth Trust, London.

Useful websites

Association of Chartered Physiotherapists in Women's Health – www.womensphysio.com
Association for Continence Advice – www.aca.uk.com
Chartered Society of Physiotherapy – www.csp.org.uk
Continence Foundation – www.continence.foundation.org.uk
International Continence Society – www.ics.org.com
Royal College of Midwives – www.rcm.org.com
Royal College of Obstetricians and Gynaecologists – www.rcog.org.com
Royal College of Physicians – www.rcplondon.ac.uk

Further training for physiotherapists in the specialty

ACPWH c/o Chartered Society of Physiotherapy, 14 Bedford Row, London WC1R 4ED

Chapter 1

Anatomy

Jeanette Haslam

CHAPTER CONTENTS

The pelvis 1
The pelvic floor and muscles of the pelvis 5
The perineum 10
The abdominal muscles 11

The breast 12
The reproductive tract 13
The urinary tract 18
The anorectal region 22

THE PELVIS

The pelvis provides a protective shield for the important pelvic contents; it also supports the trunk, and constitutes the bony part of the mechanism by which the body weight is transferred to the lower limbs in walking, and to the ischial tuberosities in sitting. The pelvis consists of the two innominate bones and the sacrum to which the normally malleable coccyx is attached. The innominates and the sacrum articulate at the symphysis pubis, and at the right and left sacroiliac joints, to form a firm bony ring. They are held together by some of the strongest ligaments in the body (Fig. 1.1). The ring of bone is deeper posteriorly than anteriorly and forms a curved canal. The inlet to this canal is at the level of the sacral promontory and superior aspect of the pubic bones. The outlet is formed by the pubic arch, ischial spines, sacrotuberous ligaments and the coccyx. The enclosed space between the inlet and outlet is called the true pelvis, with the plane of the inlet being at right angles to the plane of the outlet.

The female true pelvis differs from the male in being shallower, having straighter sides, a wider angle between the pubic rami at the symphysis and a proportionately larger pelvic outlet. The ideal or gynaecoid pelvis is recognised by its well-rounded oval inlet and similarly uncluttered outlet (Fig. 1.2c).

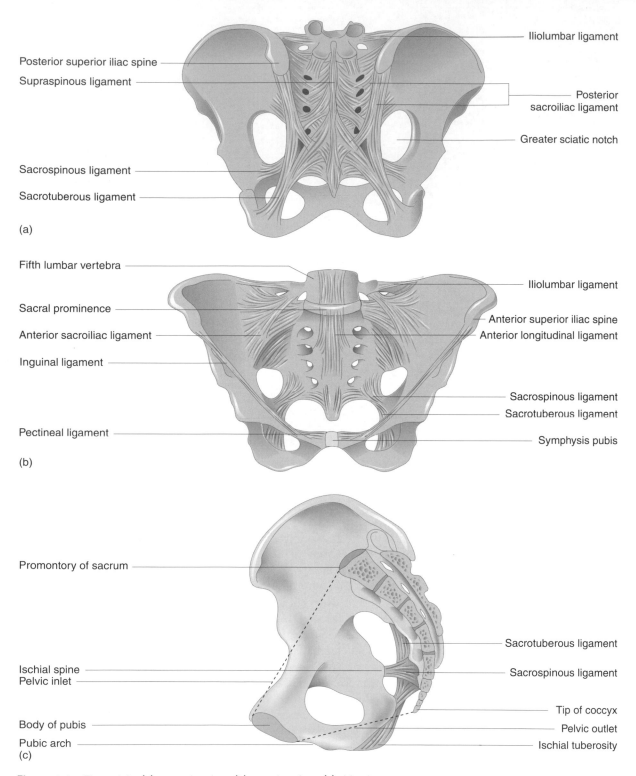

Figure 1.1   The pelvis: (a) posterior view; (b) anterior view; (c) side view.

Table 1.1 The diameters of the gynaecoid true pelvis

	A/P (cm)	Oblique (cm)	Transverse (cm)
Inlet	28	30.5	33
Midcavity	30.5	30.5	30.5
Outlet	33	30.5	28

Figure 1.2 Pelvic inlet, four types.

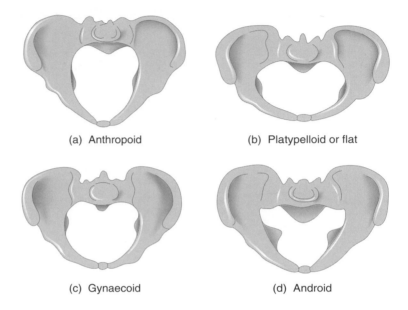

(a) Anthropoid   (b) Platypelloid or flat

(c) Gynaecoid   (d) Android

The inlet has its longest dimension from side to side, whereas at the outlet the longest dimension is anteroposteriorly (Table 1.1). The foetal skull is longest in its anteroposterior dimension. Most commonly in labour the head enters the inlet of the maternal pelvis transversely placed (i.e. long axis to long axis), rotates in mid-cavity and leaves by the outlet with its longest dimension lying anteroposteriorly (see p. 63).

Some other possible pelvic shapes are shown in Figure 1.2. Difficulties can be experienced in childbirth from such adverse features as protuberant ischial spines, a heart-shaped inlet produced by an invasive sacral prominence, or an asymmetrical pelvis (e.g. as a result of rickets or trauma). It is also possible for the inlet or outlet to be too small to allow the foetal head to pass through (cephalopelvic disproportion, see p. 77). It has recently been demonstrated that a narrow suprapubic arch is associated with a consequential prolonged labour and postpartum anal incontinence (Frudinger et al 2002).

The wedge-shaped sacrum is virtually suspended between the innominates by the exceptionally tough interosseous and posterior sacroiliac ligaments, which in the cadaver detach themselves from their periosteal junction rather than tear when the bones are forcibly separated (Meckel 1816, Sashin 1930). However, the ventral sacroiliac ligament is less substantial and is thought to tear during childbirth (Shelly et al 2002). The upper sacrum is stabilised by the illiolumbar ligaments via its attachment to the fourth and fifth lumbar vertebra and the lower sacrum by the

Figure 1.3   Rotation of sacrum under loading.

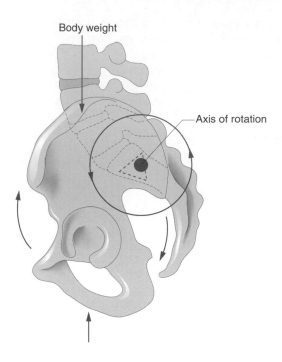

Body weight

Axis of rotation

sacrospinous and sacrotuberous ligaments attachments to the posterior iliac spines and ischial tuberosities. The sacrum supports the weight of the trunk and upper limbs; usually loading of it pushes the sacral prominence down and forward, producing a complex and individual series of changes, rotating the sacrum about a generally transverse axis (Fig. 1.3). This causes the connecting ligaments to tighten, so drawing the undulating and irregular articular sufaces of the ilia into firmer approximation with those of the sacrum. Thus loading of the sacral prominence (e.g. in pregnancy) is often, but not invariably, accompanied by lumbar lordosis and its associated adaptations, hip and knee flexion, thoracic kyphosis and cervical extension with a forward-thrusting chin. It should be noted that in this case it is the sacrum that moves on the ilia and that the pelvis as a whole does not tilt forward to produce the lumbar lordosis. The pelvic tilt may well remain constant (Bullock et al 1987).

The range of movement at the two sacroiliac joints and the symphysis pubis is normally small; however, movement at one joint can affect the other two joints in a variety of ways. During pregnancy, the elevated levels of oestrogen, progesterone and relaxin play a major role in increasing the laxity of the pelvic girdle joints (Ostergaard 1997). The hormonal levels do return to normal in the weeks following childbirth, but the time taken will also be affected by breastfeeding (Prather 2000). By 3 to 6 months postnatal, the pelvic girdle should return to its prepregnant state; it may need external stabilisation during this period (Lee 1999).

As a result of the generalised increased joint laxity in pregnancy it has been shown by sonographic assessment at the upper margin of the symphyseal joint of 49 pregnant women that there was a symphyseal width of up to 6.3 mm with a vertical shift of up to 1.8 mm at 35 weeks of pregnancy (Björklund et al 1999). However, the degree of distension did not correlate with the severity of pelvic pain either during or after childbirth. Previously, an increase has been found in the width of the symphysis pubis from 4 mm to 9 mm in asymptomatic women on X-ray (Abramson et al 1934). Lindsey et al (1988) claimed that separation of less than 1 cm should be considered normal, a greater separation being considered a partial or complete rupture; this may be up to 12 cm. It has been suggested that, where hypermobility, permissive configuration of opposing uneven iliac and sacral surfaces and appropriate stress coincide, one or both ilia may rotate backwards (i.e. the sacrum rotates forwards/sacral nutation) or forwards on the sacrum (i.e. the sacrum rotates backwards/counter-nutation), resulting in tension and pain at the sacroiliac joints or symphysis pubis, or both. However uncomfortable this increased mobility may be in pregnancy, the benefit in parturition of the bony ring of the pelvis having some 'give' is obvious. There is no doubt that the possibility of greater forward rotation and 'shuffling' movements (Grieve 1981) of the sacrum on the ilia provides at delivery a means by which inclination of the ilia and the distance between the posterior portions of the ilia can be changed to increase the transverse diameter of the pelvic outlet. The consequent posterior movement of the apex of the sacrum and the coccyx lengthens the anteroposterior diameter. This occurs particularly in the full squatting position; it has been estimated that the area of the outlet can be increased by as much as 28% in this way (Russell 1969). In squatting, the femora apply pressure to the ischial and pubic rami, thus producing separation outward at the symphysis pubis and an upward and backward rotation of the ilia on the sacrum.

THE PELVIC FLOOR AND MUSCLES OF THE PELVIS

The pelvic floor acts as a dynamic platform that spans the outlet of the pelvis to support the abdominal and pelvic organs; it is composed of muscle, fascia and ligaments. Zacharin (1980) used the term the 'pelvic trampoline' to suggest the characteristics of the pelvic floor. The layers of the pelvic floor from deepest to superficial are as follows:

- The *endopelvic fascia* is a fibromuscular tissue composed of collagen, elastin and smooth muscle fibres. The endopelvic fascia is that which connects the pelvic organs to the pelvic side-walls. Its structure depends on its specific positioning and purpose. The major ligaments are the cardinal (transverse cervical) and uterosacral ligaments. The downwards extensions of the cardinal and uterosacral ligaments are known as the pubocervical and rectovaginal fasciae, which attach the middle third of the vagina to the pelvic side-walls (DeLancey 1994a). The fascia is not under stress when the levator ani muscles are functioning normally.

- The *levator ani* muscles (Fig. 1.4), otherwise known as the pelvic diaphragm or pubovisceralis (pubococcygeus) and iliococcygeus, are

Figure 1.4 The hammock hypothesis. (From DeLancey 1994b, with permission.)

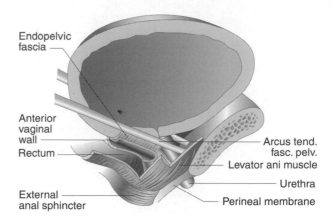

composed of striated muscle fibre. They are covered by fascia on their superior and inferior aspects. The anterior midline cleft in the muscles is known as the urogenital hiatus, through which the urethra, vagina and anorectum pass. The pubococcygeus and ileococcygeus muscles comprise the levator ani and are described below.

- The *perineal membrane* is sometimes called the urogenital diaphragm, or the triangular ligament. It lies inferior to the levator ani at the level of the hymenal ring and attaches the edges of the vagina to the ischio-pubic ramus, provides lateral attachments for the perineal body and assists in the support of the urethra. It is suggested that it has a greater supportive function when the levator ani muscles are relaxed. The external anal sphincter lies posteriorly. Anteriorly, the compressor urethrae and urethrovaginal sphincter are associated with the membrane and act to compress the distal urethra.

- The *external genital muscles* (Fig. 1.5), comprising the ischiocavernosus, bulbocavernosus (also known as bulbospongiosus) and transverse perineal muscles, are thought to be of sexual importance.

- The *external genitalia and skin*.

The chief function of the pelvic floor is support for the abdominal and pelvic viscera, but in addition the pelvic floor muscles (PFMs) contribute to the maintenance of continence of urine and faeces, while also allowing voiding, defaecation, sexual activity and childbirth.

The endopelvic fascia (see p. 5), the levator ani muscles and the perineal membrane, together with the external anal sphincter, are considered to be the supportive layers (DeLancey 1994a). Of these, the levator ani muscles have particular relevance for the physiotherapist. The *pubovisceralis* arises from the posterior aspects of the pubic bones on either side of the symphysis pubis and the anterior part of the arcus tendineus. The more medial portion is known as *pubovaginalis*, which attaches to the lateral side-walls of the vagina, the mid portion the *puborectalis*, which loops around the rectum to form the anorectal angle, and the lateral the *pubococcygeus* proper, which attaches to the anococcygeal raphe and into the

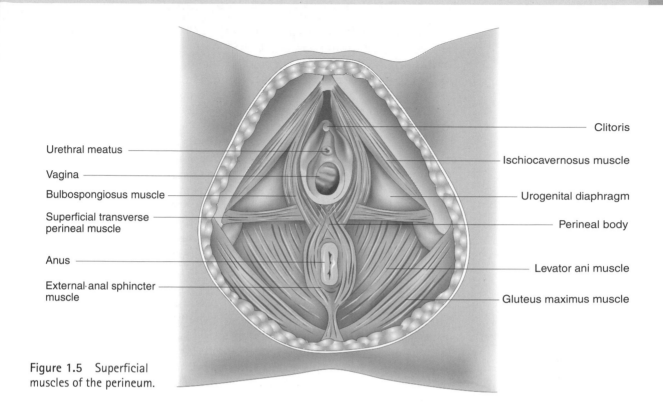

Clitoris

Ischiocavernosus muscle

Urethral meatus

Vagina

Bulbospongiosus muscle

Superficial transverse
perineal muscle

Urogenital diaphragm

Perineal body

Anus

Levator ani muscle

External anal sphincter
muscle

Gluteus maximus muscle

Figure 1.5 Superficial
muscles of the perineum.

anterior and lateral sides of the coccyx. The *iliococcygeus* originates from the arcus tendineus and passes inferiorly to the midline to interdigitate in front of the anococcygeal raphe. At other times the pubovisceral muscles are known as the puboperineus and pubococcygeus (Lawson 1974, Peschers & DeLancey 2002).

Other muscles that are intimately concerned with the PFM are the ischiococcygeus, obturator internus and piriformis. However, none of these muscles has any direct connection with the vagina or anal sphincter. The *ischiococcygeus* (sometimes known as coccygeus) finds its origin on the spine of the ischium and sacrospinous ligaments and travels medially to insert into the lower sacrum and upper coccyx. They both provide pelvic contents support and assist in the stability of the sacroiliac joint. The coccygeus has been largely dismissed in the past as having a passive role. However, its importance is increasingly known as it has been shown that PFM activity can influence the sacroiliac joint (Tichy et al 1999), and this joint may be implicated in urinary symptoms (Dangaria 1998).

The obturator internus and piriformis are the major muscles of the pelvic side-walls. The *obturator internus* finds its origin in the bony margins of the obturator foramen, the obturator membrane and rami of the pubis and ischium to converge into a tendon, leaving the pelvis via the lesser sciatic foramen to be inserted into the greater trochanter of the femur. The *piriformis* helps to form the posterior boundary originating from the anterolateral sacrum, travelling through the greater sciatic foramen and also finding insertion in the greater trochanter.

The arcus tendineus fascia of the pelvis (ATFP) is a linear fascial thickening of the obturator fascia attached anteriorly to the pubic bone and posteriorly to the ischial spine and is believed to be of great importance in the continence mechanism as a connection between the iliococcygeus and the endopelvic fascia. The endopelvic fascia surrounds the vagina and finds its attachment laterally to the ATFP. The endopelvic fascia is also thought to act as a connection between the bladder neck and urethra to the ATFP. As the iliococcygeus also finds its origin at the ATFP, during a contraction of the iliococcygeus, it is proposed that force is transmitted through the endopelvic fascia and anterior vaginal wall to assist in supporting the urethra and bladder neck (Freeman 2002). This 'hammock hypothesis' was first proposed by DeLancey (1994b) (Fig. 1.4).

There have been many names given to the component parts of the levator ani, and the reader must be aware of these when reading the literature. The levator ani were subdivided by Ashton-Miller & DeLancey (2002) into the puboperineus, the pubococcygeus, the puborectalis and the iliococcygeus. The puboperineus is that part arising lateral to the pubic symphysis and inserting into the perineal body in front of the rectum. The pubococcygeus and puborectalis both arise from the pubic bone either side of the midline. The puborectalis has some attachment to the lateral vaginal walls, and inserts partially into the rectum between the internal and external sphincter while other fibres continue to form a sling by passing behind the anorectal junction. The pubococcygeus inserts partially into the anal canal, behind the rectum and into the coccyx. Contraction of these medial fibres pulls the rectum, vagina and urethra forward toward the pubic bones thus compressing their lumens. Furthermore, the loop behind the rectum forms a sling which, by its resting tension, results in the rectum joining the anal canal at a 90° angle. This angle is considered to be a factor in the maintenance of faecal continence.

As the variety of names given to the constituent parts of the levator ani muscles can be confusing, Figure 1.6 has been constructed in an attempt to assist the reader. If both strong and coordinated, the levator ani muscles, enveloped in fascia on both surfaces, form an efficient muscular sling or 'trampoline' giving caudal support and adapting appropriately to posture, position and activity.

The levator ani is a somatic muscle, so has the possibility of voluntary control, and is supplied by the perineal branch of the pudendal nerve (S2–S4). However, recent observations on fresh-frozen female cadavers suggest that the female levator ani muscles are not innervated by the pudendal nerve but rather by an innervation originating from the sacral nerve roots (S3–S5) travelling on the superior surface of the levator ani (Barber et al 2002).

Histochemical and electron microscopic examination of levator ani muscle (Gilpin et al 1989, Gosling et al 1981) showed that it was made up of large diameter type I (slow twitch) and type II (fast twitch) striated muscle fibres, with muscle spindles observed. Type I fibres are highly fatigue resistant and consequently can produce contraction over long periods although the power of the contraction tends to be of a relatively low order. Muscle activity may be recorded by electromyograph (EMG)

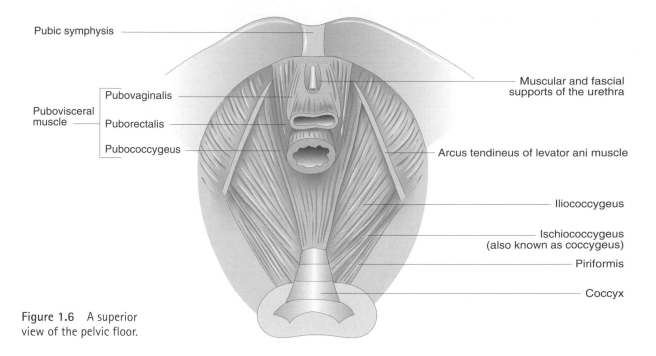

Pubic symphysis

Pubovisceral muscle

Pubovaginalis

Puborectalis

Pubococcygeus

Muscular and fascial supports of the urethra

Arcus tendineus of levator ani muscle

Iliococcygeus

Ischiococcygeus (also known as coccygeus)

Piriformis

Coccyx

Figure 1.6 A superior view of the pelvic floor.

from the levator ani muscle 'at rest' and even in sleep; presumably the type I fibres are responsible for this. By contrast, type II fibres are highly fatiguable but produce a high order of power on contraction. All these facts support the contention that the levator ani muscle is a skeletal muscle adapted to maintain tone over prolonged periods and equipped to resist sudden rises in intra-abdominal pressure, as for example on coughing, sneezing, lifting or running. It has been shown that there is reflex activity such that a fast-acting contraction occurs in the distal third of the urethra, which contributes to the compressive forces of the proximal urethra during raised intra-abdominal pressure (Constantinou & Govan 1982).

It has been reported that there are two subgroups of fast twitch fibres IIa and IIx (previously known as IIb), where IIa are fast twitch oxidative fibres and are relatively more fatigue resistant but produce slightly less power than IIx (fast twitch glycolytic). A reason for lack of standardisation of exercise may be individual differences in response to that exercise, perhaps due to genetic factors (Bruton 2002). Further research needs to be done to determine any more exacting principles regarding optimal load, frequency or repetitions in the exercise prescription to maintain normal function or improve it (Bruton 2002). Table 1.2 shows the percentage of type II fibres found by Gilpin et al (1989) in the pubococcygeus muscle.

The perineal membrane (Fig. 1.4) lies superficially (i.e. inferior to the levator ani muscle) and spans the pelvic outlet anteriorly between the descending ischiopubic rami. It is a fibrous layer and the urethra and vagina pass through it. It is intimately connected with the distal portion of the urethra and its musculature, with the medial side-walls of the vagina and with the perineal body. It is reinforced by some smooth and

Table 1.2 The percentage of
type II fibres found in pubococcygeus muscle

	Type II fibres (%)	
	Anterior pubococcygeus	Posterior pubococcygeus
Asymptomatic women	33	24
Symptomatic women	39	10

striated muscle fibres including the deep transverse perineal muscles (DeLancey 1994a). The perineal body is a central cone-shaped fibromuscular structure which lies just in front of the anus (Fig. 1.5). The cone is about 4.5 cm high and its base, which forms part of the perineum, is approximately 4 cm in diameter. Anteriorly it fuses with the vaginal wall, and some fibres of the bulbospongiosus (Fig. 1.5), the superficial transverse perineal muscles, the perineal membrane and the levator ani muscles insert into it. The perineal body also affords support to the posterior wall of the vagina and thus indirectly to the anterior wall, for in an upright posture one lies against the other. The integrity of the perineal body and its connections have been thought to be of considerable importance in the support-ive role of the pelvic floor. This explains the concern that obstetricians and midwives have had for the welfare of the perineal body in labour, particularly in the second stage when, toward delivery, the pelvic floor stretches considerably and provides a gutter to guide the foetal head towards and down the birth canal. However, some authorities (DeLancey 1994a) are now suggesting that the perineal body 'is relatively unimportant' and that the role of the levator ani muscles is paramount in support.

Attached to erectile tissue either side of the vaginal introitus, the small, thin bulbospongiosus and ischiocavernosus muscles (Fig. 1.5) are inserted into the pubic arch and clitoris. When they contract in sexual activity they pull the clitoris down, compressing its venous drainage and facilitating erection. It is suggested that these muscles and the levator ani, if strong, also have bulk and this enables them to support the vaginal wall as well as provide a sphincteric action to both vagina and urethra, which would favour urethral closure and continence, and increase satisfaction in intercourse for both partners. It is plausible that the blood supply associated with strong muscles and their activity will promote the health of epithelium in the area, encouraging adequate vaginal lubrication, increasing resistance to infection and delaying atrophic changes of ageing.

THE PERINEUM

The external genitalia are shown in Figure 1.7. At either side of the entry to the vagina (introitus) are the Bartholin's glands, which are activated mainly in sexual arousal to produce mucoid secretions; they are normally about the size of a pea. The skin and structures of the perineum are supplied by the pudendal nerve (S2–S4). It has been shown in a study of 224 primagravid women going into spontaneous labour that a short perineum of less than 4 cm resulted in significantly more episiotomies, perineal tears and instrumental deliveries (Rizk & Thomas 2000).

Figure 1.7   External genital organs.

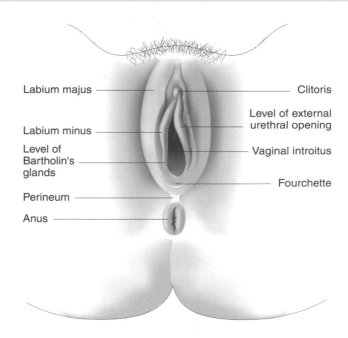

Labium majus

Labium minus

Level of Bartholin's glands

Perineum

Anus

Clitoris

Level of external urethral opening

Vaginal introitus

Fourchette

THE ABDOMINAL MUSCLES

The anterior and lateral abdominal wall is formed by the abdominal muscles (Fig. 1.8). The deepest of the group is the transversus abdominis muscle, which lies internally to the internal and external oblique muscles. From each side these three muscles insert into a broad aponeurosis, which connects with its fellow at the linea alba. This tendinous raphe, which is wider above the umbilicus than below (*Gray's Anatomy* 1989), is formed by decussating aponeurotic fibres. The aponeurosis is reinforced by the two rectus abdominis muscles, which run in sheaths formed in the aponeurosis on either side of the linea alba. Of particular relevance is the fact that the sheaths are elastic longitudinally and less so transversely. Each rectus abdominis muscle has three transverse fibrous intersections, which are firmly attached to the anterior wall of the enclosing sheath. The lowest intersection is about the level of the umbilicus, and the sheaths are deficient posteriorly in the lowest portion.

The oblique and transversus muscles are innervated by the lower six thoracic nerves, and the iliohypogastric and ilioinguinal nerves. The recti are innervated by the lower six thoracic nerves. The abdominal muscles are vascularised by the superior epigastric vessels from above (branches of the internal thoracic or mammary vessels) and the inferior epigastric vessels from below (branches of the external iliac artery and vein).

It is now believed that it is important to recognise that the PFMs are part of an abdominal capsule together with the deeper muscles of the abdomen, spine and diaphragm. These muscles are all affected by respiration and posture and as such it would seem appropriate to consider them as a complete unit when considering muscle training of any one

Figure 1.8 Abdominal muscles dissected to show deeper muscles on the right.

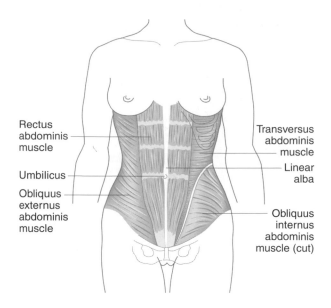

Rectus abdominis muscle

Umbilicus

Obliquus externus abdominis muscle

Transversus abdominis muscle

Linear alba

Obliquus internus abdominis muscle (cut)

part. However, there is still more work necessary to demonstrate all the muscle interactions (Sapsford 2001). The PFM timing of recruitment when there is any rise in intra-abdominal pressure may be considered crucial (Deindl et al 1993) and as such it is essential to consider any other muscle groups that may be involved.

THE BREAST

The female breast (Fig. 1.9) consists of fat and glandular tissue, overlying the pectoralis major muscle. It is roughly circular with an axillary tail extending up and laterally to the axilla. The breasts undergo two bursts of hormonally mediated growth: one in puberty, the second in pregnancy. In addition, many women notice fullness and tenderness directly related to stages in the menstrual cycle.

It has always been believed that the breast has 15–25 secreting lobes each composed of very many lobules. Each lobe has its own duct with an opening on to the nipple area. Just proximal to each opening there is a widened portion in the duct (the lactiferous sinus), which, when milk is being produced, acts as a temporary reservoir. The nipple is said by some to be the origin of 15–25 lactiferous ducts (Tot et al 2002), but others believe that there are far fewer, many of the previously quoted ducts being sebaceous glands (Love 2000). It is not disputed that the nipple has some muscle to form erectile tissue when cold, sexually stimulated or breastfeeding. The surrounding loose, pigmented skin is known as the areola and has modified sweat glands that present as small swellings known as Montgomery's tubercules. They may enlarge during pregnancy and breastfeeding. The nipples are normally slightly raised but in some women they are flat or even inverted. A baby may experience difficulty suckling where the nipples are inverted but with skilled help this can be overcome.

Figure 1.9   The breast.

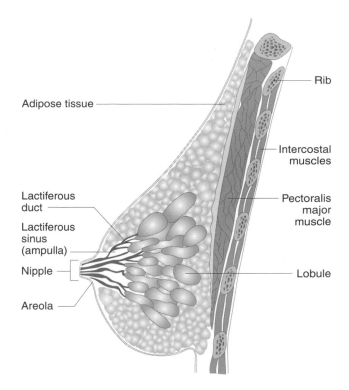

Adipose tissue

Rib

Intercostal
muscles

Lactiferous
duct

Pectoralis
major
muscle

Lactiferous
sinus
(ampulla)

Nipple

Lobule

Areola

Around the time of the menopause or earlier the breast tissue under-goes involution; this results in a decrease in number of lobules and ducts. The fibrous or fatty involution may be in varying combinations (Tot et al 2002). It is the decreasing density of breasts that make them more amenable to mammographic examination. Hormone replacement therapy (HRT) can confound the interpretation of mammograms by increasing the breast tissue density but this is rapidly reversible when HRT is discontinued (Silva & Zurrida 2000).

The blood supply to the breast is via the axillary, internal thoracic and second to fourth intercostal arteries; the breast is drained by accompanying veins. The lymphatic drainage is of some importance because of the possible development of carcinoma in breast tissue and its subsequent dissemination via the lymphatic system. There is an anastomosing network of channels, 95% of which drain to the anterior axillary nodes (Bundred et al 2000), but the medial part of the tissue is drained to the internal thoracic nodes. The nerve supply is from the anterior and lateral cutaneous branches of the fourth to sixth thoracic nerves.

THE REPRODUCTIVE TRACT

The female reproductive tract (Fig. 1.10) consists of highly specialised organs whose structure is elegantly functional: two ovaries and fallopian tubes, the uterus and the vagina.

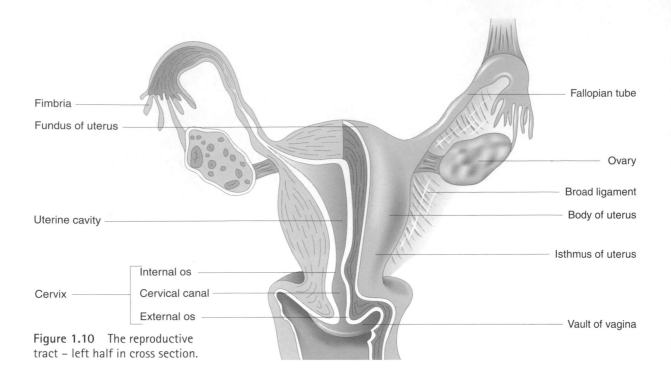

Figure 1.10 The reproductive tract – left half in cross section.

OVARIES

The ovaries produce ova, and also secrete oestrogens and progesterone under the direction of the anterior pituitary gland. In the cortex of these two pinkish-grey structures the size and shape of almonds, lie thousands of primary follicles, each consisting of an immature ovum and a single layer of stroma cells. At birth the ovaries contain about 2 million follicles; by 7 years of age there has been some wastage and weeding out of imperfect cells to reduce this number to about 300 000, a process that continues throughout life. From puberty through the reproductive years, a number of follicles develop but usually only one follicle ripens fully every month.

The ovum in this follicle develops in size and in maturity and the stroma cells differentiate so as to be able to secrete oestrogens and progesterone in increasing amounts. At ovulation the ovum is ejected from the surface of the ovary into the peritoneal cavity, to be directed by the fimbria into the fallopian tube. After ovulation the follicle collapses and undergoes a further phase of development to become a corpus luteum, so called because it is yellow in appearance. It continues to produce oestrogens and progesterone and then, if fertilisation of the ovum does not occur, shrivels after about 10 days. If pregnancy occurs the corpus luteum enlarges and continues to be active for 4 months; it probably then degenerates. Thus, over the years the initially smooth ovarian surface becomes increasingly wrinkled and puckered, and in a woman in her late 40s there are just a few hundred follicles left at most.

FALLOPIAN TUBES

The two fallopian or uterine tubes connect the ovaries with the uterus. The outer end of the tube is funnel shaped and fimbriated; one fimbria is longer than the others and is attached to the ovary. The tentacle-like processes of the fimbria are able to move, apparently stimulated in some way to search for and facilitate the passage of ova into the tube. The proximal end gains access to the uterine cavity either side of the uterine fundus. The tubes themselves are about 10 cm long. A coat of smooth involuntary muscle, consisting of an outer longitudinal layer and an inner circular layer, is responsible for peristaltic waves, which pass towards the uterus; the lining of the tubes is both ciliated and secretory. Thus, once in the tube, an ovum is not only propelled but also nourished as it passes along. It seems likely that conception most commonly occurs in the vicinity of the junction of the distal third and the proximal two-thirds of the relevant tube. The tubal secretions contain the essential ingredients to condition the sperm and ovum for fertilisation, a process known as *capacitation*. An ectopic pregnancy occurs when the fertilised ovum is implanted outside the uterine cavity, usually in the fallopian tube.

UTERUS

The uterus (womb) consists of the fundus, the body, the isthmus (which is no more than 5 mm in depth but develops into the lower segment during pregnancy) and the cervix (neck). The uterus is the shape of an inverted pear and in the nulliparous adult it measures approximately 9 cm long, 6 cm wide and 4 cm thick; it weighs about 50 g. It is a potentially hollow organ with a thick muscular wall (myometrium) lined with lush, highly vascular endothelium (endometrium), whose thickness varies with the menstrual cycle but is approximately 1.5 mm. This mucous membrane is shed at each menstruation, and consists of columnar epithelium, connective tissue and many tube-like uterine glands. After implantation of the ovum, the endometrium is called the *decidua* because it is shed following delivery. It is a rich source of prostaglandins.

The muscle fibres of the myometrium are smooth and involuntary, swathing the fundus and body and encircling the isthmus (Fig. 1.11). These fibres manifest unique properties in pregnancy and in labour. In pregnancy they grow and stretch to accommodate the foetus. In labour they systematically contract and relax, relaxing each time to a length just less than they were before. This shortening is called *retraction* and it is the means by which the uterine cavity becomes progressively smaller and the foetus is expelled. The fibres are supported on a collagenous connective-tissue base. The body of the uterus lies against the superior surface of the bladder and moves as the bladder fills and empties.

Congenital malformations of the uterus occur, resulting for example in the uterus being in two separate halves to a greater or lesser extent (bicornuate uterus). For some individuals this may become evident only in pregnancy or labour, whereas for others it may be considered to be the reason for infertility. There has been a recent case reported in which a woman with a uterus didelphys (in which bilateral müllerian ducts develop side by side rather than fusing) delivered twins successfully (Nohara et al 2003). Twin one was delivered by caesarean section at 25 weeks of pregnancy with a

Figure 1.11 Diagrammatic representation of the muscle fibres of the uterus.

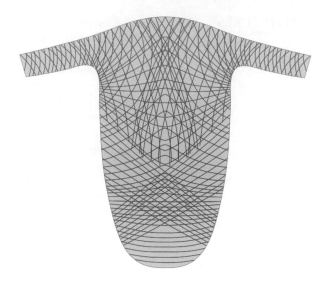

spontaneous delivery of the second twin at 35 weeks of pregnancy; they were later discharged without complications.

The cervix or neck of the womb forms a fusiform or spindle-shaped canal at the junction of the main body of the uterus with the vagina. It consists chiefly of fibrous, collagenous and elastic connective tissue, but contains some circularly disposed muscle fibres (10%) in the proximal part or internal os. The distal two-thirds protrudes into and forms the vault of the vagina – the lowest portion is called the *external os*. The canal is lined with columnar epithelium which produces mucoid secretions. At the external os there is a change to squamous epithelium, which is continuous with the lining of the vagina. The mucoid secretions from the cervix moisten the lower part of the genital tract, and their downward movement, together with the constrictive nature of the cervix, acts as a deterrent to rising infection.

Following conception there are dramatic changes in vascularity, and consequently in the colour and texture of the cervix, and this can be used in the diagnosis of pregnancy. Until recently the cervix was credited with a largely passive role in childbearing, simply being dilated in labour in response to uterine forces. However, it is now recognised that a very active 'ripening' process occurs.

VAGINA

The vagina is about 7.5 cm long and passes upwards and backwards, parallel with the pelvic floor, towards the rectum from its opening on the perineum. Most commonly it meets the longest axis of the uterus at about 90°. The vagina connects with the uterus via the cervix, which projects into its vault. The vagina is a highly elastic channel capable of considerable distension. Within its wall is a layer of smooth muscle, the fibres of which are placed both longitudinally and circularly, and the lining is of stratified squamous epithelium. The vagina is positioned posteriorly to the urethra and the base of the bladder, and anteriorly to the rectum. The urethra is embedded in the anterior vaginal wall and is therefore vulnerable to trauma during childbirth, pelvic surgery and even occasionally during sexual intercourse. There are no glands in the vagina so the vaginal moisture is composed of transudate, which seeps through the vaginal epithelium together with mucus from cervical glands and some secretion from the uterine endometrium. It should be noted that there is direct access for infection from the atmosphere to the abdominal cavity via the female genital tract. The mucoid and serous exudates from the endometrium, cervix and through the vaginal wall have a significant role in opposing any upward tracking of infection by their gravitational downward movement, and by their acidity (pH 4), which prevents the multiplication of most pathogens. Infections of the vagina can spread to the urethra (urethritis) and bladder (cystitis), or to the uterus (endometritis) and so to the tubes (salpingitis), or to the peritoneal cavity (peritonitis).

CIRCULATION AND NERVE SUPPLY

The true pelvis is a highly vascular area. The arterial blood supply to the female reproductive tract is via the left and right internal iliac arteries; branches supply the ovaries, the uterine tubes, the uterus and vagina. There is considerable overlap between these arteries so that where bleeding occurs it may well be considerable and difficult to control. The uterine arteries develop greatly in pregnancy to serve the enlarging uterus and placenta. There is a highly developed lymphatic system with many nodes within the pelvic cavity, apparently providing a good defence to infection but unfortunately facilitating the spread of carcinoma. The veins return blood via the internal iliac vessels and so to the inferior vena cava. The uterine muscle is innervated by the autonomic nervous system via the pelvic plexuses, and both parasympathetic (S2–S4) and sympathetic (T10–L1) efferents are found. Sensory nerve endings are more numerous in the cervix and the isthmus (which develops in pregnancy into the lower uterine segment) than in the rest of the uterus, and pain impulses such as those arising from labour are relayed via the hypogastric plexus to enter the spinal cord through the posterior roots of T10–L1. The cervix is sensitive to stretch whereas the isthmus is sensitive to both pressure and stretch. Sensation from the perineum is conveyed via the pudendal nerve to the spinal cord (S2–S4).

SUSPENSORY LIGAMENTS

The female reproductive tract is loosely suspended across the midline of the true pelvis, enfolded within the double layer of the slack, flimsy broad ligament, which is attached either side to the lateral inner surface of the pelvis. The ovaries are attached to the posterior layer of this ligament, and to the posterior aspect of the uterus by a fibromuscular cord. The uterine round ligaments are attached anteriorly to either side of the fundus of the uterus; they are lax, and pass forward via the deep inguinal ring and the inguinal canal to insert into the subcutaneous tissue of the labia majora. The round ligaments help to keep the uterus anteverted and anteflexed (see also p. 283).

Figure 1.12 The ligamentous support of the cervix.

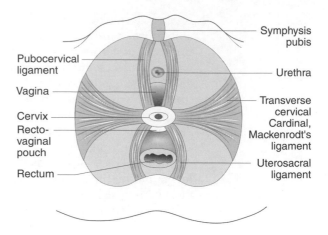

However, both the broad and round ligaments permit considerable movement of the uterus, tubes and ovaries before becoming taut, allowing adaptation to the constantly changing volumes of bladder and rectum. Furthermore, it is probable that hormonal influence enables them to increase in elasticity to adapt to the changing size of the pregnant uterus as it gradually rises to become a temporary abdominal organ.

The lower fringe of the connective tissue of the broad ligament condenses to form the more substantial transverse cervical ligaments also known as the cardinal and Mackenrodt's ligaments – connecting the cervix to the lateral walls of the pelvis (Fig. 1.12). Two bands of connective tissue – the pubocervical fascia – pass anteriorly either side of the neck of the bladder anchoring the cervix to the posterior surface of each pubis. In addition, two moderately strong fibromuscular bands of fascia – the uterosacral ligaments – connect the cervix and the upper part of the vagina to the lower portion of the sacrum. Both the transcervical and uterosacral ligaments contain some smooth muscle fibres and elastic fibres. Thus the cervix is suspended and located by 'guy ropes' on the four aspects; these risk being traumatised in labour. This support is supplemented by the lifting support of the PFMs, which form the base of the pelvic cavity.

THE URINARY TRACT

The urinary system comprises two kidneys, which excrete urine at an average of 1 ml per minute with a range of ½ to 5 ml per minute (Cardozo et al 1993), two ureters, which conduct urine to the bladder where it is stored, and the urethra, which channels urine to the outside of the body.

THE KIDNEY

The kidney is the size of the owner's fist and of a shape so typical that it is used as a descriptive term. The indentation on its medial aspect is called the *hilum*, and here the ureter and renal vein leave and the renal artery enters. The kidneys have a huge blood supply via two branches directly from the aorta, and returning to the inferior vena cava. The kidneys are placed posteriorly in the loin associated with the first lumbar vertebra; the left kidney is a little higher than the right because of the wedge-shaped liver lying superiorly on the right side. The kidney consists of a fibrous capsule, a cortex, medulla, and major and minor calyces or collecting ducts, which channel urine into the pelvis of the kidney and so to the ureter.

THE URETER

Each ureter is about 25 cm long and is a hollow muscular canal about the diameter of a small drinking straw; it is lined with transitional epithelium, as is the whole urinary tract. Contraction in peristaltic waves of the smooth muscle in the wall of the ureter assists the movement of urine down to the bladder – even when a person is supine. As the ureter enters the pelvis it lies in front of the sacroiliac joint, separated from it by the bifurcation of the common iliac artery. At the level of the internal os, it is 1 cm from the cervix and passes through the transverse cervical ligaments. The ureter enters the thick muscular wall of the bladder obliquely at each of the upper corners of the trigone of the bladder about 2 cm away from the urethrovesical junction; this arrangement results in closure of these two orifices and the prevention of reflux of urine when the detrusor muscle of the bladder contracts. However, a high pressure in the bladder may cause reflux and subsequent kidney damage.

THE BLADDER

The bladder is a hollow sac of three layers of smooth muscle, corporately called the *detrusor muscle*, whose fibres are arranged in a complex meshwork. When the detrusor muscle is in its filling phase, it is said to be compliant and acts as a reservoir; when it contracts it becomes a pump. It is lined with transitional epithelium and the outer surface is covered with connective tissue composed of collagen and elastic fibres. The detrusor muscle has outermost muscle fibres lying predominantly longitudinally, an intermediate layer lying obliquely and circular, with an innermost plexiform layer (Wall et al 1993); they are in an ideal arrangement to reduce the lumen of the bladder in all directions when they contract in unison. There is no specific polarity as there is with the uterus. The bladder is roughly boat shaped when empty, and lies directly behind the pubic symphysis. It becomes oval and rounded as it fills and rises out of the true pelvis and into the abdomen. The posterior part of the superior surface is related to the anteflexed uterus. A little further posteriorly the bladder is related to the cervix and vagina, and here a triangular, flattened portion is called the *trigone*; the apex of the triangle points downward and the base is uppermost. The trigone is acontractile, thicker than the rest of the bladder, with an internal lining that is very smooth and particularly richly innervated. The ureters enter at the two corners of the base and the urethra leaves at the apex of the trigone. The bladder is connected to the urethra by way of the bladder neck, and the trigone contributes to its funnel shape. In this zone the detrusor muscle fibres are progressively replaced by elastic and collagen fibres and by urethral smooth muscle fibres, all of which are arranged obliquely and longitudinally to the urethra in such a way that when the muscle component is relaxed, the bladder outlet is passively drawn together, closed and watertight. When the muscle component contracts the bladder neck opens. The ability of the bladder neck to be closed during bladder filling is considered to be a positive factor for continence. The angle made posteriorly between the bladder and the urethra is called the *urethrovesical angle*; it is usually about 100° and appears to be an important factor in the maintenance of continence. The medial fibres of both puborectalis sections of the levator ani muscle blend with the fascia surrounding the urethra and vagina. They pull the vagina and urethra forward when they contract, favouring this angle.

The bladder is loosely held in position by ligaments; it is joined to the anterolateral fascia of the pelvis by the fibroareolar lateral ligaments of the bladder. Anteriorly the pubovesical ligaments tether it to the pubes and a fibrous cord, the median umbilical ligament (the urachus), connects the bladder apex to the umbilicus in some people. Posteriorly there are thickenings in the pelvic fascia attached to the bladder, which also carry the internal iliac vessels supplying the bladder. The wall of the bladder is richly supplied with stretch receptors, and impulses from these pass in afferent nerves to the micturition centre in the spinal cord, S2–S4. The motor innervation of the detrusor muscle is by parasympathetic fibres in the pelvic splanchnic nerves (S2–S4). In addition there is also sympathetic innervation via the hypogastric nerve (T11–L3).

THE URETHRA

The female urethra is a fibromuscular tube of approximately 3–4 cm in length. It is embedded in the anterior wall of the vagina and lies behind the symphysis pubis. It is the connection between the bladder and the anterior opening on the perineum, and its function is to convey and control urine. It should be noted that the shortness of the female urethra makes urinary infections more likely and the fitting of incontinence devices more problematical in women than in men. The epithelial lining of the urethra is hormone sensitive and covers a rich vascular submucosa. The intermediate layer is of smooth muscle whose fibres are longitudinally and obliquely placed and whose function is probably to shorten the urethra during micturition.

The outer layer of the urethra is composed predominately of the striated urogenital sphincter muscle, also called the external urethral sphincter or rhabdosphincter, which is from 20–80% of urethral length from the internal to external meatus (DeLancey 2002). The urethral sphincter (Fig. 1.13) consists of two parts. The upper part is the urethral sphincter proper. This band, external to the smooth muscle in the urethral wall, is a circularly disposed band of type I (slow twitch) striated muscle fibres; it is thicker anteriorly and incomplete posteriorly where it lies against the vagina. It contains no muscle spindles, and the individual fibres are very narrow, about one-third of the diameter of the usual slow twitch skeletal muscle fibres (Gosling et al 1981). The lower part of the striated urogenital

Figure 1.13 Diagrammatic representation of the urethral sphincter. The vesicle neck is the first 20% of the proximal urethra and the distal sphincteric mechanism is along the next 20–80%. (From DeLancey 1994a, with permission.)

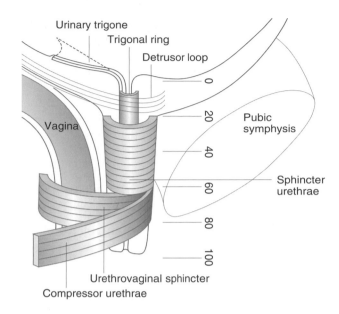

sphincter muscle is made up of two striated muscle bands that arch over the anterior aspect of the urethra. One band arises from the vaginal wall on each side – the urethrovaginal sphincter; the other extends along the inferior pubic ramus, above the perineal membrane – the compressor urethrae (DeLancey 2002). These three portions of muscle work as a single entity and are thought to be important in the maintenance of continence, particularly when the intra-abdominal pressure is raised (Fig. 1.13). Voluntary muscle contraction increases the urethral constriction whenever there is any rise in intra-abdominal pressure; proximally it constricts the lumen and distally it compresses the urethra from above (DeLancey 2002). The sphincter is believed to be responsible for one-third of resting urethral closure pressure (Rud et al 1980). Blaivas (2003) reports, however, that there are a myriad of names suggested for the support mechanism of the urethra; but at surgery he states he can only discriminate the pubourethral ligament.

The urethral smooth muscle is present in the upper four-fifths of the urethra and is a continuation of the detrusor muscle but is different to it on various accounts. It is composed of a more prominent inner longitudinal layer, which may help to shorten and funnel the urethra, and an outer thinner circular layer, which is thought to assist with reducing the lumen (DeLancey 2002).

The blood supply to the urethra is carried in a highly vascular submucosal layer. The source is via branches of the internal iliac arteries, and drainage is via the venous plexuses in that region to the internal iliac veins. The vascular plexus assists in forming the watertight closure of the mucosal surface. It also appears to be hormonally sensitive, as does the urethral mucosa.

It was long held that somatic efferent fibres via the pudendal nerves supplied the striated urogenital sphincter, but it now seems possible that it is supplied via the pelvic splanchnic nerves (S2–S4), travelling with the fine, easily damaged parasympathetic fibres to the smooth muscle of the urethra (Hilton 1989). However, there is still controversy as to whether the actual motor supply to the sphincter is somatic or autonomic, or both. Because the fibres are striated, a somatic nerve supply is most logical. Whatever is the fact, it appears likely that, like the levator ani muscle, there is electrical activity within the sphincter even in sleep. There is also sympathetic innervation to the smooth muscle of the urethra.

THE ANORECTAL REGION

The descending colon is about 25 cm long and passes down inside the left lateral aspect of the trunk to enter the pelvis posterior to the anterior superior iliac spine. At the pelvic inlet it is continuous with the sigmoid colon, a 25 cm long loop of gut that passes medially and posteriorly to the anterior aspect of the sacrum. From the level of the third sacral vertebra it is called the *rectum*; for about 13 cm, it follows the curve of the sacrum and coccyx posterior to the vagina. The rectum has a muscle wall composed of a layer of longitudinal fibres outside a layer of circularly disposed smooth muscle. There is a lining of mucous membrane which falls into three very specific transverse folds, two on the left wall and one on the right. On piercing the pelvic floor approximately 2.5 cm anterior to the coccyx it continues as the *anal canal* to the external outlet. At the junction of the rectum and the anal canal, the puborectalis portion of the levator ani muscle forms a sling, which pulls the junction anteriorly to create the anorectal angle, otherwise known as the rectoanal flexure. The puborectalis has no posterior attachment. The peritoneum reflects across from the upper two-thirds of the rectum to the uterus, dropping a little between the two structures to produce the pouch of Douglas. The lining of the upper half of the anal canal is composed of columnar epithelium, which lies in vertical folds called *anal columns*. By contrast, the lining of the lower half of the canal is of squamous epithelium, which is continuous with the skin surrounding the anus. Just behind the anus and below the coccyx is a mass of fibrous tissue called the *anococcygeal body*.

The anal canal (Fig. 1.14) is about 4 cm long and joins the rectum with the anus; it is kept firmly closed by the pull of the puborectalis portion of the levator ani muscles and the internal and external anal sphincters.

The *internal anal sphincter* (IAS) is composed of an inner circular layer of smooth muscle with an outer longitudinal muscle layer as a continuation of the smooth muscle of the rectum. The IAS is thickened in comparison with that of the rectum and is an involuntary muscle under the control of the autonomic hypogastric plexus. The function of the IAS is to maintain resting pressure of the anal sphincter, which has a normal value of 70 cm H_2O using a microballoon system (other systems have the resting pressure between 60–160 cm H_2O). Using the microballoon system a pressure of less than 45 cm H_2O is found with daily faecal leakage.

Figure 1.14 Anatomy of the anal canal and rectum.

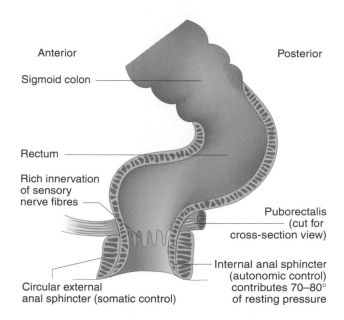

Anterior

Posterior

Sigmoid colon

Rectum

Rich innervation
of sensory
nerve fibres

Puborectalis
(cut for
cross-section view)

Internal anal sphincter
(autonomic control)
contributes 70–80°
of resting pressure

Circular external
anal sphincter (somatic control)

The *external anal sphincter* (EAS) has muscle fibres that surround the IAS; it is under voluntary control and has been reported as being comprised of a series of three loops (Bogduk 1996):

- an upper loop composed of the deepest part of the external sphincter encircling the anal canal and that butts with the puborectalis at its upper edge
- the middle loop composed of the mid part of the external sphincter and which is attached posteriorly to the coccyx
- the most superficial circumferential basal loop that is also penetrated by the tendinous fibres of the conjoint longitudinal layer.

The EAS is composed of both slow and fast fibres: the slow for tonic contractions and the fast for phasic contractions. These are capable of doubling the squeeze pressure (by a further 70 cm of H_2O) when there is a need for a powerful contraction to avoid the passing of wind or to delay bowel emptying to a socially acceptable place. If there is an inability to generate more than 50 cm H_2O the person may be clinically presenting with faecal urgency and soiling. (See also Ch. 12.)

The blood supply to both the rectum and the anal canal is via the rectal vessels. The nerve supply to the rectum and the smooth muscle of the upper half of the anal canal is via the inferior hypogastric plexuses, and responds only to stretch. It was thought at one time that there were sensory stretch receptors in the lining, and that these relayed the sensation of fullness to consciousness. It is now known that the stretch receptors within the levator ani muscle are stimulated by change in volume and pressure of the distending rectum (Parks 1986). The nerve supply to the lining of the lower half of the canal and the external anal sphincter is from the pudendal nerve and the perineal branch of the fourth sacral nerve. Thus this area responds to pain, temperature, touch and pressure.

References

Abramson D, Roberts S M, Wilson P D 1934 Relaxation of the pelvic joints in pregnancy. Surgery in Gynaecology and Obstetrics 58:595.

Ashton-Miller J A, DeLancey J O L 2002 The functional anatomy of the female urethral support and sphincteric closure systems. In: MacLean A B, Cardozo L (eds) Incontinence in women. RCOG Press, London, p 14–28.

Barber M D, Bremer R E, Thor K B et al 2002 Innervation of the female levator ani muscles. American Journal of Obstetrics and Gynecology 187(1):64–71.

Björklund K, Nordstrom M L, Bergstrom S 1999 Sonographic assessment of symphyseal joint distension during pregnancy and post partum with special reference to pelvic pain. Acta Obstetrica et Gynecologica Scandinavica 78:125–130.

Blaivas J G 2003 The emperor's new clothes. Neurourology and Urodynamics 22.

Bogduk N 1996 Issues in anatomy: the external anal sphincter revisited. Australian and New Zealand Journal of Surgery 66:626–629.

Bruton A 2002 Muscle plasticity: response to training and detraining. Physiotherapy 88(7):398–408.

Bullock J, Jull G, Bullock M et al 1987 The relationship of low back pain to postural changes during pregnancy. Australian Journal of Physiotherapy 33:10.

Bundred N J, Morgan D A L, Dixon J M 2000 Management of regional nodes in breast cancer. In: Dixon M (ed.) ABC of breast diseases, 2nd edn. BMJ Books, London, p 44–49.

Cardozo L, Cutner A, Wise B (eds) 1993 Basic urogynaecology. Oxford Medical Publications, Oxford, p 11–12.

Constantinou C E, Govan D E 1982 Spatial distribution and timing of transmitted and reflexly generated urethral pressures in healthy women. Journal of Urology 127(5):964–969.

Dangaria T R 1998 A case report of sacroiliac joint dysfunction with urinary symptoms. Manual Therapy 3(4):220–221.

Deindl F M, Vodusek D B, Hesse U et al 1993 Activity patterns of pubococcygeal muscles in continent nulliparous women. British Journal of Urology 72:46–51.

DeLancey J O 1994a Functional anatomy of the pelvic floor and urinary continence mechanism. Ch 1 in: Schussler B, Laycock J, Norton P, Stanton S (eds) Pelvic floor re-education. Springer-Verlag, London, p 9–21.

DeLancey J O 1994b Structural support of the urethra as it relates to stress urinary incontinence: the hammock hypothesis. American Journal of Obstetrics and Gynecology 170:1713–1723.

DeLancey J O L 2002 Anterior pelvic floor in the female. In: Pemberton J H, Swash M, Henry M M (eds) The pelvic floor: its function and disorders. W B Saunders, London, p 13–28.

Freeman R 2002 The effect of pregnancy on the lower urinary tract and pelvic floor. In: MacLean A B, Cardozo L (eds) Incontinence in women. RCOG Press, London, p 331–345.

Frudinger A, Halligan S, Spencer J A D et al 2002 Influence of the suprapubic arch angle on anal sphincter trauma and anal incontinence following childbirth. British Journal of Obstetrics and Gynaecology 109:1207–1212.

Gilpin S A, Gosling J A, Smith A R B et al 1989 The pathogenesis of genitourinary prolapse and stress incontinence of urine. A histological and histochemical study. Journal of Obstetrics and Gynaecology 96:15–23.

Gosling J A, Dixon J S, Caitchley H O D, Thompson S 1981 A comparative study of the human external sphincter and periurethral levator ani muscles. British Journal of Urology 53:35–41.

Gray's anatomy 1989 37th edn. Myology. Ch 5 in: Williams P, Warwick R, Dyson M, Bannister L (eds) Churchill Livingstone, Edinburgh/London, p 603.

Grieve G P 1981 Common vertebral joint problems. Churchill Livingstone, Edinburgh, p 53.

Hilton P 1989 Mechanisms of urinary continence. Abstracts of First International Congress on the Pelvic Floor, Cannes, p 17–21.

Lawson J O N 1974 Pelvic anatomy 1: pelvic floor muscles. Annals of the Royal College of Surgeons of England 54:244–252.

Lee D 1999 Biomechanics of the lumbo pelvic hip complex. Ch 5 in: Lee D (ed.) The pelvic girdle. Churchill Livingstone, London, p 43–72.

Lindsey R W, Leggon R E, Wright D G et al 1988 Separation of the symphysis pubis in association with childbearing. Journal of Bone and Joint Surgery 70A(2):289–292.

Love S M 2000 The breast and its development. Ch 1 in: Dr Love's breast book. Perseus, Massachusetts, p 3–32.

Meckel J F 1816 Handbuch der Menschlichen Anatomie, vol 2, 2nd edn. Halle, Berlin.

Nohara M, Nakayama M, Masamoto H et al 2003 Twin delivery in each half of a uterus didelphys with a delivery interval of 66 days. British Journal of Obstetrics and Gynaecology 110:331–332.

Ostergaard H C 1997 Lumbar back and posterior pelvic pain in pregnancy. In: Vleeming A, Mooney V, Dorman T, Snijders C, Stoeckart R (eds) Movement stability and low back pain. Churchill Livingstone, Edinburgh, p 411–420.

Parks A G 1986 Faecal incontinence. Ch 4 in: Mandelstam D (ed.) Incontinence and its Management, 2nd edn. Croom Helm, London, p 76–93.

Peschers U M, DeLancey J O L 2002 Anatomy. In: Laycock J, Haslam J (eds) Therapeutic management of incontinence and pelvic pain. Springer, London, p 7–16.

Prather H 2000 Pelvis and sacral dysfunction in sports and exercise. Physical Medicine and Rehabilitation Clinics of North America 11(4):805–836.

Rizk D E, Thomas L 2000 Relationship between the length of the perineum and position of the anus and vaginal delivery in primigravidae. International Urogynecological Journal 11:79–83.

Rud T, Anderson K E, Asmussen M et al 1980 Factors maintaining the intraurethral pressure in women. Investigation in Urology 17:343–347.

Russell J G B 1969 Moulding of the pelvic outlet. Journal of Obstetrics and Gynaecology of the British Commonwealth 76:817–826.

Sashin D 1930 A critical analysis of the anatomy and pathological changes of the sacro-iliac joints. Journal of Bone and Joint Surgery 12:891.

Sapsford R 2001 The pelvic floor: a clinical model for function and rehabilitation. Physiotherapy 87(12):620–630.

Shelley B, Knight S, King P et al 2002. Anatomy. In: Laycock J, Haslam J (eds) Therapeutic management of incontinence and pelvic pain. Springer, London, p 161–165.

Silva O E, Zurrida S 2000 Breast cancer a practical guide. Elsevier, Oxford, p 374–375.

Tichy M, Malbohan I M, Otahal M et al 1999 Pelvic muscles influence the sacro-iliac joint. Journal of Orthopaedic Medicine 21(1):3–6.

Tot T, Tabar L, Dean P B 2002 Practical breast pathology. Thieme, Stuttgart, p 1–23.

Wall L L, Norton P A, DeLancey J O L 1993 Practical urogynaecology. Williams & Wilkins, Baltimore, p 6–40.

Zacharin R F 1980 Pulsion enterocele: review of functional anatomy of the pelvic floor. Obstetrics and Gynecology 55:135–140.

Further reading

Barnes J, Chamberlain G 1988 Lecture notes on gynaecology, 6th edn. Blackwell, Oxford.

Fry D 1999 Perinatal symphysis pubis dysfunction: a review of the literature. Journal of the Association of Chartered Physiotherapists in Women's Health 85:11–18.

Gosling J A, Harris P F, Humpherson J R et al 1985 Atlas of human anatomy. Churchill Livingstone, Edinburgh.

Govan A D T, Hodge C, Callander R 1989 Gynaecology illustrated, 4th edn. Churchill Livingstone, Edinburgh.

Lee D 1999 The pelvic girdle, 2nd edn. Churchill Livingstone, Edinburgh.

Love S M 2000 Dr Love's breast book. Perseus, Massachusetts.

Pemberton J H, Swash M, Henry M M (eds) 2002 The pelvic floor: its function and disorders. W B Saunders, London.

Schiff Boissonnault J, Kotarinos R K 1988 Diastasis recti. In: Wilder E (ed.) Obstetric and gynecologic physical therapy. Churchill Livingstone, Edinburgh, p 63–82.

Schussler B, Laycock J, Norton P et al (eds) 1994 Pelvic floor re-education. Springer-Verlag, London.

Snell R S 1986 Clinical anatomy for medical students, 3rd edn. Little, Brown, Boston.

Chapter **2**

Physiology of pregnancy

Jeanette Haslam

CHAPTER CONTENTS

Menstruation 27
Pregnancy and foetal development 29
The physical and physiological changes of
    pregnancy 31
Complications of pregnancy 43

MENSTRUATION

A diagrammatic representation of the events and hormonal control of the menstrual cycle is shown in Figures 2.1 and 2.2. A normal, regular menstrual cycle pattern is sensitive to changes in body health and environment; it can certainly be disturbed by drug abuse (Sheridan 1997), polycystic ovaries, disease, and also by such life changes as travel, extreme shock or stress, excessive activity and severe loss of weight. For example, anorexic females suffer from amenorrhoea, as do ballet dancers (Kaufman et al 2002) and marathon runners (Tomten 1996). It is thought that this results from changes in the hormonal balance. Endocrinologists have suggested that the hormonal control of the human body is like a major orchestra, a large number of instrumentalists working together to perform a great orchestral work. As knowledge increases, so does the concept of the size of the orchestra and the complexity of the work being played. Although much has yet to be fully understood, this appears to be particularly true of the menstrual cycle, pregnancy, labour and the puerperium, where changes within the reproductive system are supported by a continuum of secondary adjustments, some of which are in other systems.

One set of changes associated with the menstrual cycle, which seems to be generally little known, concerns the normal cyclic changes in vaginal

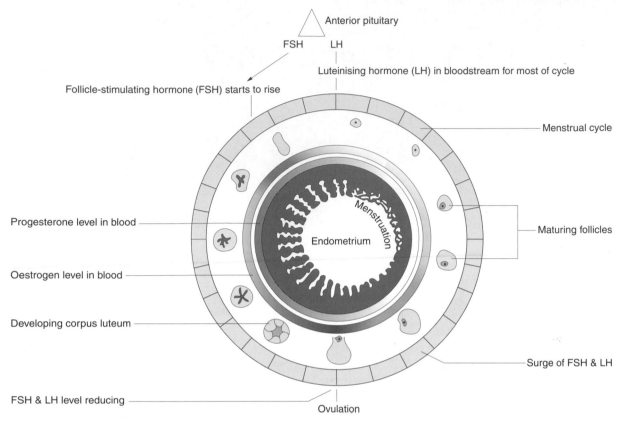

Figure 2.1   Diagrammatic representation of the menstrual cycle.

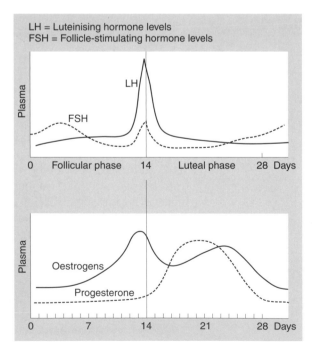

Figure 2.2   Hormonal secretions in relation to the menstrual cycle.

secretions. Indeed there are women who, in ignorance, fear that they signify some pathology. Following menstruation, women usually experience several 'dry days' when there is little or no obvious secretion within the vagina. The first noticeable mucus is scant but opaque, white, thick and sticky. After one or more days the mucus begins to thin, is still cloudy but feels progressively more slippery. By about the 7th or 8th postmenstrual day the mucus is watery, clear, more profuse and very slippery. Women may have an impression of being wet. This state is associated with ovulation and thus the peak of fertility. Over the remaining days, prior to the next menstruation, the mucus quickly becomes thicker, opaque and more sticky, and then there are several further dry days. This sequence gives the woman the information she needs about her own fertility, and can even be the basis for natural, non-invasive family planning, this being known as the Billings ovulation method. In addition, sexual arousal increases secretions to the vagina, and also from the Bartholin's glands.

PREGNANCY AND FOETAL DEVELOPMENT

Following fertilisation the ovum begins to divide, and over the next 8 days the group of cells is nourished by secretions from the fallopian tube as it is propelled along towards and into the uterine cavity. From possibly the day of conception the outer layer (trophoblast) of this increasing group of cells (morula) produces human chorionic gonadotrophin (HCG) to prevent menstruation and involution of the corpus luteum in the ovary. For 8 weeks the corpus luteum is the principal producer of the hormones progesterone, several oestrogens and relaxin. If the morula is to survive, implantation must occur in order to develop a more permanent nutritional supply line and additional hormone production. The outer cells become lined with a second layer, and together these two layers are called the chorion.

The spherical ball of cells is now called a blastocyst; it is hollow, with an inner mass of cells to one side which will develop into the embryo. The chorion divides to produce a myriad little tongue-like processes or villi all over the outer surface of the blastocyst. These burrow into the uterine endometrium, or decidua as it is also known in pregnancy. It is these chorionic villi that can be sampled between 8 and 10 weeks to detect inherited disease (see p. 101). The villi actually penetrate the decidual blood sinusoids, and maternal blood washes over them. The blastocyst is thus embedded within the decidua; however, as it grows it protrudes into the uterine cavity, stretching the covering surface of decidua. The villi atrophy over this portion, but not where the blastocyst remains in contact with the inner part of the decidua. The innermost site develops into the placenta from about the 6th week.

The disc-shaped placenta grows through pregnancy, and at term measures about 20 cm in diameter, is 3 cm thick and weighs about 500–700 g, approximately one-sixth of the baby's weight. It maintains the foetal circulation, which is entirely separate from that of the mother, and is responsible for the vital exchange functions of respiration, absorption of nutrition and excretion; it acts as both lungs and gut to the foetus. The placenta also becomes a major hormone-producing structure in pregnancy, producing progestogens and oestrogens. By raising the maternal levels of these hormones, menstruation continues to be inhibited. Early in pregnancy the placenta also produces HCG, which reaches a peak around 8–10 weeks and then declines by 18 weeks to a much lower level that is maintained until after delivery. HCG has been implicated in 'morning sickness' (Masson et al 1985). It has been suggested that the corpus luteum may remain active throughout pregnancy as a source of relaxin, but Bigazzi et al (1980) and Bryant Greenwood (1982) report human decidua as another production site.

It used to be thought that the placenta acted as a barrier to substances in the maternal blood that could be detrimental to the foetus, for example viruses and drugs (including nicotine and alcohol). This is now known not to be the case, and a simple principle to follow is that if a substance is in the maternal blood then it is also in the foetal blood. Furthermore, the foetal tissues are more sensitive to the effect of drugs as the foetal liver is immature, metabolism of drugs hardly occurs, so there may be an accumulation over time of a particular drug bound to plasma proteins. This is why great care must be taken in both the use of over-the-counter (OTC) drugs and the prescription of medicinal drugs for pregnant women.

A human pregnancy is calculated as usually lasting about 40 weeks or 280 days. If the date on which the last menstrual flow commenced is known, the estimated date of delivery (EDD) can be calculated by adding 7 days to the date and then adding 9 months; for example:

Date of commencement of last menstrual flow = 8 January
8 January + 7 days = 15 January
15 January + 9 months = 15 October
EDD = 15 October

Alternatively, add 7 days to the date of the last menstrual flow and then deduct 3 calendar months. This method of calculating the EDD is known as *Naegele's rule*. Pregnancy is divided for the purpose of description and discussion into three 3-month periods or trimesters: it culminates in labour and the delivery of the foetus and placenta, and is followed by the puerperium, a period of 6–8 weeks during which time the remaining changes of pregnancy revert.

For the first 8 weeks it is usual to call the developing baby an *embryo*; thereafter to delivery it is called the *foetus*. The foetus grows within a thin semitransparent sac (the amnion), is bathed in amniotic fluid and is attached to the placenta by the umbilical cord. The fluid is secreted by the placenta, amnion and cord. The foetus drinks it and excretes it as urine; it is said to be replaced every 3 hours. It is of interest that where foetal kidneys are absent or the urethra is blocked there is less fluid than normal (oligohydramnios), and where the foetus has atresia of the oesophagus there may be increased fluid (polyhydramnios). The volume of fluid normally increases throughout pregnancy to its maximum of about a litre at

Table 2.1 Basic pattern of foetal growth

Weeks	Detail	Length (cm)	Weight (g)
3	Embryo has primitive circulation	0.2	
4	Head, trunk, tail differentiated	0.7	
6	Limb buds growing	1.5	
8	Now called a foetus; has eyelids, ears, external genitalia	4	
12	Fingers, toes, nails, bones, cartilage forming	9	
16	Moving quite strongly	16	
20	Hair erupting, vernix depositing	21	500
28	Essential development complete	35	1250
36	Greatly increasing in bulk	43	2500
40	Term	50	3500

around 38 weeks of gestation. It contains a variety of substances including proteins, sugars, oestrogens, progesterone, prostaglandins and cells from foetal skin. This is the fluid withdrawn at amniocentesis. Table 2.1 gives a basic outline of foetal growth.

A baby is said to be 'full term' at a gestational age of 37 or more weeks, providing it weighs more than 2500 g. Survival is good over 34 weeks and is poorer under 28 weeks, although survival following birth at 23 weeks' gestation has now been achieved. The morbidity associated with the shorter gestational age baby is due to the lungs and respiratory centre not being fully developed, little or no immunity to infection, immaturity of the liver leading to clotting defects, and feeding difficulties.

A baby is said to be of low birthweight if it weighs less than 2500 g at birth. Very low birthweight infants (VLBW) are those below 1500 g at birth and extremely low birthweight infants (ELBW) as less than 1000 g at birth (Halliday 1992, cited in Lindsay 1997). A 'preterm' baby is one when the gestational age is less than 37 weeks. The term 'extremely preterm' is used for those born at or before 26 weeks (Rutter 1995). A baby will be judged 'small for gestational age (SFGA)' where the birthweight is below the 10th centile for its gestational age. Of all neonatal deaths 75–90% are due to pre-term births (Amon 1992, cited in Lindsay 1997).

THE PHYSICAL AND PHYSIOLOGICAL CHANGES OF PREGNANCY

The changes of pregnancy are chiefly the direct result of the interaction of four factors: the hormonally mediated changes in collagen and involuntary muscle, the increased total blood volume with increased blood flow to the uterus and the kidneys, the growth of the foetus resulting in consequent enlargement and displacement of the uterus, and finally the increase in body weight and adaptive changes in the centre of gravity and posture. The demands that these changes must make upon a woman should never be underestimated.

ENDOCRINE SYSTEM

The changes of pregnancy are orchestrated by hormones and much concerning their action and interaction has yet to be elucidated. However, progesterone, oestrogens and relaxin seem to be the most important for the physiotherapist. Increased joint laxity has been demonstrated in pregnancy (Marnach et al 2003); however, in this study the changes in peripheral joint laxity did not correlate well with maternal oestradiol, progesterone or relaxin levels. It has, however, been suggested that relaxin might have a role relating to continence in pregnancy (Kristiansson et al 2001).

Progesterone is produced first by the corpus luteum, then by the placenta. The output of the corpus luteum reaches a maximum of about 30 mg per 24 hours at about 10 weeks of pregnancy and thereafter declines. The placenta begins an increasing production from about 10 weeks, which at first supplements that from the corpus luteum and then completely takes over the role. The amount produced rises steeply from about 75 mg per 24 hours at 20 weeks to 250–300 mg per 24 hours at 40 weeks. Three progestogens are produced in the placenta but the chief one is progesterone.

Oestrogens are produced first by the corpus luteum; as with progesterone, this supply is gradually taken over by the placenta, reaching an output of about 5 mg per 24 hours at 20 weeks and 50 mg per 24 hours at 40 weeks. Several oestrogens are produced in the placenta; one of these (oestriol) is produced in considerable quantities and excreted in the maternal urine. The amount excreted in this way in 24 hours was formerly used as a measure of foetal well-being. In the developed world biophysical assessment, for example foetal growth by ultrasonography, has replaced this biochemical test. There is evidence to show that the maternal and foetal adrenal glands and the foetal liver also contribute towards oestrogen synthesis in pregnancy (Fransden 1963). Relaxin is produced in the theca and luteinised granulosa cells in the corpus luteum (Verralls 1993) and later in the decidua (Bigazzi et al 1980, Bryant Greenwood 1982, Yki-Jarvinen et al 1983, Zarrow & McClintock 1966). Research suggests that it is produced as early as 2 weeks of gestation, is at its highest levels in the first trimester and then drops by 20% to remain steady (O'Byrne et al 1978, Weiss 1984).

Effects of progesterone

1. Reduction in tone of smooth muscle:
   (a) food may stay longer in the stomach; peristaltic activity is reduced
   (b) water absorption in the colon is increased leading to tendency to constipation
   (c) uterine muscle tone is reduced; uterine activity is damped down
   (d) detrusor muscle tone reduced
   (e) dilatation of the ureters favouring urine stasis with elongation to accommodate the increasing size of the uterus; this may contribute to the likelihood of urinary tract infections
   (f) urethral tone reduced, which may result in stress incontinence
   (g) reduced tone in the smooth muscle of the blood vessel walls leading to dilation of blood vessels, lowered diastolic pressure.
2. Increase in temperature (0.5–1°C).
3. Reduction in alveolar and arterial P_{CO_2} tension, hyperventilation.

4. Development of the breasts' alveolar and glandular milk-producing cells.
5. Increased storage of fat.

Effects of oestrogens

1. Increase in growth of uterus and breast ducts.
2. Increasing levels of prolactin to prepare breasts for lactation; oestrogens may assist maternal calcium metabolism.
3. May prime receptor sites for relaxin (e.g. pelvic joints, joint capsules, cervix).
4. Increased water retention, may cause sodium to be retained.
5. Higher levels result in increased vaginal glycogen, predisposing to thrush.

Effects of relaxin

1. Gradual replacement of collagen in target tissues (e.g. pelvic joints, joint capsules, cervix) with a remodelled modified form that has greater extensibility and pliability. Collagen synthesis is greater than collagen degradation and there is increased water content, so there is an increase in volume.
2. Inhibition of myometrial activity during pregnancy up to 28 weeks when women become aware of Braxton Hicks contractions.
3. May have a role in the remarkable ability of the uterus to distend and in the production of the necessary additional supportive connective tissue for the growing muscle fibres.
4. Towards the end of pregnancy, rising levels of relaxin effect softening of the collagenous content of the cervix (Verralls 1993).
5. May have a role in mammary growth.
6. Affects relaxation of the pelvic floor muscles (Verralls 1993).

REPRODUCTIVE SYSTEM

Amenorrhoea is one of the first signs of pregnancy for most women, although it is not uncommon to experience a slight bleed, for 1–2 days, at the time at which menstruation would be expected if conception had not occurred. Within a few days of conception the cervix, if viewed with a speculum, will be seen to have changed in colour from pink to a bluish shade. From a firmly closed structure, which increases in depth early in pregnancy, the cervix changes by a gradual but accelerating process, which in the final weeks involves the softening, greater distensibility, effacement and eventually dilation (collectively called ripening) of the cervix. It has been described as changing from feeling firm like the cartilage of the nose, to feeling soft like the lips. These changes can be felt on digital examination and are produced by the endocrine-controlled restructuring of collagen and other tissues. As pregnancy progresses a plug of thick mucus forms in the cervical canal, sealing the uterus. The Bishop score is the accepted method of calculating the degree of ripeness of the cervix before labour. Nine points or more is considered favourable (see p. 54).

The growing uterus rises out of the pelvis to become an abdominal organ at about 12 weeks' gestation, increasingly displacing the intestines and coming to be in direct contact with the abdominal wall as pregnancy proceeds. The average fundal height related to gestation is shown in

Figure 2.3 Fundal heights in relation to gestation in weeks.

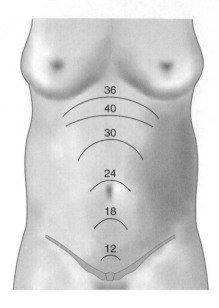

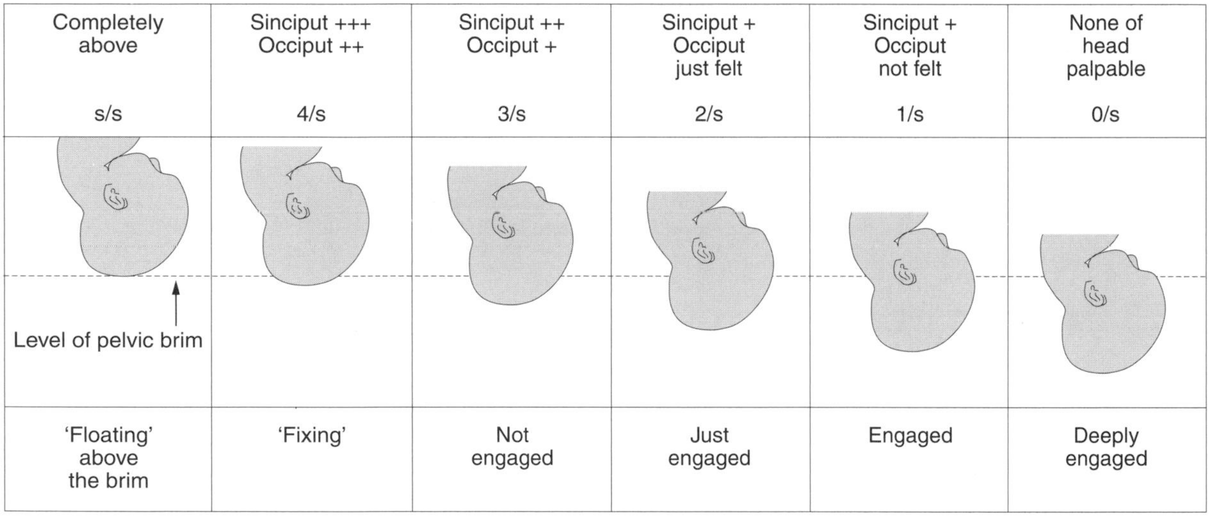

Completely above	Sinciput +++ Occiput ++	Sinciput ++ Occiput +	Sinciput + Occiput just felt	Sinciput + Occiput not felt	None of head palpable
s/s	4/s	3/s	2/s	1/s	0/s
Level of pelvic brim					
'Floating' above the brim	'Fixing'	Not engaged	Just engaged	Engaged	Deeply engaged

Figure 2.4 Descent of the foetal head. (From Llewellyn-Jones 1990, with permission of Faber.)

Figure 2.3. It can be seen that in the final 2–3 weeks the fundal height drops; this is because the foetal head has entered the pelvic inlet, which may cause an increased frequency of micturition. The head will be said to be 'engaged' when its greatest diameter has passed through the brim of the pelvis. This drop in fundal height is particularly noticed by the primigravida; in multigravidae the foetal head may not engage until labour begins owing to lax uterine and abdominal muscles (Sweet 1997a). At the end of pregnancy abdominal palpation is used to determine how much of the foetal head remains above the pelvic brim. This is estimated in fifths (Fig. 2.4) or by using the terms 'unengaged', 'engaging', 'engaged'.

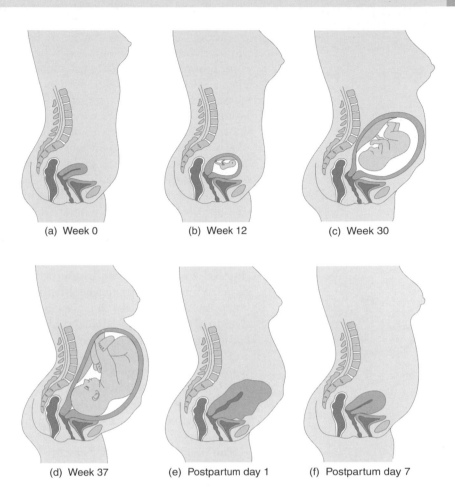

(a) Week 0   (b) Week 12   (c) Week 30

(d) Week 37   (e) Postpartum day 1   (f) Postpartum day 7

Figure 2.5 Diagrammatic representation of the physical changes of pregnancy.

The uterus increases in size dramatically, as does its blood supply (Fig. 2.5). The weight of the uterine tissue itself increases from about 50 g to 1000 g at term. The muscle fibres of the fundus and body are exceptional in their ability to increase in length and thickness throughout pregnancy to accommodate the growing foetus; it has even been suggested that new fibres may develop. The collagenous tissue, on and by which the muscle fibres are supported, increases in area and elasticity through pregnancy under hormonal influence. It has been said that in the nulliparous woman the uterus would hold about a quarter of a teaspoon of fluid, whereas the gravid uterus at term would contain 10 pints. As pregnancy progresses the isthmus develops to become the lower uterine segment, and by term it accounts for approximately the lower 10 cm of the uterus above the cervix. The musculature is not highly developed in this area and towards term it becomes soft and stretchy, allowing the foetus to sink lower in the uterus and into the true pelvis.

The muscle fibres of the uterus increase in activity, and coordinated contraction of the uterus can be detected by the woman by about 20 weeks' gestation. Bursts of irregular, short, usually painless contractions become progressively more evident and systematic. They are called Braxton Hicks contractions; they facilitate the blood flow through the placental site and play a part in the development of the lower uterine segment. At some stage regular and increasingly painful contractions establish and labour is said to have begun; however, in the mean time some women experience considerable sequences of contractions of variable length (20 seconds to 4 minutes), the intensity of which may or may not be painful. Terms such as 'false labour' or 'prelabour' have been used for this; it is more common in the multigravid woman.

There has been a recent increase in research interest in the effects of exercise on the pregnant woman and on the foetus, whether continuing or starting an exercise regimen. Maternal hyperventilation resulting from maternal activity – particularly that using large muscle groups – reflects an increased demand for oxygen, and risks the possibility of blood flow being shunted from the uterus to the active skeletal muscles. This should be borne in mind by women's health physiotherapists when advising women. It supports the view that it is wise for women to be advised to reduce their workload later in pregnancy when foetal demand is at its greatest. However, it is believed that mild to moderate exercise will not be harmful and will most probably be beneficial provided that care is taken for the woman not to become overheated or exhausted, and the supine position is avoided after the 16th week of pregnancy (Sharp 1993). Supervised water-based exercise is deemed beneficial owing to the weight-reducing effect of water buoyancy. It has also been shown that exercise in pregnancy can promote a psychological and a social sense of well-being (Lee 1996).

The foetal heart can be heard using a Sonic-aid from about 14 weeks' gestation, and by a Pinard stethoscope at about 24–26 weeks. Foetal movements are usually felt by the multigravida somewhere between 16 and 18 weeks and by the primigravida between 18 and 20 weeks. This sensation is sometimes called 'quickening'. The outline of the foetus can be palpated from about 24 weeks' gestation.

CARDIOVASCULAR SYSTEM

The blood volume increases by 40% or more to cope with the increasing requirements of the uterine wall with the placenta as well as servicing the other demands placed on the body, for example weight gain – both supplying the greater bulk and the increased power needed to move it. There is a greater increase in plasma than in red cells; consequently the haemoglobin level falls to about 80%. This effect is variously called 'dilution anaemia' or 'physiological anaemia of pregnancy,' and is one cause of women experiencing tiredness and malaise from quite early in pregnancy.

Progesterone acts on the smooth muscle of blood vessel walls to produce slight hypotonia, and causes a small rise in body temperature; therefore pregnant women generally have a good peripheral circulation and do not feel the cold. The heart increases in size and accommodates more blood, so the stroke volume rises and the cardiac output increases by 30–50%; there is a progressive small increase in heart rate through pregnancy. These changes begin to occur quite early, and it must be appreciated by physiotherapists involved in training programmes that a standard amount of exercise will produce a greater increase in cardiac output in pregnant women than in non-pregnant ones. This situation is further compounded as a woman gains bulk and weight. Blood pressure may even fall a little through the second trimester of pregnancy, so women may easily feel faint from prolonged standing; care should also be taken when getting up from a lying position. In the third trimester the weight of the foetus may compress the aorta and inferior vena cava against the lumbar spine when the woman is lying supine, causing dizziness and even unconsciousness; this is called the 'pregnancy hypotensive syndrome'. The infallible remedy is to turn the woman on to her side. Vigorous activity or other sympathetic stimulation will result in a redistribution of the cardiac output to the working muscles and away from the abdominal organs – including the placenta. With the upsurge of interest in antenatal exercise in water it is important for the physiotherapist to take account of the physiological effects of immersion (see p. 118), the differences in muscle groups being used and the effects of change in body position on the cardiovascular system. In general it is known that the stroke volume increases but the heart rate and blood pressure after an initial rise show a small decline in water. The response of pregnant women seems to be similar to that in the non-pregnant state (McMurray et al 1988). However, exercise in heat should be avoided because of the possible teratogenic effect of a raised core temperature, particularly in the early weeks; for this reason a pregnant woman should avoid saunas and hot pools (Tikkenhan & Heinonen 1991).

Slight vascular hypotonia, downward pressure of the enlarging uterus, weight gain, raised intra-abdominal pressure, and progesterone and relaxin-mediated changes in collagen all predispose to varicose veins, particularly in the legs, and to gravitational oedema. Varicosities of the vulva and anus (haemorrhoids, piles) may also occur. Oestrogens may be responsible for fluid retention generally in the body tissues. Some women can no longer wear hard contact lenses because their eye shape changes.

As a result of the increased peripheral circulation and hormonal stimulation, the mucous membranes (e.g. nasal, vaginal) become more active and lush. This can result in symptoms such as 'stuffy' nose and increased vaginal discharge. Consequently prolongation of coughs and colds may be experienced, also nose bleeds and vaginal thrush.

RESPIRATORY SYSTEM

The increased circulating progesterone levels of pregnancy further sensitise the respiratory centre in the medulla to carbon dioxide; this and the increasing demand for oxygen act as mild stimulants to ventilation. The resting respiratory rate goes up a little, from about 15 to about 18 breaths per minute, and there is a lowering by some 2% of the maternal blood carbon dioxide tension; consequently women notice breathlessness on activity. Tidal volume increases gradually by up to 40%, and alveolar ventilation also rises. The vital capacity seems to stay much as it was, so it is the expiratory reserve that is reduced. By the third trimester in many pregnant women, the enlarging uterus increasingly impedes the descent of the diaphragm. Towards term it may actually displace the diaphragm upwards, often by 4 cm or more. The displacement is most significant where the foetus is large or the abdominal component of the maternal torso is short, or both. The upward pressure of the foetus also affects the ribs causing them to flare (see p. 154). Maternal lower costal girth is increased, often by as much as 115 cm, as is the subcostal angle. Because of this the respiratory excursion is limited at the lung bases and greater movement is observed in the mid-costal and apical regions, and women frequently experience considerable breathlessness on even modest exertion towards the end of the pregnancy.

It seems probable that the hormone relaxin softens the costochondral junctions and renders them more mobile. Women complain of costal margin pain or rib ache, and of the foetus kicking the diaphragm and ribs; some have evidence of bruising and of disruption of costochondral joints.

BREASTS

As early as 2–4 weeks of pregnancy, unusual tenderness and tingling may be experienced in the breasts and enlargement begins soon, with the breasts becoming nodular and lumpy. The rise in oestrogens is responsible for the growth of the duct system and progesterone for that of the alveoli (Sweet 1997b). This growth continues through pregnancy and results in an increase of total breast weight of some 400–800 g. There is an increase in blood supply (veins may become visible on the chest) and in the number, size and complexity of the ducts. At about 8 weeks, sebaceous glands in the pigmented area around the nipples become enlarged and more active, appearing as nodules (Montgomery's tubercles). The sebum secreted assists the nipple to become softer and more pliable. By 12 weeks of pregnancy the nipples and an area around them (the primary and secondary areolae), become more pigmented and remain so for as much as 12 months after parturition. This pigmentation is thought to be due to the stimulation of melanin production by the anterior pituitary. As early as the 12th week a little serous fluid may be expressed from the nipples and by about the 16th week colostrum can be expressed. Human milk 'comes in' about the 3rd or 4th postpartum day. Nipple stimulation results in the release of oxytocin from the posterior pituitary (Irons et al 1994). This can be used in labour to increase uterine contraction and assist dilation of the cervix. It has been suggested that it could even be used to encourage labour to start (Adewole et al 1993, Elliott & Flaherty 1984, Kadar et al 1990); however, Crowley (2002) reported in a Cochrane database systematic review that there is not enough evidence to evaluate the effects of breast and nipple stimulation.

SKIN

The pigmentation of the areolae increases and is more pronounced in brunettes. The effects of pigmentation are also seen as darkening of the skin of the vulva, nipples and face; blotches which sometimes occur on the forehead and cheeks are called 'chloasma' or the 'mask of pregnancy'. In later pregnancy the pigmentation may also form a dark line in the skin overlying the linea alba. Striae or 'stretch marks' can develop over buttocks, abdomen and breasts and may become pigmented. These striae are a consequence of rupture of the dermis; the overlying epidermis is stretched and the resulting scar is therefore visible and permanent. Striae are caused by the need for skin to stretch rapidly over the enlarging body but may be aggravated by the hormonally mediated softening of collagen and by unnecessary weight gain. Some individuals appear to be more prone to striae than others so a genetic predisposition has been suggested. Certainly the application of oils with or without massage is unlikely to be effective in prevention or cure; however, they may ease the sensation of tight and stretching skin.

There is an increase in blood flow to the skin, which increases the activity of sebaceous and sweat glands, and so increases evaporation. Pregnant women may be expected to drink more to compensate. Fat is laid down, particularly in the second and third trimesters, on the thighs, upper arms, abdomen and buttocks, and is said to be a store which is subsequently called on in breastfeeding, provided a woman does not 'eat for two' in the puerperium.

GASTROINTESTINAL SYSTEM

Nausea and vomiting, thought now to be the response of some to HCG, is not necessarily restricted to the early morning, nor does it always cease by the 16th week. It can be aggravated by certain foods, even by their odours, and by iron tablets, and if inappropriately managed in severe cases (hyperemesis gravidarum) can lead to maternal dehydration, malnutrition and weight loss. Gross et al (1989) showed a higher risk for foetal growth retardation and possible foetal anomalies amongst sufferers with weight loss. The gut musculature becomes slightly hypotonic and the motility is decreased. The inevitable sequelae of this are prolongation of gastric-emptying time and a slower passage of food. Delay in the large bowel results in increased absorption of water and a consequent predisposition to constipation because the faeces are dry and hard. The reduced speed of oesophageal peristalsis, a hormonally mediated slackness of the cardiac sphincter, displacement of the stomach and an increased intra-abdominal pressure as pregnancy progresses, all favour the gastric reflux or 'heartburn' of which so many women complain. There is softening and hyperaemia of the gums, and bleeding may occur from quite minor trauma. Salivation may be increased.

It has been estimated that a pregnancy involves an energy expenditure of about 1000 kJ (239 kcal) per day (Durnin 1989, Hytten & Leitch 1971); however, since most women reduce or adapt their activity because of fatigue or the restrictions of their increased size and weight, and also because metabolism becomes more efficient (Van Raaij et al 1987), it is rarely necessary in the UK to increase intake, but only to encourage a well-balanced diet with plenty of fibre. The average weight gain is between 10 and 12 kg (Hytten & Chamberlain 1980) and is distributed as shown in Figure 2.6. Although obesity is associated with hypertension, diabetes and the need for caesarean section, pregnancy is not the time to commence a weight-reducing diet (Moore 1997).

Figure 2.6 To show how an average weight gain of 10–12 kg may be distributed.

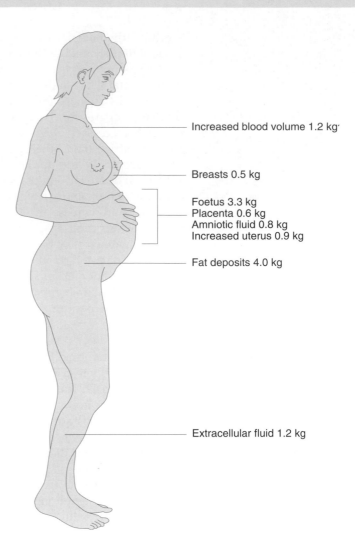

Increased blood volume 1.2 kg·

Breasts 0.5 kg

Foetus 3.3 kg
Placenta 0.6 kg
Amniotic fluid 0.8 kg
Increased uterus 0.9 kg

Fat deposits 4.0 kg

Extracellular fluid 1.2 kg

NERVOUS SYSTEM

Mood lability, anxiety, insomnia, nightmares, food fads and aversions, slight reductions in cognitive ability and amnesia are all well substantiated and common accompaniments of pregnancy. Recent work has shown a real decrease in brain size in pregnancy (Holdcroft 1997, Oatridge et al 2002) How this and alterations in emotional, cognitive and sensual function are brought about is not known, but they are presumably hormonally mediated phenomena.

Water retention quite frequently causes unusual pressure on nerves, particularly those passing through canals formed of inelastic material like bone and fibrous tissue (e.g. the carpal tunnel), with resulting neuropraxia. This can be relieved by the use of lightweight splints (Wand 1990). Occasionally pregnant women complain of symptoms indicating traction on nerves, which can be due to increased weight, for example water retention in the arm increasing its weight and producing depression of the shoulder, and paraesthesia in the hand.

URINARY SYSTEM

The presence of HCG in the urine early in pregnancy forms the basis of the pregnancy test; the level falls after 12 weeks of pregnancy. Throughout pregnancy there is an increase in blood supply to the urinary tract in order to cope with the additional demands of the foetus for waste disposal. There is an increase in size and weight of the kidneys, and dilation of the renal pelvis. The musculature of the ureters is slightly hypotonic so that they are a little dilated, and also seem to elongate to circumvent the enlarging uterus; the possible result of these factors may be vesicoureteral reflux (Mikhail & Anyaegbunam 1995) or kinking with possible pooling and stagnation of urine; this may predispose to urinary tract infections. There is an increased urinary output, and small changes in tubular resorption caused by the pregnancy may result in excretion of significant amounts of sugar and protein. Diabetes may be first diagnosed in pregnancy because pregnancy is one of the factors that may precipitate its onset in women genetically predisposed to the condition. This usually regresses after delivery (gestational diabetes).

As the pregnancy progresses the bladder changes position to become an intra-abdominal organ, is pressed upon and even displaced by the increasingly large and heavy uterus. Thus the urethrovesical angle may be altered and the intra-abdominal pressure raised; the smooth muscle of the urethra may become slightly hypotonic, and it seems possible that supportive fascia and ligaments of the tract and pelvic floor may become more lax and elastic (Landon et al 1990). What is certain is that many women complain of frequency in early pregnancy, which has often resolved by the time they come to the booking clinic. This may be due to an early rise in urinary output (Francis 1960a) and to subsequent adjustments to this. Later in pregnancy, particularly towards term, there may be urge and stress incontinence. The latter is said to occur in 50% of primigravida and the majority of multipara (Francis 1960b). This led Francis (1960b) to suggest that it was pregnancy rather than parturition that caused subsequent incontinence problems in women. However, it is now well established that delivery can damage the urethral closure mechanism (Snooks et al 1984) and be a cause of pudendal nerve damage (Smith et al 1989). The cause of changes in continence in pregnancy is more likely to be multifactorial, as discussed above. Caesarean section appears to be only partially protective (Wilson 2002).

MUSCULOSKELETAL SYSTEM

The influences of pregnancy on the musculoskeletal system are the ones that involve the physiotherapist most directly, first to attempt to prevent disorders arising and then, where problems do arise, to treat them.

There is a generalised increase in joint laxity, and so in joint range, which is hormonally mediated. Oestrogens, progesterone, endogenous cortisols and particularly relaxin seem to be responsible for this. Research (Calguneri et al 1982) has shown that there is a greater increase in joint range, and therefore in the degree of laxity, in a second pregnancy than the first, but that subsequent pregnancies produce no greater degree. Generally joint laxity returns postpartum to near its prepregnancy state, but this may take up to 6 months. Histological animal studies suggest that the laxity is made possible by a gradual breakdown of collagen in the target tissue and its replacement with a remodelled modified form which has higher water content and which has greater pliability and extensibility. The volume of the remodelled tissue is greater. Relaxin receptor sites have been reported in a variety of tissues, for example rat uterus, mouse symphysis pubis fibrocartilage, guinea pig cervix and human skin (MacLennan 1981). Some women experience greater degrees of relaxation of the pelvic girdle joints, apparently more so in the Scandinavian countries. It was thought that it may be a susceptibility to relaxin contributing to the problem (MacLennan 1991). However, Hansen et al (1996) found in a study of 38 women with symptom-giving pelvic girdle relaxation in pregnancy that there were no differences in serum relaxin concentrations throughout pregnancy and after delivery. They therefore concluded that relaxin does not have an important role in symptom-giving pelvic girdle relaxation in pregnancy.

During pregnancy it is usually necessary for a woman to adapt her posture to compensate for her changing centre of gravity. How a woman does this will be individual and will depend on many factors, including muscle strength, joint range, fatigue and role models. Physiotherapists are in no doubt that for most women the lumbar and thoracic curves are increased. Until recently it was thought that the greater lumbar lordosis was due to an increase in the pelvic tilt; however, work by Bullock et al (1987) brings this into question. What is certain is that about 50% of pregnant women experience back pain (Östgaard et al 1991) (see p. 142). The increased body weight must result in more pressure through the spine, and increased torsional strains on joints. Women become clumsier and are inclined to trip and fall. These factors, together with joint laxity and fatigue (see p. 161), particularly in the first and third trimester, must make pregnant women more prone to injury. Multiple pregnancies tend to have exaggerated minor symptoms. Brisk walking has all the benefits and fewer of the risks of running, and exercising excessively or to the point of fatigue does no good to mother or foetus. The current recommendations from the Centers for Disease Control and Prevention and the American College of Sports Medicine (CDC-ACSM) for the health and well-being of non-pregnant women is 30 minutes of exercise on most days. Artal & O'Toole (2003) state that pregnant women could adopt the same recommendations in the absence of either medical or obstetric complications. Kramer (2003) undertook a systematic review of 10 trials regarding aerobic exercise during pregnancy for the Cochrane review. It was concluded that regular aerobic exercise during pregnancy appears to maintain or even improve physical fitness and body image. However, the data were insufficient to infer important risks or benefits for the mother or infant.

The changing centre of gravity is chiefly made necessary by the distending abdomen. How the abdominal wall adapts to the required degree of distension is worth considering. The muscle fibres permit stretch, but the collagen components – the aponeurosis, fibrous sheaths and intersections, and the linea alba – probably undergo hormonally mediated structural change to provide the necessary temporary extra extensibility. The girth of a woman or the distance from xiphisternum to symphysis pubis can be used as a guide to foetal growth. The distance between the two rectus abdominis muscles can be seen to widen throughout a pregnancy and the linea alba may even split under the strain (diastasis recti), and this may lead to poorer mechanical function. It is of interest that Booth et al (1980) showed some altered function in the abdominal muscles of pregnant women, in that the muscles were recruited in movements in which they do not usually participate. Other muscles have increasing loads to lift and, if not encouraged to gain strength by daily use, may on occasion be overwhelmed. For example, unless a woman makes a habit early in pregnancy of using her hips and knees when bending down to pick things up, weight gain may render it impossible until after parturition.

In the third trimester there is increased water retention, which may result in a varying degree of oedema of ankles and feet in most women, reducing joint range. The oedema can also cause pressure on nerves, as in carpal tunnel syndrome where oedema in the arms and hands causes paraesthesia and muscle weakness affecting terminal portions of the median and ulnar nerve distributions (see p. 155).

With so much active growth and adaptation occurring within and supported by the body, the healthier a woman is before pregnancy, the better. Women's health physiotherapists are the health professionals best equipped to assess and advise on physical health before, during and between pregnancies. They are also well able to judge the effects of particular occupations and sports, and the wisdom of continuing them through pregnancy both in general and for a specific individual.

COMPLICATIONS OF PREGNANCY

ANAEMIA

Anaemia is very common in pregnancy, and is accepted to be significant at a haemoglobin level of less than 10.5 g/100 mL or less and is due in most cases to an iron deficiency. The majority of the depletion of the maternal stores are due to the increasing demands of the pregnancy. However, in migrants from Europe, S E Asia, or Africa, thalassaemia or sickle cell anaemia may be the cause (see p. 49). Although the majority of those with mild anaemia are asymptomatic as the haemoglobin levels fall, pallor, dyspnoea and oedema are more likely. Severe anaemia is said to be present if the haemoglobin levels fall below 6.5 g/100 mL. Oral iron is the usual method of treatment, parenteral therapy being used if the woman fails to respond to the oral preparations.

ANTEPARTUM HAEMORRHAGE

Antepartum haemorrhage (APH) is a serious complication, defined as bleeding from the genital tract at any stage from 24 weeks' gestation to the birth. Bleeding during labour is often called 'intrapartum haemorrhage'. Bleeding can occur and be contained within the site (concealed), but more often it escapes per vaginam. Where the placenta has embedded low on the uterine wall, close to or even across the isthmus and cervix (placenta praevia) it is easy to understand how increasingly intense contractions of the uterine muscle might tear fringe vessels. However, the reason why in other cases the placenta totally or partially detaches (placental abruption) is not well understood (see p. 77).

ASSOCIATED PATHOLOGY

Although it is ideal for a mother to be thoroughly healthy prior to and during pregnancy, women with, for example, diabetes mellitus, asthma, cystic fibrosis, hemiplegia, rheumatoid arthritis, systemic lupus erythematosus, multiple sclerosis, uterine fibroids, tumours and organ transplants have been successfully delivered of healthy children; however, some disorders may be aggravated by the pregnancy. Society is becoming increasingly prepared to provide the additional support necessary to enable those with disabling conditions to achieve and enjoy parenthood. Patients with rheumatoid arthritis and multiple sclerosis tend to go into remission during pregnancy, but may well suffer exacerbations after delivery. Subjective evidence suggests that being pregnant does not protect women from contracting most of the diseases suffered by their peer group. However, delaying a first pregnancy until after the age of 30 years results in twice the likelihood of breast cancer of those women having their first child before the age of 20 (McPherson et al 2000). Pregnant women can have all the conditions and pathology of their peer group. The skilled team caring for the women can all contribute towards her health care and by having good communication with one another can play a part in her general well-being.

BREECH POSITION

Many foetuses lie in breech position at some time during pregnancy. However, the majority have turned into a vertex presentation by the 34th week of pregnancy. A breech lie is predisposed by: some uterine anomalies, oligohydramnios, placenta praevia, fibroids, a contracted pelvis, some foetal anomalies, polyhydramnios and multiple pregnancy. The condition is diagnosed by abdominal palpation but is sometimes missed. Ultrasound examination should be considered if there is any doubt in the examiner's hands and has the added advantage of determining whether the foetus is suitable for external cephalic version (ECV). There are possible problems with ECV: foetal distress, premature rupture of membranes, premature separation of the placenta and preterm labour. The operator must therefore be both skilled and able to manage any presenting problems. Positioning for spontaneous cephalic version has also been suggested (see Further Reading, p. 52). If version is unsuccessful or contraindicated, the condition and the possibility of caesarean section must be discussed with the woman.

CARDIAC DISEASE

Cardiac output increases by 30–50% during pregnancy. Therefore any woman with an underlying cardiac condition must be closely monitored. Obstetricians will then determine whether they have a low, moderate or high risk condition and treat them accordingly. It is of prime importance that any pregnant woman with a cardiac condition has adequate rest, avoids any infections and has antibiotic cover during labour (Symonds 1992). There is also a risk of cardiac decompensation, especially during labour and in the 4 days following parturition. Those with a valve replacement may require anticoagulant therapy.

DIABETES MELLITUS

Pregnant women with diabetes mellitus need careful supervision, as even well-controlled diabetes may become unstable in pregnancy. The total or relative lack of insulin can result in dehydration, hyperglycaemia, ketosis, polyuria and polydipsia. Ultimately, in someone untreated, the result can be acidosis, coma and even death. In addition the risk of perinatal death remains relatively high for the offspring of diabetic mothers; the incidence of pre-eclampsia, of foetal abnormalities and of intrauterine death are also higher. Type I diabetics are insulin dependent whereas type II may be controlled by diet alone or oral hyperglycaemic agents. Those at increased risk of diabetes are those with a family history of diabetes, a previous baby weighing more than 4.5 kg, a previous unexplained perinatal death, polyhydramnios, obesity, a history of a baby with congenital abnormalities or glycosuria on two occasions in the antenatal clinic (Bewley 1997). Babies of diabetic mothers have a greater risk of being macrosomic, weighing more than 4.00 kg. The maternal hyperglycaemia stimulates foetal insulin production and this in turn favours protein and fat deposition in the foetus. A macrosomic foetus is at greater risk of birth trauma especially brachial plexus lesion due to shoulder dystocia (Bewley 1997). However, some of the babies are very small owing to placental dysfunction. Diabetic mothers are often admitted to hospital early (30 weeks) for careful surveillance, and then for early induction for those who are most stable, or for elective caesarean section at 37–38 weeks for those who are not.

ECTOPIC PREGNANCY

The fertilised ovum occasionally implants outside the uterus, most commonly in the fallopian tube at the ampulla or the isthmus – the junction of the tube with the uterus. The ovum burrows into the blood vessels of the tubal musculature; there being no decidua, this can cause surrounding necrosis. As the pregnancy develops, distension of the tube results in pain, and if left untreated, eventual rupture of the tube or bleeding leads in some patients to shock and even maternal collapse. More recently the development of immunoassays using monoclonal antibodies to β-HCG and high-resolution ultrasound scanners means that there can be a diagnosis of ectopic pregnancy before any significant haemorrhage occurs (Bhatt & Taylor 1995). Treatment options can then be considered; these may be surgical, medical or observation and monitoring.

FIBROIDS

Fibroids of the uterus (see p. 278) are more common in older and in Afro-Caribbean women. Acute abdominal pain may be caused by degenerative changes resulting from altered blood supply or from pressure and tension as the uterus hypertrophies and stretches. They may also obstruct labour and lead to an abnormal lie of the foetus.

GENITAL HERPES

Herpes simplex virus can cause facial sores (usually HSV-1) or genital sores (usually HSV-2). Either type can affect a newborn baby. If the HSV virus is present in the birth canal during delivery it can be transmitted to the infant. Neonatal herpes is a rare but life-threatening disease in which there can be damage to the infant's skin, eyes, mouth, central nervous system and internal organs and it can cause mental retardation or even death. It is, however, quite rare in the UK, with an incidence of 1.65/100 000 live births (Tookey & Peckham 1996). A genitourinary physician should be involved with the care of the mother with acyclovir being the usual treatment. Delivery by caesarean section is recommended for those mothers with an active HSV-2 infection. Women's health physiotherapists must be aware of the risk of neonatal transmission from active HSV lesions.

GESTATIONAL DIABETES

This is a temporary condition associated with pregnancy. Those women that develop hyperglycaemia (detected with an impaired glucose tolerance test during pregnancy) may have an adverse neonatal outcome if left untreated. Even small degrees of maternal hyperglycaemia can affect foetal outcomes (Hod et al 1991).

INTRAUTERINE DEATH

Even apparently light-hearted comments by pregnant women that foetal movements have substantially reduced or appear to have ceased should be taken seriously, for a foetus can become compromised and even die in utero. A women's health physiotherapist should arrange immediate referral to a midwife or doctor, and steps should be taken to monitor the foetal heart. Placental insufficiency and eclampsia can cause foetal death, but often the cause is obscure.

HUMAN IMMUNODEFICIENCY VIRUS (HIV)

The HIV virus is a retrovirus affecting human lymphocytes and other cells of the central nervous system. There are different descriptors for the level of HIV infection: asymptomatic, persistent generalised lymphadenopathy (PGL), AIDS-related complex (ARC), acquired immune deficiency syndrome (AIDS) and neurological HIV. Initially the HIV infection is asymptomatic with a variable incubation period. The transmission of the virus can be sexual, blood borne or maternal to foetus or infant. In those women with HIV there is a greater risk of preterm labour and also low birthweight babies. Foetal AIDS manifests itself as intrauterine growth retardation (IUGR), microcephaly, a prominent forehead and blue sclerae (Symonds 1992). The maternal transmission of HIV can be transplacental, by ingestion or inoculation at birth or by breastfeeding (Murray 1997). In treating an HIV positive woman it is essential to treat the woman as someone that is HIV positive rather than someone who is pregnant (Kotler

2003). A women's health physiotherapist must practise universal infection control policies with all patients, regardless of their condition.

INTRAUTERINE GROWTH RETARDATION

Foetal growth retardation may result from impaired placental function. Progressive hypoxia affects growth with eventually the foetal organs beginning to fail, the placenta ageing, renal blood flow falling with a decrease in amniotic fluid. Anoxia of the central nervous system results in decreased movement, tone and foetal heart rate variability. The condition is poorly understood, but can be due to pre-eclamptic toxaemia, hypertension, small placental separations, infarctions, failure of the placenta to develop or premature reduction in its function. Foetal growth may be accurately assessed by serial ultrasound scan measurement of the biparietal diameter of the foetal skull and abdominal width. External cardiotocograph of the foetus and Doppler studies may also be carried out.

MULTIPLE PREGNANCIES

There is increased physical and emotional strain upon the mother with multiple pregnancies, and as might be expected an increased likelihood of the occurrence of the other complications of pregnancy. Obviously the stretch on the structures of the abdominal wall will be greater than in a singleton pregnancy. In addition, possibly due to the proportionately larger content of the uterus at each stage in gestation, there is a predisposition to pregnancy-induced hypertension (PIH) and premature labour.

OLIGOHYDRAMNIOS

Oligohydramnios is a rare condition where the liquor amnii is much reduced and milky. It appears to be associated with abnormalities in the urinary tract, such as renal agenesis (Potter's syndrome). It is said to cause foetal abnormalities (e.g. talipes, torticollis) owing to the lack of space for movement. The baby's skin is very dry and leathery.

PLACENTA PRAEVIA

Normally the placenta implants and develops high up on the uterine wall. However, occasionally implantation occurs lower down, close to or over the cervix. Associated factors include multiparity, multiple pregnancy, older mothers, a scarred uterus, smoking and placental abnormality. There are four degrees:

- *Type I* – the major part of the placenta is in the upper uterine segment but encroaches on the lower segment; vaginal delivery is possible.
- *Type II* – part of the placenta is in the lower uterine segment reaching but not covering the internal os; vaginal delivery is possible, particularly if the placenta is anterior.
- *Type III* – the placenta is to one side over the internal os when it is closed, but not completely on dilatation; vaginal delivery should not be allowed.
- *Type IV* – the placenta is sited centrally over the internal os; vaginal delivery will not be allowed.

Placenta praevia will probably be diagnosed ultrasonically in pregnancy. Types I and II may improve during the course of pregnancy, the placenta being drawn upwards to a safer level as the upper uterine segment thickens and the lower uterine segment develops.

POLYHYDRAMNIOS

Polyhydramnios is the presence of an abnormally large quantity of amniotic fluid so that the uterus is tense and distended to a degree inconsistent with the gestation dates, and it may be impossible to palpate the foetus. It may be an indication of foetal abnormality, e.g. oesophageal atresia, open neural tube defect; it may be associated with multiple pregnancy and diabetes mellitus.

PREGNANCY-INDUCED HYPERTENSION (PRE-ECLAMPTIC TOXAEMIA) AND ECLAMPSIA

Pregnancy-induced hypertension is the most common and potentially serious complication of pregnancy for both mother and foetus. Estimates put the incidence at 10% of all pregnancies. It is more common amongst the least privileged, primigravid women and in twin pregnancies. The cause is unknown, and the patient may be unaware and uncomplaining. It is usually treated with hypertensive medication. For many years the cardinal signs of this syndrome were considered to be raised and rising blood pressure, oedema and proteinuria; however, oedema is a normal feature of pregnancy. Pre-eclampsia is a multisystem disorder in which there is hypertension and major abnormalities occurring in the kidneys, liver, brain and coagulation systems (Brown & Whitworth 1999). Pre-eclamptic toxaemia (PET) has been further defined by a threshold diastolic pressure of 90 mmHg, with proteinuria serving to distinguish severe cases from mild ones (Nelson 1955). Redman & Jefferies (1988) have suggested that a combination of a high maximum diastolic pressure with a large increase from the early pregnancy baseline is an even better criterion for identifying the 'at risk' group. This is not to say that all new complaints of puffy hands and face, as well as swollen ankles, malaise, nausea, headaches or of seeing flashing lights, should not be investigated at once. The women's health physiotherapist is a member of the caring team who must share in the careful monitoring of pregnant women. It is better to take the blood pressure and find it normal than to miss a substantial rise, although care is needed not to cause unnecessary alarm. The more severe forms of pre-eclampsia and eclampsia may occur in the second trimester, although they most often occur in the third trimester (Symonds 1992).

In cases of severe pre-eclampsia the HELLP syndrome (haemolysis, elevated liver enzymes and low platelet count) may rarely occur with progressive liver function deterioration arrested only by delivery (Goldberg et al 1989). Untreated PET may progress to eclampsia, a rare life-threatening state complicating fewer than 1 in 1000 deliveries (Redman 1988). Eclampsia is the term used to describe convulsions during pregnancy, labour or within 7 days of delivery not caused by epilepsy or any other convulsive disorder, and, if combined with high blood pressure, it can result in kidney damage, cerebral haemorrhage, cardiac arrest and maternal death. It has an incidence in the UK of 4.9/10 000 maternities (Douglas & Redman 1994). The maternal case fatality rate is 1.8% with 35% of women having at least one complication (Douglas & Redman 1994). It is considered a preventable condition, as it is a result of failing to recognise the deterioration of pre-eclampsia (Symonds 1992). Impaired utero–placental blood flow can cause foetal growth retardation or intrauterine death (Brown & Whitworth 1999). Early diagnosis is vital, and termination of pregnancy – usually by delivery – will alleviate the condition, although postpartum eclampsia occasionally occurs. Alternatively bed rest, sedatives and diuretics may contain the situation long enough to allow a pregnancy to continue to a more auspicious gestational stage. It is believed that no pregnancy should be allowed to continue after term in the presence of even the mildest hypertension (Symonds 1992).

SICKLE CELL DISEASE (SCD)

The ethnic origins of people with SCD are mainly Africa, the Caribbean, eastern Mediterranean, the Middle East and Asia. Those with SCD have sickle haemoglobin, such that when the haemoglobin gives up the oxygen to the tissues it forms long rods inside the cell, making the cells rigid and sickle shaped. This affects the viscocity of the blood causing local stasis and transient vascular occlusion. Chorionic villus sampling (CVS) at around the 9th or 10th week or amniocentesis between the 16th and 18th weeks of the pregnancy can determine whether the foetus is affected. Hypertension has been found to be the most common complication for pregnant women with SCD with one-fifth of the pregnancies producing preterm deliveries and SFGA infants (Smith et al 1996). Therefore close monitoring throughout pregnancy is essential. During labour, cardiac function can be compromised because of chronic hypoxemia and anaemia. Cord blood saved from a non-affected child can be banked for use in the case of a further sibling suffering with the condition.

THE THALASSAEMIAS (ALSO KNOWN AS COOLEY'S ANAEMIA)

These genetic disorders are associated with a decrease in the production of one or more of the globulin chains of haemoglobin. The two main types are alpha thalassaemia and beta thalassaemia and are more common in populations from the Mediterranean countries, India and SE Asia. If all four alpha-controlling genes are inherited, a baby will be stillborn, if three, the baby is live but severely anaemic, if two, hypochromic anaemia is common, and if one, the alpha-controlling gene is deleted and the baby is a clinically undetected carrier. Those women with the condition will need repeated transfusions during their pregnancy. They are also at greater risk of pregnancy-induced hypertension and urinary tract infections. Thalassaemia in the foetus can be determined by CVS early in pregnancy, or by sampling the foetal blood in the umbilical cord later in the pregnancy.

UNSTABLE LIE, TRANSVERSE LIE

Towards term, if the longitudinal axis of the foetus is repeatedly changing within the uterus, it is said to be unstable. This occurs almost exclusively in grand multiparae, that is those with four or more viable past pregnancies, but is also associated with polyhydramnios, fibroids, foetal abnormality and lax abdominal muscles. Occasionally the foetus comes to rest more permanently transversely across the pelvic inlet (transverse lie). In these cases, elective caesarean section is frequently considered as being safest for the foetus.

References

Adewole I F, Franklin O, Matiluko A A 1993 Cervical ripening and induction of labour by breast stimulation. African Journal of Medical Science 22(4):81–85.

Amon E 1992 Premature labour. In: Reece E, Hobbins J, Mahoney M, Petrie R (eds) Medicine of the fetus and mother. J B Lippincott, Philadelphia, p 1398–1429.

Artal R, O'Toole M 2003 Guidelines of the American College of Obstetricians and Gynecologists for exercise during pregnancy and the postpartum period. British Journal of Sports Medicine 37:6–12.

Bewley C 1997 Medical conditions complicating pregnancy. In: Sweet B, Tiran D (eds) Mayes' midwifery, 12th edn. Baillière Tindall, London, p 548–568.

Bhatt A N, Taylor D J 1995 Advances in the treatment of ectopic pregnancy. In: Bonnar J (ed) Recent advances in obstetrics and gynaecology, no. 19. Churchill Livingstone, London

Bigazzi M, Nardi E, Bruni P et al 1980 Relaxin in human decidua, Journal of Clinical Endocrinology and Metabolism 51(4):939–941.

Booth D, Chennelle M, Jones D et al 1980 Assessment of abdominal muscle exercises in non-pregnant, pregnant and postpartum subjects using electromyography. American Journal of Physiology 26(5):177.

Brown M A, Whitworth J A 1999 Management of hypertension in pregnancy. Clinical and Experimental Hypertension 21(5–6):907–916.

Bryant Greenwood G D 1982 Relaxin as a new hormone. Endocrine Review 3(1):62–90.

Bullock J, Jull G, Bullock M 1987 The relationship of low back pain to postural changes during pregnancy. Austrian Journal of Physiotherapy 33:10–17.

Calguneri M, Bird H A, Wright V 1982 Changes in joint laxity occurring during pregnancy. Annals of Rheumatic Disease 41:126–128.

Crowley P 2002 Interventions for preventing or improving the outcome of delivery at or beyond term (Cochrane Review). In: The Cochrane Library, Issue 4. Update Software, Oxford.

Douglas K A, Redman C W G 1994 Eclampsia in the United Kingdom. British Medical Journal 309:1395–1400.

Durnin J V 1989 Energy requirements of pregnancy. Lancet ii:895–900.

Elliott J P, Flaherty J F 1984 The use of breast stimulation to prevent postdate pregnancy. American Journal of Obstetrics and Gynecology 149:628–632.

Francis W 1960a Disturbance of bladder function in relation to pregnancy. Journal of Obstetrics and Gynaecology of the British Empire 67:353–366.

Francis W 1960b The onset of stress incontinence. Journal of Obstetrics and Gynaecology of the British Empire 67:899–903.

Fransden V A 1963 The excretion of oestriol in normal human pregnancy. Munksgaard, Copenhagen.

Goldberg I, Hod M, Katz I et al 1989 Severe preeclampsia and transient HELLP syndrome. Journal of Obstetrics and Gynaecology 9:299–300.

Gross S, Librach C, Cecutti A 1989 Maternal weight loss associated with hyperemesis gravidarum: a predictor of fetal outcome. American Journal of Obstetrics and Gynecology 160:906–909.

Halliday H 1992 Prematurity. In: Calder A, Dunlop W (eds) High risk pregnancy. Butterworth Heinemann, Oxford, p 332–354.

Hansen A, Jensen D V, Larsen E et al 1996 Relaxin is not related to symptom-giving pelvic girdle relaxation in pregnant women. Acta Obstetrica et Gynecologica Scandinavica 75(3):245–249.

Hod M, Merlob P, Friedman S 1991 Gestational diabetes mellitus – a survey of perinatal complications in the 1980s. Diabetes 4(suppl):74–78.

Holdcroft A 1997 MRI brain changes. Modern Midwife 7(8):5.

Hytten F E, Chamberlain G (eds) 1980 Clinical physiology in obstetrics. Blackwell, Oxford.

Hytten F E, Leitch I 1971 The physiology of human pregnancy. Blackwell, Oxford.

Irons D W, Sriskandabalan P, Bullough C H 1994 A simple alternative to parenteral oxytoxics for the third stage of labour. International Journal of Gynaecology and Obstetrics 46(1):15–18.

Kadar N, Tapp A, Wong A 1990 The influence of nipple stimulation at term on the duration of pregnancy. Journal of Perinatology 10:164–166.

Kaufman B A, Warren M P, Dominguez J E et al 2002 Bone density and amenorrhea in ballet dancers are related to a decreased resting metabolic rate and lower leptin rates. Journal of Clinical Endocrinology and Metabolism 87(6):2777–2783.

Kotler D P 2003 Human immunodeficiency virus and pregnancy. Gastroenterology Clinics of North America 32(1):437–448.

Kramer M S 2003 Aerobic exercise for women during pregnancy. In: The Cochrane Library, Issue 1. Update Software, Oxford.

Kristiansson P, Samuelsson E, von Schoultz B et al 2001 Reproductive hormones and stress urinary incontinence in pregnancy. Acta Obstetricia et Gynecologica Scandinavica 80(12):1125–1130.

Landon C R, Crofts C E, Smith A R et al 1990 Mechanical properties of fascia during pregnancy: a possible factor in the development of stress incontinence of urine. Contemporary Reviews in Obstetrics and Gynecology 2:40–46.

Lee G 1996 Exercise in pregnancy. Modern Midwife 6(8):28–33.

Lindsay P 1997 Preterm labour. In: Sweet B, Tiran D (eds) Mayes' midwifery, 12th edn. Baillière Tindall, London, p 603–609.

Llewellyn-Jones D 1990 Antenatal care. In: Fundamentals of obstetrics and gynaecology, 5th edn. Faber, London, p 66.

MacLennan A H 1981 Relaxin – a review. Australian and New Zealand Journal of Obstetrics and Gynaecology 21:195–202.

MacLennan A H 1991 The role of relaxin in human reproduction and pelvic girdle relaxation. Scandinavian Journal of Rheumatology 88(suppl):7–15.

McMurray R G, Katz V L, Berry M J, et al 1988 Cardiovascular responses of pregnant women during aerobic exercises in water; a longitudinal study. International Journal of Sports Medicine 9:443–447.

McPherson K, Steel C M, Dixon J M 2000 Breast cancer – epidemiology, risk factors and genetics. In: Dixon M (ed) ABC of breast diseases, 2nd edn. BMJ Books, London, p 26–32.

Marnach M L, Ramin K D, Ramsey P S et al 2003 Characterization of the relationship between joint laxity and maternal hormones in pregnancy. Obstetrics and Gynecology 101(2):331–335.

Masson G, Anthony F, Chau E 1985 Serum chorionic gonadotrophin (HCG), Schwangerschafts protein 1 (SP1) progesterone and oestrodiol levels in patients with nausea and vomiting in early pregnancy. British Journal of Obstetrics and Gynaecology 92(3):211–215.

Mikhail M S, Anyaegbunam A 1995 Lower urinary tract dysfunction in pregnancy: a review. Obstetrics and Gynecology Survey 50(9):675–683.

Moore J 1997 Preconception care. In: Sweet B, Tiran D (eds) Mayes' midwifery, 12th edn. Baillière Tindall, London, p 171–184.

Murray L 1997 Sexually transmitted diseases. In: Sweet B, Tiran D (eds) Mayes' midwifery, 12th edn. Baillière Tindall, London, p 570–577.

Nelson T R 1955 A clinical study of preeclampsia. Journal of Obstetrics and Gynaecology of the British Empire 62:48–57.

O'Byrne E, Carriere B, Sorensen L et al 1978. Plasma immunoreactive relaxin levels in pregnant and non-pregnant women. Journal of Clinical Endocrinology and Metabolism 47:1106.

Oatridge A, Holdcroft A, Saeed N et al 2002 Change in brain size during and after pregnancy: study in healthy women and women with preeclampsia. American Journal of Neuroradiology 23(1):19–26.

Ostgaard H C, Andersson G B, Karlsson K 1991 Prevalence of back pain in pregnancy. Spine 16(5):549–552.

Redman C W G 1988 Eclampsia still kills. British Medical Journal 296:1209–1210.

Redman C W G, Jefferies M 1988 Revised definition of pre-eclampsia. Lancet i:809–812.

Rutter N 1995 The extremely preterm infant. British Journal of Obstetrics and Gynaecology 102:682–687.

Sharp C 1993 Physiological aspects of pregnancy and exercise. Journal of the Association of Chartered Physiotherapists in Obstetrics and Gynaecology 73:8–13.

Sheridan V 1997 Health promotion and education. In: Sweet B, Tiran D (eds) Mayes' midwifery, 12th edn. Baillière Tindall, London, p 285–297.

Smith A R, Hosker G L, Warrell D W 1989 The role of partial denervation of the pelvic floor in the aetiology of genito-urinary prolapse and stress incontinence of urine. British Journal of Obstetrics and Gynaecology 96:24–28.

Smith J A, Espeland M, Bellevue R et al 1996 Pregnancy in sickle cell disease: experience of the cooperative study of sickle cell disease. Obstetrics and Gynecology 87:199–203.

Snooks S J, Swash M, Setchell M et al 1984 Injury to innervation of the pelvic floor sphincter musculature in childbirth. Lancet ii:54550.

Sweet B 1997a Antenatal care. In: Sweet B, Tiran D (eds) Mayes' midwifery, 12th edn. Baillière Tindall, London, p 208–238.

Sweet B 1997b The anatomy of the breast. In: Sweet B, Tiran D (eds) Mayes' midwifery, 12th edn. Baillière Tindall, London, p 457–459.

Symonds E M 1992 Antenatal disorders. In: Symonds E M (ed) Essential obstetrics and gynaecology. Churchill Livingstone, London, p 99–113.

Tikkenhan J, Heinonen O 1991 Maternal hyperthermia during pregnancy and cardiovascular malformations in the offspring. European Journal of Epidemiology 7(6):628–635.

Tomten S E 1996 Prevalence of menstrual dysfunction in Norwegian long-distance runners participating in the Oslo Marathon games. Scandinavian Journal of Medical and Sports Science 6(3):164–171.

Tookey P, Peckham C S 1996 Neonatal herpes simplex virus infection in the British Isles. Paediatric Perinatal Epidemiology 10:432–442.

Van Raaij J M A, Vermaat-Miedema S H, Schouk C M et al 1987 Energy requirements of pregnancy in the Netherlands. Lancet ii:953–955.

Verralls S 1993 Anatomy and physiology applied to obstetrics, 3rd edn. Churchill Livingstone, London.

Wand J 1990 Carpal tunnel syndrome in pregnancy and lactation. Journal of Hand Surgery 15-B:93–95.

Weiss G 1984 Relaxin. Annual Review of Physiology 46:42.

Wilson D 2002 Pregnancy and incontinence 1. Discussion in: MacLean A B, Cardozo L (eds) Incontinence in women. RCOG Press, London, p 366–367.

Yki-Jarvinen H, Wahlstrom T, Seppala M 1983 Immuno-histochemical demonstration of relaxin in the genital tract of pregnant and non pregnant women. Journal of Clinical Endocrinology 57(3):451–454.

Zarrow M X, McClintock J A 1966 Localisation of 131-I-labelled antibody to relaxin. Journal of Endocrinology 36:377–387.

Further reading

Artal R, Wiswell R, Drinkwater B C 1991 Exercise in pregnancy, 2nd edn. Williams & Wilkins, Baltimore.

Sutton J, Scott P 1995 Understanding and teaching optimal foetal positioning. Birth Concepts, Tauranga.

Sweet B, Tiran D (eds) 1997 Mayes' midwifery. A textbook for midwives, 12th edn. Baillière Tindall, London.

Symonds E M 1992 Essential obstetrics and gynaecology, 2nd edn. Churchill Livingstone, London.

Symonds E M, Macpherson M B A 1997 Diagnosis in color. Obstetrics and gynecology. Mosby-Wolfe, London.

Useful addresses

Action on Pre-eclampsia (APEC)
84–88 Pinner Rd, Harrow, Middlesex HA1 4HZ
Website: www.apec.org.uk

Cooley's Anemia Foundation
Website: www.thalassemia.org

National Childbirth Trust (NCT)
Alexandra House, Oldham Terrace, Acton, London W3 6NH
Website: www.nctpregnancyandbabycare.com

Pre-Eclampsia Society
c/o Dawn James, Rhianfa, Carmel, Caernarfon, Gwynedd LL54 7RL
Website: www.dawnjames.clara.net

Pre-Eclamptic Toxaemia Society
33 Keswick Avenue, Hullbridge, Essex SS5 6JL

Sickle Cell Society
54 Station Road, London NW10 4UA
Tel 020 8961 7796
Website: www.sicklecellsociety.org

UK Thalassaemia Society
19 The Broadway, Southgate Circus, London N14 6PH
Website: www.ukts.org

Thalassaemia International Federation
Po Box 28807, Nicosia 2083, Cyprus
Website: www.thalassaemia.org.cy

Chapter **3**

Physical and physiological changes of labour and the puerperium

Jeanette Haslam

CHAPTER CONTENTS

Introduction   53
Physical and physiological changes   53
The process of normal labour   56
Management of normal labour   68

Complications of labour   73
Interventions in labour   79
The puerperium   84

INTRODUCTION

Labour is part of an ongoing and integrated physiological process starting at conception and completed some weeks after the baby is born. Normally, between 36 and 42 weeks of gestation, labour commences, culminating in the delivery of the foetus. Some women have the misapprehension that labour begins at a specific, easily determined point in time. However, it is difficult to identify the beginning of labour other than retrospectively; the midwifery criteria are regular painful contractions accompanied by cervical dilatation. For the purpose of description, labour is divided into three stages, but it is helpful also to consider a period of prelabour.

PHYSICAL AND PHYSIOLOGICAL CHANGES

PRELABOUR

Enzymes released from 36 weeks' gestation onwards affect the collagen of the cervix to effect cervical softening prior to labour (Granstrom et al 1989). This effacement or taking up of the cervix occurs in the final 2 or 3 weeks of the pregnancy. The Bishop score (Table 3.1) calculates the degree of ripeness of the cervix; a score of nine or more is considered favourable. The position of the foetus at the start of labour is significant because it has a crucial impact on the mechanics of labour. Usually (97% of the time) the

Table 3.1 Bishop score of cervical changes

Score	Length	Dilation	Consistency	Position	Level of presenting parts
0	3 cm	Closed	Hard	Posterior	>3 cm above ischial spines
1	2 cm	1–2 cm	Intermediate	Intermediate	2–3 cm above spines
2	1 cm	3–4 cm	Soft	Anterior	<2 cm above spines
3	Fully effaced	5 cm	–	–	Below spines

foetus presents head down to the cervix (cephalic presentation). In most cases the foetus lies with the back and occiput to the maternal left; this is described as left occipitolateral (LOL). If the spine is slightly more anterior this is known as left occipitoanterior (LOA). Where the foetal occiput and spine are positioned in line with the mother's spine this is known as left occipitoposterior (LOP). Alternatively if the foetus is lying towards the right then the terms ROL, ROA and ROP are used. Likewise the degree of flexion or extension of the foetal head, which is recognised by the position of the fontanelles on vaginal examination, will affect the progress of labour.

THE STAGES OF LABOUR

First stage

First stage of labour is said to be established when there are regular painful contractions with effective descent of the foetus and dilatation of the cervix. A multiparous woman may have a dilated cervix of 3 cm without being in labour, whereas a primiparous woman may be in established labour at a lesser cervical dilatation. The midwife is skilled to assess each presenting woman to determine when the first stage of labour is established. When the regular uterine muscle contractions are established, they become progressively longer, stronger and closer together. For most women these contractions are painful and many require some form of analgesia. Within the uterus, the uterine contractions exert an intermittent upward pull on the lower segment of the uterus and cervix, while at the same time applying downward pressure on the foetus. This combination opens the cervix, pushing the foetus against and through it (Fig. 3.1). It has been compared to pulling a polo-neck sweater over the head. In addition the uterine cavity becomes progressively smaller. The first stage is almost always the longest stage. It is said to be complete when the cervix has reached full dilatation – about 10 cm diameter depending on the size of the foetal head – to allow the foetal head through to proceed down the vagina.

Second stage

There is often a noticeable change in the tempo of contractions; they may become more widely spaced and even a little shorter, while still remaining intense. This continued action of the uterine muscle further reduces the size of the uterus and expels the foetus from it into the vagina. This process is accompanied in most women by a compelling urge to bear down. The diaphragm and the abdominal muscles are brought into

Figure 3.1 Dilatation of the cervix.

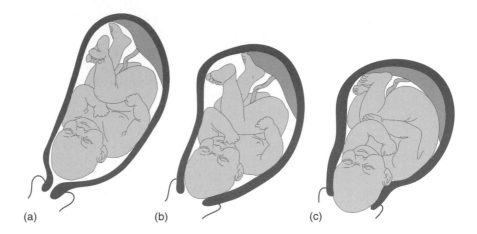

(a)   (b)   (c)

action to help push the foetus out. The pelvic floor distends under the pressure, the puborectalis and pubococcygeus muscles are parted and pushed aside and outward, and the soft tissues of the perineum extend to form a canal, which gutters forwards from the coccyx. This canal protrudes and is directed anteriorly. It takes time for the perineum to stretch sufficiently to allow the foetus through, and performing an episiotomy may accelerate its delivery. The second stage is normally much shorter than the first, ending with the birth of the baby.

Third stage

The third stage is the delivery of the placenta once it has detached from the uterine wall. It is usually the shortest phase.

SIGNS THAT THE START OF LABOUR MAY BE IMMINENT

1. Late in pregnancy the mucoid '*show*' – often blood stained – is passed per vaginam down the cervical canal; this may be considered a sign that labour is imminent. The purpose of this mucous plug during pregnancy is to act as a barrier to upward-moving infection. Ripening of the cervix and increased uterine muscle activity results in it being released sooner or later. Except where there is any measurable loss of fresh blood, women are advised to note the event but take no other special action.

2. '*Ruptured membranes*' or the '*breaking of the waters*'. This is a rupture of the amniotic sac resulting in a sudden or gradual loss of amniotic fluid. It may be difficult for a woman to discriminate between gradual, slight amniotic fluid loss, and loss of urine due to stress or urge incontinence. Where the foetus presents head first in labour, and the head is beginning to fit snugly into the lower segment and cervix, a small bulging portion of the sac filled with fluid may be in front of the head (the forewaters), and it is essentially cut off from the remainder (the hindwaters). Thus when it is suspected that the membranes have ruptured, the amount lost may be some guide to the position of the foetal head. Where the head is high and not well applied to the cervix a larger

amount is lost than when the head is firmly applied. A gradual dripping would suggest a small puncture in either the fore- or hindwaters. Women are advised to report suspected loss of amniotic fluid, particularly if it is considerable, as it is possible for the umbilical cord to prolapse downwards through the ruptured sac and already dilating cervix, ahead of the presenting part where this is not well engaged. If this is the case then subsequent uterine contractions will plunge the foetus downwards and might compress the cord. Should this happen the resulting vascular occlusion could compromise the foetus and lead to distress or death. Any sign of umbilical cord prolapse requires immediate medical care. It should be remembered that amniotic fluid production will continue until delivery so that, even when large amounts are lost, further dripping will occur.

3. *Contractions*. Braxton Hicks contractions increase in frequency and strength as pregnancy progresses, to eventually become regular and lasting 20–30 seconds at 20–30-minute intervals as a herald of the uterine contractions of established labour. Labour is said to be established when the uterine muscle contraction of the fundus and body become increasingly apparent and settle into a regular, continuing and increasingly intense and painful pattern.

These three signs are commonly presented in the literature and parent-craft classes as heralds of labour. There is, however, wide individual variation, for example a 'show' and 'ruptured membranes' may occur well in advance of or during labour, and intermittent sequences of strong, painful contractions can be experienced without labour becoming established (Braxton Hicks contractions). Therefore the only really reliable signs that labour is established are regular, painful and continuing contractions, and a progressively dilating cervix.

THE PROCESS OF NORMAL LABOUR

Labour is only part of the ongoing physiological process starting at conception and completed some weeks after the baby is born. What actually initiates the onset of labour is still not fully understood, but it is almost certainly triggered by a combination of factors; the following have been suggested.

1. *A rise in the oxytocin level*. It has also been shown that there is an increase in nocturnal myometrial activity from 24 weeks of pregnancy. The plasma concentrations of oxytocin have been shown to have nocturnal peaks between 37 and 39 weeks (Moore et al 1994). The physical size and pressure of the growing foetus on the ripening cervix may stimulate a neurogenic reflex which causes the posterior pituitary to release more oxytocin. In addition, or alternatively, the maturing foetus may produce increasing amounts of oxytocin, which cross the placenta. Oxytocin is known to cause the uterine muscle to contract.

2. *Prostaglandin production.* The uterine wall has the potential, like many other tissues, to produce prostaglandins. These are fatty acids which in 1930 were first found in semen and shown to cause smooth muscle to contract. They have a short life because they are rapidly metabolised, and therefore have local effects. It is known that oestrogens could trigger the release of myometrial prostaglandins. It is also known that the disruption of decidual cells, such as occurs when the amniotic sac is artificially ruptured, would cause prostaglandin release. It has been suggested that stretching of the uterine wall by the growing, kicking foetus has a similar effect. The prostaglandins in semen may be the explanation for the circumstantial evidence that intercourse appears to stimulate the start of labour in some cases. However, Kavanagh et al (2001) completed a systematic review of the literature for the Cochrane database and concluded that the role of sexual intercourse for the induction of labour is uncertain. However, it was also stated that it would be difficult in any trials to standardise sexual intercourse as a possible intervention for meaningful comparison with other methods of induction.

3. *Foetal adrenal hormones.* Studies in animals (Currie et al 1973, Liggins 1974) have shown a rapid increase in the production of foetal cortisols a few days before the onset of labour. These high concentrations act at the placenta to reduce the secretion of progesterone and increase the secretion of oestrogens. A marked rise in oestradiol is associated with a prostaglandin being produced in the placenta. It is suggested by some (Shearman 1986) that a similar set of changes must be operative to enable the human foetus to control the onset of labour.

Late in pregnancy and continuing in early labour, the lower part of the uterus – the isthmus – responds to the contraction of the muscle of the fundus and body by stretching and thinning to form the lower uterine segment. It is thought that uterine contractions are normally initiated around the openings to the fallopian tubes, spread to the fundus and then down the body of the uterus. Ideally there is a gradient pattern in these contractions, with the fundus dominant and the lower uterine segment less active; this is called normal uterine polarity.

The early signs, symptoms and circumstances are highly individual to each labour but contractions usually settle into a regular pattern. Often, initially, these are short in length (about 30 seconds) and some distance apart (15–20 minutes), but progressively become longer, stronger and closer together until they are about 1–1.5 minutes in length and occur every 2–5 minutes. Occasionally women notice only the longer, stronger contractions.

Further tension on the lower uterine segment causes the cervix to be 'taken up' or effaced, so eventually the cervical canal becomes part of the containing uterine wall. It is then gradually opened or dilated. Thus ultimately it is effacement and dilatation that releases the plug of mucus or 'show' if it has not occurred earlier. As labour progresses there is an increase in oxytocin release by the posterior pituitary, which causes contractions to become stronger. This output is enhanced and continued by a positive feedback from the dilating cervix and the distending vagina to the hypothalamus and so to the posterior pituitary.

In labour the uterine muscle of the fundus and body acquire the unique ability to retract systematically, by alternately contracting firmly, then relaxing, but to a shorter and thicker length each time. Thus the uterine cavity becomes progressively smaller, the uterine muscular wall increases in thickness from about 6 mm to 25 mm, and the foetus and other uterine contents are expelled.

During contractions the shape of the abdomen may be seen to alter, particularly as they become longer and stronger. The fundus moves forwards so that the long axis of the uterus and the thrust of the muscle are brought into the appropriate line and meet the cervix and the vagina at the best angle (drive angle) to propel the foetus into the vagina. This forward tilt (anteversion) occurs more easily if the woman is upright or lying on her side, for gravity opposes it in the supine position (Figs 3.2, 6.1 on p. 178). It is of interest that women instinctively tend to lean forward. Supine position may result in vena caval compression (Abitol 1985).

The first stage of labour can be subdivided into two phases. The latent phase is calculated from the onset of labour to 3 cm of cervical dilatation, and commonly lasts 4–6 hours in the primigravida, although it can be much longer. The active phase extends from 3 cm to full dilatation of the cervix; in this phase the contractions are stronger, more frequent and more painful, and the cervix opens more rapidly – about 1 cm per hour in the primigravida and 1.5 cm per hour in multigravidae. Cervical dilatation is measured by palpation and estimation of the diameter of the opening in centimetres by a digital vaginal assessment. The midwife determines how often this examination takes place, and this is normally:

- on admission to confirm the onset of labour and to exclude cord prolapse

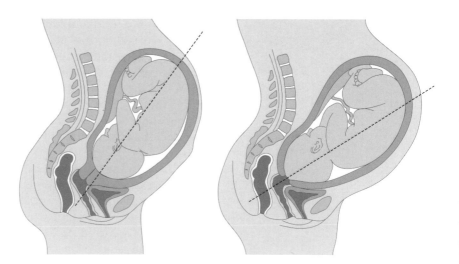

Figure 3.2 To show the forward movement of the drive angle.

- prior to sedation if the membranes rupture when the foetal head is not well engaged
- if the woman wishes to push when there is nothing visible
- if there is undue delay in the second stage of labour
- to rupture the membranes if necessary.

Vaginal examination is kept to a minimum because of the risk of introducing infection and also it is a particularly uncomfortable investigation in labour. There must always be an explanation for and description of the procedure in order for the women to give informed consent. Many units vaginally examine women at 4 hourly intervals during labour for plotting on a partogram. The descent can be measured by how much of the foetal head – in fifths – is still palpable above the pelvic brim or is below the ischial spines as palpated vaginally (see Fig. 2.4 on p. 34).

The second stage contractions vary from those in the first stage, in that there is not only a uterine contraction creating force, but also a bearing down caused by the contraction of the diaphragm and abdominal muscles of the woman to aid expulsion. This stage can also be considered to have two phases: the phase of descent in which the foetal head descends down on to the perineum, and the perineal phase in which the perineum stretches, adaptively remodels to form an extended passage and allows the head through. It is now appreciated that a prolonged active second stage may be dangerous for both child and mother, causing foetal distress or maternal pelvic floor neuropathy. Therefore most labour suites have their own criteria for deciding when assistance such as intravenous infusion of oxytocic drugs, episiotomy, vacuum extraction or forceps should be considered to accelerate delivery.

Following delivery, the uterus continues to contract, constricting the placental vascular sinuses and causing the placenta to sheer away from the wall and separate. The contraction and retraction of uterine muscle has the effect of ligating the maternal blood vessels within the placental attachment site and controlling the considerable risk of serious haemorrhage when the placenta eventually detaches. Further contractions and, in most units, an intramuscular injection of ergometrine and oxytocin given after delivery of the shoulders with continuous cord traction, normally result in the delivery of the placenta. It is known that nipple stimulation, for example when an infant suckles, causes the posterior pituitary to produce oxytocin. Some midwives utilise this fact by encouraging the newly delivered infant to begin suckling in the third stage of labour to enhance uterine contractions and speed the separation and delivery of the placenta. Some even manually stimulate nipples in the first and second stage where contractions seem to be failing.

THE PAIN OF LABOUR

Pain has been defined as 'an unpleasant sensory and emotional experience associated with actual or potential tissue damage, or described in terms of such damage' (Mersky 1979). Parturition pain is an experience that is shared by women at every level of civilisation (Melzack et al 1981), and it has been mentioned since the recording of history began. Although cultural, socioeconomic, psychological and emotional aspects must have a place in the intensity of the pain experienced and women's reactions to it, and even though current evidence and research have increased understanding about the physical causes and the individual perception of labour discomfort, questions still remain as to the purpose of childbirth pain. Labour is the normal physiological continuation of pregnancy, but in other circumstances pain is usually regarded as a warning that something is malfunctioning or is being damaged within the body. Could the reason for what many women perceive and record as the most intense pain they will ever experience, be simply an alarm system for the protection of the incredibly helpless new young human being?

The body does have its own way of dulling pain; it has been shown that there is a rise of plasma endorphins through pregnancy (Newnham et al 1983), possibly in preparation for labour. There is a further rise in labour in response to stress; where epidural analgesia is given there is a significant drop in plasma endorphin levels (Abboud et al 1983, 1984). Women's reactions to labour pain are influenced by their personalities, their previous experiences and also by how they feel at the time; women who feel safe and secure as they labour, and who understand what is happening, will almost certainly record lower pain scores than they would if they were fearful and apprehensive. For very many new mothers the first sight of their baby blots out all memories of pain; unfortunately there will also be those who will say, even many years later, that they have never got over it.

Causes of labour pain

The main cause of pain during the first stage of labour is thought to be directly associated with dilatation of the cervix and distension of the lower uterine segment around the descending presenting foetal parts (Fig. 3.1). The sensory nerve supply from these two areas of the uterus is greater than that from the fundus or uterine body (see p. 17). Other suggested causes of first stage labour pain include ischaemia of the myometrium and cervix, pressure on sensory nerve endings in the uterine body and fundus, inflammatory changes in the uterine muscles, and reflex contraction of the cervix and lower uterine segment due to the 'fear–tension–pain' cycle (Wall & Melzack 1984); however, these have not been substantiated by research. Brown et al (1989) compared the pain experienced at two stages of dilatation in the first stage of labour: 2–5 cm and 10 cm. As cervical dilatation increased, there were significant increases in self-reported and observed pain. Using words from the McGill pain questionnaire, pain was characterised as 'discomforting' during early dilatation and as 'distressing, horrible, excruciating' as labour progressed. Green (1993) states that anxiety regarding pain is a strong predictor of negativity regarding labour and birth, together with poor postnatal emotional well-being.

In common with pain from other viscera, first stage pain is referred to the dermatomes supplied by the same spinal cord segments (T10–L1) that receive input from the uterus and cervix (Fig. 3.3). As labour progresses and the intensity and frequency of the contractions increase, the

Figure 3.3 The nervous pathways involved in labour pain.

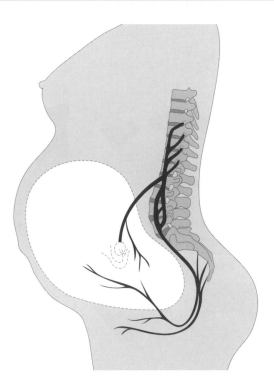

pain zones enlarge and become more diffuse (Fig. 3.4). At the end of the first stage of labour some women experience aching, burning and cramping discomfort in the thighs. This is due to stretching of, and pressure on, pain-sensitive structures (uterine and pelvic ligaments and fascia, bladder, urethra and rectum) and pressure on the lumbar and sacral nerve roots. Once the cervix is fully dilated the nature and distribution of pain changes.

In the second stage and during delivery the pain is felt chiefly in the soft tissues of the perineal region (S2–S4) as they stretch, distend and even tear; in addition, pain may be experienced as the pelvic outlet is pushed open by the foetus, affecting the symphysis pubis, sacroiliac and sacrococcygeal joints. An effort has been made to describe the areas of pain distribution as labour progresses (Bonica 1984), but a tremendous variability should be expected. Some women will experience widespread discomfort, and others will have more discrete painful areas.

The obstetric team must never underestimate the intensity of labour pain. Using the McGill pain questionnaire, some scores as low as 10 (very mild pain) were recorded by Melzack (Table 3.2), but at the top end of the scale scores as high as 62 (extremely severe pain) were registered (Melzack 1984). Primiparae tend to experience higher levels of pain than multiparous women, and, although those women who have received childbirth training record lower levels of pain than the untrained (Melzack et al 1981), it is still greater during a first labour than subsequently.

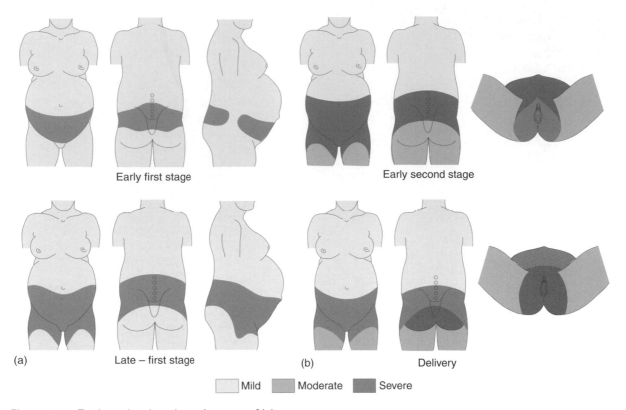

Figure 3.4   To show the changing pain zones of labour.

Table 3.2   Pain scores in labour using the McGill questionnaire (possible maximum 80)

Pain scores (%)	Very mild to mild 2–11 and 12–21	Moderate 22–31	Severe 32–41	Extremely severe 42–62
Primiparae	9.2	29.5	37.9	23.4
Multiparae	24.1	29.6	35.2	11.1

Individuals vary greatly in the way they perceive, interpret and respond to pain (Noble 1983), and a vast range of factors, both physical and emotional, will play their part in the severity of pain felt during labour. Research by Wuitchik et al (1989) investigated the intensity of pain experienced and the women's thoughts – as to whether they were distress related or not – in three phases of labour. A positive correlation was found between the two parameters – pain and distress-related thoughts – in the latent phase of the first stage of labour and the subsequent duration of labour. They were also prognostic of obstetric outcome. The inference is drawn that the latent phase is critical and it is suggested that pain and distress-related thoughts could actually contribute to labour inefficiency and poor outcome, for example the foetus needing paediatric assistance. If this is so, the implications for childbirth educators and the labour team are important. Childbirth educators have an undoubted responsibility to prepare women realistically and positively for the possibilities that may confront them at the time of birth. Whichever 'coping strategies' are taught (Brayshaw & Wright 1994), women and their partners must realise that their 'ideal' birth, and the way they wish to handle it, may be unattainable – particularly if it is a first labour or the mother falls into a 'high-risk' category. Some women with no preparation find labour entirely manageable; others who attend antenatal classes and acquire pain-relieving skills (relaxation, breathing awareness, massage, movement, positioning, etc.) may find these offer sufficient relief. However, because labour is often still painful even after antenatal training, very many women will need the extra assistance of analgesia and anaesthesia (Charles et al 1978, Melzack et al 1981). It may be important for this to be commenced early to avoid distress-related thoughts. It is imperative that the women's health physiotherapist does not make women who use any of the currently available pain-relieving drugs feel failures, especially if they have not been able to cope with labour without additional help.

NORMAL LABOUR AND DELIVERY

The mechanics of labour

In 38% of cases, labour starts with the foetal head in the left occipito-lateral (LOL) position; that is the foetus is facing the right maternal ilium. A further 24% are in the right occipitolateral position. In either case the long axis of the foetal head is on the long axis of the maternal pelvic inlet (see p. 3). Initially the upper part of the head is the presenting portion; however, as labour progresses the head flexes and descends so that the upper and more posterior part of the head (the vertex) leads.

As the descent into the pelvis continues the foetal head rotates through 90° until the face is towards the sacrum and coccyx, and the occiput is below the symphysis pubis. All the diameters in mid-cavity are similar (see p. 3); this allows a corkscrew action with the body following, ending with the long axis of the foetal head in the long axis of the maternal pelvic outlet. In addition the foetus has to negotiate a 'corner' in its route as the pelvic inlet is at right angles to the outlet.

Further descent produces extension of the foetal neck beneath the symphysis pubis. Usually at delivery the baby's head faces posteriorly; the shoulders are still oblique but turning. As the shoulders descend, their greatest width comes to lie anteroposteriorly in the long axis of the outlet, and the baby's head, which is by now delivered, turns to face the mother's right leg (restitution). The anterior shoulder slips under the symphysis pubis first, and is usually quickly followed by the other shoulder and the rest of the body.

The effect of labour on maternal and foetal physiology

Both the mother and the foetus will experience modest stress even during a perfectly normal and straightforward labour, and levels of the catecholamines, adrenaline (epinephrine) and noradrenaline (norepinephrine) are raised, producing the familiar 'fight or flight' response. In both mother and foetus this will result in the shunting of blood to vital organs such as the heart and lungs, so making more oxygen available, and in the mobilisation of energy stores. It must be appreciated, however, that excessive stress is detrimental to both mother and foetus. For example, it may result in shunting of blood from the contracting uterus and placenta, leading to slowing of contractions and foetal distress.

The foetus There is still a great deal that is not fully understood, but it is known that the particular stress of the second stage and delivery on the foetus results in a surge of catecholamines, predominantly noradrenaline (norepinephrine), which facilitates normal breathing, and helps the baby maintain body heat and survive adversity – particularly low oxygen conditions – in the first few hours of independent life. Compression of the foetal thorax in both first and second stages squeezes out fluid that normally fills the lungs, but absorption of the remaining lung liquid and the release of sufficient surfactant appears to be dependent on an increase in plasma catecholamines immediately at birth to prevent the neonate from drowning.

The mother **Cardiovascular system** In response to contraction of the large uterine musculature there is a small progressive rise in heart rate, which is accelerated by anxiety, pain and dehydration, and cardiac output is increased. Blood pressure may also rise modestly in the first stage but more specifically in the second stage, when it tends to swing up with expulsive pushing and then fall between contractions. The latter is aggravated by prolonged breath holding with bearing down (the Valsalva manoeuvre), raising the intrathoracic and intra-abdominal pressure, which compresses veins and impedes the return of blood to the heart. The result is a fall in cardiac output and thus in blood pressure.

Respiratory system The mild hyperventilation of pregnancy becomes more noticeable in labour, when during strong first stage contractions of uterine muscle, both respiratory rate and depth increase in response to the increased oxygen requirement. Some decrease in arterial P_{CO_2} tension appears to be normal, but in severe cases of overbreathing, the woman experiences numbness and tingling of the lips and extremities owing to the blood becoming relatively alkalotic, leading to calcium ionisation, which affects nerve conductivity. Maternal alkalosis results in oxygen being more tightly bound to the haemoglobin, and consequently it is given up less easily. Occasionally this will mean that, at the placenta, the foetal circulation may not obtain as much oxygen as it would normally, and this can be compounded by the fact that acute maternal hyperventilation may cause uterine vasoconstriction and reduce placental blood flow. Insufficient oxygen to the foetus may force it to metabolise anaerobically; this can result in foetal acidosis and distress (see p. 73).

Gastrointestinal system There is a reduction in peristalsis and absorption, and towards the end of the first stage, nausea and vomiting may occur.

The wisdom of eating and drinking in labour is a controversial subject. Those against the practice cite the risk of eating and drinking followed by any need for a general anaesthetic causing aspiration of gastric contents; this is known as Mendelson's syndrome (Mendelson 1946). The acidic gastric juice is highly irritant and, if inhaled, causes bronchospasm, dyspnoea, cyanosis and pulmonary oedema. Therefore it was previously advocated that nothing should be taken orally during labour; this belief continued for many decades. However, others believe that a lack of nutrition in labour may lead to dehydration and ketosis with an increased consequential need for intervention. Those who advocate feeding in normal labour suggest the ingestion of frequent light meals that are low in fat and roughage and easily absorbed; fluids should be allowed as desired. This is generally considered reasonable provided that there is no suggestion that there will be a need for general anaesthesia or that narcotic analgesia has been given. Speak (2002) reviewed the available literature and concluded that guidelines dating from 1946 should not be used to determine the management of women in labour; also that women in labour should be given the choice. There is insufficient research evidence to dictate a policy of no food or drink in labour; further research is required.

Temperature   The strong muscle activity results in heat production; there may be a slight rise in temperature, and women feel hot and perspire. However, redistribution of blood often results in the feet being very cold. The midwife monitors the temperature in labour as a raised temperature may also indicate infection or ketosis; if either is suspected appropriate action must be taken.

The effect of labour on the pelvic floor and perineum

As the foetal head descends it follows the curve of the sacrum and coccyx to reach the pelvic floor. It exerts pressure, which dilates the vagina, stretches the perineum, and separates and displaces the levator ani muscles sideways and downwards. The bowel is compressed, and the urethra is stretched as the bladder is pulled up above the symphysis pubis by virtue of its attachment to the cervix and uterus. This makes more space in the pelvis. The stretching, lengthening and consequent thinning of the posterior portion of the pelvic floor and perineum, ahead of the foetus, form the birth canal, and enable the vaginal opening to be turned and directed more anteriorly. Physiotherapists should note that it is this stretching, bowing and thinning of the pelvic floor, particularly when aggravated by the use of instruments needed for assistance (e.g. forceps) that is thought to be a cause of pudendal nerve damage. This has been shown to be associated with faecal and urinary incontinence postpartum (Allen et al 1990, Snooks et al 1984, Sorensen et al 1988, Sultan et al 1994a). It can also cause vascular damage resulting in haematoma, or more general bruising and oedema. Fascia may be overstretched and muscle fibres torn.

The stretching and thinning takes time in the second stage of labour and may result in a tearing of the vaginal opening. Previously it was believed that judgement should be used to determine, first, whether foetal and maternal welfare are best served by waiting for the natural stretching to occur or by accelerating the delivery process with an episiotomy and, secondly, whether an episiotomy is needed to avoid an uncontrollable tear, perhaps involving the anal sphincter. However, there is now evidence that using an episiotomy to prevent tears does not result in less trauma, improve healing or decrease incontinence and dyspareunia (Sleep et al 1984, Sleep & Grant 1987). Furthermore in a study of 697 low-risk randomised women, it was shown that perineal and pelvic floor morbidity was greatest amongst women receiving median episiotomy compared with those remaining intact or with spontaneous tears (Klein et al 1994).

The duration of labour

Each labour is individual, even in the same woman, and there are wide variations in duration, particularly between primigravidae and multigravidae. Statistics seem to indicate that modern obstetric practices, particularly induction, acceleration, sedation, ambulation and the greater use of caesarean section, have resulted in labours on average being shorter now than formerly. In many centres it is general policy to try to ensure that 24 hours is the outside limit for a labour, it being considered more than enough for all parties involved. A prolonged labour may cause maternal distress, with a rise in temperature, pulse and blood pressure; dehydration, oliguria and ketosis also develop, perhaps accompanied by vomiting (O'Brien 1997). Other possibilities cited by the author are intrauterine infection, the risk of ruptured uterus if there is an undetected cephalopelvic disproportion, and of operative intervention, anaesthesia and postpartum haemorrhage. There is also the possibility of intrauterine hypoxia of the infant with all the ensuing problems that may occur as a result.

Nesheim (1988), in a sample of 9703 labours in Norway, found a median duration of 8.2 hours for nulliparae and 5.3 hours for multiparae, whereas Morrin (1997a) quoted in primigravidae 12–14 hours for the first stage and 1 hour for the second stage, and in multigravidae 6–10 hours for the first stage and a second stage of up to 30 minutes. Nesheim (1988) showed that induced labours were shorter than those with spontaneous onset, 1.9 hours shorter in nulliparae and 1.4 hours in multiparae, and also that tall women had quicker labours than short women. Maternal age did not seem to influence duration, but the weight of the baby, maternal weight gain in pregnancy and the prepregnancy weight all correlated positively with longer labours. The implications in health education are clear: that women should be encouraged to achieve an optimum weight for their height preconceptually and then control their weight gain during pregnancy. Interestingly, Nesheim (1988) found that, whereas in nulliparae the occipitoposterior positions and failure of the head to flex prolonged labour, breech presentations did not. In multiparae, none of these presentations prolonged labour.

Positioning in labour

Considerable research effort has been expended on determining whether there is advantage, as logic would suggest, in the upright positions in labour, for example sitting, standing or forward-leaning, and kneeling. Caldeyro-Barcia (1979), Flynn et al (1978), Mendez Bauer et al (1975) and Mitre (1974) seem to show a shorter first stage correlating with being upright and ambulant, but McManus & Calder (1978) and Williams et al (1980) could find no statistical difference whether a labouring woman remained recumbent or was actively encouraged to be upright and move around. It is agreed, however, that the labouring woman's contractions are stronger in the upright position (Flynn et al 1978, Read 1981). Positional change also has a positive effect on the efficiency of uterine contractions (Roberts et al 1983). Over one hundred years ago, Clark (1891) reported that 'The effectiveness of uterine pains has been increased by change in posture, especially after a patient has maintained for a long time a constrained position.' The other, very important, aspect of this issue is how the women judge being upright and mobile in the first stage of labour. Most of the researchers cited above reported greater maternal satisfaction and comfort where women were free to move and rest as they wished; Flynn et al (1978) found the need for analgesia to be significantly reduced for those who were ambulant. Any suggestion that ambulation might compromise the foetus appears to be unfounded for the majority of women with appropriate foetal monitoring, and where proper exclusion criteria are applied (e.g. women at risk for cord prolapse). In addition, there is now the inference that good pain control and alleviation of thoughts of distress and fear in the latent phase of the first stage may be critical in encouraging an effective shorter labour (Wuitchik et al 1989). A study of 58 women has shown that the sitting position offers a relief of both continuous and intermittent back pain between 6 and 8 cm dilatation compared with the supine position (Adachi et al 2003).

Sosa et al (1980) found that labouring women who were empathetically cared for by a lay female supporter (a *doula*) also had shorter labours. More recently Hodnett (2001) concluded that continuous support of a woman in labour has a beneficial effect on both the maternal and infant outcomes without any associated risks.

For the second stage, sitting, standing, kneeling and squatting have advantages over the supine and side-lying positions by resulting in stronger, more efficient contractions (Caldeyro-Barcia 1979) and more effective use of gravity. In squatting particularly, there is also an increase in the size of the pelvic outlet (Russell 1982), which may be important. Supported squatting (see Fig. 6.4, p. 180) is helpful for women who find the full squat impossible, uncomfortable or tiring (Poschl 1987). In the 1990s those supporting the theory of optimal foetal positioning (Sutton & Scott 1995) suggested that a supported squat position should be flat footed and straight backed with the bottom at least 45 cm above the floor – allowing the woman to assist the passage of the foetus. See p. 177 for further information regarding positioning in labour.

Human support with skin contact is often preferred, but special birthing chairs, cushions (Gardosi et al 1989), stools and beds have been devised. Squatting can hasten the onset of the urge to bear down, whereas the 'all-fours' position, by taking pressure off the cervix, can be used to control this urge (especially if the prone kneel fall position is adopted, see p. 180), and also eases backache and assists with the anterior rotation of a posterior position (Grant 1987, Scruggs 1982). However, Sutton & Scott (1995) also suggest that kneeling on the hands and knees assists in the self-delivery of the baby's head in second stage.

Epidural anaesthesia always used to mean a recumbent or semirecumbent mother. However, the more recent 'mobile' epidural techniques have been shown to be both effective and to have a beneficial impact on delivery mode (Wilson et al 2002).

The third stage usually lasts not more than 30 minutes. The mother is normally so involved with the baby that, if all goes well, she is unaware of the process. The woman intuitively adopts a resting posture with the baby; many midwives prefer the supine position for the third stage because the uterus is more easily observed and cord traction, if needed, can be applied more effectively. It is said that there is also less danger in this position of air reaching the blood sinuses in the placental site, which could cause an air embolism.

MANAGEMENT OF NORMAL LABOUR

Most maternity units now have written protocols regarding the management of the labouring woman, with set criteria for intervention. These predetermined consensus guidelines have the advantage of overcoming, to some extent, the problems posed by several consultants serving one unit, each with their own management preferences. Such protocols can be of benefit also to midwives where the shift system and staff changes can make continuity of care and communication difficult. However, it is clear that management of the labouring woman does vary from place to place as evidenced by the variation from one UK health region to another of the caesarean section rate. Extremes of philosophy can be found, by which one unit will routinely monitor women for a short period on admission but intervene only where it is suspected that maternal or foetal well-being are threatened, whereas another unit will apply a very active management from the start, monitoring continuously and intervening immediately if progress deviates from a set norm.

THE START OF LABOUR

When a woman decides that labour may be starting she will alert her carers, who will either go to her at home, or await her at a maternity unit. In either case the midwife will be concerned to establish immediately that both foetus and mother are well, and so will check the foetal heart rate and the maternal temperature, pulse and blood pressure. The midwife will then palpate the lie of the foetus and the presenting part, and palpate and monitor the quality and frequency of any contractions. A vaginal examination determines the state of the cervix and confirms the level of the foetal head. From all these data, in time, it will be possible to determine whether labour is established. Urine will be tested for protein, glucose and ketones.

RECORDING THE PROGRESS OF LABOUR

In most consultant units the progress of labour is now recorded on a partogram (Fig. 3.5), a combination of charts on which the pattern of uterine contractions, the descent of the presenting part, cervical dilatation and medication, together with measures of maternal well-being such as blood pressure and pulse rate, are graphically recorded against time, and thus are easily evaluated. There is a recognised norm, and this visualisation highlights early evidence of labour failing to progress and allows consideration of appropriate action.

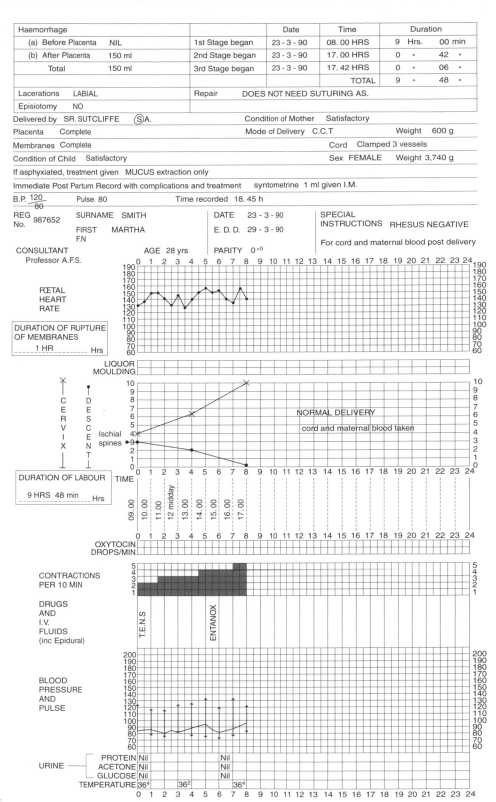

Figure 3.5   A partogram.

Medical and midwifery staff may monitor the foetal heart rate intermittently using a Pinard stethoscope or a simple Sonic-aid. More continuous surveillance requires a foetal heart monitor; this uses an ultrasound transducer on the woman's abdomen, and produces a printout, as well as signalling the foetal heart rate via a flashing light or an audible bleep. Alternatively the foetal heart rate may be recorded through an electrode attached to the foetal scalp. The same machine, a cardiotocograph (CTG), will also give a printout of uterine activity by means of a maternal tocograph. For this, either a very delicate pressure gauge is strapped externally to the woman's abdomen, or a modified gauge may be passed vaginally to monitor contractions more accurately internally. A recent Cochrane report (Thacker et al 2003) concluded that the only clinically significant benefit of continuous monitoring was the reduction of neonatal seizures. They also stated that the decision determining whether continuous or intermittent auscultation be used during labour should be made jointly between the clinician and the woman. Furthermore, MacLennan (1999) states that the evidence regarding electronic monitoring does not show that it prevents cerebral palsy.

FIRST STAGE OF LABOUR

Early in labour, unless there are special circumstances, women should be encouraged to continue with rest or gentle activities appropriate to the time of day and consistent with the philosophy of conserving energy. It is a disadvantage to go into labour tired. Management in the first stage consists chiefly of regular monitoring of foetal and maternal well-being, and relief of fear and pain by, in the first instance, ensuring that the labouring woman has sympathetic and empathetic companionship. Blood pressure is initially measured every 2–4 hours, then hourly as labour advances (Morrin 1997a). Sosa et al (1980) reported a small study using a supportive lay woman, a doula; this showed major perinatal benefits for the supported group, including shorter labours. Women should be encouraged to be as physically and mentally comfortable as possible, moving or staying still as feels best, as discussed previously. So for many women the first stage is passed with periods of walking around, periods of sitting in chairs or beanbags, and periods of resting, even dozing on a sofa or bed. Pleasant surroundings (Chapman et al 1986), music and a warm bath (Lenstrup et al 1987) or shower may be invaluable. Changes of position are important (Roberts et al 1983) in assisting progress. A woman should try to empty her bladder at 2 hourly intervals (Morrin 1997a), as a full bladder may increase pain and delay progress. The fluid input and output is recorded to assist in maintaining a fluid balance. If a woman becomes ketotic or dehydrated then intravenous fluids and dextrose will be required. Ideally the decision regarding additional pain relief is one made jointly by the mother and the midwife. Cool flannels for sponging, sucking ice, and massage to the back and abdomen are soothing to some. Women have for very many years heeded the advice to have a warm bath in the first stage of labour to assist with relaxation and hence pain relief. Some maternity units also offer the option of a woman labouring and perhaps delivering her baby in a birthing pool; women having a home birth may also elect to hire a birthing pool for their own use at home. The birthing pool is said to assist relaxation, aid pain relief and enhance cervical dilatation. This is thought to be due to the effects of buoyancy, reduction of anxiety and conservation of energy. However, concern has been expressed regarding the passing of infection to the mother and baby, water embolism and perineal trauma (Morrin 1997b). It is therefore essential that strict protocols should be adhered to regarding the suitability of the labouring mother and the procedures to be followed (see pp. 95, 190).

SECOND STAGE OF LABOUR

The management of the second stage of labour consists of caring for the mother and foetus from the time of the full dilatation of the cervix until the delivery of the baby. There are a variety of positions in which it is possible for a woman to deliver her baby (see Fig. 6.4 on p. 180). The prime considerations are the baby's safety, the mother's comfort and the position which enables her to respond best to the bearing-down reflex. Difficulties can arise if a midwife finds it impossible to monitor and control the delivery in the position selected by the labouring woman. However, where the conventional reclining posture has been chosen but the mother is not pushing effectively or the urge to bear down is weak, she should be encouraged, even temporarily, to change position, perhaps into some adaptation of squatting if this is possible and safe. It has been suggested for some time that lying on the back for prolonged periods in the second stage could adversely affect the foetus by reducing placental perfusion; left-side lying has been shown to reduce the problem. Johnstone et al (1987) showed that even a tilt of 15° to the left, effected by using a firm pillow or towels under the right hip, was effective in this regard. During the second stage of labour, contractions become longer, stronger and more frequent to aid expulsion. The pressure of the foetus, about 1 centimetre above the ischial spines, stimulates nerve receptors in the pelvic floor increasing the urge to bear down; this is known as Ferguson's reflex (Morrin 1997b).

As the foetal head descends the perineum distends, the anus dilates and the vagina opens progressively with contractions; however, some regression may be seen between contractions. The midwife controls the head at 'crowning' to allow the vaginal opening gently to complete the extreme distension needed; the mother may be asked at this point to refrain from pushing and to pant instead. The foetal head is encouraged into extension under the pubic arch and the neck explored to locate the cord. Once delivered, the baby's head turns to face the maternal right leg. The head is laterally flexed towards the anus to assist the delivery of the right shoulder, then to the symphysis pubis to ease out the second shoulder; the body usually follows easily. The baby may need nasal and mouth suction to clear the airways but is laid either between the mother's legs or on her abdomen. If active management of the third stage is adopted, an injection of ergometrine and oxytocin is given into the mother's thigh once the shoulders are delivered, and the cord is clamped.

The accepted method of assessment and recording the baby's condition is by the Apgar score (Table 3.3) at 1, 5 and 10 minutes after delivery.

Table 3.3 Apgar: a score for neonatal assessment

	0 points	1 point	2 points
Colour	Blue, pale	Pink body, blue extremities	Pink
Respiratory effort	Absent	Gasping	Sharp, cry
Heart rate	Absent	Less than 100 beats/min	More than 100 beats/min
Reflex activity	Absent	Grimace	Cry
Muscle tone	Low	Some limb flexion	Active movement

A score of less than 7 requires immediate paediatric assistance. It has been found that babies with low Apgar scores followed by signs of cerebral depression, despite not having cerebral palsy, have an increased risk of neurodevelopmental impairment and learning difficulties (Moster et al 2002).

THIRD STAGE OF LABOUR

The third stage is the time from after the delivery of the baby until there has been the expulsion of the placenta and membranes. There is difference of opinion regarding clamping of the umbilical cord, cited in Morrin (1997c). Inch (1985) believes that the cord should remain unclamped for the unhindered compression of the placenta and retraction of muscle fibres, whereas Prendiville & Elbourne (1989) state that early clamping of the cord can reduce the length of third stage of labour. In a rhesus negative woman there should never be a delay in cord clamping, otherwise there is an increased risk of fetomaternal transfusion. Unless there is an individual reason not to, common practice is to clamp the cord after it has stopped pulsating. If the mother puts the baby to the breast, the release of oxytocin will assist the physiological process of separation and delivery of the placenta. Management, which may be passive or active, consists of ensuring the complete separation and safe delivery of the placenta, and monitoring and controlling haemorrhage where necessary.

Passive management (otherwise known as expectant or physiological management) allows the natural physiological changes to take their course, and excludes the use of oxytocic drugs. This usually takes 15–30 minutes. Strong uterine contractions enable the midwife to feel the fundus of the uterus. Initially it will usually be above the umbilicus, and feels bulky owing to the presence of the placenta. Once the placenta has separated completely, further contractions assist it into the lower uterine segment, thus enabling the uterus to contract down progressively further, until the placenta is expelled. The mother may be asked to assist with expulsive effort. The midwife may prefer the mother to adopt a standing, kneeling or squatting posture rather than lying back, to utilise both gravity and intra-abdominal pressure in helping the process.

Active management requires an intramuscular injection of an oxytocic drug after the shoulders are delivered. The midwife places one hand above the symphysis, and when the uterus contracts, pressure is applied on the fundus in an upward direction toward the umbilicus to prevent the uterus from being drawn down, while the other hand exerts steady downward controlled traction on the cord. If the placenta is not delivered, then controlled cord traction is tried again after 2–3 minutes during a contraction. The sequence may have to be repeated. The chief objective is to avoid inverting the uterus where complete separation has not yet occurred. The mother is usually sitting back with her knees bent, to allow the uterine pressure to be applied.

Active management of the third stage of labour has been recommended by WHO (1994) in order to reduce the incidence of postpartum haemorrhage. However, in the UK this poses less of a problem, hence women tend to be able to make an informed choice as to which method they prefer. Once delivered, the placenta is weighed and examined for completeness, and the total amount of blood loss is estimated.

COMPLICATIONS OF LABOUR

FAILURE TO PROGRESS

The phrase 'failure to progress' is used to indicate that labour has stopped proceeding from phase to phase as expected, and the presenting part is not descending and rotating any further as time passes. There are a variety of possible causes; for example, contractions may be insufficiently strong or long, the pelvis may be too small for the size of the foetus (cephalopelvic disproportion) or the cervix may fail to dilate. The experienced midwife will quickly recognise a deviation from normal on the partogram, and most centres now have their own set criteria for appropriate active intervention.

FOETAL DISTRESS

Uterine contractions are a normal stress to the foetus, compressing it and producing a temporary reduction in the oxygenated blood supply through the placental site. A healthy term foetus with a normal CTG has a normal baseline foetal heart rate of 110–150 beats per minute with a normal baseline variability of 10–25 b.p.m. Accelerations are transient increases in foetal heart rate of 15 b.p.m. or more lasting 15 seconds or more. Two accelerations recorded in a 20-minute period are termed 'reactive' and indicate optimal foetal health. Decelerations are transient reductions in the foetal heart rate from the baseline by more than 15 b.p.m. and lasting more than 15 seconds; these indicate foetal distress (Varma et al 2000). At best the foetal heart rate is unaffected by the contractions, or there is only a slight deceleration coincident with the peak of contractions (early decelerations) and the rate then picks up. In the absence of other adverse signs, a drop of not more than 40 b.p.m. is often acceptable, but foetal hypoxia must be suspected if:

1. the decelerations are by more than 40 b.p.m.
2. the time taken for recovery to the higher rate is increasing
3. there is generalised slowing of the heart rate
4. the maximum deceleration occurs after the peak of the contraction (late decelerations).

Foetal hypoxia is the most common cause of foetal distress and may be due to pressure on the cord, premature separation of the placenta, hypertonia of the uterine muscle or hypertonia of maternal blood vessels. The passing of foetal meconium per vaginam may also be a serious sign, indicating the possibility that foetal hypoxia has induced anal sphincter muscle hypotonia. Hypoxia can be confirmed by foetal scalp blood sampling and testing the blood pH value. Normally foetal blood is more acid (pH 7.25–35) than maternal blood (pH 7.44), but in the presence of hypoxia the pH value falls, a pH of less than 7.20 being an indicator of foetal distress.

MATERNAL DISTRESS

Previously labour was classed as prolonged when exceeding 24 hours; however, it is now believed that the acceptable limit is 12 hours (O'Brien 1997). This has reduced the number of women suffering from exhaustion. In a normal labour there is rarely any cause for real anxiety about the mother's physical condition; however, a constant watch is kept. A distressed woman in labour shows signs of both mental and physical exhaustion; there is an increase in pulse rate, temperature and blood pressure with the development of oliguria, ketosis and dehydration. Therefore the mother's urine is regularly checked for protein and ketones.

The emotional distress which some women experience is associated with fear, pain and apparent lack of progress. Good antenatal preparation, together with continuity of care in labour, sensitive support and companionship, adequate appropriate pain relief, skilled attention to comfort and regular realistic progress reports and reassurance, go a long way towards preventing the labouring woman experiencing excessive emotional distress.

MALPRESENTATION

When the presenting part is other than the vertex, for example the buttocks, arms or face, it is categorised as a malpresentation. The most common of these, the breech, is discussed here; suggestions for further reading are given at the end of the chapter.

BREECH PRESENTATION

The presenting part of the foetus is the buttocks, i.e. the 'breeches' end. Approximately 3% of foetuses present buttocks first at term. In the middle trimester it is much more common, owing apparently to there being more room to move at this stage, but the majority eventually turn to become cephalic presentations. A breech presentation is potentially dangerous because of the severe intermittent pressure on the after-coming head from the dominant part of the uterus. In addition the foetal head, which is the largest part, will not have been moulded to the bony birth canal so there could be the risk of cephalopelvic disproportion. There is also some anxiety that the cervix might close on the foetal neck and obstruct the passage of the head; forceps may therefore be used to protect and guide the after-coming head. It is now believed that the major cause of intracranial haemorrhage in a breech delivery is anoxia (Sweet 1997). Other dangers of breech delivery include fractures, dislocations, brachial plexus lesions, rupture of abdominal organs and genital oedema and bruising (Sweet 1997). The American College of Obstetricians and Gynecologists (ACOG 2002) reported and recommended, as a result of the large and well-controlled Term Breech Trial, that:

- obstetricians continue to reduce breech deliveries in singleton pregnancies by applying ECV whenever possible
- planned vaginal delivery of a singleton breech may no longer be appropriate
- if breech vaginal deliveries are pursued then it must be with great caution
- those with persistent breech presentation at term singleton gestation should undergo a planned caesarean section
- a planned caesarean delivery does not apply to:
  - those in advanced labour with a breech presentation in whom delivery is imminent
  - those in whom a second twin is in a non-vertex position.

For many the choice will lie between external cephalic version and elective caesarean section (Young & Johanson 2001). Meanwhile the best mode for preterm breech is unclear (Mukhopadhyay & Arulkumaran 2002). Vaginal delivery will be unavoidable in certain circumstances but as a consequence of the Term Breech Trial, progressively fewer midwives and junior doctors will gain the experience and confidence to conduct a vaginal breech delivery. It may be that regular teaching using video clips or mannequins will be necessary to preserve skills (Mukhopadhyay & Arulkumaran 2002).

There are three types of breech:

1. *fully flexed* – both legs are flexed and drawn up on the abdomen, most common in multigravidae
2. *extended* – legs are flexed at the hips but extended at the knees, and the feet are in contact with the baby's shoulders, most common in primigravidae
3. *footling* – one or both feet present first (below the buttocks) with the hips and knees extended.

MALPOSITION

When the vertex is less than optimally placed there is said to be malposition. The most common malposition is the occipitoposterior; for other possibilities see Further Reading, p. 91.

Occipitoposterior position

When the foetal head enters the pelvis or turns midcavity, so that the occiput is toward the maternal sacrum rather than the maternal symphysis pubis, it is said to be in the occipitoposterior position (OP). Commonly the occiput will be toward the right side of the sacrum (ROP), and less often to the left (LOP). The head will eventually rotate in a majority of cases to present at the pelvic outlet in the OA position as previously described. OP labours tend to be longer as there may be slower descent of the foetal head and hence slower dilatation of the cervix. If there is failure of the head to flex sufficiently, the longer diameter of the foetal head is presented; therefore cervical dilatation may have to be greater and the perineum is more greatly distended. An episiotomy is more than likely to be required. Severe backache is a frequent problem, probably because of the pressure of the occiput on the sacrum, and epidural anaesthesia may be appropriate. If rotation of the foetus becomes obstructed it is called a 'transverse arrest', and most probably an emergency caesarean section becomes necessary.

Prolapse or presentation of the cord

For the cord to prolapse into the vagina or to appear at the vulva, the amniotic sac must have ruptured (see p. 55), and the presenting part is likely to be high or ill fitting for some reason (e.g. malpresentation, multiparity). Subsequent pressure on the cord from the head during contractions, traction, or simply the colder environment, outside the amniotic sac may cause the foetal blood supply to be obstructed, so early delivery is imperative. It is possible for the cord to rest alongside and even ahead of the main presenting part within an intact amniotic sac. This is a serious state which can cause foetal distress, and which requires constant vigilance to diagnose. Medical help must be immediately summoned at the first observation of any umbilical cord prolapse. An American review of 65 cases identified from 26 545 deliveries determined that cord prolapse continues to be associated with poor perinatal outcomes despite emergency delivery (Prabulos & Philipson 1998). Furthermore, a Turkish study has shown that abnormal foetal presentation and multiparity are associated with an increased risk of umbilical cord prolapse (Uyger et al 2002). It has also been reported that umbilical cord prolapse is a possible complication of external cephalic version in patients with rupture of membranes and oligohydramnios (Berghella 2001).

KNOTS OF THE UMBILICAL CORD

A true knot of the umbilical cord is caused by the movement of the foetus knotting the cord prior to birth. A false knot may be due to the cord blood vessels being longer than the cord or other irregularities and node formation (Morrin 1997c). In a large study population of 69 139 singleton deliveries (Hershkovitz et al 2001), true knots of the cord resulted in significantly higher foetal distress with a higher proportion of meconium-stained amniotic fluid. Furthermore there was an increased likelihood of caesarean delivery and a fourfold higher rate of antepartum foetal death among these foetuses (Hershkovitz et al 2001). The obstetric factors significantly correlated with true knots were gestational diabetes, hydramnios, patients undergoing genetic amniocentesis and male foetuses. Any patient attending for physiotherapy who mentions that there is a diminution of foetal activity should be checked by a midwife or doctor.

INCOORDINATE UTERINE ACTIVITY

The ideal pattern of uterine polarity (see p. 57) does not always occur. Disordered uterine action, which is painful yet unproductive, occurs most commonly (96%) in primigravid labours, with hypertonia of the lower segment, alterations in polarity so that fundal dominance is lost, and parts of the uterus contracting independently or out of sequence (colicky uterus). This condition prolongs labour and may require active intervention if it does not speedily resolve. Cervical dystocia is a rare condition in which the cervix fails to dilate owing to some structural abnormality, with the result that vaginal delivery is impossible; a caesarean section then needs to be performed (O'Brien 1997).

HAEMORRHAGE

Because of the hugely enhanced blood supply to the uterus, which has developed through pregnancy, haemorrhage at any stage of labour is extremely serious and emergency steps to expedite delivery must be taken, possibly by caesarean section. Where haemorrhage is uncontrollable, a hysterectomy may be necessary; mercifully this is very rare.

CONTRACTED PELVIS AND CEPHALOPELVIC DISPROPORTION

There are some women who have a normally shaped but small gynaecoid pelvis; small hands and feet correlate with this. Women with an android pelvis have pelvic walls that converge so that the outlet is narrow and the ischial spines may be very prominent (see p. 3). In women with a flat pelvis the inlet is narrow and difficult for the foetal head to pass through; there are yet others whose pelvis has been affected by trauma or disease. When one of the diameters of the true pelvis (see p. 3) is 1 cm less than the ideal gynaecoid pelvis, it is called a 'contracted pelvis'. In addition, some babies are large in proportion to their mothers. A woman's pelvis is not routinely assessed in pregnancy. Ultrasound assessment is used to determine foetal size in comparison with the woman's size. Where apparently the foetal head is physically unable to go through there is said to be cephalopelvic disproportion (CPD). A decision is usually made toward the end of a pregnancy, where there is a potential problem, either to deliver by elective caesarean section or to allow a 'trial of labour' with or without early induction. However, despite reasonable antenatal care, CPD can arise spontaneously in labour and is a reason for failure to progress.

A 'trial of labour' usually indicates that CPD is suspected, but it is hoped that moulding of the foetal head during labour and the maximum flexibility of the maternal pelvis at that stage may allow a normal vaginal delivery. Very careful monitoring of the descent of the head will soon indicate delay, and caesarean section can be carried out where necessary. Induction at earlier than 40 weeks' gestation will mean the baby is smaller (see Table 2.1, p. 31).

PLACENTAL ABRUPTION

Occasionally partial or complete separation of the placenta occurs before the birth of the baby. Blood may be retained at the site or drain out through the vagina. Where it is retained it may seep into the myometrium, causing marked damage (Coulevaire uterus). Any tendency for placental separation is a critical situation requiring immediate delivery of the baby by the most expeditious means.

MULTIPLE BIRTHS

Twin pregnancy is the most common to come to delivery; in more than 80% of cases the first baby will present by the vertex, and there is an almost equal chance of the second baby being vertex or breech. There is an increased risk of premature labour owing to the bulk of the pregnancy, possibly because uterine muscle has a finite limit of stretch at which labour contractions start and the cervix begins to open.

Where there are more than two babies it is usual for them to be delivered preterm by elective caesarean section.

PERINEAL TRAUMA

Labial lacerations

Labial lacerations are a common occurrence in the childbirth process. However, evidence-based management of minor tears has yet to emerge from the scientific literature (Arkin & Chern-Hughes 2002). They may bleed profusely and be painful but are generally superficial. Usually they are not sutured but kept dry and clean with analgesia as appropriate.

Haematoma

Stretching of the vagina and labia at delivery may result in rupture of veins. The resulting haematoma can be quite large, cause great pain, and may require aspiration. Vaginal haematoma can be a consequence of delivery in which there is shoulder dystocia.

Perineal tears

Perineal tears may occur spontaneously at delivery, or tearing may extend an episiotomy. It has been shown that perineal massage in the last 5–6 weeks of pregnancy is an effective method to increase the likelihood of an intact perineum for women undergoing a first vaginal delivery, but not for women with a previous vaginal delivery (Labrecque et al 1999). An English study (Shipman et al 1997) also showed benefits from antenatal perineal massage. They found that the best effect was in the age group of 30 years and above. It has also been concluded that perineal massage during the second stage of labour does not decrease the likelihood of an intact perineum or reduce the risk of pain, dysparenia or urinary and faecal problems (Stamp et al 2001).

Perineal tears are classified according to the structures involved and are almost exclusive to the posterior perineum:

1. *First degree* – involves the skin only, i.e. the fourchette.
2. *Second degree* – is deeper and affects any or all of the superficial perineal muscles and the pubococcygeus; the tear may extend up both sides or one side of the vaginal wall.
3. *Third degree* – as above, plus anal sphincter involvement; the tear may extend up the rectal wall.
4. *Fourth degree* – indicates a very severe third degree tear, extending into the anal mucosa.

First and second degree tears will be repaired following infiltration with lidocaine (lignocaine) 1% unless there is an epidural block in progress. A midwife or doctor may perform the repair. Third and fourth degree tears may require a general anaesthetic and will be performed by an obstetrician or rectal surgeon. There is considerable debate concerning the best suture material (Grant 1987, Grant et al 1989). It is also important that the thread is not pulled tight, to allow for the inevitable oedema (see p. 221).

RETAINED PLACENTA AND PLACENTA ACCRETA

The placenta may have separated normally from the uterine wall but still need assistance to leave the uterus. Allowing the baby to suckle to stimulate oxytocin production and uterine contraction, or rubbing the abdomen to stimulate contractions and firmly pressing upward on the fundus while applying gentle traction on the cord, is often sufficient (see p. 73) for it to be delivered.

Where separation appears to be incomplete, or is not occurring at all, there is an increase in the possibility of haemorrhage or shock. The manual removal of the placenta takes place under epidural, spinal or general anaesthesiae depending on the individual circumstances. In rare instances the placental chorionic villi have invaded the myometrium (placenta accreta) to such an extent that separation is very difficult and may cause life-threatening haemorrhage; in this case a hysterectomy may be the only safe course to take.

INTERVENTIONS IN LABOUR

TO INITIATE LABOUR IN THE FIRST STAGE

Prostaglandins

If for some reason induction of labour is being considered and the normal ripening of the cervix has not yet occurred, then prostaglandin pessaries or gel applied to the cervix may produce the required effect. Sometimes this is sufficient in itself to encourage the uterus to begin contracting, and labour to commence. Prostaglandin E_2 is thought to be superior to other forms and is the most commonly used. Oral administration of Prostaglandins need multiple doses over a longer time and can be associated with maternal gastrointestinal side-effects.

Oxytocin

Synthetic oxytocin via an intravenous drip causes uterine contractions; it works best where the cervix is ripe (favourable) and the membranes have been ruptured. Artificial rupture of membranes (ARM) will be performed when using oxytocin if the membranes have not spontaneously ruptured. Oxytocin may also be used to re-establish or accelerate labour at any stage when contractions have weakened or stopped altogether. However, as there are few oxytocin receptors in the cervix, it is not always as successful as anticipated.

Amniotomy

Amniotomy or ARM is sometimes called a surgical induction and is an irrevocable intervention. It may be used in association with oxytoxic drugs either to initiate or to accelerate labour. An amnihook, or forceps, is used to rupture the amniotic sac, as a result of which prostaglandins appear to be released and contractions may begin or be accelerated.

TO ASSIST DELIVERY IN THE SECOND STAGE

Episiotomy

Episiotomy involves an incision in the perineum equivalent to a second degree laceration. The perineum should be infiltrated with a lidocaine (lignocaine) solution (0.5 or 1%) before the episiotomy. The incision to enlarge the vaginal opening may be mediolateral or median (Fig. 3.6). Local anaesthetic should be used, although a well-distended perineum is said to have little sensation. The objective is usually to speed delivery or avoid excessive stretching or tearing of the surrounding tissues. Episiotomy used in conjunction with forceps or vacuum extraction allows more space for introduction of the instruments into the vagina. The incision is sutured after delivery is complete. A woman should have the possibility of an episiotomy discussed with her when she is completing her birth plan with her midwife. If at the time of delivery it is considered necessary to have an episiotomy, regardless of her earlier decision, the reason for episiotomy must be given and informed consent gained before the procedure.

Forceps delivery

Assistance with forceps may be necessary in the second stage:

- when progress is nil or very slow
- for foetal distress to speed delivery
- for maternal distress, exhaustion or where minimum maternal effort is desirable, e.g. in cardiac failure, severe pre-eclampsia, cystic fibrosis or hypertension
- to protect a preterm baby or during a breech delivery to protect the after-coming head.

Forceps should not be used if the head is not engaged, if there is a malpresentation of the face or brow, if the baby's position cannot be defined, if the head is above the ischial spines, in foetal macrosomia, if there has been a foetal death with postmortem changes or by someone lacking training or experience (Dennen 1994).

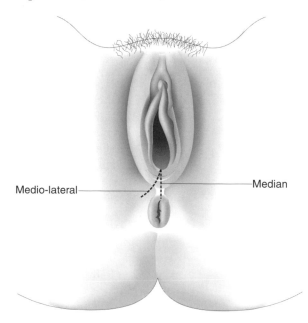

Medio-lateral ———— Median

Figure 3.6   To show the position of episiotomy.

Local, pudendal, spinal or epidural anaesthesia is required, and the woman will most commonly be placed in the lithotomy position.

High-cavity forceps (Kielland's) have longer, straighter handles and are used to assist the head at a higher level within the pelvis (e.g. for deep transverse arrest or OP positions) where rotation of the head or even downward traction to encourage rotation is needed; a large episiotomy is required. These forceps are rarely used in common practice.

Mid-cavity forceps (Neville Barnes) are the most commonly used forceps for exerting traction without rotation.

Low-cavity forceps (Wrigley's) are short, light forceps designed for use when the foetal head is low on the perineum – hence the term 'low forceps'. They have curved blades to receive the head and also have curved shafts to match the curve of the birth canal. They are now rarely used other than when performing a caesarean section.

Vacuum extraction or ventouse delivery

The indications for vacuum extraction are similar to those for forceps and are the common method of choice for an assisted delivery. A suction cup of an appropriate size is introduced into the vagina and applied to the foetal scalp posteriorly. Suction is used to draw the scalp up into the cup. Careful traction can then be given during uterine contractions. The success of the ventouse delivery can be dependent on the expertise of the operator. At delivery the baby will have a raised, red imprint of the cup on its head (chignon), which will persist for some days. This method of giving assistance has taken longer to gain acceptance in the UK than in other parts of the world (Chalmers & Chalmers 1989), but has continued to increase in popularity (Johanson et al 1993).

There has been considerable discussion as to whether vacuum extraction has a lesser morbidity of the maternal anal sphincter than does forceps delivery. Work by Sultan et al (1994b) showed vacuum extraction to be associated with fewer third degree tears than forceps delivery. However, although MacArthur et al (1997) found that instrumental delivery was associated with the development of faecal incontinence, there was no significant difference between forceps and vacuum extraction.

CAESAREAN SECTION

Delivery of the infant through incisions in the abdominal and uterine wall may be classified as 'elective', indicating that this mode of delivery has been chosen for specific reasons ahead of labour, or 'emergency', where it is decided on safety grounds to terminate labour. It may be carried out under either epidural (see p. 196) or general anaesthetic, at any stage of labour.

Reasons for an elective caesarean section are:

- contracted pelvis or CPD
- diabetes
- eclampsia
- serious illness or injury to the mother
- previous caesarean section

- placenta praevia
- multiple births of more than two babies
- malpresentation (breech presentations may or may not be caesarean deliveries depending on the complications presenting)
- peri- and postmortem delivery if appropriate
- active genital herpes
- previous vaginal reconstructive surgery
- previous incontinence surgery
- pelvic tumours
- severe intrauterine growth retardation
- foetal macrosomia
- some foetal abnormalities
- 'precious babies', history of infertility, etc.
- maternal request.

Reasons for an emergency caesarean section are:

- antepartum haemorrhage
- foetal or maternal distress
- failed trial of forceps
- prolapse of the umbilical cord
- failure to progress.

Many caesarean deliveries are done under spinal or epidural anaesthesia; the mother is then able to see and hold her baby immediately after delivery. Often emergency caesarean deliveries have to be done under general anaesthesia as speed is of the essence; general anaesthesia takes less time to take effect than epidural or spinal anaesthesia. There are two types of caesarean section. One is the classical section, consisting of a longitudinal incision in the upper uterine segment, via a paramedian incision. It is used for very premature babies where no lower segment has been formed. The other type is the lower segment section; this is the more common today and is favoured by women for its good cosmetic result. A Pfannenstiel (bikini line) incision, with separation of the recti, and a transverse incision into the lower uterine segment are used. These heal well, and do not usually preclude repeated caesarean section for future pregnancies or subsequent normal vaginal deliveries.

Caesarean section now has low risk of morbidity and mortality in comparison with former years (Jibodu & Arulkumaran 2000). Many women perceive benefit from a caesarean section, but the issues are complicated and far reaching. Decisions regarding the mode of delivery may ultimately be based after full discussion on preference rather than statistics (Jibodu & Arulkumaran 2000). Edwards & Davies (2001) enquired of 344 women attending a routine antenatal clinic as to which mode of delivery they would prefer in an uncomplicated pregnancy. Of the women surveyed, 14.5% elected for caesarean section. The main reasons given were the avoidance of a prolonged labour, maternal trauma and foetal well-being. The researchers concluded that it is hard to refuse a well-informed woman an elective caesarean section on request even if this results in an additional rise in the caesarean section rate.

Procedure for lower segment section

An incision is made through the skin and subcutaneous tissue in the natural fold just above the pubic hair. Transverse incisions are made in the anterior part of the rectus sheath on each side, the linea alba is divided, and these are blended into one transverse incision which can be stretched manually (the posterior portion of the rectus sheath is deficient at this level). The rectus sheaths are mobilised to expose the rectus muscles, which are then retracted laterally to gain access to the abdominal cavity.

The peritoneum is exposed and is opened with a transverse incision. The bladder is located and retracted away from the lower uterine segment, which is excised transversely and the wound further extended by manual stretching and tearing. This minimises bleeding and avoids the risk of instrumental damage to the foetal head. The head is eased out first, either manually or with Wrigley's forceps, and then the body. The cord is clamped and the baby held head down, while suction is used to clear mucus and liquor from the upper respiratory tract.

Active management of the third stage includes intravenous ergometrine given to effect placental separation; when this has occurred, the placenta can be gently withdrawn. The incision in the uterus is then closed with two layers of sutures, followed by closure of the peritoneum. The two recti are approximated and held together by three or four lightly tied sutures. The sheaths of the recti and the skin are then closed. A drain may be inserted.

Postoperative complications

Immediate complications may include haemorrhage, abdominal wind causing acute discomfort, wound infection, deep vein thrombosis, pulmonary embolism, abdominal adhesions and pelvic infection. Occasionally women experience urine retention, and it must be appreciated that neurological damage is possible, as is perforation of the bladder or ureters, particularly in emergency caesarean sections.

There are other possible long-term implications to future childbirth cited in the worldwide literature. The following studies presented are from the UK, Finland, USA, Israel and Hong Kong.

Fertility In 1989, Hall et al found that, in a large cohort of 22 948 women, of those having a caesarean section, 23.2% fewer had a further pregnancy than those who had had a spontaneous delivery. This difference was not accounted for by early sterilisation, maternal height or social status, and only partly attributable to age. Lowered fertility was also reported in a review concerning the impact of caesarean section by Hemminki (1996). It was found by Jolly et al (1999) that, in a study of 750 women, caesarean section and instrumental delivery left women frightened about further childbirth and was a factor not only in voluntary infertility but also in involuntary infertility.

Miscarriage Hall et al 1989 found that miscarriage was more common in women who had been previously delivered by caesarean section, and Hemminki (1996) also stated that it may be a factor in future miscarriage.

Placenta praevia and placenta accreta McMahon et al (1997) reviewed a population of 342 women with placenta praevia and 1082 randomly selected controls. They found that women with a history of caesarean section or parity of three or more births were at increased risk of having placenta praevia as a complication in a further pregnancy. Scheiner et al (2001) found that a previous caesarean section was found to be independently correlated with the occurrence of placenta praevia. In a review of 50 485 deliveries, To & Leung (1995) confirmed that there was an association between caesarean section and placenta praevia and placenta accreta. Furthermore they suggested that those women with a diagnosis of placenta praevia who have had a previous caesarean section should be considered at high risk for developing placenta accreta in a future pregnancy. Miller et al (1997) comment that placenta praevia and placenta accreta have caesarean section as an independent risk factor. Furthermore, Lachman et al (2000) remark that the increased rate of caesarean sections in recent years has resulted in an increase of placenta accreta. They also state that there is a direct correlation between placenta accreta and placenta praevia. The authors further state that placenta accreta should always be considered when performing a caesarean section for placenta praevia.

Ectopic pregnancy   Hemminki (1996) reported that an ectopic pregnancy is more likely after a caesarean delivery.

THE PUERPERIUM

The puerperium is the final phase in the childbearing continuum, and is the period of 6–8 weeks following delivery in which the woman's genital tract returns to a non-pregnant state. The process by which this occurs is called 'involution', and it commences as soon as the placenta is expelled. Once the placenta separates from the uterus, placental hormone production ceases, causing a dramatic decline in maternal blood levels of oestrogens and progesterone, and consequently in the physiological effects of these on maternal respiration, cardiovascular system, digestion and metabolism (see p. 31).

THE UTERUS

By the end of labour the uterus has considerably reduced in size, and this reduction continues by three processes. First, uterine contractions continue after delivery, becoming intermittent. Suckling by the baby at the breast stimulates the posterior pituitary to release more oxytocin, which causes further bursts of uterine contraction. Even the sight, sound or smell of the baby can have this effect, which causes labour-type pain to be felt in the lower abdomen; it may also be referred to the lumbar region. More multiparous women experience this than primiparae, in a ratio of 2:1 (Murray & Holdcroft 1989); it is described as throbbing, cramping or aching. For some women the pain is considerable – moderate to severe as scored on the McGill pain questionnaire – and is referred to as 'after pains'.

Secondly, there is an actual reduction in uterine tissue: retraction of the uterine muscle has the effect of controlling haemorrhage, and also gradually reduces the blood supply to the muscle tissue to a point where the additional muscle and supportive collagen required for pregnancy can no longer be maintained. Consequently a degrading process (autolysis) is set in motion, whereby the excess material is liquefied and absorbed into the bloodstream to be excreted via the kidneys.

Thirdly, for 2 to 3 weeks a parturient woman experiences a diminishing discharge called the lochia, similar to a heavy period, which consists of blood and necrotic decidua. The lochia is alkaline and organisms flourish in it more readily than in the normal vaginal secretions, which are acid, so there is an increased risk of infection. Much of the endometrium is regenerated in a fortnight; only the placental site takes longer. In the first few hours after delivery the cervix remains flaccid and open, but then gradually closes. The parous cervix has a permanently different appearance to a nulliparous one, the opening at the external os being a slit rather than a tiny circle.

One sign that the uterus is involuting (i.e. returning to a non-pregnant state), will be found in the gradual drop in the fundal height, which can be palpated. On the first postpartum day it is usually just above the umbilicus, by 6 days it is midway between the umbilicus and the symphysis, and by 10 days has disappeared down behind the symphysis. However, the parous uterus is always a little bigger than it was when nulliparous.

THE VAGINA AND PERINEUM

In the first few hours women often experience numbness of the perineum whether or not local anaesthesia was used. At first the vagina is very lax and women may notice air held within it, being released when they move, sit down or take a bath. In addition trauma such as labial tears, episiotomy, oedema and haematoma causes pain and takes time to heal. There may be pain inhibition of PFM contractions; actual trauma to the nerve supply to the pelvic floor musculature may manifest itself in difficulty in contracting the PFM and in bowing of the pelvic floor on straining.

There is a noticeable increase in the amount of urine passed in the first few days as the body releases the excess fluid retained in pregnancy. It has high nitrogen content owing to the autolytic process in the uterus; women often complain of frequency. Continence is sometimes disturbed in the puerperium and women experience variously: urgency, pain on micturition, stress incontinence, retention of urine and occasionally faecal incontinence. Trauma to the urethra, to supportive ligaments in the pelvis and to the muscle in the area and its nerve supply account for this. It is of great importance that those women having epidural anaesthesia understand that they must attempt to micturate as soon as leg sensation has returned and they are mobile. Bladder sensation can take up to 8 hours to return after the last top-up (Cutner 1997). If micturition is delayed for this time, the bladder will have become overly distended with the possibility of long-standing or even permanent damage. Vigilance is necessary to ensure good bladder care especially for those at risk. For this reason it is advocated that those women having an epidural for delivery should have a catheter inserted to remain in position for 12 hours after the last top-up (Cutner 1997).

LACTATION

The level of prolactin produced by the anterior pituitary rises steadily throughout pregnancy, but its effect on the milk-producing cells of the breast is inhibited by the placental hormones (particularly oestrogen). As the placental hormones decline, a point is reached – usually about the 3rd or 4th postpartum day – when prolactin is free to act and milk production begins. Up until that time the suckling child will obtain colostrum. Milk is produced by glandular cells and stored in the alveoli of the 15–20 lobes of each breast. Suckling, and eventually, by a conditioned reflex, even the sight, sound or smell of the baby, stimulates the posterior pituitary to release oxytocin, which, in addition to its effects on uterine muscle (see p. 84), causes myoepithelial cells around the alveoli to contract. This contraction propels the milk with variable force into the lactiferous sinuses ready for removal by the baby, and is called the 'let-down' or milk ejection reflex. Some women feel sharp pains and experience actual spurting out of the milk, whereas others sense only tingling and find the milk just dripping from their nipples.

It is important for the physiotherapist to understand the physical process by which the baby gains the milk. This is well described in the booklet *Successful Breastfeeding* produced by the Royal College of Midwives (RCM 2002). In addition to the 'let-down' reflex, milk is transferred from the breast by the baby taking the whole nipple and some of the areola well into the mouth so that it lies over the length of the tongue. The baby then squeezes the milk-filled sinuses behind the nipple by compression of the lower jaw and tongue against the upper jaw and hard palate (see pp. 13 and 208).

Human breast milk is unique, and, although an infant does apparently thrive on other available milks, there is no question but that 'breast is best' for babies, with very rare exceptions. It is the recommendation of the RCM (2002) that babies should be exclusively breast-fed until they are at least 4 months (and preferably 6 months) old. Regrettably, although 64% of women in the UK choose to breastfeed (OPCS 1985), only 26% are still fully breastfeeding at 4 months. Fisher (1989) documents the subtle and critical differences that make colostrum and then human breast milk so infinitely superior to anything else for babies. Research continues to show that breast milk has value other than nutritional benefit (Coppa et al 1990, Goldman 1993). Breast milk not only contains the right nutrients in the correct proportions for all aspects of human development, it also contains enzymes to help digest them appropriately, and important anti-infective agents such as macrophages, neutrophils, IgA and lysozyme, as well as antiallergic factors, to protect the growing child.

Very few women are physically unable to breastfeed if they really want to, and very few babies are best fed by anything other than their mother's milk. The establishment of breastfeeding is therefore one of the most important matters in the early puerperium, and a person prepared to give the unhurried, skilled, consistent help to women to achieve this ranks very highly in value to both mother and baby. The length of each feed should not be restricted because it has been shown (RCM 2002) that the calorific content of the later or hindmilk is higher than the foremilk.

MANAGEMENT IN THE PUERPERIUM

It is usual to encourage women to rest quietly for the first 2–6 hours, even after the most straightforward labour, to allow clotting over the placental site to occur and to give the body time to adapt to the substantial changes that have taken place. Thereafter a pleasant, relaxed, protected environment, whether in a maternity unit or at home, is required, which provides a woman with a little breathing space and any guidance she wants before she takes up full responsibility for her life again. Most women appreciate having their own basic needs supplied for a few days and being free to follow their instincts in feeding and caring for the baby, sleeping and pottering as they feel inclined. Where partners are able to be at home, they find this supportive role can be hugely rewarding and an excellent start to active fathering.

Women vary greatly in the amount and type of help and direct guidance they need. Those who have had a long, traumatic labour, an assisted delivery or a caesarean section will need more help and rest, and primiparae may require more guidance in baby feeding and baby care than multiparae. All women should be given relaxed opportunities to talk and ask questions about the labour, ideally with one of the professionals who attended them.

In the UK there is provision for individual packages of care for every mother under the supervision of a midwife during the first 10 days postpartum; whether or not there are complications. The midwife is concerned to monitor the fundal height, the amount and colour of the lochia and the condition of the perineum, as well as the general physical wellbeing of the mother and infant. Whether the child is being breastfed or bottle-fed, it is important to ensure that feeding proceeds satisfactorily and that the baby is thriving. The midwife is also well placed to observe any early evidence of postnatal depression, as well as encouraging the mother and, where necessary, instructing her in childcare. When the circumstances require it the midwife may continue in attendance for up to 28 days. Thereafter the continuum of care is the responsibility of the health visitor.

COMPLICATIONS IN THE PUERPERIUM

Postpartum haemorrhage

All recently delivered women are at risk of postpartum haemorrhage (PPH), which is defined as a loss of blood following delivery in excess of 500 ml within the first 24 hours. After that time it is termed secondary PPH. The usual cause is uterine atonia; the uterus fails to contract and control the bleeding from the placental site for some reason (e.g. uterine exhaustion). The uterus may also be prevented from contracting down where the placenta has not completely separated or placental fragments remain. If the blood loss is rapid and severe the woman may collapse very quickly; immediate medical aid must be summoned. Where light bleeding continues well into the puerperium or recurs, placental fragments may be suspected and ergotamine tablets prescribed to stimulate further uterine contractions in the hope of dislodging what may well be only a very small tag of placenta.

Venous thrombosis, pulmonary embolism

Superficial and deep venous thrombosis are not common conditions despite the potential risks of trauma, stasis and infection and heightened activity of the body's coagulation system in the puerperium. However, pulmonary embolism continues to be a cause of maternal death. The physiotherapist is an important member of the caring team in monitoring and preventing any such problems.

Gravitational oedema

Many women have experienced gravitational oedema up to delivery and this must be encouraged to disperse postpartum. A few women develop oedema of the feet and ankles for the first time after delivery; this is not easily explained except in terms of vascular damage.

Puerperal infection

Puerperal infection usually refers to infections of the genital tract; but pyrexia may be due to infection anywhere in the body (e.g. chest or urinary tract). Endometritis, salpingitis, pelvic cellulitis (parametritis) and even peritonitis are all possible. Such conditions were the scourge of childbearing until this century and, although they are rarely seen now in developed countries, physiotherapists, particularly those working in the Developing World, should be aware of them. Treatment is by administration of the appropriate antibiotic.

Vesicovaginal fistula

Although vesicovaginal fistula is rarely seen in the UK, it has become apparent that in less developed countries, women delivering without proper assistance may sustain serious tearing of the perineum and even high vaginal tears which are then not sutured. Prolonged second stage or sheer obstruction can result in ischaemia and necrosis, causing tissue breakdown and a vesicovaginal or urethrovaginal fistula. The result is that from delivery onwards a substantial number of women suffer from incontinence of urine and faeces; they are disabled and ostracised, and are often too poor to pay the high fees required by doctors to effect a repair (Tahzib 1989).

References

Abboud T K, Sarkis F, Hung T T et al 1983 Effects of epidural anaesthesia during labour on maternal plasma beta endorphin levels. Anesthesiology 59(1):1–5.

Abboud T K, Goebelsmann U, Raya J et al 1984 Effect of intrathecal morphine during labor on maternal plasma beta-endorphin levels. American Journal of Obstetrics and Gynecology 149:709–710.

Abitol M M 1985 Supine position in labor and associated fetal heart changes. Obstetrics and Gynecology 65:481–486.

ACOG committee opinion 2002 Mode of singleton breech delivery, No 256. International Journal of Gynecology and Obstetrics 77(1):65–66.

Adachi K, Shimada M, Usui A 2003 The relationship between the parturients positions and perceptions of labor pain intensity. Nursing Research 52(1):47–51.

Allen R E, Hosker G L, Smith A R B et al 1990 Pelvic floor damage and childbirth: a neurophysiological study. British Journal of Obstetrics and Gynaecology 97:770–779.

Arkin A E, Chern-Hughes B 2002 Case report: labial fusion postpartum and clinical management of labial lacerations. Midwifery Womens Health 47(4):290–292.

Berghella V 2001 Prolapsed cord after external cephalic version in a patient with premature rupture of membranes and transverse lie. European Journal of Obstetrics, Gynecology and Reproductive Biology 99(2):274–275.

Bonica J J 1984 In: Wall P, Melzack R (eds) Textbook of pain. Churchill Livingstone. Edinburgh, p 337–392.

Brayshaw E, Wright P 1994 Teaching physical skills for the childbearing year. Books for Midwives Press, England, p 53–64.

Brown S T, Campbell D, Kutz A 1989 Characteristics of labour pain at two stages of cervical dilation. Pain 38:289–295.

Caldeyro-Barcia R 1979 The influence of maternal position on time of spontaneous rupture of membranes, progress of labour, and fetal head compression. Birth Family Journal 6:7.

Chalmers J A, Chalmers I 1989 The obstetric vacuum extractor is the instrument of first choice for operative vaginal delivery. British Journal of Obstetrics and Gynaecology 96:505–509.

Chapman M G, Jones M, Springs J E et al 1986 The use of a birthroom: a randomized controlled trial comparing delivery with that in the labour ward. British Journal of Obstetrics and Gynaecology 93(2):182–187.

Charles A G, Norr K L, Bloch C R et al 1978 Obstetric and psychological effects of psychoprophylactic preparation for childbirth. American Journal of Obstetrics and Gynecology 131:44–52.

Clark A P 1891 The influence of position of the patient in labor in causing uterine inertia and pelvic disturbances. Journal of the American Medical Association 16:433.

Coppa G V, Gabriella O, Giorgi P et al 1990 Preliminary study of breast feeding and bacterial adhesion to uroepithelial cells. Lancet 335:569–571.

Currie W B, Wong M F, Cox R I et al 1973 Hormonal changes in ewes and their fetuses at parturition. Journal of Reproduction and Fertility 32:333–334.

Cutner A. 1997 The urinary tract in pregnancy. In: Cardozo L. (ed) Urogynecology. Churchill Livingstone, London, p 417–442.

Dennen P 1994 Forceps delivery. In: James D K, Steer P J, Weiner C P et al (eds) High risk pregnancy. W B Saunders, London, p 1129–1144.

Edwards N J, Davies G 2001 Elective caesarean section – the patient's choice? Journal of Obstetrics and Gynaecology 21(2):128–129.

Fisher C 1989 Feeding. In: Bennet V R, Brown L K (eds) Myles textbook for midwives, 11th edn. Churchill Livingstone, Edinburgh, p 491–503.

Flynn A M, Kelly J, Hollins G et al 1978 Ambulation in labour. British Medical Journal 2:591–593.

Gardosi J, Hutson N, Lynch C B 1989 Randomised, controlled trial of squatting in second stage of labour. Lancet ii:74–77.

Goldman A S 1993 The immune system of human milk: antimicrobial, anti-inflammatory and immunomodulating properties. Paediatric Infections Disease Journal 12:664.

Granstrom L, Ekman G, Ulmsten U et al 1989 Changes in connective tissue of corpus and cervix uteri during ripening and labour in term pregnancy. British Journal of Obstetrics and Gynaecology 96:1198–1202.

Grant A, Sleep J, Ashurst H et al 1989 Dyspareunia associated with the use of glycerol-impregnated catgut to repair perineal trauma. Report of a 3 year follow up study. British Journal of Obstetrics and Gynaecology 96:741–743.

Grant J 1987 Reassessing second stage. Journal of the Association of Chartered Physiotherapists in Obstetrics and Gynaecology 6:230.

Green J M 1993 Expectations and experiences of pain in labour: findings from a large prospective study. Birth 20(2):65–72.

Hall M H, Campbell D M, Fraser C et al 1989 Mode of delivery and future fertility. British Journal of Obstetrics and Gynaecology 96(11):1297–1303.

Hemminki E 1996 Impact of Caesarean section on future pregnancy – a review of cohort studies. Paediatric and Perinatal Epidemiology 10(4):366–379.

Hershkovitz R, Silberstein, Sheiner E et al 2001 Risk factors associated with true knots of the umbilical cord. European Journal of Obstetrics, Gynecology and Reproductive Biology 98(1):36–39.

Hodnett E D 2001 Caregiver support for women during childbirth. Cochrane Database System Review 2001(1):CD000199

Inch S 1985 Birthrights. Hutchinson, London.

Jibodu O, Arulkumaran S 2000 Caesarean section on request. Journal of the Society of Obstetrics, Gynecology and Childbirth 22(9):684–689.

Johanson R B, Rice C, Doyle M et al 1993 A randomised prospective study comparing the new vacuum extractor policy with forceps delivery. British Journal of Obstetrics and Gynaecology 100:524–530.

Johnstone F D, Aboe Imagel M S, Haruny A K 1987 Maternal posture in second stage and fetal acid base status. British Journal of Obstetrics and Gynaecology 94:753–757.

Jolly J, Walker J, Bhabra K 1999 Subsequent obstetric performance related to primary mode of delivery. British Journal of Obstetrics and Gynaecology 106(3):227–232.

Kavanagh J, Kelly A J, Thomas J 2001 Sexual intercourse for cervical ripening and induction of labour. Cochrane Database System Review 2:CD003039.

Klein M C, Gauthier R J, Robbins J M et al 1994 Relationship of episiotomy to perineal trauma and morbidity, sexual dysfunction, and pelvic floor relaxation. American Journal of Obstetrics and Gynecology 171(3):591–598.

Labrecque M, Eason E, Marcoux S et al 1999 Randomized controlled trial of prevention of perineal trauma by perineal massage during pregnancy. American Journal of Obstetrics and Gynecology 180:593–600.

Lachman E, Mali A, Gino G et al 2000 Placenta accreta with placenta previa after previous Caesarean sections – a growing danger in modern obstetrics. Harefuah 16 138(8):628–631.

Lenstrup C, Schartz A, Berget A et al 1987 Warm tub bath during delivery. Acta Obstetrica et Gynecologica Scandinavica, 66:709–712.

Liggins G C 1974 Parturition in the sheep and the human. Basic Life Science 4:423–443.

MacArthur C, Bick D E, Keighley M R B 1997 Faecal incontinence after childbirth. British Journal of Obstetrics and Gynaecology 104:46–50.

MacLennan A for the International Cerebral Palsy Task Force 1999 A template for defining a causal relation between acute intrapartum events and cerebral palsy: an international concensus statement. British Medical Journal 319:1054–1059.

McMahon M J, Li R, Schenk A P et al 1997 Previous Caesarean birth. A risk factor for placenta previa? Journal of Reproductive Medicine 42(7):409–412.

McManus T J, Calder A A 1978 Upright posture and efficiency of labour. Lancet i:72–74.

Melzack R 1984 The myth of painless childbirth. Pain 19:321–337.

Melzack R, Taenzer P, Feldman P et al 1981 Labour is still painful after prepared childbirth training. Canadian Medical Association Journal 125:357–363.

Mendelson C L 1946 The aspiration of stomach contents into the lungs during obstetric anaesthesia. American Journal of Obstetrics and Gynecology 52:191–205 (cited by Speak, 2002).

Mendez Bauer C, Arroyo C, Garcia-Ramos C et al 1975 Effects of standing position on spontaneous uterine contractility and other aspects of labor. Journal of Perinatal Medicine 3:89–100.

Mersky H 1979 Pain terms: a list of definitions and notes on usage. Pain 6:249–252.

Miller D A, Chollet J A, Goodwin T M 1997 Clinical risk factors for placenta previa–placenta accreta. American Journal of Obstetrics and Gynecology 177(1):210–214.

Mitre I 1974 The influence of maternal position on duration of the active phase of labor. International Journal of Gynecology and Obstetrics 12:181.

Moore T R, Iams J D, Creaset R K et al 1994 Diurnal and gestational patterns of uterine activity in normal human pregnancy. Obstetrics and Gynecology 83(4):517–523.

Morrin N A 1997a Midwifery care in the first stage of labour. In: Sweet B, Tiran D (eds) Mayes' midwifery, 12th edn. Baillière Tindall, London, p 355–384.

Morrin N A 1997b Midwifery care in the second stage of labour. In: Sweet B, Tiran D (eds) Mayes' midwifery, 12th edn. Baillière Tindall, London, p 385–402.

Morrin N A 1997c Midwifery care in the third stage of labour. In: Sweet B, Tiran D (eds) Mayes' midwifery, 12th edn. Baillière Tindall, London, p 402–417.

Moster D, Lie R T, Markestad T 2002 Joint association of Apgar scores and early neonatal symptoms with minor disabilities at school age. Archives of Disease in Childhood, Fetal and Neonatal Edition 86:F16–21.

Mukhopadhyay S, Arulkumaran S 2002 Breech delivery. Best Practice Research in Clinical Obstetrics and Gynaecology 16(1):31–42.

Murray A, Holdcroft A 1989 Incidence and intensity of postpartum lower abdominal pain. British Medical Journal 289:1619.

Nesheim B 1988 Duration of labor. Acta Obstetrica et Gynecologica Scandinavica 67:121–124.

Newnham J P, Tomlin S, Ratter S T et al 1983 Endogenous opioid peptides in pregnancy. British Journal of Obstetrics and Gynaecology 90:535–538.

Noble E 1983 Childbirth with Insight. Houghton Mifflin, Boston: p 51.

O'Brien W 1997 Prolonged labour and disordered uterine action. In: Sweet B, Tiran D (eds) Mayes' midwifery, 12th edn. Baillière Tindall, London, p 623–630.

OPCS 1985 Infant feeding. Department of Health HMSO, London.

Poschl U 1987 The vertical birthing position of the Trobrianders, Papua New Guinea. Australian and New Zealand Journal of Obstetrics and Gynaecology 27:120–125.

Prabulos A M, Philipson E H 1998 Umbilical cord prolapse. Is the time from diagnosis to delivery critical? Journal of Reproductive Medicine 43(2):129–132.

Prendiville W J, Elbourne D 1989 Care during the third stage of labour. In: Chalmers I, Enkin M, Keirse M (eds) Effective care in pregnancy and childbirth, vol 2. Oxford University Press, Oxford, p 1145–1169.

RCM 2002 Successful breastfeeding, 3rd edn. Churchill Livingstone, Edinburgh.

Read J A 1981 Randomized trial of ambulation versus oxytocin for labor enhancement. American Journal of Obstetrics and Gynecology 139:669.

Roberts J E, Mendez-Bauer C, Wodell D A 1983 The effects of maternal position on uterine contractility and efficiency. Birth 10:243–249.

Russell J G B 1982 The rationale of primitive delivery positions. British Journal of Obstetrics and Gynaecology 89:712–715.

Scheiner E, Shoham-Vardi I, Hallak M et al 2001 Placenta previa: obstetric risk factors and pregnancy outcome. Journal of Maternal and Fetal Medicine 10(6):414–419.

Scruggs M 1982 Personal communication quoted by Grant J 1987 Reassessing second stage. Journal of Associated Chartered Physiotherapists in Obstetrics and Gynaecology 60:20–30.

Shearman R P 1981 Endocrine changes during pregnancy. In: Dewhurst J (ed) Integrated obstetrics and gynaecology for postgraduates. Blackwell, Oxford, p 135–145.

Shipman M K, Boniface D R, Tefft M E et al 1997 Antenatal perineal massage and subsequent perineal outcomes: a randomised controlled trial. British Journal of Obstetrics and Gynaecology 104(7):787–791.

Sleep J, Grant A 1987 West Berkshire perineal management trial: three year follow up. British Medical Journal 295:749–751.

Sleep J, Grant A, Garcia J et al 1984 West Berkshire perineal management trial. British Medical Journal 289:587–590.

Snooks S J, Setchell M, Swash M et al 1984 Injury to innervation of pelvic floor sphincter musculature in childbirth. Lancet ii:546–550.

Sorensen S M, Bondesen H, Istre D et al 1988 Perineal rupture following vaginal rupture. Acta Obstetrica et Gynecologica Scandinavica 67:315–318.

Sosa R, Kennell J, Klaus M et al 1980 The effect of a supportive companion on perinatal problems, length of labour and mother–infant interaction. New England Journal of Medicine 303:597–600.

Speak S 2002 Food intake in labour: the benefits and drawbacks. Nursing Times 98(21):42–43.

Stamp G, Kruzins G, Crowther C 2001 Perineal massage in labour and prevention of perineal trauma: a randomised controlled trial. British Medical Journal 322:1277–1280.

Sultan A H, Kamm M A, Hudson C N 1994a Pudendal nerve damage during labour: prospective study before and after childbirth. British Journal of Obstetrics and Gynaecology 101:22–28.

Sultan A H, Kamm M A, Hudson C N et al 1994b Third degree obstetric anal sphincter tears: risk factors and outcomes of primary repair. British Medical Journal 308:887–891.

Sutton J, Scott P 1995 Understanding and teaching optimal foetal positioning. Birth Concepts, New Zealand.

Sweet B R 1997 Malpresentations. In: Sweet B, Tiran D (eds) Mayes' midwifery, 12th edn. Baillière Tindall, London, p 639–657.

Tahzib F 1989 An initiative on vesico-vaginal fistula. Lancet i:1316–1317.

Thacker S B, Stroup D, Chang M 2003 Continuous electronic heart rate monitoring for fetal assessment during labor

(Cochrane Review). In: The Cochrane Library, Issue 1. Update Software, Oxford.

To W W, Leung W C 1995 Placenta previa and previous Caesarean section. International Journal of Gynecology and Obstetrics 51(1):25–31.

Uyger D, Kis S, Tuncer R et al 2002 Risk factors and infant outcomes associated with umbilical cord prolapse. International Journal of Gynecology and Obstetrics 78(2):127–130.

Varma R, Smith C, Arulkumaran S 2000 Cardiotocograph interpretation: essential knowledge for paediatricians. Current Paediatrics 10(2):85–91.

Wall P D, Melzack R 1984 Textbook of pain. Churchill Livingstone, Edinburgh, p 378.

WHO 1994 Mother–baby package. Implementing safe motherhood in developing countries. Maternal Health

and Safe Motherhood programme, Division of family health, WHO, Geneva, WHO/FHE/MSM/94:11.

Williams R M, Thom M H, Studd J W 1980 A study of the benefits and acceptability of ambulation in spontaneous labour. British Journal of Obstetrics and Gynaecology 87:122–126.

Wilson M J, Cooper G, MacArthur C et al 2002 Comparative obstetric mobile epidural trial (COMET) study group UK. Anaesthesiology 97(6):1567–1575.

Wuitchik M, Bakal D, Lipshitz J 1989 The clinical significance of pain and cognitive activity in latent labor. Obstetrics and Gynecology 73(1):352.

Young P F, Johanson R B 2001 The management of breech presentation at term. Current Opinion in Obstetrics and Gynecology 13(6):589–593.

Further reading

Alexander J, Levy V, Roth C (eds) 1996 Midwifery practice – core topics 1. MacMillan, London.

Alexander J, Levy V, Roth C (eds) 1997 Midwifery practice – core topics 2. MacMillan, London.

Alexander J, Levy V, Roth C (eds) 2000 Midwifery practice – core topics 3. MacMillan, London.

Chamberlain G, Stewart M 1987 Walking through labour. British Medical Journal 295:802.

Graham I D 1997 Episiotomy. Challenging obstetric interventions. Blackwell Science, London.

Lagercrantz H, Slotkin T 1986 The stress of being born. Scientific American 4:100.

Lupe P J, Gross T L 1986 Maternal upright posture and mobility in labor a review. Obstetrics and Gynecology 67:727.

Sweet B, Tiran D (eds) Mayes' midwifery, 12th edn. Baillière Tindall, London.

Chapter 4

The antenatal period

Jo Fordyce

CHAPTER CONTENTS

Introduction 93
Antenatal care options 95
Routine antenatal care 97
Antenatal screening 100
Preconceptual care 102

Antenatal classes 104
Diet and weight gain in pregnancy 119
Planning and leading labour and parentcraft classes 126

INTRODUCTION

In spite of the fact that pregnancy is a normal physiological process usually experienced by a healthy woman, the number of professions involved in the caring team continues to proliferate in the UK. In the sequence of involvement, the team often consists of general practitioners, midwives, obstetricians, ultrasonographers, phlebotomists, women's health physiotherapists, dentists, dieticians, health visitors and paediatricians. Where necessary, other medical consultants, radiographers and social workers may also be part of the team. It is essential that all personnel are aware of the very special needs of pregnant women and respond to them accordingly. Increasingly, pregnant women turn also to practitioners of alternative therapies or activities (e.g. yoga, Pilates, swimming, acupuncture, hypnotherapy).

At the opposite end of the spectrum, in less developed countries, most women go through pregnancy and give birth without ever meeting a medical professional. Every year there are 600 000 known maternal deaths (WHO 1997) with over 99% occurring in developing countries. The main causes are haemorrhage, sepsis, hypertensive diseases of pregnancy, prolonged labour and complications of abortion. Because women in Africa and Asia have larger families (an average of four to six children, compared with fewer than two in Europe), the risk of maternal mortality during pregnancy may be as high as 1 in 15 in a developing country. Additionally, contraction of some diseases such as tuberculosis, malaria and human immunodeficiency virus (HIV) may be aggravated by pregnancy and poor nutrition, and lack of access to clean water may increase complications. Discrimination against women in society and the home, and levels of abuse and violence (Murray 1999), can also affect mortality rates.

For every maternal death there are at least a further 30 women (approximately 15 million per year) damaged through childbirth so as to never regain their full health. Furthermore, it is important to consider that for every woman who dies or who is damaged by pregnancy or childbirth, a family is greatly affected too. One of the worst consequences of childbirth is vesicovaginal fistula (see p. 88), which is often caused by prolonged, obstructed labour. This results in continuous leakage of urine and sometimes faeces. Women suffering from this horrific condition, which is particularly endemic in the sub-Saharan region of Africa (Tahzib 1989), often become rejected social outcasts. Tragically the restorative surgery which could transform their lives is largely unavailable except in specialist centres.

Women's health physiotherapists working in affluent Western countries where women are increasingly demanding a better quality of birth must never forget their less fortunate sisters for whom simply surviving pregnancy and giving birth to a healthy baby who grows into adulthood may be all that matters. The 'Safe Motherhood Initiative' is a global effort begun in 1987 aiming to reduce these maternal mortality and morbidity rates using the following objectives: to ensure women's access to health services, and raise awareness of them; to provide family planning services and increase the numbers and training for health-care providers, thereby promoting women's rights to whether and when to have children (www.rcm.org.uk).

The current UK maternal mortality rate is given as 11.4 per 100 000 deaths. This is a combination of both direct deaths (medical conditions exacerbated by pregnancy) and indirect deaths (deaths from conditions that directly arise from pregnancy). The latter category outweighs that of deaths from direct causes and includes a high number of suicides (Lewis 2001). Higher-risk groups are women from lower socioeconomic classes, very young girls, specific ethnic groups and those from the travelling community.

The aims of modern antenatal care are:

1. to promote and maintain optimal physical and emotional maternal health throughout pregnancy
2. to recognise and treat correctly medical or obstetric complications occurring during pregnancy
3. to detect foetal abnormalities as early as possible
4. to prepare for and inform both parents about pregnancy, labour, the puerperium and the subsequent care of their baby
5. the overriding goal is that pregnancy will result in a healthy mother and a healthy infant.

ANTENATAL CARE OPTIONS

Women should be informed of the options available to them and have an opportunity to discuss these in order to make an informed choice (see *Place of Birth* leaflet in Further Reading, p. 138). Legally a woman is entitled to choose the place of delivery and the type of care she would prefer. Usually there are several models of care available, which should enable the woman to choose the options that best suit her needs. For most women this will be National Health Service (NHS) care, but it is possible to arrange private care for any part of the time.

WATER BIRTHS

The use of water for labour or birth is an increasingly popular choice of delivery for women (RCM 2000a, see also p. 190). Currently, an estimated 50% of maternity units offer this facility, with between 15 and 60% of the women delivering at those units using the service (RCM 2000a). However, a survey in England and Wales between April 1994 and March 1996 identified only 0.6% of births occurring in water, of which 9% were home births (Tookey & Gilbert 1999). The facilities for water birth (see AIMS in Useful Addresses, p. 138) are limited within the NHS but pools can be hired for use at home or in hospital. Potential benefits of immersion in warm water include relaxation, pain relief and less perineal trauma, with adverse consequences including infection, water inhalation by the baby and decreased mobility. Nikodem (2003), when reviewing the above benefits and risks for water birth, concluded there was not enough evidence to evaluate the use of immersion in water. More research is needed in this area, as suggested by Alderdice et al (1995), but they concluded from their survey that there was no evidence not to continue with water immersion as an option. To support this, although Schorn et al (1993) found no improvement regarding progression of labour using water immersion, no evidence was found of increased maternal, neonatal or infectious morbidity. (For more information see Further Reading, p. 138.)

HOME BIRTH

If a woman decides that she would like to have her baby at home, in the UK she does not need to have the permission of her general practitioner (GP) or an obstetrician. However, there is a statutory obligation on the part of the local Supervisor of Midwives to provide midwifery care antenatally, during labour and delivery, and postnatally.

The UK home birth rate is about 2% but has large geographical variations from 1 to 20% (Macfarlane et al 2000). Home birth should be understood as mainstream maternity care and offered as a realistic and positive option. This can be promoted by selecting low-risk women and providing adequate infrastructure and support (Springer & Weel 1996). Hospital birth is still perceived as a safer option than home delivery even though there is no evidence that this so (RCM 2002).

TEAM/CASELOAD MIDWIFERY/DOMINO (DOMICILIARY MIDWIFE IN AND OUT)

Midwifery-led care should be promoted as an appropriate choice for women experiencing normal pregnancy and birth (Tyler 2001). This option enables the pregnant woman to be cared for throughout her pregnancy, delivery and postpartum period by the same community-based team of midwives (ideally six per team), thus providing a continuity of care so often lacking in hospital-based obstetrics. The mother calls her midwife when she considers labour to have begun, and is ideally then delivered by a known midwife. With the domiciliary model of care the midwife accompanies her to hospital, delivers the baby and brings the mother home again 6–7 hours after the birth.

GP/MIDWIFERY SHARED CARE

GPs who have undertaken appropriate training may offer a service with midwives based at the local surgery. Delivery may be at home or in hospital.

MIDWIFERY-LED UNITS

These are stand-alone units which have a midwifery-managed model of care. These have been implemented into the maternity services to provide a service which fulfills the individuals' needs. A study carried out in Glasgow completed a randomised controlled trial (RCT) of 1299 women comparing midwifery-led care with the more traditional shared care (i.e. doctor and midwife), in terms of clinical efficacy and patient satisfaction (Turnbull et al 1996). The results showed a similar level of intervention, or lower, for the midwifery-led unit. There were less episiotomies and reduced induction of labour with the midwifery-led model, and only 32.8% needed to transfer from this care to involve an obstetrician in labour. Women using both services expressed satisfaction with care, but the midwifery-led model scored significantly higher in all aspects from the antenatal to the postnatal period. Other studies comparing the two models of care have also found no major differences between the two in terms of outcome for the women and babies (Campbell et al 1999). The current opinion is that these units are clinically effective for healthy women and are to be advocated, but integrated with existing services.

GENERAL PRACTITIONER UNITS

General practitioner obstetric units may exist independently in a district general hospital or may stand alongside a consultant unit. They are increasingly uncommon.

CONSULTANT CARE

Women identified as high risk during pregnancy, that is with a risk of thrombosis, thromboembolism, gestational diabetes, or hypertensive disease, or with a poor obstetric history, will probably be based under the care of the consultant obstetrician having hospital-based visits on a more frequent basis. Their care may be shared with their GP or midwives.

CONSULTANT OBSTETRIC UNITS

These larger units are usually based in district or regional centres, although a few still exist as independent entities. They should all have access to up-to-date diagnostic procedures, and be able to call upon staff of many disciplines. These will usually have a paediatric/neonatal intensive care unit attached. Women often complain of an impersonal, fragmented, 'conveyor belt' approach; very few such units seem able to provide continuity of care for all their clients.

PRIVATE OBSTETRIC CARE/INDEPENDENT MIDWIVES

A woman may decide to use the private sector for all her antenatal care and delivery, using private hospitals and having much more input by their obstetrician. Alternatively, she may opt to have all her care under an independent midwife, delivering at home or in a private unit. Presently, due to the increasing litigation culture that is being adopted, insurance companies are reluctant to insure this group, or are charging huge insurance premiums which are financially difficult to meet. Many independent midwives therefore currently work without the protection of insurance, which has potential risks for both themselves and their clients.

For further information on what options are available geographically in the UK visit www.birthchoice.

ROUTINE ANTENATAL CARE

Following confirmation of pregnancy by their GP, women are usually referred to a booking clinic, either at their local hospital or GP's surgery, or visited at home. This ideally occurs between 12 and 14 weeks' gestation, but realistically ranges from 9 to 16 weeks.

BOOKING VISIT

Usually, women are reviewed by a midwife, unless medical risks are identified and involvement by the obstetrician is necessary. To ensure every woman has an antenatal care plan tailored to her individual needs, details of the woman's social, family, medical, psychological and past obstetric history are taken. This also assesses her health and attempts to uncover any factor that may adversely affect childbearing.

All mothers should have their body mass index (BMI) calculated at the time of booking. A BMI of more than 30 indicates obesity, a risk factor for thromboembolism, gestatational diabetes and pre-eclampsia (PET – see p. 48). If the BMI is low, this may indicate an eating disorder resulting in the woman being undernourished. There may also be emotional implications regarding the expected weight gain of pregnancy.

This first visit provides an ideal opportunity to provide advice and education regarding general lifestyle, for example diet, exercise, alcohol and smoking. All pregnant women should also be given advice about the correct use of car seatbelts as soon as possible (see p. 107). Routine blood tests will be taken and antenatal screening options discussed.

Violence against women encompasses physical, psychological, sexual and emotional abuse. It can often start (30%) or escalate during pregnancy (Lewis 2001, Mezey 1997, RCM 1999). It is associated with both maternal and foetal death, severe morbidity, miscarriage, depression, suicide as well as substance abuse. In the last confidential inquiry into maternal deaths, 12% of the women whose death was reported had voluntarily admitted to violence during their pregnancy. As health professionals working in this field, all should be aware of the prevalence and the probable under-estimation of the problem. It is now advocated to develop routine questioning and screening of women during antenatal visits with appropriate networks in place to support them once a problem is identified.

SUBSEQUENT VISITS

The pattern of visits has been reviewed in recent years to ascertain whether the frequency, which is based largely on tradition, could be replaced by a more evidence-based model of care. Currently the National Institute for Clinical Excellence (NICE) is reviewing guidelines for antenatal care to be published in October 2003. The schedule of care will vary in each Trust and allow for flexibility with each woman, but after the first attendance it is usual for the next visit to follow the 'anomaly scan' at 20 weeks. Monthly visits from 24–26 weeks, fortnightly visits from 32–34 weeks to 40 weeks and weekly visits until delivery are usual. Any anxieties or problems the woman may have should be discussed at these visits. In addition the following are always recorded: blood pressure, urine, presence of oedema, fundal height and 'lie' of the foetus, foetal movements and foetal heart rate.

Blood pressure

Although there is an increase in blood volume and cardiac output during pregnancy, this is not normally accompanied by a rise in blood pressure; in fact there may even be a slight drop during the middle trimester, which is probably due to the hormonally mediated dilatation of blood vessels. Blood pressure is taken at each antenatal visit, and it is important to record a baseline blood pressure early in pregnancy as a rise can be the first sign of a potentially serious complication such as pregnancy-induced hypertension.

Urine

Urinalysis is carried out at each visit for protein content; colour and odour are also noted. Increased proteinurea may indicate pregnancy-induced hypertension or the possibility of infection, or both. The latter may be diagnosed by laboratory testing of an MSU (mid-stream specimen of urine).

Weight

It is inadvisable for a woman to allow her pregnancy weight gain to become excessive – an average of 12.5 kg (25–35 lb) is acceptable.

Oedema

The hands and lower limbs are checked for the presence of oedema, and for other indications of fluid retention, which may be another sign of pregnancy-induced hypertension and PET (e.g. paraesthesia, see p. 48).

Fundal height and the 'lie' of the foetus

The level of the fundus of the uterus is noted and compared with the gestational stage (see p. 34). Intrauterine growth restriction (IUGR) may be suspected if the fundal height is lower than expected. Multiple pregnancy or polyhydramnios could cause an increase in fundal height. Early in pregnancy the foetus will frequently change position. By 36 weeks more than 95% will be in a cephalic presentation – the remainder will be breech or other variations (see p. 44). Women with breech presentations at term may be offered the application of external cephalic version; where this fails caesarean section may be advised (ACOG 2001).

Foetal movements

Although foetal movements are usually noticed by the mother, at some time between 16 and 22 weeks' gestation, the foetus has in fact been moving from 8 weeks. Until the uterus has risen out of the pelvis and is actually in good contact with the anterior abdominal wall, the woman is unaware of movements because the uterus is insensitive to touch. In a second or subsequent pregnancy she will probably notice her baby moving earlier, possibly because she recognises the sensation. As pregnancy advances, foetal movements may be used as a measure of the baby's well-being. All women should realise that a decrease or cessation of normal movement for any length of time might have serious implications. The women's health physiotherapist must be constantly alert to this possibility and pick up even the mildest expression of maternal anxiety. It takes only a few moments of the midwife or doctor's time to listen for the foetal heart, or it can be monitored using a CTG. 'Kick' charts are an easily used monitoring device. If a foetus moves less than 10 times in an average day, the pregnancy is likely to be assessed more carefully.

Foetal heart rate

Although foetal movements reported by the mother can be a good indication of the baby's well-being, most midwives and doctors will also record the foetal heart rate. Although the foetal heart can be seen to be functioning as early as 8–10 weeks using ultrasound scanning, it is not usually possible to hear the heart beat before 16 weeks using a Sonic-aid monitor. The normal rate will vary between 110 and 150 b.p.m. A Pinard stethoscope, largely replaced by the electronic Sonic-aid monitor, will pick up the heart rate from about 20 weeks. Fathers may like to put an ear against their partner's abdominal wall in order to hear this exciting sound. Alternatively the cardboard tube from a toilet roll can substitute for a stethoscope!

Other tests

Blood tests

Blood tests are used to detect haemoglobin levels, the presence of sexually transmitted infection, blood group, blood sugars, rubella antibodies and haemoglobinopathies.

Haemoglobin levels

A decrease is normal during pregnancy because of the increased blood plasma volume (see p. 36). Women showing signs of anaemia may be prescribed iron supplements in either tablet or liquid form as well as being advised about dietary input to help address the problem.

Sexually transmitted infection

All pregnant women should be given information on HIV and its transmission from mother to child. HIV testing should be recommended as part of routine antenatal care (RCM 1998). Transmission of HIV from mother to child can be reduced by effective drug medication during pregnancy, delivery by caesarian section and avoiding breastfeeding (Dunn et al 1992).

The Venereal Disease Research Laboratory (VDRL) slide test is used to detect syphilis. Where a woman appears to be at risk of suffering from other sexually transmitted infections, appropriate tests will be carried out. She will also be routinely screened for hepatitis B.

Blood group   The woman's blood grouping will be determined, as will her Rhesus status. If a Rhesus negative status is identified, prophylactic anti-D injections would be given at 28 and 34 weeks' gestation. (NICE 2002) Anti-D is administered in order to prevent the mother from developing antibodies to the Rhesus factor during pregnancy. These antibodies, although rare, may cause significant foetal anaemia.

Haemoglobinopathies   Tests for the haemoglobinopathies (e.g. sickle cell disease and thalassaemia), may be carried out when one of the parents is of non-Northern-European descent (see p. 49).

ANTENATAL SCREENING

A woman during her pregnancy today now expects to have some form of antenatal screening for foetal abnormality but there remains a wide variation in options and practices used.

Down's syndrome occurs in approximately 1:800 births; the risk increases with maternal age. Down's syndrome is the most common chromosomal problem found at birth (a disorder where the affected person has an extra copy of chromosome 21). Routine screening aims to detect this and other foetal abnormalities, either by maternal serum screening or by nuchal translucency (NT) measurement (see ultrasound screening).

MATERNAL SERUM SCREENING

As well as measuring the alpha fetoprotein (AFP) level, screening may also record additional hormone levels. Depending on how many markers are used, this is termed the double, triple or quadruple test. These levels are combined with maternal age to provide a risk estimate of the foetus having Down's syndrome. Currently, the UK National Screening Committee (NSC) suggests that the cut-off level for an increased risk should be around 1:250 at term, and by using ultrasound scans to accurately date the pregnancy, the test should yield a detection rate of about 60% for a 5% false positive rate (NSC 2002). It is usually performed between 15 and 18 weeks of pregnancy, and if women have a screen positive result (i.e. above the cut-off value) then they will be referred for further invasive diagnostic procedures such as chorionic villus sampling (CVS) or amniocentesis.

High levels of AFP may also indicate neural tube defects (NTDs) such as spina bifida or anencephaly, but multiple pregnancies will also produce high levels.

ULTRASOUND SCANNING

This valuable diagnostic technique has become increasingly more sophisticated and, since the 1990s, has been developed to measure the nuchal translucency, an area of subcutaneous fluid at the nape of the foetal neck. Increased thickness may indicate Down's syndrome as well as other chromosomal and structural abnormalities (Hyett et al 1999, Snijders et al 1998). The optimal time to perform this test is between 11 and 14 weeks of pregnancy and it is combined with maternal age to give a risk estimate which, if high, will lead to the offer of CVS procedure or amniocentesis.

In 2001, a survey in England found that 72% of women were offered serum screening only, 15% NT screening and 13% a combination of both, with 87% of women who were offered screening having an ultrasound scan to date pregnancies accurately prior to the tests (NSC 2002). Although the NSC recommends that all pregnant women should be offered second trimester serum screening, it is aware of the need to standardise interpretation of results throughout the country, thereby improving accuracy of detection rates. In turn, offering invasive diagnostic procedures only to women who really need them reduces unnecessary anxiety and cost levels to the service.

In the UK most pregnant women will have at least one anomaly scan at around 20 weeks' gestation, and this is used for detection of certain abnormalities (e.g. spina bifida, anencephaly and cardiac abnormalities). Where pregnancies are complicated by problems such as pregnancy-induced hypertension (PIH), IUGR and antepartum haemorrhage, or where there is more than one foetus, a series of scans may be carried out.

CHORIONIC VILLUS SAMPLING

Chorionic villus sampling is a technique which is carried out transabdominally. Fragments of placental chorionic villi are removed under ultrasound guidance and inspected for genetic foetal abnormalities such as Down's syndrome. Although the benefit of this technique is that it can be performed early in pregnancy (between 11 and 13 weeks' gestation), it carries a risk of about 1% miscarriage in experienced hands.

AMNIOCENTESIS

In this test a small amount of amniotic fluid is withdrawn transabdominally, with the assistance of ultrasound monitoring. Culture of the cells shed by the foetus within this fluid is used to give an indication of genetic abnormalities such as Down's syndrome. Foetal sex can also be determined and will be important where there is a familial history of sex-linked disorders such as haemophilia or Duchenne muscular dystrophy. The drawbacks of amniocentesis are: it is performed after 15 weeks' gestation, there is a longer delay than with other tests before results are available, and – once again – it carries the approximate 1% risk of triggering a miscarriage.

ACCEPTABILITY OF ANTENATAL TESTING

As screening becomes more universal, diagnostic tests and procedures are applied to all rather than just the small number of women in whom it is deemed necessary by virtue of specific signs, symptoms and facts.

Because of the speed with which the medical profession has adopted procedures such as ultrasound investigations during pregnancy, it has become increasingly routine. More research regarding its effects and clinical effectiveness is needed including the psychological and social consequences (Bricker 2001).

Although most parents enjoy the reassurance and connection of seeing their baby during a scan, respect for a woman's wishes must be given if she declines screening. Further provision regarding explanation of all antenatal screening and potential outcomes need to be addressed, with support in place for negative outcomes. Furthermore, if a woman is not prepared to consider the termination of her pregnancy, there is no point in suggesting CVS, amniocentesis or any other test that may show abnormalities.

PRECONCEPTUAL CARE

Although many babies are still conceived accidentally, more and more hopeful parents-to-be and their medical advisers are becoming aware of the benefits of dealing with health problems and attaining optimal physical and mental well-being prior to pregnancy. Both partners may decide to prepare for conception by giving thought to their diet, alcohol consumption, smoking habits, exercise routines, occupation and drug (medicinal or social) intake. Today, one in seven couples (Chambers 1999) will experience difficulties with conceiving and will need specialist help, but may, by addressing all of the above, improve their chances of success.

Every organ system within the mother's body will alter and adjust according to the demands made upon it by the growing foetus (see p. 31). Therefore, the woman who begins pregnancy feeling fit and comfortable is more likely to be able to cope with the physical and emotional changes during the subsequent 9 months. Östgaard et al (1994) found that women who were exercising weekly prepregnancy had reduced back pain during pregnancy. Women who have been taking the contraceptive pill are usually advised to discontinue its use 3 months before the hoped-for pregnancy.

Where such conditions as spina bifida and anencephaly have previously occurred, folic acid will be recommended (see p. 120). Genetic counselling should be available to parents with a family history of hereditary disease. Renal disorders, as well as identified risk factors for maternal morbidity and mortality (e.g. cardiac disorders, diabetes and hypertension) should be treated and stabilised before conception. Essential drug regimens and their possible teratogenic effects should be considered.

Many of today's women, including those with disabilities, are aware of their responsibility in asserting control over their own health and bodies, and are very open to preconception advice. However, women in lower socioeconomic groups may understandably be primarily concerned with finance, accommodation and food, and might give preconceptual planning, exercise and antenatal classes little priority. Even so, it is still possible for the women's health physiotherapist whilst on the postnatal wards to teach the principles of good 'body care' between pregnancies (see p. 210). The women's health physiotherapist should be the member of the postnatal team who, with enthusiasm and knowledge, can create good body awareness during the childbearing years, which will benefit mothers and their families throughout life.

Some women attempt to become superfit overnight preconceptually by means of overvigorous activity such as aerobics, jogging or weight training. Taken to its extremes, this could lead to amenorrhoea. Such overzealous enthusiasm can be channeled into safer activities by the women's health physiotherapist; swimming, Pilates, yoga, cycling and walking, for example, are less likely to cause injuries. Assessment and treatment of back problems before the physiological ligamentous changes begin, and imprinting the concept of good back care, could prove invaluable in the months of pregnancy and later. The women's health physiotherapist can give advice regarding urinary disorders (e.g. stress incontinence, urgency or frequency) and begin pelvic floor and abdominal muscle education or re-education using exercise and possibly biofeedback. All women, but particularly those who are attending infertility clinics, will benefit from stress-reducing techniques, including relaxation and positive thinking. Women with physical impairment or pathologies such as multiple sclerosis, rheumatoid arthritis or the effects of a cerebrovascular accident would benefit from the specialised skills and support of the women's health physiotherapist to empower them for the marathon of pregnancy and motherhood.

INFERTILITY/ SUBFERTILITY

Ninety per cent of couples having unprotected sex will conceive within a year, 50% of them in the first 3 months (Chambers 1999). The causes of infertility can be divided into male or female factors, or a combination of the two, with a third of couples no factor is identified. Treatment options are varied, but within the NHS investigations and availability can be limited and necessitate a frustrating wait for couples in an already stressful situation.

The causes of infertility are varied, as are the treatment options. Hormonal treatment may be advocated for a woman failing to ovulate as with polycystic ovaries (PCO). Clomifene is commonly used, either alone or with gonadotrophins; however, there is an increased risk of multiple pregnancies and ovarian hyperstimulation syndrome (OHSS).

If a woman has tubal disease, then in vitro fertilisation (IVF) is one of the first options, with success affected by duration of infertility, woman's age and previous pregnancies. Multiple pregnancies are more likely. There are many other assisted-conception techniques including intracytoplasmic sperm injection (ICSI), where the egg is again fertilised before being transferred to the uterus (as in IVF), but where one sperm is injected directly into the cytoplasm of the egg. This may be used where the sperm count is low. For more details of assisted conception see Chambers 1999.

Pregnancy, especially for primiparous women, can be a combination of incredible excitement at the prospect of being a mother combined with anxieties regarding the health of their baby, carrying them to full term and the labour itself. If a couple has been through assisted conception to achieve this pregnancy, they will probably have all of the above emotions, plus not surprisingly, increased worries regarding a positive outcome. Whether the women's health physiotherapist is treating the mother for a musculoskeletal condition or the couple as part of an antenatal class, appropriate sensitivity to their needs has to be demonstrated.

EARLY PREGNANCY

The entire female organism adapts to preserve and nourish the fetus growing within the uterus and with the anabolic metabolism comes a mental tranquillity and somnolent beauty.

(Llewellyn-Jones, 1969)

This somewhat romantic statement encapsulates the process of pregnancy – practically every system within the pregnant woman's body automatically changes during the 9 months. There is also the notion that the foetus is able to manipulate its environment to suit itself!

Once pregnancy is diagnosed and established, a women's health physiotherapist's input should be available. An early introduction to ergonomic back-care education, understanding of stress and its control, and an appreciation of the importance of physical health (with particular reference to strength and endurance) is essential. Activities for the pelvic floor and abdominal muscles, legs and arms can usefully be included. Different centres will have different ways of introducing appropriate information, and this will depend to a large extent on the clientele and the individual Trust's provision of services. It is most important not to overburden women, whether primigravid or multigravid, with any regimen without first taking into account the individual's lifestyle. Those engaged in strenuous activity will need to devote more time to rest and stress control; those leading a more leisurely life will benefit from a considered programme of exercise.

ANTENATAL CLASSES

In practically every NHS centre involved with the care of pregnant women, antenatal classes of some sort or another are offered. These may be held in hospitals, but increasingly are held in the community. Wide variation in content, presenting personnel and style of teaching is found around the country. Ideally midwives, women's health physiotherapists and health visitors should work closely together to provide a comprehensive programme at a time and in a place which is convenient and accessible to the parents. This was the ideal, as envisaged in the joint statement agreed by the three professions in 1987 and updated in 1994 (see p. xix).

Antenatal 'preparation for parenthood' classes must be designed to fulfil the parents' expressed needs, and should never simply be a forum for professionals to impart the sort of information *they* think their audience requires. In fact, the didactic lecturer/student image should be avoided at all costs and replaced with a more appropriate adult teaching approach, encouraging self-learning and problem solving. Antenatal education is most successful when it is parent centred, with everyone involved contributing fully. It is vital that all aspects of this service are flexible and regularly reviewed and evaluated. Rigidity and routine are anachronistic, and are to be condemned, and the continuity of professional personnel is as important as their ability and expertise in fulfilling this very special role. The antenatal class is no place for the inexperienced physiotherapist, midwife or health visitor. The precise details of course organisation and planning must vary with local needs, and each women's health physiotherapist should be sensitive to these. Apart from NHS classes, organisations such as the National Childbirth Trust (NCT), the Active Birth movement and occasionally private individuals offer courses in preparation for parenthood.

The earliest antenatal education was primarily concerned with hygiene and nutrition, in an attempt to lower maternal and infant mortality rates. Later, teachers began to be concerned with presenting skills to help women prepare for and cope with labour pain. Today, the brief is much wider:

- Couples should be helped to check and increase their knowledge of the physiological changes of pregnancy, labour and the puerperium.
- They should be shown ways that may be useful for coping with the physical changes of pregnancy and their associated discomforts.
- They should be guided towards a realistic understanding of labour and the assembly of a 'tool kit' of coping skills.
- Couples should be encouraged to consider the profound change in lifestyle that parenthood brings, and the emotional maturity necessary to manage successfully their additional responsibilities.
- They should be encouraged to talk and air any fears, ask questions, and be helped to obtain satisfactory answers in an open environment.

Although the best antenatal classes in the world probably could not prepare expectant couples for the full reality of parenthood, they aim to improve a couple's confidence and knowledge regarding labour and give some insight into their new roles as parents. People who attend these classes tend to have different sociodemographics compared with non-attenders: they tend to be older, more educated, middle class women (Nichols 1995) and partners are likely to attend. Current literature is very focused at identifying the clients' needs, especially for the fathers attending, and this includes covering parenting rather than predominantly the labour itself (Hallgren et al 1999).

'EARLY BIRD' CLASSES

Some centres are offering sessions directly after the initial booking visit when interest and motivation are often at its highest. Although it is appreciated that some women may miscarry, the support that such a group offers outweighs the disadvantages. Women are encouraged to bring their partners or some other person of their choice. The classes will probably be shared by physiotherapists with midwives, dieticians, health visitors, dentists and, possibly, doctors. The antenatal screening options offered within the particular Trust may also be discussed. Prioritisation and quality of presentation are of prime importance for the physiotherapist, and practical participation by all class members is imperative! It is essential that the following subjects be included in the physiotherapist's part of the sessions.

Pregnancy back care

Postural, hormonal and weight changes, ergonomic education involving sitting and working positions, bending, lifting and household activities should all be considered (Figs 4.1–4.5) Ideally, no woman should go home without an individual posture check, instruction in using seatbelts in pregnancy (Fig. 4.6), and information regarding access to further help if she is experiencing back pain or other physical discomfort (see p. 142).

Symphysis pubis dysfunction (SPD)

Although the true incidence of this pregnancy-related condition has not yet been identified, it is a common occurrence usually beginning in the antenatal period. Many women may experience the signs and symptoms

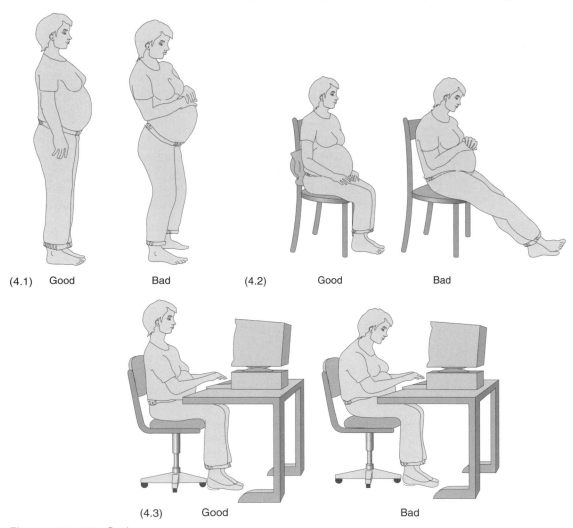

(4.1)   Good   Bad   (4.2)   Good   Bad

(4.3)   Good   Bad

Figures 4.1–4.3   Back care.

of SPD but are unaware of its management; indeed not all health professionals are familiar with it. It is therefore important to flag this up during the antenatal class to enable the woman to seek further help during both pregnancy and labour (see p. 153). National guidelines for this condition

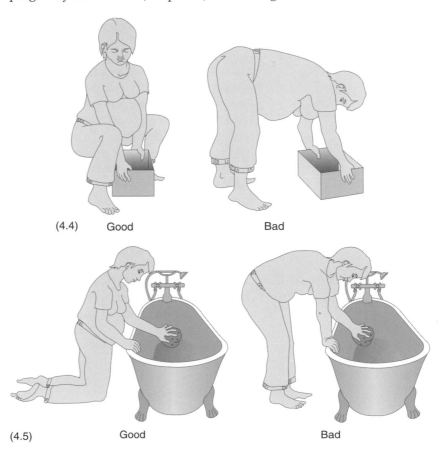

(4.4)   Good   Bad

Figures 4.4–4.5   Back care.   (4.5)   Good   Bad

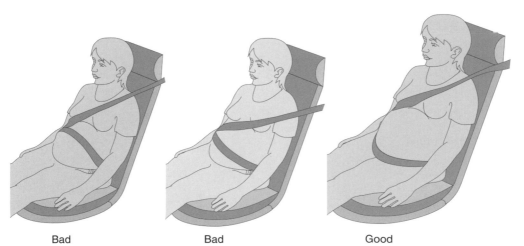

Bad   Bad   Good

Figure 4.6   Seatbelts and pregnancy – 'above and below the bump, not on it'.

are available from the Chartered Society of Physiotherapists (CSP 1994) and were devised by the Association of Chartered Physiotherapists in Women's Health (ACPWH; see Further Reading, p. 138).

Pelvic floor and pelvic–tilting exercises

A brief explanation of the role of the pelvic floor using a model of a pelvis should be given by the women's health physiotherapist teaching pelvic floor muscle (PFM) contractions. Mason et al (2001) showed that women who had learnt and practised PFM contractions during pregnancy experienced less urinary incontinence postpartum than those who had not learnt the skill antenatally. A study comparing PFM ability with a nulliparous group and a group of women at 10 months postpartum with no incontinence symptoms demonstrated the former had increased muscle power and endurance, again indicating the importance of exercising this muscle during the postpartum period (Marshall et al 2002). Where the group is large, pelvic tilting can be demonstrated while sitting on the edge of a chair (Fig. 4.7). The group should understand that this exercise can be helpful for maintaining abdominal muscle strength (particularly the transversus abdominis muscle), correcting posture and easing backache, and that it can be done in a standing position (Fig. 4.8) as well as crook lying, side lying and prone kneeling (Fig. 4.9).

Exercises for circulation and cramp

An explanation should be given as to how pregnancy can affect leg circulation, and women who travel long distances and have sedentary jobs should especially be encouraged to carry out frequent foot and ankle exercises.

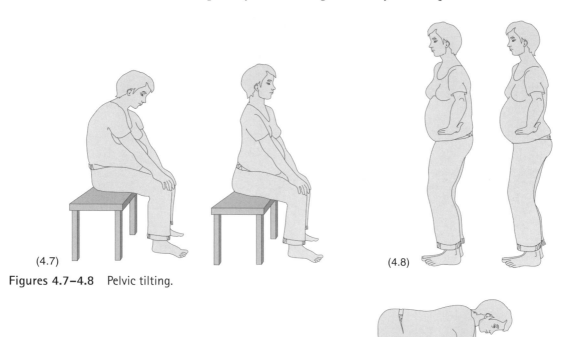

(4.7)

(4.8)

Figures 4.7–4.8   Pelvic tilting.

Figure 4.9   A good position to practise transversus abdominis contractions.

Ankle dorsiflexion and plantar flexion, and foot circling carried out for 30 seconds regularly, should be suggested; women should be advised not to cross the knees when sitting. The technique of stretching in bed with the foot dorsiflexed and not plantar flexed for preventing and easing calf cramp should also be shown. Additional suggestions for cramp relief include avoiding long periods of sitting, a pre-bedtime walk, calf stretches, a warm bath, and foot and ankle exercises in bed before going to sleep.

Fatigue

Many women who are pregnant for the first time (and their partners) are completely overwhelmed by the intense tiredness that they experience in the first trimester. Sometimes this is so severe that they feel totally unable to function when evening comes. This fatigue is sometimes aggravated by 'evening sickness'. The assurance that for most of them this will pass, and advice on coping strategies and relaxation techniques are reassuring and helpful.

The effects of stress on body and mind

An attempt should be made to elicit the causes and the effects of stress from the group itself. The Mitchell method of physiological relaxation (see Further Reading, p. 138) is ideally suited for teaching informally and can be reinforced by a handout. Other stress-coping strategies, such as music, a warm bath or shower, a walk or exercise, dancing and massage, should be discussed (see p. 167).

Emotional reactions

The session will not be complete without some discussion of the amazing range of possible psychological and emotional responses to the recently confirmed pregnancy experienced by both partners.

Advice on lifestyle

Work and how long to continue it, adaptations and alterations in lifestyle if necessary, sport and exercise should all be discussed. Plenty of opportunity should be given for questions and discussion.

At the end of these 'early bird' sessions, the supply of supporting leaflets reinforcing the main points and providing contact details of the women's health physiotherapist is desirable. The ACPWH leaflet *Fit for Pregnancy* covers many of the above topics (see Further Reading, p. 138).

STRESS AND RELAXATION

The changing roles of women in the early twenty-first century, combined with a materialistic and more mobile society and its search for wealth and possessions, as well as the loss of close family support, impose pressure on all and especially on young women and their partners embarking on parenthood. Women today are often delaying motherhood while they pursue their careers; the mean age of first time mothers in 2000 was 27, with the average age of all mothers being 29, part of a continuing upward trend (Botting 2001). In England and Wales the survey showed in 1997–1999 only 38% of women were under the age of 25 when they had their first baby, compared with 49% between 1988 and 1990. While women have more choices compared with previous generations, the downside to this is often the juggling described in order to combine both career and motherhood. Life crises will always take their toll, and pregnancy and becoming a parent for the first time is certainly one of these.

Unemployment is not unusual in today's working population and the woman in the partnership may find herself the sole breadwinner as well as the childbearer. It is not uncommon for the woman to be the higher wage earner, and this has financial implications regarding maternity leave, return to work and childcare choices/provision.

On average, women in the UK now work longer into their pregnancies, with 37% in 1996 going beyond 34 weeks' pregnancy compared with 15% in 1988. Also, women are returning to work earlier after the birth, with 81% restarting within 28 weeks compared with 75% in 1988 (Press notice July 1997 www.dwp.gov.uk). The above changes in working patterns may exacerbate the everyday stresses already being experienced by a couple. Many women during the early weeks of pregnancy experience extreme fatigue and nausea; to this may be added unsympathetic and demanding employers, moving to larger accommodation and anxieties about finance. Supporting women in the antenatal period presents the women's health physiotherapist with a valuable opportunity to enable them to understand the causes and physiological effects of stress; to become aware of it in themselves and others, and to be able to control, manage and dissipate it throughout their lives and whenever it threatens to reach harmful levels.

There is a variety of ways in which the subject of stress can be introduced. Women quickly identify with such experiences as going to the dentist, a job interview, commuting and traffic jams and will have no difficulties in describing their physiological response. Similarly, after a moment's thought they can describe the appearance of someone who is angry, grieving, frightened or in pain.

Physiological effects of stress

The body's response to threat, whether physical or mental, real or imagined is essentially that of 'fight or flight'. The physical manifestations include increased heart rate, raised blood pressure, rapid respiration or breath holding. Blood is drained from areas of low priority, such as the gastrointestinal tract and the skin, and diverted to skeletal muscle. The mouth dries, the pupils dilate, the liver releases its glycogen store, blood coagulation time decreases and the spleen discharges additional red blood cells into the circulation. Sometimes the bladder and bowel may be affected, causing frequency and diarrhoea. There are certain similarities in joint and muscle response whatever the causative stress. A common theme runs through the positions adopted which combine to produce a posture of tension.

These include hunched shoulders, flexed elbows and adducted arms, clenched or clutching hands, and flexed head, trunk, hips, knees and ankles. The face contorts to express the relevant emotion. In anger, the brow is furrowed, the chin juts forward; in grief, pain or fear, it is drawn in and down to the chest. The jaw is frequently clenched together.

Table 4.1 Stress caused by change in lifestyle on a scale of 0–100 (Holmes & Rahe 1967)

Score	Event	Score	Event
100	Death of spouse	29	Son or daughter leaving home
73	Divorce	29	Trouble with in-laws
65	Marital separation	28	Outstanding personal achievement
63	Jail term		
63	Death of close family member	26	Wife begins or stops work
53	Personal injury or illness	26	Begin or end school
50	Marriage	25	Change in living conditions
47	Fired at work	24	Revision of personal habits
45	Marital reconciliation	23	Trouble with boss
45	Retirement	20	Change in work hours or conditions
44	Change in health of family member	20	Change in residence
40	Pregnancy	20	Change in schools
39	Sex difficulties	19	Change in recreation
39	Gain of new family member	19	Change in church activities
39	Business adjustments	18	Change in social activities
38	Change in financial state	17	Mortgage or loan less than $10 000
37	Death of close friend		
36	Change to different line of work	16	Change in sleeping habits
35	Change in number of arguments with spouse	15	Change in number of family get-togethers
31	Mortgage over $10 000	15	Change in eating habits
30	Foreclosure of mortgage or loan	13	Vacation
29	Change in responsibilities at work	12	Christmas
		11	Minor violations of the law

Examples of stress-causing life events and their suggested rating are shown in Table 4.1.

Teaching neuromuscular control

The Mitchell method of physiological relaxation

This method utilises knowledge of the typical stress/tension posture and the reciprocal relaxation of muscle – whereby one group relaxes as the opposing group contracts. Thus, stress-induced tension in the muscles that work to create the typical posture may be released by voluntary contraction of the opposing muscle groups. Proprioceptive receptors in joints and muscle tendons record the resulting position of ease, and this is relayed to and registered in the cerebrum. Laura Mitchell, who developed this beautifully simple and elegant technique (Mitchell 1987), devised a series of very specific orders which are given to the areas of the body affected by stress: for example, for hunched shoulders – 'Pull your shoulders towards your feet. *Stop*. Feel your shoulders are further away from your ears – your neck may feel longer.' Because of the simplicity and the physiological basis of this method it is suitable for all levels of intellect. Physiotherapists would be wise to use the exact instructions prescribed, which have been developed after many years of trial and error. A leaflet form of this method is available from the ACPWH (see Further Reading, p. 138).

Contrast method

The contrast method stems from the work of Edmund Jacobson and involves alternately contracting and relaxing muscle groups progressively round the body to develop recognition of the difference between tension and relaxation (Jacobson 1938). Although this technique has been taught extensively for many years, some people find that it increases a feeling of tension, which makes it of doubtful benefit for those feeling tense and tired.

Visualisation and imagery

This method encourages a person to think in pictures as opposed to words, using all of the senses (Payne 1998). Imagining a pleasant and warm environment of their own choice, such as a favorite country walk or sunny day at the beach, can be used to induce a feeling of calm and enhance the relaxation methods described.

Touch and massage

All physiotherapists will naturally appreciate the physiological potentials of massage in inducing relaxation and relieving pain. Simple touch can communicate a sense of companionship, caring and sharing, particularly when received from a loving partner. Soothing stroking, effleurage or kneading to appropriate areas may be used with good effect when properly taught.

Breathing

Expiration frequently accompanies the spontaneous release of tension, for example a sigh of relief. The outward breath is the relaxation phase of the respiratory cycle; this fact can be utilised to enhance the relaxation response. The very rhythm of slow, easy breathing and its predictability is reassuring and calming. Women who may not remember more complex techniques will almost always be able to rely on this approach.

Whichever method is used, thought must be given to the position in which it is taught. Initially the woman should be comfortable and fully supported in lying, side lying or sitting (Fig. 4.10). As she becomes more

Figure 4.10 Women should be encouraged to practise relaxation in a variety of positions.

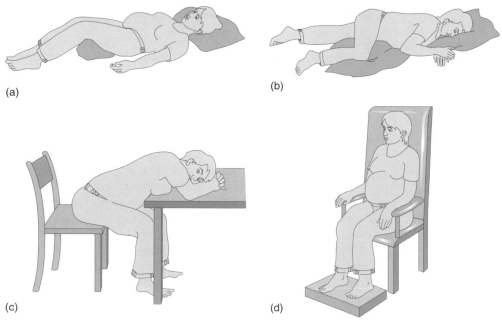

(a)

(b)

(c)

(d)

proficient she should be able to adapt the concepts to less supported postures, even standing. However, the women's health physiotherapist must be aware that as pregnancy progresses prolonged periods of supine lying are to be avoided owing to supine hypotensive syndrome (see p. 37). Right side lying is a favourable alternative.

Through the course of antenatal classes, it is hoped that women and their partners will become increasingly able to identify the effects of stress in those around them, and more particularly in themselves. This recognition is an essential part in the development of 'body awareness', and enables women to know when to use the appropriate stress-reducing techniques to induce a relaxation response. It should be emphasised that this approach is not limited to pregnancy and labour, but should become a lifelong philosophy and skill. It must also be emphasised that a formal relaxation technique is not the only way to manage stress. Yoga, movement, music, aromatherapy, warm baths and countless other alternative coping strategies all have a place. People should be guided and encouraged to seek their own individual solutions.

EXERCISE AND PREGNANCY

It has long been suggested that women whose lives were filled with hard active work and who were consequently physically fit tended to have easier labours than those with a more sedentary lifestyle. (Exodus 1 : 19; Vaughan 1951). Until the twentieth century, however, most women were grateful simply to survive the multiple hazards of pregnancy, labour and the puerperium; a healthy baby was an additional bonus! With the environmental and medical advances that have led to safer childbirth and a substantial drop in the maternal and foetal mortality rates has come an enormous change in expectations of parturient women. Some, particularly middle-class professionals, approach childbirth as they would a job or an examination – they study, prepare and *train* for it. Others, conscious of being relatively 'unfit' (in the athletic sense of the word), feel that they ought to improve their strength, flexibility, stamina and endurance in preparation for pregnancy and childbirth – or actually during the months after their pregnancy has been confirmed. All these women probably hope that exercise will give them an easier pregnancy and a shorter labour, and enable them to cope more efficiently with the exhausting early days of new motherhood.

It is not possible to set strict guidelines for women wanting to exercise during pregnancy as there are too many variables, such as individual fitness levels, the intensity and type of exercise and the individual factors affecting each pregnancy. With exercise and activity now being encouraged as part of a healthy lifestyle, more women are likely to be exercising before and during pregnancy. This increase in the number of women wishing to be active during pregnancy means the women's health physiotherapist will be involved in educating and encouraging exercise in many different situations. These range from leading antenatal exercise groups, advising women who are habitual exercisers and are wishing to continue with exercise, pregnant women who wish to become more active but do not regularly exercise, and about the use of suitable home exercise videos.

The physiological changes that occur when a woman exercises, particularly in aerobic exercise, are primarily to maintain the woman's internal homeostasis during the exercise period. When assessing effects of exercise in the pregnant woman, concerns will be related to the physiological effects on the mother and effect on foetal well-being.

Maternal risks

1. There is a greater risk of musculoskeletal trauma because of connective tissue laxity owing to the secretion of the hormone relaxin. This causes an increase in joint laxity with an increased range of movement; thus joint integrity can be compromised. Postural changes due, in part, to the increasing size and orientation of the uterus may also impair balance and coordination as the centre of gravity alters. This may be compounded by changes in perception and reduced coordination. The anatomical and physiological changes associated with pregnancy have the potential to increase the risks from sport and exercise, but with good exercise prescription and advice these can be reduced (Carpenter 1994; Heckman & Sassard 1994).

2. There will be increased demands on a cardiovascular system already altered by pregnancy which include an increase in blood volume, cardiac output and resting pulse and a decrease in the systemic vascular resistance. After the first trimester the supine position should be avoided as it may cause supine hypotension (see p. 37).

3. There will be a small increase in the number of calories per day needed during pregnancy and this is mostly significant in the last trimester; if a woman is exercising this will also increase the amount needed. Hypoglycaemia may arise with maternal exercising, which could lead to foetal hypoglycaemia.The pregnant woman has a reduced fasting blood sugar compared with the non-pregnant woman, and also metabolises carbohydrates faster. Hypoglycaemia is more likely to happen during a resting and fasting state, so the pregnant, exercising woman has to ensure her calorific intake is adequate when exercising.

4. Thermoregulation – there is an increase in both basal metabolic rate and heat production during pregnancy with the foetal temperature approximately 1°C higher than the maternal temperature. Hyperthermia can cause teratogenic effects to the foetus, a maternal temperature of 39.2°C being the possible threshold for neural defects within the first trimester of pregnancy (Milunsky et al 1992) and IUGR during later pregnancy. During moderate to vigorous activity most energy from the increased metabolism is transformed into heat, which is dispersed by redirecting blood flow to the skin where some of the heat is stored and hence results in an increase in core temperature. Pregnancy is thought to induce an enhanced response to heat production via a more sensitive thermoregulation response, thereby minimising the effect of heat. A study by Jones et al (1985) showed that women exercising at a self-imposed rate did not experience huge increases in their core temperatures and were within safety limits (<38°C) indicating that

women may well self-regulate to a level (i.e. moderate rather than vigorous exercise), thereby not rendering their foetus vulnerable to hyperthemia.

5. Respiratory changes – there is an increase in minute ventilation by almost 50%, which is mainly due to an increase in tidal volume. There is an increase in oxygen uptake with an increase in oxygen consumption of 10–20%. The increase in resting oxygen requirement is due to the mechanical effect of the uterus upon the diaphragm, which will reduce the availability of oxygen available for aerobic-type exercise. As moderate activity is advocated, the supply of oxygen should not impose difficulties.

Foetal risks

1. Foetal distress could occur during vigorous and prolonged exercise because of the selective redistribution of blood flow away from the splanchnic organs, including the shunting away of the uteroplacental blood flow towards the working muscles by up to 50%. In the normal healthy woman and during mild and moderate exercise this will only rarely be a problem. The effects of vigorous activity by the pregnant woman on the foetal heart rate have shown an increase of 5–15 beats per minute. The exercise intensity of up to 70% of maternal aerobic power for short time periods does not affect foetal heart rate.

2. Foetal growth and development – studies have shown maternal exercise to increase, decrease and have no effect on birthweight. Magann et al (2002) studied the significance of exercise on maternal and foetal outcome on low-risk healthy pregnant women. They were divided into four groups ranging from no exercise to heavy exercise (exercising voluntarily at more than 28 weeks and continuing until 28 weeks gestation or throughout their pregnancy). The women who exercised to a moderate to heavy level delivered babies who were 86 g on average smaller than the group of non-exercisers. No adverse consequences were identified in the lower-birthweight babies.

3. Foetal malformations, arising from the teratogenic effects of a raised maternal core temperature during the first trimester, are possible (see thermoregulation).

4. Preterm labour, with or without delivery, is a concern, especially in the last trimester; the concern is that exercise may trigger uterine contractions. When Hatch et al (1998) conducted a study investigating maternal exercise and time of delivery, no association was found between low to moderate exercise and gestational length. Alderman et al (1998) found, using a sample of 291 women, that moderate to vigorous physical activity for 2 hours per week or more in any month was associated with a reduced risk of a large birthweight baby for gestational age, and there was no significant effect or risk for small infant size. Artal & Sherman (1999) support this view. Indeed, a study comparing aerobic exercise in the first two trimesters of pregnancy and type of delivery found that sedentary women were more likely to deliver by caesarean

delivery than active women. Even though not statistically significant, it was suggested that regular activity in the first two trimesters may be associated with a reduced risk for delivery by caesarean in primiparous women (Bungum et al 2000).

Contraindications

Currently there are three main bodies which offer recommended guidelines and contraindications for exercise in pregnancy; the American College of Obstetrics and Gynecology (ACOG 1994b, 1995), American College of Sports Medicine (ACSM 1991) and the Society of Obstetrics and Gynaecology of Canada (SOGC 1995). There is some disagreement as regards interpretation of current research to optimise safety of mother and foetus but Table 4.2 gives some guidance (see also the ACASC position paper in Further Reading, p. 138).

Women in these categories tend to be aware of their limitations; there is no reason, however, why routine antenatal exercises for leg circulation, pelvic floor muscles and gentle movements to maintain good posture and back comfort (e.g. pelvic tilting) should not be taught and practised regularly (see Early Bird Class p. 105). Activities that may be contraindicated include competitive and contact sports, and activities such as horse riding, skiing, waterskiing and scuba diving carry far greater risks when a woman is pregnant.

Guidelines for women exercising during pregnancy

- Jerky, bouncing, ballistic movements and activities should be avoided.
- Regular mild to moderate exercise sessions, at least three times a week, are safer than intermittent bursts of activity.

Table 4.2 Contraindications to vigourous exercise in pregnancy

Absolute	Relative
• Cardiovascular disease • Acute infection • A history of recurrent spontaneous abortion (miscarriage) • Preterm labour in current or previous pregnancy • Multiple pregnancy • Vaginal bleeding or ruptured membranes • Incompetent cervix • Pregnancy-induced hypertension • Suspected IUGR or foetal distress • Thrombophlebitis or pulmonary embolism • Chronic hypertension, active thyroid, cardiac, vascular or pulmonary disease • Diabetes type 1 uncontrolled	• Women unused to high levels of exertion • Blood disorders such as sickle cell disease and anaemia • Thyroid disease • Diabetes – however, a carefully supervised programme of *gentle* exercising may actually benefit some patients • Extreme obesity or underweight • Breech presentation in third trimester

- A careful 'warm-up' should precede vigorous exercise, which must always be followed by a 'cool-down' or gradual decline in activity.
- Flexibility and mobility follow the warm-up section, avoiding ballistic stretching. All main muscle groups should be included and positions stretching at the extreme range of movement avoided.
- Strenuous exercise must be avoided in hot, humid weather, or when the pregnant woman is pyrexial.
- The maternal heart rate should not exceed 140 b.p.m. and vigorous exercise should not continue for longer than 15 minutes.
- Fluid must be taken before, during and after exertion to avoid dehydration, and energy intake must be sufficient for the needs of pregnancy as well as the exercise.
- As with women beginning exercise outside pregnancy, it is essential that those accustomed to a sedentary lifestyle should start with low-intensity physical activity. Walking, swimming, stationary bicycling or yoga are probably ideal, with gradual increases in activity levels according to a woman's own individual tolerance capacity.
- An aerobic component should be in the mode best suited to the individual, using large muscle groups and being rhythmical in nature, i.e. brisk walking, cycling, aerobic dance – all avoiding high impact.
- Avoid supine positions after the first trimester.
- Avoid standing motionless for long periods of time.
- Exercise should be decided by the limitations imposed by pregnancy. The competitive element must be excluded.

Traditionally, monitoring and intensity of aerobic exercise was by heart rate, but during pregnancy, it is too limited as the heart rate alters (ACSM 1995). Women should be encouraged to use the BORG rating of perceived exertion (RPE) aiming between 12 and 14 or the 'talk test' (Borg 1970).

The following list of signs and symptoms from the ACSM (1995) are considered significant and, if apparent, would need medical review:

- any signs of bloody discharge from the vagina
- any 'gush' of fluid from the vagina (premature rupture of membranes)
- sudden swelling of ankles, hands or face
- persistent, severe headaches or visual disturbance, or both; unexplained spell of faintness or dizziness
- swelling, pain and redness in the calf of one leg
- elevation of pulse rate or blood pressure that persists after exercise, excessive fatigue, palpitations and chest pain
- persistent contractions (>6–8 hours) that may suggest onset of premature labour
- unexpected abdominal pain
- insufficient weight gain (<1.0 kg/month during the last two trimesters)
- absence of or reduced foetal movements.

The women's health physiotherapist will be able to advise and encourage women wishing, with the consent of their doctors, to continue or begin appropriate physical activity. For the uncomplicated pregnancy the specific symptoms and discomfort of pregnancy will often dictate for the woman an adaptation in the mode of exercise, as well as changes in the intensity, frequency and duration (Sternfeld 1997). However, it must always be appreciated that many women do not wish to participate in group activities and are not interested in exercising formally on their own. They should *not* be made to feel guilty. Where it is obvious that a woman's daily workload is minimal, it may be possible to persuade her to walk a reasonable distance regularly, or to use an exercise bicycle. It is worth reminding women that the discomforting symptoms of pregnancy have been shown to reduce with exercise including less nausea, backache, round ligament pain and fatigue (Sternfeld et al 1995). The improvements in personal well-being that are associated with exercise are also pertinent during pregnancy, including a reduced frequency of somatic symptoms, decrease in insomnia and anxiety and a higher level of pyschological well-being (Goodwin et al 2000).

Although exercise has undoubted physical and psychological benefits at all times, it has yet to be proved that a particular regimen has any effect on the length or ease of labour and delivery. What is indisputable is the fact that physically fit, athletic women recover more rapidly after the birth than those who have a less active pregnancy and who are athletically unfit.

Swimming and water exercise in pregnancy

Swimming is possibly the perfect pregnancy exercise. Even non-swimmers can benefit from a programme of exercise and relaxation in a pool. The buoyancy of the water supports the mother's increasing body weight, enabling her to continue with the excellent toning and strengthening activity which increases her physical fitness and endurance, as well as promoting her sense of well-being. In addition, exercise in water offers several physiological advantages to the pregnant woman (Katz 1996).

As well as being a form of exercise, a study involving a group of women from 18 weeks' gestation to the 1st week postpartum, randomised to either water gymnastics once a week or to a control group, found a significant reduction in intensity of back or low back pain in the first group as well as a decreased number of women on sick leave due to back pain (Kihlstrand et al 1999). The regular swimmer should be encouraged to continue with her normal routine, adapting her strokes and the distance of her swims to her advancing pregnancy; as with all other sports, she should be warned to 'listen to her body' and slow down accordingly. A woman with SPD needs to avoid breaststroke as the hip abduction can exacerbate the condition; front crawl can be suggested as an alternative. Care should be taken with either stroke not to exaggerate the lumbar lordosis, which can happen if a woman is not submerging her head under water.

Women should 'warm up' prior to their main swim, and 'cool down' following it. A session of relaxation aided by the buoyancy of the water can be most therapeutic, particularly in the final trimester. For non-swimmers a programme of suitable exercises can be suggested, including activities for the legs, arms and trunk, as well as 'water walking' and relaxation. Many swimming pools and leisure centres now provide special sessions for pregnant and postnatal women, but the women's health physiotherapist interested in running this sort of class and who does not have a hydrotherapy qualification should consider observing and taking advice from specialist colleagues. The books *Aquarobics* by Glenda Baum (1998) and *Swimming Through Your Pregnancy* (1983) and *Water Fitness During Your Pregnancy* (1995) by Jane Katz are useful texts and the ACPWH Aquanatal guidelines (1995) will also be helpful (see Further Reading, p. 138).

Yoga

Yoga is an increasingly popular activity during pregnancy. Although there are many similarities between some yoga positions and exercises traditionally used by physiotherapists, the emphasis placed on stretch and mobility may not be appropriate for all women. It is unwise for health-care professionals to incorporate aspects of this philosophically different approach to their classes without proper training in yoga. Women who express interest in this form of exercise should be directed to properly accredited teachers.

Pilates

Pilates is currently enjoying vast popularity, but was initially developed by its master Joseph Pilates back in the mid twentieth century. The Pilates method encompasses an holistic approach to exercise, developing body awareness and general fitness, which starts from a central core of stability concentrating on abdominal and pelvic floor muscles. Hence, this gentle form of exercise can be employed by the pregnant and postnatal exercising woman to help maintain and retrain these muscles in both stages, as well as focusing on posture and coordination. However, it is important to ensure that women are directed to classes led by instructors who have had the appropriate training.

DIET AND WEIGHT GAIN IN PREGNANCY

That 'we are what we eat' is undoubtedly true, but the assertion that pregnant women need to 'eat for two' in terms of quantity is now quite out of date. During pregnancy, the body works more efficiently, saving energy by adjustments in physical activity and adapting its metabolic rate. The average woman needs only an extra 300 calories per day in the second and in the third trimester when the baby is growing at its fastest rate. What is important is the nutritional intake in the first trimester, as this is when the formation of the foetus is occurring and major influences will be the uterus, placental structure and the mother.

A normal weight gain of 11–15 kg (25–35 lb) is expected, but will vary according to prepregnancy weight, height, age, and whether the woman has had a baby previously. The approximate distribution can be seen from Figure 2.6 (see p. 40). If a woman's BMI is high, she will be encouraged to aim for a weight gain towards the lower end of the scale; the opposite will apply to those with low BMI. Maternal weight gain or loss is also a poor indicator of foetal well-being – another reason why routine weighing of women has stopped. Women should eat according to appetite, adopt the habits of a healthy diet, and be advised that pregnancy is not the time to start dieting. Current evidence suggests that a single birth results in a 2–3 kg increase in average body weight (Gunderson & Abrams 1999), with postpartum weight retention more likely with a higher gestational weight gain, especially if the weight is gained earlier in the pregnancy (Muscati et al 1996, To & Cheung 1998).

Breastfeeding is often advocated to help lose weight retained postpartum. A study comparing the effect on mothers' weight of breastfeeding or bottle feeding from birth to 18 months postpartum did find a significant positive association with breastfeeding (Janney et al 1997). Similar findings were found by Dewey et al (1993), the weight loss being significantly higher in breastfeeding mothers at 12 months postpartum (by 2 kg) compared with mothers using formula feeding. The accumulative effect of breastfeeding was emphasised, that is, to gain the benefit of the weight loss postpartum, women needed to breastfeed for at least 6 months.

If a healthy diet is adopted preconceptually and maintained throughout pregnancy, this should give a good balance of the nutrients needed to maintain the mother's health during pregnancy, as well as helping her baby grow and develop normally. The five basic food elements are proteins, fats, carbohydrates, fruit and vegetables and dairy products.

NUTRIENTS

Particular attention is paid to the following nutrients.

Folic acid

This helps in the prevention of neural tube defects such as spina bifida (Garcia-Morales et al 1996). It is found in vegetables (cauliflower, frozen peas, tomatoes), oranges, breakfast cereals and yeast extract. It is recommended that a daily supplement of folic acid (0.4 mg/day) is taken by all women both preconceptually and in the first trimester of pregnancy.

The following vitamins and minerals can all be acquired in the appropriate amounts with diet and without additional supplements:

Calcium

This is needed for bone, teeth and gum formation. It is found in dairy products, sardines and dried fruit. The foetus takes the quantities required by absorbing it from the mother's stores; it is important therefore to maintain intake. Vitamin D helps with absorption of calcium.

Omega–3 fatty acids (e.g. fish oils)

These are important for development of the baby's brain and neural development. They are found in mackerel, salmon, sardines and other oily fish, as well as flaxseed.

Iron

This is to combat anaemia common in pregnancy. It is found in red meat, beans, nuts and green vegetables. As well as iron supplements, it can also be increased via the diet. To ensure good absorption, the woman should eat it with vitamin C (orange juice) and avoid combining eating with caffeine (this can reduce absorption).

Dietary fibre

This is to help prevent the constipation common in pregnancy. It is found in fruit, vegetables, nuts and pulses, wholemeal bread and cereals. It is important to be taken in combination with high water intake.

Diet and healthy eating should be discussed at the initial booking visit with the midwife, with written information also available. The following websites are helpful: www.shef.ac.uk/pregnancy_nutrition, www.Babycentre.co.uk, www.babycenter.com.

FOODS TO AVOID

Women's immunity is lowered during pregnancy, so they are more open to infection. It is thus worthwhile advising on the foods that should be avoided despite the relatively small risk they pose in terms of infection and potential damage to the unborn baby.

Listeria

This bacterium is rare, occurring only in 1/20 000 pregnancies (University of Sheffield 1999). It can cause flu-like symptoms in mothers, miscarriage in early pregnancy, premature labour and stillbirth. It has been associated with certain foods, and the following guidance is recommended:

- **Avoid** soft mould-ripened soft cheeses (e.g. Brie, Camembert), blue-veined cheeses (e.g. Stilton, Roquefort) and unpasteurised goats/sheep cheeses.
- **Avoid** meat, fish and vegetable pate.
- **Avoid** soft-whip ice cream.
- Reheat thoroughly cook-chill foods and cooked poultry.
- Take care with prepacked salads – always use within date and wash before use.

Salmonella

This is a common cause of food poisoning, causing sickness and diarrhoea in the mother. It rarely harms the baby during pregnancy, but it is best to avoid a severe infection. As it is associated with raw eggs and poultry, women should be recommended to:

- **Avoid** mayonnaise, mousses made with raw eggs.
- Always defrost poultry and cook thoroughly.

Toxoplasmosis

This is caused by an organism found in raw meat and cat faeces and, although very rare, infecting 1/50 000 (University of Sheffield 1999), it can have serious effects on the foetus if caught during pregnancy. If transferred to the foetus it may cause hydrocephalus, epilepsy, hearing or visual problems, even blindness. A multicentre study to determine the highest environmental risk factors, found eating undercooked beef or game, contact with soil, and travel outside Europe, the USA and Canada were most strongly predictive. Contact with cats was not a risk factor in this study (Cook et al 2000). The following guidance is given:

- Wash hands after handling raw meat. Always cook thoroughly.
- Wash salads and vegetables thoroughly.
- **Avoid** unpasteurised sheep and goat dairy products.

- Wear gloves when emptying a cat tray or gardening. Wash hands after handling cats/kittens.
- Pregnant women should not help with lambing or milk ewes recently delivered, as sheep may carry toxoplasmosis, *Listeria* or *Chlamydia*.

Liver

Excessive amounts of vitamin A in the retinol form have been associated with congenital malformations, therefore the advice should be:

- **Avoid** liver and liver products.

Dark fish

Dark fish (e.g. swordfish, shark, tuna or marlin) contain high levels of mercury, which can affect the development of the foetal nervous system; therefore it should not be eaten frequently. It is currently recommended to limit consumption to two portions per week.

Peanuts

The number of children with allergies, including peanut allergy, has been increasing over the years and the reason for this is unclear. However, it is thought that they may develop during pregnancy. As peanut allergy can be life threatening the current recommendation is that if a woman or her partner has a known peanut allergy, or suffers from asthma, eczema, hay fever or other food allergies, she should avoid peanuts both during pregnancy and whilst breastfeeding.

Caffeine

This does not need to be avoided during pregnancy, but it is suggested to limit it to 300 mg/day. It is found in tea, coffee, cola drinks and chocolate. High levels of caffeine consumption have been associated with low-birthweight babies and miscarriage (Rasch 2003). However, other studies have found no association with IUGR, low birthweight or preterm delivery with moderate caffeine consumption (Bracken et al 2003, Clausson et al 2002, Grosso et al 2001). Women who drink large amounts of coffee (more than eight cups/day) double the risk of stillbirth compared with non-caffeine-drinkers (Wisborg et al 2003).

Alcohol

What is a unit/measure of alcohol? This is as follows according to the leaflet *Sensible Drinking* by the Health Education Authority:

- 1 single pub measure of spirits
- 1 small glass of sherry or fortified wine
- 1 small glass of table wine
- ½ pint of ordinary lager, beer or cider
- ¼ pint of strong lager, beer or cider.

The effects of maternal drinking on foetal development have been the aim of many research projects. However, it is difficult to isolate the effects of alcohol from those due to other associated effects (i.e. smoking, drug abuse, socioeconomic status and diet). Further research is needed to identify what level and pattern of drinking becomes dangerous to the foetus. Currently, drinking one or two units once or twice a week has shown no evidence of foetal harm and is the UK guideline. Little or no evidence of foetal harm has been found if women are drinking up to 10 units a week, but to give consistency the lower level is recommended. Some countries are even more conservative, suggesting no alcohol consumption at all during pregnancy.

Excessive and binge drinking causes a condition known as foetal alcohol syndrome (FAS), which can present as IUGR craniofacial abnormalities or severe learning difficulties as well as cognitive, hearing and visual disabilities (*Alcohol in Pregnancy*, see Further Reading, p. 138). In the first trimester, when organ development is occurring, heavy drinking can cause organ damage, whereas growth and neurobehavioural development are more affected in the second and third trimesters. A healthy woman who has one occasion of drinking heavily in the early stages of pregnancy (i.e. before she is aware of being pregnant) should not worry that she will have a damaged baby and then be advised accordingly of the safe limits.

From the above list, it is easy to see why some women worry about what they should and should not be eating or drinking to avoid harming their baby, so perspective must be maintained that the above infections are relatively unlikely. If common sense and basic food hygiene are maintained all should be well. The women's health physiotherapist must keep abreast of current guidelines and, if unsure, be able to direct women to the appropriate professional or information resource.

SMOKING IN PREGNANCY AND LATER

There is strong evidence to show that maternal smoking, and possibly maternal passive smoking, is harmful to the foetus, and that it can affect the pregnancy and the subsequent development and health of children after they are born. It is accepted that there is a direct link between maternal smoking and low birthweight, as well as an association with exposure to environmental tobacco smoke (Windham et al 2000). Smoking is also associated with foetal hypoxia, IUGR, placental abruption, premature rupture of membranes, miscarriage, premature delivery (Wisborg et al 1996) and low Apgar scores. It has been demonstrated ultrasonically (Pinette et al 1989) that there is an acceleration of placental maturation and therefore of premature senescence and calcification leading to poor function in smokers. Wisborg et al (2001), using a cohort of 25 102 singleton children, found an increased risk of stillbirth associated with mothers who smoked and an infant mortality of almost double the risk, compared with a child of a non-smoking mother. Yet, if women stopped by 16 weeks' gestation, their risks became comparable with non-smokers throughout the pregnancy. The problems do not cease with the birth of the baby.

Postnatally, the consequences of smoking during pregnancy continue with smoker's children having three times the risk of sudden infant death syndrome (SIDS) than those of non-smokers, the risk increasing with the number of cigarettes smoked (Wisborg et al 2000). When children are brought up in families where smoking continues, long-term after-effects have been reported including increased childhood mortality, postnatal growth retardation and chronic respiratory illnesses.

Stopping smoking is one of the most effective steps a woman can take to improve her baby's health and that of her own. In the last UK survey, 35% of women smoked before or during their pregnancy, but the figure reduced to 20% for women continuing throughout the pregnancy (DOH 2002). Although this figure does not indicate what proportion of women stopped smoking independently, professional advice and support can achieve significant cessation rates. As the risks of maternal and paternal smoking continue into the baby's infancy and childhood, the women's health physiotherapist should be able to direct motivated women to the relevant groups, and resources to help stop the habit.

MEDICATION IN PREGNANCY

Since the thalidomide disaster in the 1960s, when an antiemetic drug given in early pregnancy to women suffering from nausea and vomiting was found to be the cause of severe limb and organ deformities in their babies, it has become obvious that the placenta does not act as a barrier to harmful chemicals. Research showing no adverse effect on animals does allow the assumption that this will be the same on humans. It is important for women who find that they are pregnant, and those likely to become pregnant, to understand that some drugs can damage the developing foetus. The most sensitive time for embryonic damage is in the first trimester; women and their partners need to realise that it is not only doctor-prescribed medicines that can damage babies, but also over-the-counter treatments.

The mother's health must be the primary consideration, but where a woman becomes ill in pregnancy, or has a pre-existing condition that obliges her to take medication, doctors will always try to use drugs with the least known risk, changing original prescriptions to substances known to be safer. Drugs with major teratogenic effects are rare, but retinoic acid (used to treat severe acne), some cytotoxic drugs and radiochemicals can cause grave damage. Pregnant women whose foetuses have been exposed to these substances are offered terminations. Tetracycline taken in pregnancy is known to cause subsequent discoloration of children's teeth, and many other drugs in common usage can cause damage of various sorts and degrees depending on the stage in the pregnancy that they were taken. Physiotherapists presently do not prescribe as part of their clinical practice but, if seeking further information on drugs which are potentially harmful to the foetus, should refer to the current British National Formulary (BNF). A patient should always be referred back to her GP or obstetrician for further clarity. It is important for women to realise that they have a responsibility in this context too; they should always remind their doctor, dentist or pharmacist that they are pregnant whenever medication is prescribed or when they buy 'over-the-counter' remedies of any kind.

Although it is probably safest to avoid unnecessary medication during pregnancy, it is estimated that over one-third of women take self-prescribed 'over-the-counter' medication during pregnancy (Jordan 2002). Paracetamol is the commonest painkiller for use both during pregnancy and breastfeeding (Byron 1995), for example for headaches or colds, and is commonly prescribed without ill effect.

Looking ahead to the puerperium, some drugs are contraindicated in breastfeeding women; most drugs, however, appear in breast milk only in quantities small enough not to be harmful to the infant (see Further Reading, p. 138).

ADDICTIVE DRUGS IN PREGNANCY

Although many centres have pockets of drug users, addiction in the UK is not as great as it is in other parts of the world. Many regular drug abusers will have other health problems and probably poor social conditions too; sadly, they are often identified as a group likely to be poor attenders regarding antenatal care so that the foetus is at risk from several sources.

Congenital abnormalities have been reported following the use of the narcotics, cocaine, lysergic acid diethylamide (LSD) and the amphetamines (including 'Ecstasy'). Placental insufficiency, IUGR and perinatal mortality are all increased where women use heroin and its derivatives. A major problem is the effect of narcotic drug withdrawal on the foetus and neonate, which can prove fatal if not very carefully managed both during pregnancy and the immediate postpartum period. However, the prognosis for the infant of the drug-addicted mother is good if the mother cooperates with antenatal care and drug control (Bolton 1987).

MULTIPLE PREGNANCIES

The rate of multiple pregnancies is increasing in many countries, largely owing to the increased use of assisted conception. Thirty per cent of couples using assisted conception will conceive twins or higher-order multiple pregnancies (www.Dartmouth.education/~obgyn/mfm/index.html). In 2000, the incidence of multiple births in the UK was 14.67 per 1000 births. An increase in maternal age is also associated with increased probability of twins.

Twins may arise from the splitting of one fertilised ovum (monozygotic or uniovular) or from the fertilisation of two ova (dizygotic or binovular). There may be a family history of twins, and the tendency for double ovulation will be passed on to other women in the family. Diagnosis is by ultrasound, or sometimes the uterus shape is much larger than expected for the stage of pregnancy.

Pregnancy discomfort and problems can be intensified due to the increased weight, and towards the end of gestation women can be extremely uncomfortable. Multiple pregnancies are associated with a higher risk of obstetric complications such as PIH, antepartum haemorrhage and delivery by caesarean section (Doyle 1996). The incidence of preterm delivery is significantly higher in twin deliveries, with a consequently higher risk of low birthweight babies and perinatal mortality (Buscher et al 2000). The average length of pregnancy for twins is 35 weeks and for triplets 33 weeks. Delivery by caesarean section is more likely with multiple pregnancy; also, because a high number of these pregnancies are associated with assisted conception, often termed 'precious pregnancies', here again the choice of delivery is often the caesarean mode.

PLANNING AND LEADING LABOUR AND PARENTCRAFT CLASSES

Lack of information has direct effects on limiting informed choice, including dependence and engendering passivity, with implications for control, fear, and lack of cognitive preparation'

(Sherr 1995)

One of the aims of parent education is empowerment of the parents, educating individuals to increase their knowledge thereby enabling them to make informed decisions. With more control regarding their choice making, this in turn will build parents' confidence and self-esteem. Parent education aims to help pregnant women (and their partners and supporters) acquire knowledge of childbirth and parenting, which historically, women gained from attending births, being involved in closer family networks. Mothers today are undervalued and unsupported by a society that is becoming ever more critical of parents, who are expected to do a job for which the only training they have is their experience of being parented (Schott 1994).

CLASS ARRANGEMENTS

When planning new antenatal courses it is imperative for the team to explore the perceived needs of the prospective clientele; these vary from area to area and can fluctuate within a community. Whether urban or rural, populations develop and change, and the ethnic and socioeconomic composition can be dramatically altered. The women's health physiotherapist needs to be flexible in her approach, adapting the classes according to the needs of the group: are the groups aimed at primiparous or multiparous women; are they couples or women only; and what provision has been made for non-English-speaking parents or those with disabilities?

A study completed by the NCT asking parents to identify what they thought the content of the classes should be, found that questionnaires completed before their classes, after them and following delivery, were all consistent in requesting more coverage regarding the changes in their lives and relationships with the arrival of a new baby (Nolan 1997) as well as the practicalities of a new baby.

The advantages of an 'early bird' class are generally recognised, and are discussed on page 105. Commonly the main antenatal course consists of four to six sessions, and usually begins around 32 weeks' gestation. The number of classes offered and which professionals facilitate them will vary widely according to the resources and preferences of individual trusts. Parent education sadly remains low on the priority list of some units, partly owing to resource implications and professional reluctance to take classes during unsociable hours. This can result in shortened courses, with the result of fewer classes being offered leading to exclusion of certain topics.

Some women, although entitled to take time to attend antenatal classes, often find it hard to commit during the working day and as mentioned previously are continuing to work until close to term. Managers within Trusts need to be sensitive to the best interests of their clients, offering classes which are community based and providing them during the evenings or at weekends. Ideally groups should consist of 8–16 people, but it should always be possible to integrate latecomers, and women should be encouraged to fit in classes as and when they can. It is recognised that, even when non-pregnant, an individual's attention span is limited. Sessions of 2–2½ hours allow for plenty of variety in teaching and learning methods, with a break in the middle for drinks and informal socialising. It is to be remembered that one aim for those attending these classes is often to form new friendships with other mothers-to-be, who potentially can become part of a vital support network in the postnatal period.

In some areas it will be possible to run regular courses of six weekly classes, whereas in other areas it may be better to present a more limited programme over 4 weeks. Women expecting their first baby may welcome a longer course; those who already have children may appreciate a more condensed programme. Although many centres have traditionally concentrated on 'women only' classes, today, with the greater involvement of men in childbearing and rearing, it is more usual to enrol the woman with her partner (do not assume though that everyone has a partner and welcome alternative companions such as mothers, sisters or friends). While there are obvious advantages, the disadvantages must not be overlooked. There may be times when women will be inhibited in their discussion by the presence of men, and vice versa. It may be helpful to split the group at some stage during the session to overcome this, which also has the advantage of encouraging peer group learning. Having two or more leaders will offer the group different styles and role models, so parents gain different aspects from the differing approaches.

Today, separate classes for teenagers are encouraged, so there is no risk of them being part of a group of clients with whom they have little in common. Instead the class for this group will be able to target their specific needs, (i.e. to return to education with a baby).

In areas with large groups of ethnic minorities, or non-English-speaking population, a specific group may well be appropriate in overcoming language difficulties whilst addressing cultural needs. However, if such a couple attends a standard class, the facilitator should aim to accommodate their needs whilst absorbing them with the rest of the group.

From time to time it may be necessary and useful to hold 1-day 'crash courses' or 'labour days' for those women and their partners who are unable, for one reason or another, to attend a full course, whatever its length. With the increasing interest in fitness, specific antenatal exercise groups including aquanatal and Pilates classes have been developed. Whether these classes should be part of the provision by the NHS or left up to the individual's responsibility is certainly debatable. However, it is most certainly in the interests of the NHS that the organisers of such classes be appropriately qualified.

Environment

Antenatal classes are frequently held in very unsuitable places such as 'nooks and crannies', basements and windowless 'cupboards'. Ideally the parentcraft accommodation should be purpose built, carpeted, light and airy, clean, and with windows looking if not on a green and pleasant environment then at least out! It must be conveniently sited for transport and ease of access, including that for wheelchair users, and be large enough to include an area for socialising, drinking tea or coffee and reading information and booklets. There should be space for exercising and relaxation, and toilets, refreshment and washing facilities and ample storage space close by. A welcoming atmosphere can be fostered by attractive curtains, pictures and plants. All furniture and other equipment, including mats, wedges, bean bags, chairs and pillows should be chosen for their durability, and with ergonomic and safety principles in mind. A long mirror is desirable. Noticeboards displaying news items of current interest, advertisements of articles for sale and photographs of baby 'graduates' complete the ideal set-up for women's health physiotherapist.

The following outline for a parent education 6-week course is intended as a guideline only, and can obviously be modified and tailored to the locality. For the purpose of description it is assumed that the women's health physiotherapists will be working alongside midwives and health visitors; less frequently they may be responsible for the entire programme, more usually if they are working in the private sector. It is also assumed that women will have attended one or more early classes. If this is not the case, earlier topics will need inclusion.

A 6-WEEK COURSE

Week 1: introductions

Class and class facilitators meet each other. Although all the people attending have one obvious thing in common, they are essentially a group of strangers to each other. 'Ice breakers' are invaluable in decreasing awkwardness and inhibition to then allow the group to gel and interact. This may be time consuming but pays dividends for the course in the long term, as anyone who has ever been faced with a situation where eliciting group participation is an uphill struggle will verify!

The first session is an ideal opportunity to tackle immediate problems and worries, for example any specific queries re back pain, SPD and general aches and pains, and other priority concerns. Encourage class attenders to take responsibility for their own learning and identify topics they want to cover during the course, so it remains very parent centred. From this a plan for each session is devised providing well-structured classes incorporating the parents' agenda, which boosts their self-esteem by valuing their opinions. A balance is needed between preparation for labour and for parenthood, with time allotted for postnatal emotional issues.

If there is time include:

- a suitable, short general programme of exercises to promote comfort, mobility and strength, including (for example) foot and ankle movements, pelvic tilting in a variety of positions, PFM exercises, wall press-ups, squatting (modified if necessary), 'tailor' sitting and posture correction and back care
- when to come into hospital (early signs of labour) and what to bring into hospital.

Week 2: stages, signs and length of labour, birth plans/choices

Include the following:

- Labour
- First stage of labour
- Relaxation – a discussion on the causes and effects of stress, and coping strategies. Detailed and leisurely instruction and practice, using a variety of positions, of one method of relaxation (e.g. the Mitchell method). If women become confident with its usage antenatally, they will understand the benefits of using it postnatally to cope with all the stresses and demands of a new baby. (Depending on the group, it may be more appropriate to introduce relaxation in the first session and focus on exercise in the second.)

Week 3: coping with the first stage of labour

Include:

- coping strategies for early stage of labour (at home): distractions including mobilising, reading, music, television, cards, scrabble; relaxation, baths, showers, light meals
- TENS (see p. 185)
- as the first stage progresses: positions, breathing awareness, massage and visualisation techniques.

Week 4: pain relief and other possibilities

Include:

- medical pain relief, including the use of Entonox, pethidine and epidurals
- discussion of the end of the first stage, transition and the second stage of labour
- positions for the second stage
- foetal monitoring, episiotomies, assisted deliveries, vacuum extraction and forceps.

Week 5: further possibilities in labour, and feeding baby

Include:

- third stage of delivery, the use of syntometrine
- induction of labour, caesarean delivery
- the first feed and the postnatal care of woman and baby in hospital
- breastfeeding, benefits of breastfeeding for babies and mothers; practical information regarding positioning, latching on, and possible hurdles; the UNICEF Baby Friendly Initiative, (see p. 134).

Week 6: parenthood and getting back into shape!

Include:

- care of the new baby, a 24-hour job
- transition to parenthood, adjustment to relationships
- postnatal depression
- postnatal exercises.

A class reunion

This encourages the formation of friends and a support network. Include discussion with a recently delivered mother and father, accompanied by their baby, their experience of labour and early postnatal problems and discomforts, and how to cope with them.

A visit to the delivery suite may be incorporated into one of the classes or offered on a separate occasion, but is a useful way to dispel fears and preconceptions parents may have regarding this place so much talked about but never actually experienced.

Some services offering daytime classes arrange a partner's evening session to include fathers unable to attend during the working day. Regrettably, in some centres, financial restraints result in classes being available mainly to primigravidae and only exceptionally to multigravidae. Ideally, any pregnant woman who wants to attend antenatal classes should be free to do so, no matter how many babies she has had. Where courses are available to multigravidae, they are often a condensed or 'refresher' version, but there are great advantages in mixing women of differing parity. The special needs of multigravidae (which can be met in any class) include talking through previous labour experiences, updating their knowledge of labour management, considering the impending changes in the family, and how to make time for the baby as well as the existing children. Relaxation becomes more important as parity increases. In some respects a multigravid woman will be more self-confident, but age and experience bring other anxieties – she may well feel that her luck is running out: Will this baby be normal? What could go wrong in this labour? Many of these feelings, problems and their solutions can be fully shared in a group of mixed parity; women can be very supportive of each other.

Although these guidelines may appear rather formal, it must be remembered that the sensitive women's health physiotherapist will be constantly alert to the day-to-day needs of the individuals in the class, and will be prepared to divert from the original course plan whenever necessary. At the same time the facilitator must be able to guide and control discussion. Although group discussion can change attitudes, and must be encouraged, women and their partners *do* come to antenatal classes to gain information and may resent the conversation being monopolised by a few vociferous participants. Antenatal educators must not fall into the trap of solely preparing their parents for the 'grand finale' of pregnancy – labour. They must always remember that labour, particularly for the primigravida, is in fact the transition to a totally new lifestyle which will gradually evolve, and time and consideration needs to be given to easing the adjustment.

The findings of studies investigating effectiveness of antenatal parent education classes vary. Hetherington (1990) found prepared couples were more likely to receive little or no pain medication, whilst Nichols (1995) found no differences when comparing attenders with non-attenders in terms of childbirth satisfaction, parenting sense of competence, and ease of transition into parenthood. However, it was suggested that further evaluation of course content is needed; rather than looking at birth outcomes as a measurement of successful parent education, studies should ascertain what information is useful to the couple during labour and birth to facilitate a positive birth experience. A group of 59 women completed a questionnaire after their birth regarding influence of their parent education classes. Although many of them enjoyed the classes, and found information gained about pain relief helpful for decision making in labour, minimal influence was shown in terms of breastfeeding and length of hospital stay (Handfield & Bell 1996).

When they are expecting their first child, many prospective parents have great difficulty in actually appreciating the changes that parenthood can bring. It is extremely important during every antenatal class to look constantly to the future, and to stimulate thought about the way the parents will care for their baby, the sort of parents they will be, and how they will reorganise their lifestyle to cope with this major life event.

ANTENATAL SELF-HELP STRATEGIES FOR GOOD MATERNAL POSTNATAL ADJUSTMENT

Advice can include:

1. Try to make friends with couples who have young children or who are also expecting.
2. Reduce housework and its importance.
3. Continue your outside interests, but reduce your responsibilities.
4. Give yourself permission to slow down as pregnancy progresses.
5. Go to parent education classes with your partner.
6. View maternity leave as a time of relaxation and rest rather than an extended holiday with large schedules and 'to do' lists.
7. Try not to move house less than 6 months before or 6 months after the birth.
8. Think about organising someone to babysit occasionally and maybe to help out at home too if possible.

THE TRANSITION TO PARENTHOOD

Why consider life after birth? Parenthood is the only job people are expected to do 24 hours a day, 7 days a week, 52 weeks a year. Yet, while in today's world most new appliances or things come with a manual, babies do not come with one to identify their specific wants and character. There are many, many baby 'experts' out there, books to read, and websites to browse. However, it is now being recognised that more help is needed to instil confidence in today's parents regarding their individual baby's development and care.

The confirmation of a pregnancy is greeted by a wide range of emotions from women and their partners: joy and satisfaction if the pregnancy is a planned and wanted one; ambivalence, which can turn to acceptance and pleasure, even if it was unplanned; despair and rejection when the pregnancy is unwanted. Even women and men who have struggled with infertility over the years, undergoing all sorts of physically and psychologically demanding treatments, may as the wildly hoped-for pregnancy progresses develop physical and emotional problems. A percentage of women will not enjoy being pregnant, for a number of reasons, and this is to be acknowledged by any health professional involved with their care. Pitt (1978), in *Feelings about Childbirth*, says that a period of adjustment is needed when even a greatly wanted object, previously unattainable, becomes a reality. Mixed feelings will be present in all expectant parents during and even after pregnancy, and both partners will have fears about what the new baby will do to their relationship and lifestyle.

For the mother there will be adjustments to her career, either halting or altering her job, a change in her exercise and social activities. With the many physical changes occurring, she will have to adjust to her pregnant 'body'. Some women thrive and 'bloom', particularly in the second trimester, but others do have body image issues and resent their pregnant state. This is not helped by the current media's obsession of projecting messages that suggest being thin and eternal youth are what is attractive. Changes in the relationship are inevitable as two becomes three and both parents will have worries over this as well as concerns over what kind of parents they will be. While the woman may have started to make changes to her lifestyle even before conception (e.g. in alcohol, smoking, diet, taking of folic acid supplements) which are then intensified and increased as pregnancy progresses, the man's life can continue much the same. The woman, because of actually carrying that baby, may often feel an intense, loving bond which can offset these normal worries.

Even though people are aware of postnatal depression (PND), it is not sufficiently appreciated that antenatal depression is just as common. A study using the Edinburgh postnatal depression scale as a measure of women's mood throughout their pregnancy and postnatally found that depression scores were higher at 32 weeks' pregnancy than at 8 weeks' postpartum. More recognition and understanding of antenatal depression is needed so effective treatment can be organised (Evans et al 2001), especially as the majority of women diagnosed with PND will probably have the onset during pregnancy.

Fathers

Although it is the woman's body that conceives, carries and gives birth to the baby, and is equipped by nature to provide everything in the way of nourishment the infant requires in the first few months of life, parenthood is usually a shared experience. Fathers too go through a sequence of changes as they leave independence or the 'cosy twosome', or face a new addition to an established family. While many men are delighted at the prospect of becoming a father, this is combined with fears and anxieties about how they will cope with the new demands that will be made on them. Within one generation there have been notable changes to the father's role, with men now much more actively involved with childrearing, rather than the traditional role of being the sole financial provider. Research has shown many benefits for involved fathers including: firstborns who have good relationships with their fathers, being much more accepting of a new sibling, and women with involved partners being less likely to suffer with postnatal depression (Martyn 2001).

In a few societies ritual *couvade* is practised by men. Special dress, confinement, restriction of activities, avoidance of polluting substances and mock labour are all said to signify magical protection of the mother and infant, symbolic expression of the bond between father and child and the acceptance of fatherhood. As has been seen, many men in our society today also complain of a variety of physical and emotional health problems during their partners' pregnancies and in the early postpartum period as well. It has been suggested that this is an expression of the father's subjective involvement in the pregnancy (Munroe & Munroe, 1971) and also an expression of profound caring for their partner and unborn child (Clinton, 1985). Also, ante- and postnatal depression is by no means restricted to women.

The women's health physiotherapist must also understand the anxieties expectant fathers may have: 'Will I be able to cope with her distress in labour?'; 'Will this enlarged, moody female ever again become the slim, happy, active girl I used to know?'; 'Will sex *ever* be the same again?' Common concerns may also include the responsibilities that come with parenting, worrying about being a good father, financial concerns providing for his family if his partner is not working, and adjusting to sharing her with the baby. These are some of the doubts and fears men have and they are often unable to express. Men have few role models and positive images of fatherhood to draw upon; attending classes which encourage discussion with other expectant fathers may help reduce worries, and a skilled facilitator can give them a realistic and practical insight into beginning to adjust to their role as father.

ANTENATAL CARE OF THE BREASTS AND PREPARATION FOR BREASTFEEDING

Grantly Dick Read when writing about breastfeeding in his book *Childbirth Without Fear* (1954) said: 'The newborn baby has only three demands: warmth in the arms of its mother, food from her breast and security in the knowledge of her presence. Breastfeeding satisfies all three.' Chloe Fisher, a senior community midwife (now retired) in Oxford, has described breastfeeding as 'a wonderful, programmed human interaction which gives the mother intense satisfaction, and her baby all it requires to sustain life for many months' (Inch 1987). Perhaps the best preparation for successful and happy breastfeeding comes long before pregnancy – during childhood in fact (RCM 2000b). Children who are brought up in a culture where babies are breastfed quite unconsciously, and by many role models, mothers, sisters or friends, will grow up aware that this physiologically normal method of nourishing the newborn can be natural, easy and pleasurable for both mother and baby (Toothill 1995). Having seen mothers breastfeeding, young women will have confidence in their own bodies being able to provide milk, and their babies knowing how to take it.

Despite the many benefits to both mother and baby regarding breastfeeding (Wilson et al 1998), the UK continues to have one of the lowest breastfeeding rates within Europe. The last British infant-feeding survey in 2000 showed that 69% of babies were initially breastfed, with a drop to 42% by 6 weeks and 28% at 4 months (DOH 2001). While this showed a small increase in the number of women who commenced breastfeeding, by 6 months the rate had dropped to 21% (the same level as for 1995), even though the WHO recommends that babies should be exclusively breastfed to that age (WHA 2001, World Health Assembly Resolution 51.2.2001).

Older mothers (over the age of 30) are more likely to have breastfed: 78% compared with 46% of teenage mothers. This is a factor well recognised in the promotion of breastfeeding. Other factors influencing the likelihood of women breastfeeding include being a first time mother, working in a professional occupation, education beyond the age of 19, and having an ethnic minority background.

Ninety per cent of women questioned who discontinued breastfeeding before 6 weeks would have liked to have continued for longer; reasons for giving up are perceived insufficient milk supply, painful breasts or nipples and the process being too long or tiring. A recent study in Australia also found maternal confidence to be a significant predictor of breastfeeding duration (Blyth et al 2002) and this should be recognised in antenatal education and care from all professionals.

To this end the UNICEF UK Baby Friendly Initiative was launched in 1992 to provide a framework for the implementation of best practice by NHS Trusts using the *Ten Steps of Successful Breastfeeding* (Henschel & Inch 2000, UNICEF UK 1992). Radford (2001) describes the initiative as crucial to breastfeeding promotion and support of a mothers' chosen feeding method.

Antenatal advice on breast care has changed a great deal in recent years, so that it is now limited to the following few main points. First, as soon as mothers are aware of their increasing breast size, they will probably feel more comfortable in a good supporting bra of the correct measurement and cup size. It is recommended during pregnancy that underwired bras are not used so there is no cutting into the increased breast tissue. Women with very heavy breasts may benefit from wearing a bra at night. Most of the increase in breast size takes place in the early months of pregnancy, so maternity bras will be needed accordingly and, although often more cumbersome and functional in appearance than non-pregnancy bras, are important for providing support; the increased weight can otherwise transmit to the thoracic spine causing backache. Simple elbow circling, and thoracic spine flexion and extension, can help relieve this problem. From 36 weeks' gestation the woman can be measured for a nursing bra.

Many young women are accustomed to being 'bra-less' these days and may not like the idea of having to be 'upholstered' during pregnancy and while breastfeeding. However, if they can understand that the breast is not a self-supporting structure, and that its increased weight could lead to drooping and sagging later in life, most will see the benefit of a good uplift.

ROLE OF THE WOMEN'S HEALTH PHYSIOTHERAPIST

As mentioned previously, the topic of breast or artificial feeding is one of the main priorities to cover within parentcraft education by the midwife. The women's health physiotherapist can provide valuable additional advice and ergonomic education regarding best feeding positions to ensure proper support of the sore perineum and spine (see p. 217).

Because the shape of the breast when the nipple is offered is all important, women must appreciate that it will be more difficult for their baby to be positioned correctly if they are leaning back, as their breasts will be flatter than if leaning forward, in which the breast assumes a more pointed shape making it easier for their baby to 'latch on'. Side lying, as well as leaning forward initially when sitting, can achieve the desired effect, with the former also being comfortable for backache. Whilst the promotion of breastfeeding for both mother and baby is to be recommended, it is necessary to remember that some women will choose not to do so or discontinue at an early stage. There are many reasons for this, for example a previous bad experience, lack of confidence regarding adequate milk supply, or a partner's negative attitude. If the woman is aware of all the benefits and support networks are in place to facilitate breastfeeding, respect for the individual's choice antenatally must be shown and incorporated into her antenatal care plan; however, there must be flexibility to allow for a change of mind.

References

ACOG (American College of Obstetricians and Gynecologists) 1994a International Journal of Gynecology and Obstetrics 45:65–70.

ACOG (American College of Obstetricians and Gynecologists) 1994b Technical bulletin no 189. Exercise during pregnancy and the postpartum period. ACOG, Washington DC: American College of Obstetricians and Gynecologists, February 1994.

ACOG (American College of Obstetricians and Gynecologists) 2001 ACOG Committee opinion: no 265 Management of term singleton breech delivery. Obstetrics and Gynecology 98(6):1189–1190.

ACSM (American College of Sports Medicine) 1991 Guidelines for exercise testing and prescription, 4th edn. Lea & Febiger, Philadelphia, PA.

ACSM (American College of Sports Medicine) 1995 Guidelines for exercise testing and prescription. Williams and Wilkins, London.

Alderdice F, Renfrew M, Marchant S et al 1995 Labour and birth in water in England and Wales: survey report. British Journal of Midwifery 3(7):376–382.

Alderman B W, Zhao H, Holt V et al 1998 Maternal physical activity in pregnancy and infant size for gestational age. Annals of Epidemiology 8(8):513–519.

Artal R, Sherman C 1999 Exercise during pregnancy: safe and beneficial for most. Physician and Sports Medicine 27(8):51–52,54,57–58.

Blyth R, Creedy D K, Dennis C-I et al 2002 Effect of maternal confidence on breastfeeding duration: an application of breastfeeding self-efficacy theory. Birth 29(4):278–284.

Bolton P J 1987 Drugs of abuse. In: Hawkins D F (ed) Drugs and pregnancy: human tetrogenesis and related problems. Churchill Livingstone, New York.

Borg G A V 1970 Perceived exertion as an indicator of somatic stress. Scandinavian Journal of Rehabilitation 2:92–98.

Botting B 2001 Trends in reproductive epidemiology and women's health. Table A. 6, p 335 in Appendix 1 Why Mothers Die 1997–1999, Lewis G ed, RCOG Press, London.

Bracken M B, Triche E W, Belanger K et al 2003 Association of maternal caffeine consumption with decrements in fetal growth. American Journal of Epidemiology 157(5): 456–466.

Bricker L 2001 Routine ultrasound screening in pregnancy – friend or foe? MIDIRS Midwifery Digest 11(4):440–444.

Bungum T J, Peaslee D L, Jackson A W et al 2000 Exercise during pregnancy and type of delivery in nulliparae. Journal of Obstetric, Gynecologic and Neonatal Nursing 29(3):258–264.

Buscher U, Horstkamp B, Wessel J et al 2000 Frequency and significance of preterm delivery in twin pregnancies. International Journal of Obstetrics and Gynecology 69(1):1–7.

Byron M 1995 Treatment of rheumatic diseases. In: Rubin P (ed) Prescribing in Pregnancy. British Medical Journal Group, London, p. 59–71.

Campbell R, Macfarlane A, Hempsall V et al 1999 Evaluation of midwife-led care provided at the Royal Bournemouth Hospital. Midwifery 15:183–193.

Carpenter M W 1994 Physical activity, fitness and health of the pregnant mother and fetus. In: Physical activity, fitness and health. Bouchard C, Shephard R J, Stephens T (eds) Human Kinetics Publishers, p. 967–979.

Chambers R 1999 Fertility problems a simple guide. Radcliffe Medical Press, Oxford.

Clausson B, Granath F, Ekbom A et al 2002 Effect of caffeine exposure during pregnancy on birth weight and gestational age. American Journal of Epidemiology 155(5):429–436.

Clinton J 1985 Couvade patterns and predictors (final report NTIS no RONU0097). Division of Nursing, US Department of Health and Human Science, Hyattsville.

Cook A J, Gilbert R E, Buffolano W et al 2000 Sources of toxoplasma infection in pregnant women: European multicentre case-control study. European Research Network on Congenital Toxoplasmosis. British Medical Journal 321:142–147.

CSP (Chartered Society of Physiotherapy) 1994 Psychophysical preparation for childbirth. Information paper no PA13. CSP, London.

Dewey K G, Heinig M J, Nommsen L A 1993 Maternal weight-loss patterns during prolonged lactation. American Journal of Clinical Nutrition 58(2):162–166.

DoH (Department of Health) 2002 Press release notice Infant Feeding Survey 2000. BMRB Social Research, London. Sue.brooker@bmrb.co.uk.

Doyle P 1996 The outcome of multiple pregnancy. Human Reproduction 11 (suppl 4):110–117; discussion 118–120.

Dunn D T, Newell M L, Ades E D et al 1992 Risk of human immunodeficiency virus type 1 transmission through breast feeding. Lancet 340(8819):585–588.

Evans J, Heron J, Francomb H et al 2001 Cohort study of depressed mood during pregnancy and after childbirth. British Medical Journal 323:257–260.

Exodus 1:19.

Garcia-Morales M A, Limon-Luque L M, Barron-Vallejo J et al 1996 Peri-conception use of folic acid in the prevention of neural tube defect. Ginecologica y Obstetricia de Mexico 64:418–421.

Goodwin A, Astbury J, McMeeken J 2000 Body image and psychological well-being in pregnancy. A comparison of exercisers and non-exercisers. Australian and New Zealand Journal of Obstetrics and Gynaecology 40(4):442–447.

Grosso L M, Rosenberg K D, Belanger K et al 2001 Maternal caffeine intake and intrauterine growth retardation. Epidemiology 12(4):447–455.

Gunderson E P, Abrams B 1999 Epidemiology of gestational weight gain and body weight changes after pregnancy. Epidemiologic Reviews 21(2):261–275.

Hallgren A, Kihlgren M, Forslin L et al 1999 Swedish fathers' involvement in and experiences of childbirth preparation and childbirth. Midwifery 15:6–15.

Handfield B, Bell R 1996 Do childbirth classes influence decision making about labor and postpartum issues? Birth 22(3):153–160.

Hatch M, Levin B, Shu X et al 1998 Maternal leisure-time exercise and timely delivery. American Journal of Public Health 88(10):1528–1533.

Heckman J, Sassard R 1994 Musculoskeletal considerations in pregnancy. Journal of Bone and Joint Surgery 76-A:1720–1730.

Henschel D, Inch S 2000 Breastfeeding: a guide for midwives. Books for Midwives, Oxford.

Hetherington S E 1990 A controlled study of the effect of prepared childbirth classes on obstetric outcomes. Birth 17(2):86–90.

Holmes T H, Rahe R H 1967 The social readjustment rating scale. Journal of Psychosomatic Research 11:213–218.

Hyett J, Perdu M, Sharland G et al. 1999 Using fetal nuchal translucency to screen for major congenital cardiac defects at 10–14 weeks of gestation: population based cohort study. British Medical Journal 318:81–85.

Inch S 1987 Difficulties in breastfeeding: midwives in disarray? Journal of the Society of Medicine 80:53–55.

Jacobson F 1938 Progressive relaxation. University of Chicago Press, Chicago.

Janney C A, Zhang D, Sowers M 1997 Lactation and weight retention. American Journal of Clinical Nutrition 66(5):1116–1124.

Jones R L, Botti J J, Anderson W M et al (1985) Thermoregulation during aerobic exercise in pregnancy. Obstetrics and Gynecology 65(3):340–345.

Jordan S 2002 Pharmacology for midwives the evidence base for safe practice. Palgrave, England.

Katz V L 1996 Water exercise in pregnancy. Seminars in Perinatology 20(4):285–291.

Kihlstrand M, Stenman B, Nilsson S et al 1999 Water-gymnastics reduced the intensity of back/low back pain in pregnant women. Acta Obstetrica et Gynecologica Scandinavica 78(3):180–185.

Lewis G 2001 Confidential Enquiries into Maternal Deaths. Why mothers die 1997–1999. RCOG Press, London.

Llewellyn-Jones D 1969 Fundamentals of obstetrics and gynaecology. Faber, London.

Macfarlane A, Mugford M, Henderson J et al 2000 Birth counts: statistics of pregnancy and childbirth, vol 2. Statistics Office, London, p 516.

Magann E F, Evans S F, Weitz B et al 2002 Antepartum, intrapartum, and neonatal significance of exercise on healthy low-risk pregnant working women. Journal of the American College of Obstetricians and Gynecologists 99(3):466–472.

Marshall K, Wlash D M, Baxter G D 2002 The effect of a first vaginal delivery on the integrity of the pelvic floor musculature. Clinical Rehabilitation 16:795–799.

Martyn E 2001 Babyshock! Vermilion, London.

Mason I, Glenn S, Walton I et al 2001 The relationship between antenatal pelvic floor muscles exercises and post-partum stress Incontinence. Physiotherapy 87(12):651–661.

Mezey G C 1997 Domestic violence in pregnancy. Ch 21 in: Bewley S, Friend J, Mezey G (eds) Violence against women. RCOG, London.

Milunsky A, Ulcickas M, Rothman K J et al 1992 Maternal heat exposure and neural tube defects. Journal of the American Medical Association 268:882–885.

Mitchell L 1987 Simple relaxation, 2nd Edn. John Murray, London.

Munroe R L, Munroe R H 1971 Male pregnancy symptoms and cross-sexidentity in three societies. Journal of Social Psychology 84:11–25.

Murray S F 1999 Maternal mortality; piecing together the jigsaw. RCM Midwives Journal 2(5):152–154.

Muscati S K, Gray-Donald K, Koski K G 1996 Timing of weight gain during pregnancy: promoting fetal growth and minimizing maternal weight retention. International Journal of Obesity and Related Metabolic Disorders; Journal of the International Association for the Study of Obesity 20(6):526–532.

NICE (National Institute for Clinical Excellence) 2002 Guidance on the use of routine antenatal anti-D prophylaxis for RhD-negative women. NICE Technical Appraisal Guidance 41. Online. Available: www.nice.org.uk/pdf/prophylaxisFinalguidance.pdf.

Nichols M R 1995 Adjustment to new parenthood: attenders versus nonattenders at prenatal education classes. Birth 22:21–26.

Nikodem V C 2003 Immersion in water in pregnancy, labour and birth. Cochrane Database of Systematic Reviews. Update Software, Oxford.

Nolan M 1997 Antenatal education:failing to educate for parenthood. British Journal of Midwifery 5(1):21–26.

NSC (National Screening Committee) 2002 Antenatal Screening Service for Down Syndrome in England: 2001. Institute of Health Sciences, Oxford. Online. Available: paward@nscdoh.fsnet.co.uk.

Östgaard H C, Zetherstrom G, Roos-Hausson E et al 1994 Reduction of back pain and posterior pelvic pain in pregnancy. Spine 19(8):894–900.

Payne R A 1998 Relaxation techniques. Churchill Livingstone, London.

Pinette M G et al 1989 Maternal smoking and accelerated placental maturation. Obstetrics and Gynecology 73:379–382.

Pitt B 1978 Feelings about childbirth. Sheldon Press, London.

Radford A 2001 Unicef is crucial in promoting and supporting breast feeding. British Medical Journal 322(7285):555.

Rasch V 2003 Cigarette, alcohol, and caffeine consumption: risk factors for spontaneous abortion. Acta Obstetrica et Gynecologica Scandinavica 82(2):182–188.

RCM (Royal College of Midwives) 2000b Successful breastfeeding, 3rd edn. RCM Press, London.

RCM (Royal College of Midwives) 2002; Position paper 25 Home birth. January. Online. Available: www.rcm.org.uk.

RCM (Royal College of Midwives) 2000a. Position paper 1a The use of water in labour and birth. October. Online. Available: www.rcm.org.uk.

RCM (Royal College of Midwives) 1999. Position paper 19 Domestic violence. Online. Available: www.rcm.org.uk.

RCM (Royal College of Midwives) 1998. Position paper 16a HIV and AIDS. October. Online. Available: www.rcm.org.uk.

Read G D 1954 Childbirth without fear. Heinemann, London, Ch 14.

Schorn M, McAllister J, Blanco J 1993 Water Immersion and the effect on labour. Journal of Nurse Midwifery 38(6):336–342.

Schott B 1994 The importance of encouraging women to think for themselves. British Journal of Midwifery 2(1):4–5.

Sherr L 1995 The psychology of pregnancy and childbirth. Blackwell Science, Oxford. Online. Available: www.harcourt.international.com/e.books/pdf/137.pdf.

Snijders R J M, Noble P, Sebire N et al 1998 UK multicentre project on assessment of risk of trisomy 21 by maternal age and fetal- nuchal translucency thickness at 10–14 weeks of gestation. Lancet 352:343–346.

SOGC (Society of Obstetricians and Gynaecologists of Canada) 1995 Policy statement. Healthy beginnings: guidelines for care during pregnancy and childbirth. November, SOGC.

Springer N P, Weel C V 1996 Home birth. British Medical Journal 313(7068):1276–1277.

Sternfeld B 1997 Physical activity and pregnancy outcomes. Sports Medicine 23(1):33–47.

Sternfeld B, Quesenberry C P J, Eskenazi B et al 1995 Exercise during pregnancy and pregnancy outcomes. Medicine and Science in Sports and Exercise 27(5):634–640.

Tahzib F 1989 An initiative on vesicovaginal fistula. Lancet i:1316–1317.

To W W, Cheung W 1998 The relationship between weight gain in pregnancy, birthweight and postpartum weight retention. Australian and New Zealand Journal of Obstetrics and Gynaecology 38(2):176–179.

Tookey P, Gilbert R 1999 Perinatal mortality and morbidity among babies delivered in water: surveillance study and postal survey. British Medical Journal 319(7208): 483–487.

Toothill B 1995 'Infant feeding in a refugee camp'. Midwives 108:150–151.

Turnbull D, Holmes A, Shields N et al 1996 Randomised, controlled trial of efficacy of midwife-managed care. Lancet 348:213–218.

Tyler S 2001 Modernising Maternity Care. A commissioning toolkit for primary care trusts in England. RCM/RCOG/NCT, London.

UNICEF UK 1992 Baby Friendly Initiative. Online. Available: www.babyfriendly.org.uk.

University of Sheffield 1999 Healthy eating before, during and after pregnancy. Wellbeing, London.

Vaughan K 1951 Exercises before childbirth. Faber, London.

WHO (World Health Organisation) 1997 Maternal health around the world (wall chart). WHO, Geneva.

Wilson A, Stewart Forsyth J, Greene S A et al 1998 Relation of infant diet to childhood health: seven year follow up of cohort of children in Dundee infant feeding study. British Medical Journal 316:21–25.

Windham G C, Hopkins B, Fenster L et al 2000 Prenatal active or passive tobacco smoke exposure and the risk of preterm delivery or low birth weight. Epidemiology 11(4):427–433.

Wisborg K, Henriksen T B, Hedegaard M et al 1996 Smoking during pregnancy and preterm birth. British Journal of Obstetrics and Gynaecology 103(8):800–805.

Wisborg K, Kesmodel U, Henriksen T B et al 2000 A prospective study of smoking during pregnancy and SIDS. Archives of Disease in Childhood 83(3):203–206.

Wisborg K, Kesmodel U, Henriksen T B et al 2001 Exposure to tobacco smoke in utero and the risk of stillbirth and death in the first year of life. American Journal of Epidemiology 154(4):322–327.

Wisborg K, Kesmodel U, Hammer B et al 2003 Maternal consumption of coffee during pregnancy and stillbirth and infant death in the first year of life:prospective study. British Medical Journal 326:422–428.

World Health Assembly 2001 WHA resolution 51.2.2001 Infant and young child feeding. Online. Available: www.ibfan.org.

Further reading

ACPWH (Association of Chartered Physiotherapists in Women's Health) 1995 under review 2003. Aquanatal guidelines. ACPWH, c/o CSP, London.

ACPWH (Association of Chartered Physiotherapists in Women's Health) Guidelines – Symphysis pubis dysfunction. Professional Affairs, London.

ACPWH (Association of Chartered Physiotherapists in Women's Health) leaflets: The Mitchell method of simple relaxation; Fit for pregnancy; Fit for birth; Fit for motherhood. Ralph Allen Press, Bath.

Artal R, Wiswell R A, Drinkwater B L 1991 Exercise in pregnancy, 2nd edn. Williams & Wilkins, Baltimore MD.

Baum G 1998 Aquarobics. WB Saunders, New York.

Brayshaw E 2003 Exercises for pregnancy and childbirth: a guide for educators. Books for Midwives Press, Oxford.

Burgess A 1997 Fatherhood reclaimed. Vermilion, London.

Callander C, Millward N, Lissenburgh S et al 1996 Maternity rights and benefits in Britain 1996. DSS Research Series (Report no 67), available from the Stationary Office.

Figes K 2000 Life after birth. Penguin, Harmondsworth.

Forth J, Lissenburgh S, Callander C et al 1996 Family-friendly working arrangements in Britain 1996. DfEE Research Series (Report no 16), available from Camberton Ltd (01700 888688)

Katz J 1983 Swimming through your pregnancy. Doubleday, London.

Katz J 1995 Water fitness during your pregnancy. Human Kinetics.

Kitzinger S 2000 Rediscovering birth. Pocket Star, Boston.

Lawrence Beech B 1996 Water birth unplugged. Books for Midwives Press, Cheshire.

Milton P 2000 Management of infertility for the MRCOG and beyond. RCOG Press, London.

Nolan M 1998 Antenatal education – a dynamic approach. Ballière Tindall, London.

Place of Birth and *Alcohol and Pregnancy*. Informed Choice Initiative leaflets for professionals produced as a result of a collaboration between MIDIRS and the NHS Centre for Reviews and Dissemination. They can be obtained from MIDIRS, 9 Elmdale Road, Clifton, Bristol BS* 1SL or email – sales@midirs.org. www.midirs.org.uk.

RCM (Royal College of Midwives) 2002 Successful breastfeeding, 3rd edn Churchill Livingstone, Edinburgh.

Schott J, Priest J 2002 Leading antenatal classes: a practical guide. Butterworth-Heinemann, Oxford.

Online Sources

www.acasc.org ASASC (American Chiropractic Association Sports Council) Position statement: exercise and athletic participation during pregnancy by D'Arcy Forbes.

www.dartmouth.education/~obgyn/mfm/index.html

www.dwp.gov.uk 1997 Press notice July.

www.midirs.org National Electronic Library for Health MIDIRS informed choice leaflets for professionals:
Place of birth
Alcohol and pregnancy.

www.rcm.org.uk/data/international/data/safe.htm.

www.shef.ac.uk/pregnancy_nutrition.

Useful Addresses

Association of Breastfeeding Mothers
PO Box 207, Bridgewater, Somerset TA6 7YT
Email abm@clara.net

Association for Improvement in the Maternity Services (AIMS)
5 Ann's Court, Grove Road, Surbiton, Surrey KT6 4BE
Website: www.aims.org.uk

Association of Chartered Physiotherapists in Women's Health
c/o Chartered Society of Physiotherapy
14 Bedford Row, London WC1R 4ED
Website: www.womensphysio.com

Down's Syndrome Association
155 Mitcham Road, London SW17 9PG
Website: www.downs-syndrome.org.uk

Fathers Direct
Herald House, Lamb's Passage, Bunhill Road
London EC1Y 8TQ
Website: www.fathersdirect.com

ISSUE (The National Fertility Association)
114 Litchfield Street, Walsall WS1 1SZ
Website: www.issue.co.uk

Foresight – proponents of preconceptual care.
26 The Paddock, Godalming, Surrey GU7 1XD
Website: www.forsight-preconception.org.uk

Maternity Alliance
3rd Floor, 2–6 Northburgh Street, London EC1V 0AY
Website: www.maternityalliance.org.uk

Multiple Births Foundation
Queen Charlotte's and Chelsea Hospital, Goldhawk Road, London W6 0XG
Website: www.mbf.org.uk

National Childbirth Trust
Alexandra House, Oldham Terrace, Acton, London W3 6NH
Websites: www.nct.org.uk; www.pregnancyand babycare.com

Royal College of Midwives,
15 Mansfield Street, London W1M 0BE
Website: www.rcm.org.uk

TAMBA (Twins and Multiple Births Association)
PO Box 30, Little Sutton, South Wirral L66 1TH
Website: www.tamba.org.uk

Useful websites

www.midirs.org.uk
www.shielakitzinger.com
www.Babycentre.co.uk

Chapter 5

Relieving the discomforts of pregnancy

Sue Barton

CHAPTER CONTENTS

Introduction   141
Back and pelvic girdle pain   142
Some common syndromes and their treatment   149

Nerve compression syndromes   155
Circulatory disorders   157
Other problems   159

INTRODUCTION

Pregnancy is often the first time in a woman's life that she will experience so many different 'feelings', both physically and psychologically. The vast majority of primigravidae will experience 'aches and pains' during pregnancy. For some, these will be many, varied and maybe disruptive to function. For some, their first experience of the hospital environment, and personnel, comes during pregnancy or the birth. Perhaps it is because of these factors, and because pregnancy and birth are 'unknown' experiences, that the so-called 'minor ailments' of pregnancy can assume major importance to the woman herself.

The majority of these discomforts can be directly related to the physical changes that take place during pregnancy, and their resultant biomechanical effects upon functional movement. The growing uterus, and its contents, can give rise to experiences of 'pulling, pressing and pushing' discomfort or pain. Some women describe 'sharp stabbing pains', or 'dropping-out' feelings. The understanding of the physical and biomechanical changes taking place is an essential part of the 'coping strategy'. Frequently, a clear explanation, and consequent understanding, of the reasoning behind the symptoms will in the majority of cases be sufficient to enable the mother-to-be to 'manage' and cope with them. Unfortunately, pregnant women with discomfort, for example backache, are still frequently told: 'What do you expect, you are pregnant, you can't expect relief until the baby is born.' Once a physiotherapeutic diagnosis has been made the woman may actually be able to 'treat' herself. 'Self-help' treatment or coping strategies may be appropriate forms of management and can be taught so that women are able to treat themselves. The teaching skills, and knowledge, of the specialist physiotherapist are invaluable here.

BACK AND PELVIC GIRDLE PAIN

More than one-third of women experience back and pelvic pain at some stage during pregnancy (Young & Jewell 2002), yet there is a danger amongst health professionals of considering these symptoms as inevitable and unimportant. The intensity and duration of the pain can fluctuate throughout the pregnancy and often from one pregnancy to the next in the same woman. There is also great variation in severity between individuals: one person may complain of minor, transient, stiffness or discomfort, while another may be totally disabled. Östgaard & Andersson (1991), in a retrospective review, showed that back pain occurs twice as often in women who had back pain before becoming pregnant, and occurs more in women who have been pregnant before. These women also tend to have symptoms for longer. Research indicates that, in about 50% of those pregnant women experiencing pain, it is of sufficient intensity and duration to affect their lifestyle in some way, and for one-third of these individuals the pain is severe (Berg et al 1988, Fast 1999, Mantle et al 1977, 1981, Nwuga 1982).

The first episode of pain in a pregnancy may occur at any stage, but for the majority it is between the 4th and 7th months (Bullock et al 1987, Fast 1999, Mantle et al 1977, 1981). In general, back pain seems to be felt at a lower level by a woman when she is pregnant than when she is not pregnant (Mantle et al 1981). Mantle et al (1977) and Fast (1999) found the majority of sufferers have low back pain; for about half of these it radiated into the buttocks and thighs, and occasionally down the legs as sciatica. The mechanical stresses from the gravid uterus, and the compensatory lordosis (Laros 1991), would support this theory. For many women the back pain is made worse by standing, sitting, forward bending, lifting – particularly when combined with twisting (Berg et al 1988) – and walking. Some complain, in addition or solely, of pain over or in the *symphysis pubis*; for a few the *thoracic* region is affected, rather than the lower back and pelvis. *Coccydynia* can also be a problem antenatally, although it is uncommon and is often linked with a previous injury.

The general population are subject to back pain and therefore it should not be automatically assumed that a pregnant woman's backache, or leg pain, is as a direct result of her pregnancy; nor need pregnancy be an adverse or prolonging factor to recovery from back problems. It is also worth noting that back pain before pregnancy does not necessarily lead to back pain during pregnancy. Some women actually experience less back pain than usual whilst pregnant. However, it is generally accepted that there are a number of factors that could account for the significantly higher incidence of back pain in pregnant women compared with that in their non-pregnant peers: fatigue, increased mobility of joints (Calguneri et al

1982) associated with hormonally induced changes in collagen (remodelled collagen has a greater volume causing pressure on pain-sensitive structures), weight gain with increased spinal loading and associated necessary adaptations in posture, and pressure from the growing foetus.

Bullock et al (1987) showed a significant increase in lumbar and thoracic curves during pregnancy, which was still evident at the end of the puerperium. However, they could not substantiate the increase in pelvic inclination propounded by many physiotherapists, nor was there any obvious correlation between the increasing spinal curves and the onset of pain.

It must be borne in mind that hormonal levels begin to change and have their effects from the time of conception; significant weight gain and postural adaptations come later. Fast (1999) has wisely suggested that the aetiology of the pain may vary with each trimester; this is probably true. Even so, it is worth remembering that Mantle et al (1981) showed that it is possible to reduce the intensity of, and even prevent, some back pain in pregnancy. The women's health physiotherapist's role is not only to treat where appropriate, but also to be the member of the obstetric team who seeks to understand the problem, who has all the latest information concerning the causes and treatment of back pain, and who leads the team in aiming, first at prevention, and, where this fails, at containing and mitigating the problem.

PREVENTION OF BACK PAIN

One of the main aims of the women's health physiotherapist antenatally is to prevent back pain. For some women back pain may well be inevitable. In this case the aim will be to prevent an increase or exacerbation of symptoms and to educate the woman to 'manage' her symptoms. A study by Östgaard et al (1994) found that pain was reduced by individual education early in pregnancy. The suggestion was that perceived pain was less as a result of understanding and knowledge of how to manage the condition. The principles of back care are the same for the pregnant woman as they would be for the non-pregnant, although the application of those principles may have to be adapted. It is good sense to encourage a woman to be aware of her own body, and to seek to understand and 'contain' any back pain she is experiencing before undertaking a pregnancy, even though there is no clear correlation between back pain before and during pregnancy.

Antenatal classes should include education in body awareness and back care, with regular reinforcement and feedback. It is essential that the health professional leads by example as a method of reinforcement. The antenatal class is an ideal avenue to providing cost-effective opportunities that, in the long term, will influence the wider community in this, and many other, health promotional aspects.

The adaptation of back-care principles in pregnancy

Lying

Lying can be very uncomfortable during pregnancy. Comfortable resting and sleeping positions are essential. Additional support may be necessary in the form of pillows, or extra mattress support, in order to gain not only a position of comfort but one that will facilitate quality 'positioning' to prevent symptoms. The altered body mechanics as a result of pregnancy can initiate musculoskeletal symptoms if positioning is not carefully thought through. There must be whole body support, with all joints in a position of 'ease'. The role of the women's health physiotherapist will be to assess the woman and advise as to the best positioning for her as an individual. A position of unsupported rotation must be avoided at all costs. Comfort in supine lying can be increased with pillows under the thighs, though long periods in this position should be discouraged later in pregnancy owing to the increased risk of supine hypotensive syndrome. There may come a time when restlessness is preventing a good night's sleep; separate beds can mean that at least one person gets a restful night!

Rolling   Rolling can be performed more efficiently, and with less risk to the sacroiliac and symphysis pubis joints, by maintaining adduction at the hips and flexion at the knees. All human movement is performed more efficiently if it is facilitated as follows:

- turning the head in the direction of 'travel' will facilitate the upper trunk to 'roll'
- folding the arms across the chest with the top arm leading in the direction of 'travel' will facilitate the midtrunk to 'roll'
- slightly flexing the outside knee and laying it on the inside leg (closest to 'travel') will facilitate the lower trunk to 'roll'.

The body weight has now 'shifted' closer to the direction of travel. A 'lead' from the arm, and flexed knee will result in an effective, safe and efficient (ESE) 'roll'.

There is potential risk involved in getting out of bed. Many women, during pregnancy, micturate during the night. It is essential that injury does not occur whilst getting out of bed. The ESE technique is to roll on to the side, push down against the bed or 'grab' the bed sheets with the 'lead' arm, and push up sideways at the same time as swinging the legs over the edge of the bed. This process should be reversed when going from sitting to lying.

Sitting   Sitting can be just as uncomfortable during pregnancy. The aim of the chair is to be of support to the user with the following criteria:

- buttocks well back on the seat
- thighs fully supported, for at least ⅔ of their length, no more than two fingers-width from the popliteal fossa, and horizontal (i.e. hips at 90°, knees at 90°)
- feet fully supported and flat on the supporting surface
- spine fully supported enabling natural spinal curvature – a small pillow in the 'lumbar hollow' may be necessary
- enabling the functional activity, e.g. writing, word processing, watching television.

These criteria are even more important during pregnancy, with everything in moderation. Women should be encouraged not to sit for too long, as the body will 'start to complain'. Humans are mechanically 'made to move' and therefore function best whilst moving, so frequent changes of position should be encouraged. Toward the end of pregnancy it may be more comfortable to sit astride a chair, facing the backrest, and lean forward for support (but *not* if suffering from symptoms of symphysis pubis dysfunction (SPD)).

Standing and walking   It is essential to maintain a good standing and walking posture at all times, not just during pregnancy. Standing posture can be maintained by the following:

- weight evenly distributed over both feet
- feet slightly apart, and slightly angled (not balletic!)
- knees off stretch, 'soft'
- spinal curves maintained, and symmetrical
- environment or tasks positioned to enable good posture, e.g. kitchen work surface at the 'right' height.

Standing for long periods should be avoided if at all possible because of the negative effects upon the circulatory system. If necessary, standing with one foot on a raised support, or transferring weight from foot to foot, may moderate the worst effects (but *not* if the woman is suffering from the symptoms of SPD).

Walking is acceptable daily exercise for most people; however, walking for too long or whilst carrying too much may provoke pain. There is a lot to be said for 'listening to the body'.

All functional activity in standing should be performed in such a way as to reduce risk:

- avoid trunk-on-hip flexion – a 'top-heavy' bend taking the trunk outside the base of support
- avoid twisting repetitively, or whilst carrying a load
- move about the knees, using the powerful quadriceps muscles to initiate movement
- 'move' up and down the spine, within the base of support.

For example, when vacuuming the floor, the vacuum cleaner should be as close to the operator as possible (avoiding a 'top-heavy' bend), the action of pushing kept in the same plane (to avoid twisting), knee extension used when pushing the vacuum cleaner (to utilise the 'power' muscles), and the spine not held rigid but allowing it to move 'with' the movement.

The mechanical effects of functional activity upon spinal structure may under normal circumstances, initiate symptoms. During pregnancy the risk is exacerbated.

Once pregnancy advances, and abdominal girth increases, it may be necessary to adapt functional activities. It will become essential to maintain the strength of the quadriceps as this is the muscle group that will enable the woman to be able to continue to get down to, and up from, the floor, chair, etc. When getting something from floor level the woman should be advised to:

- avoid squatting unless fitness and stamina 'prevail'. This is not a stable position unless the feet are flat on the floor and the weight is within the base of support. The knee extensors are much less efficient in raising the body up against gravity, when the knees are flexed beyond 90°
- go down on one knee so that both knees are at 90°, feet on the floor with as large a surface area as possible, knees in line with hip joints …
- to kneel (with both knees) if staying down there, e.g. cleaning the bath
- go back to one knee when ready to raise up
- put the hand to knee/stool/bath and push through at the same time as …
- push through the floor, equally with both legs, to extend the knees.

Lifting   Heavy lifting should be avoided or shared. To be efficient, and minimise risk, loads should be held close to the centre of mass. This will become increasingly more difficult as pregnancy progresses. Any load carrying *must* maintain good posture (e.g. using two shopping bags, one in each hand) rather than one causing side flexion of the trunk. Joint laxity during pregnancy will also increase risk during load handling. Planning of tasks will be essential as pregnancy progresses.

The women's health physiotherapist is the professional best equipped to educate the woman with regard to ESE functioning. The education should be appropriate to the individual, and include all 'baby' activities (i.e. bathing, nappy changing, feeding, equipment buying, equipment carrying, etc.). Every opportunity should be taken to 'inform' mothers-to-be, with leaflets, posters, demonstrations and videos, all aimed at reducing risk and developing a 'body awareness'.

MANAGEMENT OF BACK AND PELVIC GIRDLE PAIN

The approach to the management of a pregnant woman with back or pelvic girdle pain must be holistic and involve the whole team. As with all such pain sufferers, a full assessment is imperative to determine whether, and what, treatment is indicated. The fact that a pain sufferer is pregnant is critical to both assessment and treatment. The approach differs from that in the non-pregnant woman when it comes to understanding the reasons for the back pain, and the differential diagnostics. The techniques used will be different as the woman, for example, may be unable to lie prone, and manual techniques will be preferable to mechanical ones because of the palpatory response to changing tissues (Sandler 1996). It is *essential* that time be allowed for a *thorough* assessment of these women. Norén et al (2002), in a prospective, consecutive 3-year study, showed that 5% of all pregnant women, or 20% of all women with back pain during pregnancy, had pain 3 years later. They suggest that the problem may be poor muscle function in the back and pelvis. There was a tendency to assume that the sacroiliac joint was the cause of 'all evil'. Sacroiliac dysfunction will sometimes be found (Berg et al 1988), but the women's health physiotherapist would be wise to heed Grieve's advice not to examine the sacroiliac joint 'until the lumbar spine, hip and lower limb examinations, including neurological tests, have been completed … one should resist the tendency to find what one would like to find' (Grieve 1981). A thorough assessment by the women's health physiotherapist, with appropriate time allowed by their manager for this, may alleviate the worrying statistics as well as result in a more accurate diagnosis.

Assessment of the patient

The physiotherapist is the expert in musculoskeletal assessment. The women's health physiotherapist must remember her 'roots', and add to this foundation knowledge her knowledge and understanding of the pregnant woman, and adapt her assessment accordingly.

Subjective examination

Patient positioning is even more important with this client group; the woman needs to be comfortable and well supported.

Routine questioning should be used constantly, linking responses to the 'problems' of pregnancy and listening for anything that might suggest necessitating referral (e.g. oedema, headaches may be indicative of preeclampsia). Throughout the process it is worth remembering that the 'status' of the woman – maybe anxious (more about the baby than themselves), stressed, tired – may heighten pain perception. Reassurance is essential.

Mandatory questions concerning the perineum and micturition should be asked. Are there any changes in perineal sensation or micturition habits? It is necessary here to discriminate between significant symptoms and the frequency and stress incontinence experienced by many pregnant women, also the pain, hyperalgia or numbness of the perineum, which may be associated with piles, haemorrhoids and venous thrombosis of the vulva, often resulting from constipation in pregnancy or from the direct downward weight of the foetus. Back pain may accompany urinary tract infections.

The *onset* of symptoms is particularly significant during pregnancy, as is the *history* of this and any previous episodes. Hormonally mediated collagen changes commence early, whereas important abdominal enlargement and weight gain are later manifestations. It is important to remember that severe backache may also be a sign of impending labour. The woman's own assessment of the cause is always worthy of note. Padua et al (2002) reported on a multicentre study of 76 women with back pain in the third trimester, and found that an evaluation of the patients' perspective of their symptoms made it possible to identify predictive factors for the occurrence of back pain. Of particular interest is a similar episode in a previous pregnancy, for there are some women who recognise conception by a recommencement of 'the backache'. Research has shown that there is a greater degree of joint laxity in second pregnancies than in first (Calguneri et al 1982), and Mantle et al (1977) and Nwuga (1982) noted the incidence and severity of back pain increased with parity. Fast (1999) found more disability caused by backache in women with prior pregnancies, and suggested changes in posture or weakness of trunk muscles as explanations. Berg et al (1988) found that low back pain in a previous pregnancy increased the likelihood of sacroiliac dysfunction in the present pregnancy.

The *general health, occupation and lifestyle* of the woman must be estimated. The philosophy of equality of the sexes, the employment climate whereby the woman may be the sole breadwinner of a partnership, the dispersal geographically of families and the belief – correct in itself – that pregnancy is a normal physiological process, can all lead to pregnant women expecting and being expected to do too much. Individual limitations must be recognised and conceded. Dramatic improvements in back pain in pregnancy have been achieved simply by discontinuing employment. In contrast, there is increasing evidence that physically fit women have fewer aches and pains in pregnancy than their unfit sisters (Hall & Kaufman 1987).

Objective examination

Positioning of the woman for stability and comfort is essential. Standing may need the support of a wall or plinth, prone lying may be possible with pillows, supine lying may require lateral tilting to avoid supine hypotensive syndrome and those with pelvic pain may find the action of getting on or off the plinth painful. Tests in lying should be completed speedily. Side lying is generally well tolerated.

Anatomical and biomechanical changes should be taken into account; for example joint mobility will be increased, trunk mobility will be reduced and joint range may be reduced if oedematous.

Routine observation should be performed in support standing with the woman appropriately undressed. Findings can then be compared with those observed as the patient moves, and with the patient in other positions as the examination proceeds. Asymmetry must be interpreted with caution as virtually all patients have bony anomalies of some sort. Waist contours and shoulder levels can also be misleading if the foetus is lying asymmetrically.

A *functional assessment* is essential. Changes produced by movement should be observed; ranges of movement, stiffness, pain, lengths/levels/contours, sensation, power and reflexes. Palpation of all appropriate areas will give the assessor more information. In a clinical specialty so prone to litigation, it is essential then to record assessment findings. Time to fulfil this requirement 'completely' should be included within the treatment time.

It is inappropriate to 'detail' hands-on techniques in this text. If the reader does not feel confident in this area it is *essential* to spend time with 'musculoskeletal' colleagues, and share knowledge and skills to the benefit of the client.

Findings then need to be interpreted to enable a treatment regimen to be decided upon and then implemented. It is essential that the patient is included in this process so that her perceived problems are addressed. Communication should also take place with the professional who is taking the 'lead' on the care of the woman: the obstetrician, GP or midwife. Safety is of paramount importance and all aspects of the pregnancy must be included in the assessment before treatment is decided upon.

Once a course of action has been decided upon it should be remembered that the pregnancy will not diminish and may even heighten the normally powerful placebo effect of any treatment given by a thoroughly competent and effective women's health physiotherapist; up to 35% success can confidently be expected *whatever* treatment is selected. Combinations of modalities have been shown to be more beneficial than a single one (Coxhead et al 1981) and patients seem to respond best where treatment is instituted early (Sims-Williams et al 1978). Young & Jewell (2002), in analysing three randomised trials looking at treatments to reduce back and pelvic pain in pregnancy, found that: exercise in water reduced pain, use of pillows improved sleep patterns, acupuncture and physiotherapy modalities reduced pain. Modalities available to the physiotherapist are many: relaxation, superficial heat, massage, manipulation (if appropriate) and mobilisation, as well as the skills of exercise, postural and back care advice.

SOME COMMON SYNDROMES AND THEIR TREATMENT

LOW BACK PAIN

It is worth remembering that there are many causes of back pain and that the pregnant woman is not immune to the 'ills' her peers are prone to. However, pregnant women are more 'at risk' as a result of physiological (e.g. joint laxity), anatomical (e.g. increased lumbar curve) psychological (e.g. inability to concentrate) and mechanical (e.g. altered centre of mass) changes taking place during pregnancy.

Treatment

It is essential that the woman be fully informed about her 'condition', and that support networks are in place to enable her to 'manage' it. There is no evidence to suggest that advice to stay active is harmful (Hilde et al 2002), but there is evidence to suggest that prolonged bed rest is. It would therefore be wise to advise the woman to remain active within her pain range. The expert with regard to human function is the physiotherapist. The women's health physiotherapist will be able to use her 'core' skills, along with her obstetric knowledge, to the benefit of the woman; this is an essential role in enabling the woman to 'manage' her symptoms – how to sit, to lie, to move with minimum effort, maximum effect and least pain.

If the symptoms are less acute, a reduction in overall activity is still advisable, but with a similar approach to 'managing' symptoms, and maintaining 'back care' and posture. Physiotherapeutic 'input' is essential in advising the woman on an appropriate course of action, and administering pain relief to enable function – gentle heat and massage have been used to effect, and maybe the use of transcutaneous electrical nerve stimulation (TENS) is indicated if the pain continues (see p. 185).

NB   *The physiotherapist is reminded to take careful note of current research with regard to the use of TENS in pregnancy. At the time of going to press there is no evidence that it might be harmful to the foetus, but there is also no evidence that it is harmless. The physiotherapist should make a professional judgment as to its use in light of a detailed assessment. If the decision is taken to use TENS, and the mother consents to its use, then the completion of a consent form is advisable.*

It is essential that all treatment be appropriate to assessment findings. An *exercise programme* – whether land or water-based – may be appropriate to maintain treatment results. Though Tulder et al (2002), when analysing 39 randomly controlled trials, found little evidence to indicate that specific exercises are effective for the treatment of low back pain, when comparing them to inactive treatments they do suggest these may be of benefit to facilitate return to daily activities.

SACROILIAC JOINT DYSFUNCTION

Pregnancy could have many possible effects on the sacroiliac joint; for example joint laxity may allow repetitive new movement at one, or both, joints causing pain, if combined with sufficient activity. The newly permitted movement could result in the uneven surfaces becoming 'fixed', therefore rendering the joint immobile and having a mechanical effect upon the other joint. Both anterior and posterior torsion, or rotation of the ilium on the sacrum, have been described, but there is disagreement as to which is the more common (Don Tigny 1985). It seems likely, however, that the complex and highly individual configuration of the sacroiliac joint allows for any number of possible directions of movement. The increased weight during pregnancy thrusts the sacrum downwards between the ilia in all upright postures, and in walking, each sacroiliac joint alternately transmits the total loading. Is there a potential for the joint to fail as a result of joint laxity? Certainly sclerosis of the sacroiliac joints (e.g. osteitis condensans ilii) is seen on X-ray after childbirth. Schemmer et al (1995), using plain film, arteriography and computed tomography (CT), found a statistically significant association of osteitis condensans ilii with parity. This usually disappears in a few months, but indicates transient stress. A support belt may provide comfort for some women.

Changes in orientation or degrees of movement at a sacroiliac joint may affect the symphysis pubis, and also the spine. It has also been shown that pain from the lumbar spine, and occasionally from the hip, may be referred to the sacroiliac region, and there is no doubt that disorders of the lumbar spine and sacroiliac joints can coexist. Thus pain experienced over a sacroiliac joint is *not* synonymous with disorder of that joint; other possibilities must be explored and other confirming or refuting signs sought. Accurate and thorough assessment is essential if treatment is to be successful.

Treatment

A careful 'gapping' of the joint, enabling it to return to a more normal approximation on release, has been shown to be effective in cases of joint 'fixation'.

Technique 1 With the woman lying supine, and the knee of the affected side flexed, the toes are hooked under the lateral aspect of the straight knee. The therapist passively takes the flexed knee across the body while holding the shoulder of the affected side against the plinth. Thus tension is applied to the affected sacroiliac joint and any slack is 'taken up'; at the end of range a single, gentle thrust is given. The woman may benefit from

Figure 5.1   A self-help position that may relieve sacroiliac joint pain.

Figure 5.2   A self-help manoeuvre that may relieve sacroiliac joint pain. (From Fraser 1976.)

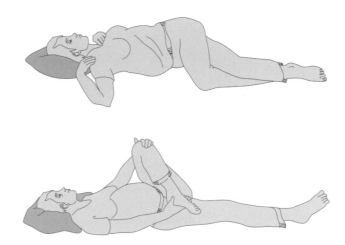

repeating this position at home (Fig. 5.1), with or without a gentle rocking movement, but minus the thrust.

Technique 2   For the left sacroiliac joint, the woman lies supine, trunk fully supported, right leg relaxed and straight, grasping the left flexed knee at the level of the tibial tubercle with the left hand. The left hip is rotated laterally sufficiently to allow the left calcaneum to be cupped in the right hand; she gently pulls the left knee towards a point just lateral to the left shoulder, and the left heel is eased toward the right groin. The pressure is then released and reapplied once or twice. It is suggested that if performed once or twice daily this will encourage normal correlation. Advocates (Fraser 1976) usually recommend that the movement is then repeated on the other side (Fig. 5.2).

Technique 3   Sit or standing (Don Tigny 1985) with the hip and knee of the affected side flexed and the foot up on a chair or bench, the woman rocks forward to the knee and back.

Technique 4   Cyriax recommended – the woman lying (on bed/plinth), crosses the leg of the affected side over the other, and rotates the lower trunk to allow the lower leg of the affected side to dangle over the side of the bed, thereby exerting traction through the leg and hip to the sacroiliac joint. The position is maintained, relaxed, for 10–20 minutes, then activity is resumed carefully.

Technique 5   Lying, a sharp longitudinal 'leg pull' is performed on the affected side, with the leg slightly abducted (Golightly 1982). Sudden traction through the capsule of the hip joint to the ilium can, in some cases, unlock the sacroiliac joint surfaces and so assist with a return to the usual alignment. This, however, is a very traumatic approach and should not be entered into lightly.

Technique 6   The author uses lying, with hips at 90°, and lower legs supported horizontally (by a solid surface) (Fig. 5.3), the woman presses with her thigh (affected side) against a firm surface, holds, and releases.

Figure 5.3   A self-help manoeuvre that may relieve sacroiliac joint pain.

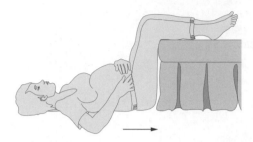

It is essential that the woman has full understanding of her 'problem', and knows how best to maintain the correction and prevent recurrence.

Side lying is usually the most comfortable resting position with a pillow between the knees or forward under the top knee. The knees should be kept together and 'crooked' when turning over in bed. Work involving leaning forward should be avoided, but when essential, placing a foot on a low stool, or equivalent, controls the anterior rotation of the pelvis to some degree (but *not* if suffering the symptoms of SPD). If the abdominal muscles are weak, and if it is realistic to attempt strengthening exercises, this should be done. A supportive belt applied following a manoeuvre may increase comfort and help avoid recurrence of the malposition. Where recurrence does happen, the therapist will have to decide how often it is wise to manipulate in this way. Repetitive reductions could encourage further joint instability, perhaps even in the longer term.

It may be that, in the early stages, rest can facilitate a reduction in inflammation and oedema, and where there is torsion then general relaxation and gentle non-weight-bearing movements in the bed may allow the joint to return naturally to its normal position.

TENS may be a useful adjunct to corrective and preventative therapy in the early, painful phase, but it is important for the patient to understand that this temporarily masks the pain rather than curing its cause.

SCIATICA

When a pregnant woman complains of sciatica, her obstetrician may possibly suggest it is the baby sitting on a nerve. However, this, unless the woman is near term, seems unlikely. Sciatica may accompany backache and sacroiliac joint dysfunction; it will rarely occur alone. The L4 and L5 component of the sciatic nerve, due to its course, would become involved in any dysfunction or inflammatory reaction at this site. An increased lumbar lordosis resulting in lying and standing would also change the lie of these roots. Increased loading may result in the spinal foramina being reduced in size with consequent root compression. Disc lesions are not unknown, and is it impossible for abdominal adhesions (e.g. following infection or surgery) to be another causative factor?

Treatment

Management of the symptoms is by far the best approach, with reduced activity levels, within pain-free range. Advice from the physiotherapist on positioning, back care, posture correction, activities of daily living and pain relief can be taken 'as read'.

SYMPHYSIS PUBIS DYSFUNCTION (SPD)

The width of the symphysis pubis has been shown to increase asymptomatically in pregnancy from about 4.8 mm to 7–9 mm (Abramson et al 1934). A study of pelvic girdle relaxation in pregnancy found that 31.7% of pregnant women reported the symphysis as a site of pain (MacLennan et al 1997). The pain is described as a 'burning' or 'bruised' feeling in and around the joint, which may also radiate suprapubically and to the medial aspect of the thigh(s). Pain varies in severity and may be of gradual onset or incidious. It may be linked to a specific activity or a traumatic incident. It is provoked by weightbearing, especially unilateral, and hip abduction. Difficult activities will include:

- getting in or out of the car or bath
- changing position in bed, particularly 'turning over'
- dressing
- walking, which is severely restricted or impossible.

The possible link with sacroiliac dysfunction has already been suggested. Clinical assessment will require *great* care as the pain is likely to be acute. Differential diagnoses should not be overlooked, for example missed urinary tract infection, or round ligament pain.

Treatment

It is essential that the woman, and if possible her partner, are made fully aware of the condition. The difficulties caused by SPD in relation to 'normal' activities can be alarming and a full understanding will help with 'coping strategies'.

Rest and reduction of non-essential 'chores' is vital, as is keeping the legs adducted and avoiding single leg standing (Fry et al 1997).

Pelvic support may reduce pain levels, for example a Tubigrip 'roll-on', trochanteric belt, SPD belt or maternity support underwear, by helping to stabilise the pelvic mechanics.

In severe cases functional aids may be required (e.g. walking aids, a 'helping hand', a slide board or turntable).

Gentle isometric contraction of hip adductors, in sitting – small cushion between the knees (whilst maintaining pelvic stability), may relieve adductor tension. Supervised exercise in water is a positive approach, though care should be taken when getting in or out of the pool, and breaststroke *must* be avoided.

COCCYDYNIA

Previous injury to the coccyx predisposes to this problem in pregnancy, but otherwise this condition is rare antenatally unless caused by a fall.

Treatment

This includes:

- *cushion* when sitting, taking pressure through ischial tuberosities and thighs
- gentle mobilisations – grasping the coccyx, using a gloved index finger, in the anus, and the thumb, posteriorly
- ice packs, heat, ultrasound and TENS.

These are all worthy of consideration, but the physiotherapist should always take careful note of current research with regard to the use of interventional modalites.

THORACIC SPINE PAIN

Some women during pregnancy complain of pain over the thoracic spine. The rib cage expands during pregnancy as a result of the growing foetus. This may well have a mechanical effect upon the costovertebral joints resulting in pain. There may be symptoms radiating to the upper limb as a result. Muscular symptoms may be the result of the increasing size and weight of the breasts.

This may also be linked with pain along the anterior margin of the lower ribs (i.e. costal margin pain (rib ache), and intercostal neuralgia).

The 'flaring' can increase the diameter of the chest by as much as 10–15 cm. 'Intercostal neuralgia' is a term sometimes used to describe the intermittent pain, usually unilateral, which can radiate around the chest and may be referred to the lateral abdominal wall.

Treatment

The following are helpful:

- mobilisations may ease costovertebral joint pain, but it is *essential* to remember that during pregnancy there is an increase in joint laxity
- posture correction (taping may assist with proprioception)
- self-mobilisation techniques
- exercises, stretching – which may address spasm and stiffness
- a well-fitting brassiere should also be considered
- 'rib lifting' techniques are helpful in dealing with rib 'flare': raise both arms over the head with the hands clasped side flexion (with arm raised) away from the pain; sit astride a chair 'backwards' (but *not* if suffering the symptoms of SPD or sacroiliac joint problems)
- hot-water bottle or an ice pack.

POSTURAL BACKACHE

Frequently the backache complained of during pregnancy will be described as a 'tired ache' in the lower back, often at the end of the day, or after particularly heavy effort. There are many comfortable positions to relieve this sort of discomfort and they can be demonstrated, and practised during antenatal classes, for relief at work and at home (Fig. 5.4).

PREGNANCY–ASSOCIATED OSTEOPOROSIS (PAO)

PAO is rare, but maybe underdiagnosed, and therefore misunderstood (Funk et al 1995). It is essential that the physiotherapist working in obstetrics is aware of its possibility when considering particularly back, hip, and rib problems in pregnant women. The highest proportion of fractures are: vertebral compression, rib and pubic ramus (Dunne et al 1993, Gruber et al 1984, Smith et al 1985, 1995). The majority of authors, including Reid et al (1992) and Dunne et al (1993), show that it appears to affect women of 27 years and above. It is seen to be rare for it to affect

Figure 5.4 Suggested coping positions for back discomfort.

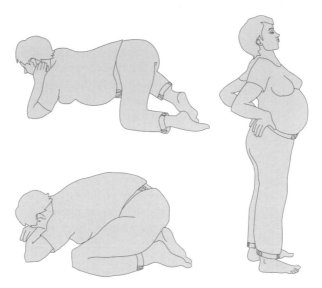

women under this age. It has been suggested (Smith et al 1985) that there may be a transient failure of the usual changes in calciotrophic hormones which prepare the maternal skeleton for the stress of childbirth. Dunne et al (1993) also suggest that there is an underlying genetic abnormality, perhaps collagen linked, that may contribute. Brayshaw (2002) followed up subjects in Dunne's (1993) study. The symptoms experienced by these women were as follows:

- *backache*, sometimes radiating around the chest wall, sudden severe backache, back 'spasm', progressing to severe incapacitating back pain
- *hip/groin pain* progressing to an inability to walk or weight-bear
- *vertebral fractures* with subsequent loss of height and consequential effect upon posture.

Back pain is a common symptom in pregnancy and therefore osteoporosis can be missed. Its awareness *must* be raised amongst health professionals. This condition has many implications for the management of pregnancy.

NERVE COMPRESSION SYNDROMES

During the third trimester of pregnancy, fluid retention can lead to oedema, which, as well as being visible in the ankles, feet, hands and face of the pregnant woman, can lead to reduced joint mobility and a variety of nerve compression syndromes.

CARPAL TUNNEL SYNDROME

Carpal tunnel syndrome, the most common of the nerve compression syndromes, is clinically recognised as impairment of sensory and sometimes motor nerve function in the hand, caused by compression of the median nerve as it passes through the narrow carpal tunnel under the flexor retinaculum at the wrist. Ekman-Ordeberg et al (1987) reported that 2.5% of a population of pregnant women had symptoms of carpal tunnel syndrome, although other authors show much higher incidence of up to 50% (Gould & Wissinger 1978, Melvin et al 1969, Voitk et al 1983). It appears to be associated with the generalized oedema suffered by some women in the final trimester of pregnancy, although a purely localised oedema can also cause the symptoms. Hand and wrist pain is the second most frequent musculoskeletal symptom of pregnancy (Heckman & Sassard 1994). A frequent complaint from a woman presenting with this condition is paraesthesia and pain, which is commonly experienced at night, disturbing much-needed sleep. It can be at its worst first thing in the morning, and sufferers may have difficulty holding objects and performing fine movements. The ulnar nerve, although it passes in front of the flexor retinaculum, may also suffer compression at the wrist or at the elbow.

Treatment

The following may all give relief:

- ice packs (a small bag of frozen peas wrapped in a wet handkerchief could be used at home)
- resting with the hands in elevation
- wrist and hand exercises
- ultrasound
- splinting limiting wrist flexion.

Positions which put the wrist joint into a position of stress should be avoided (e.g. prone kneeling) – taking weight through the wrist and arm could be adapted to taking weight through the knuckles or forearm. Although the syndrome usually resolves spontaneously following delivery (Heckman & Sassard in 1994 found that 95% had complete relief 2 weeks post partum), decompression surgery may occasionally be necessary.

BRACHIAL PLEXUS PAIN

Some women complain of pain and paraesthesia in the shoulder and arm. Fluid retention and postural changes are thought to cause this, but a familial factor has been noted which could be associated with some anomaly such as a cervical rib.

Treatment

The following may prove helpful:

- exercises – shoulder girdle
- stretching
- elevation of the arm.

MERALGIA PARAESTHETICA

Generalised fluid retention can result in compression of the lateral femoral cutaneous nerve of the thigh as it passes under the inguinal ligament. Symptoms of meralgia paraesthetica – burning paraesthesia over the anterolateral aspect of the thigh, together with mild sensory loss to light touch and pin-prick – can vary from mild to severe. This condition may occur as early as 25 weeks' gestation.

Treatment

- TENS: Fisher & Hanna (1987) placed electrodes along the course of the nerve and found it to be highly successful, non-invasive, non-neurolytic and to carry no foetal risk.

The physiotherapist is reminded to take careful note of current research with regard to use of interventional modalities.

POSTERIOR TIBIAL NERVE COMPRESSION

Ankle oedema can compress the posterior tibial nerve as it passes behind the medial malleolus. This will lead to paraesthesia of the sole of the foot and the plantar aspect of the toes.

Treatment

The following may be used to relieve discomfort:

- resting with the legs in elevation
- foot and ankle exercises
- ice packs
- ultrasound.

CIRCULATORY DISORDERS

VARICOSE VEINS IN THE LEGS

The hormonally induced hypotonia of the walls of the veins and raised intra-abdominal pressure, an increase in blood volume, together with the presence of incompetent valves, lead to unsightly and often uncomfortable varicosities.

Treatment

Attention to leg circulation is important, maintaining blood flow by working the muscle pump. The following advice is helpful:

- Avoid standing or sitting for long periods, with the legs dependent, or the knees crossed.
- Frequent and *vigorous* ankle dorsiflexion and plantar flexion may be performed (for at least 30 seconds) though it is doubtful as to whether it really has an effect.
- Brisk walking is far more advantageous in promoting efficient venous return.
- Elevate feet when sitting or lying.
- Support tights, or elastic support stockings, may be worn and should be put on in bed *before* getting up in the morning.

VULVAL VARICOSE VEINS

The causes of these are identical to varicose veins in the legs, but fortunately they are less common in the vulval region. They are incredibly painful and restricting.

Treatment

The following may give relief:

- rest with the foot of the bed raised
- keeping sanitary pad in situ (creating pressure)
- frequent pelvic floor muscle contractions
- avoiding prolonged standing
- avoiding constipation and therefore 'straining'.

HAEMORRHOIDS

Together with the venal hypotonia, here there is a relative relaxation of the intestinal smooth muscle, resulting in a slowing of faecal material through the gut, consequent increased fluid absorption and harder stools, often leading to constipation. Straining to move the bowels can cause ballooning of the veins in and around the anus; these are called haemorrhoids or piles. The increase in uterine weight and resultant pressure on the bowel and the pelvic veins may also be contributing factors. Haemorrhoids are a frequently unmentioned source of discomfort.

Treatment

The following may give relief:

- pelvic floor muscle contractions to improve perineal and anal circulation
- a small ice pack for pain relief
- pad for equalising pressure
- teaching of defaecation techniques may prevent the constipation worsening (see p. 387)
- use of a pressure-relieving cushion may increase comfort in severe cases
- dietary advice, and maybe pain relief, may be given in consultation with the multi-disciplinary team.

MUSCLE CRAMP

Different theories as to the cause have been suggested – calcium deficiency, ischaemia and nerve root pressure among them. Towards term, increased fluid retention together with reduced activity, particularly in the evenings, may be an additional factor. Many women suffer from cramp during pregnancy. The most common site is the calf, the cramp frequently being triggered by the stretching in bed and plantarflexing at the ankle. This painful problem can also occur in the feet and thighs.

Treatment

The following may give relief:

- calf stretches to relieve muscle spasm
- knee extension with dorsiflexion will release calf cramp
- massage – deep kneading
- vigorous foot exercises, to prevent the bruise-like pain which often follows a cramp 'event'
- a pre-bedtime brisk walk, vigorous foot exercises, and a warm bath may be prophylactic.

THROMBOSIS AND THROMBOEMBOLISM

Thrombosis is not common in pregnancy, but is significant because of the possibility of thromboembolism. The raised level of fibrinogen together with a slowing of venous blood flow, particularly in the legs, as pregnancy progresses, predisposes to this condition. Pulmonary embolism, rare but potentially fatal, may be the result.

Treatment

This includes:

- use of antiembolic stockings
- anticoagulant treatment (e.g. heparin) in severe cases
- physiotherapy consisting of an antithrombotic regimen, including foot and leg exercises and deep breathing.

OTHER PROBLEMS

CHONDROMALACIA PATELLAE

Because of the increased ligamentous laxity, slightly wider pelvis and femoral torsion, chondromalacia of the patella can occasionally be a problem. The woman will complain of aching at the front of her knee, which is exacerbated by prolonged sitting or by knee flexion or extension activities. Although symptoms may disappear after the baby is born, it is possible that the increase of knee flexion, with the necessity to squat or kneel when picking up toddlers, can lead to a recurrence of this troublesome condition months later.

Treatment

This includes:

- ice packs two or three times per day
- a strengthening routine for the knee extensor group of muscles
- avoiding the double squat postion by 'going down' on one knee and maintaining 90° flexion (and no more) at both joints.

RESTLESS LEG SYNDROME

The restless leg syndrome is an unpleasant 'creeping' sensation, deep in the lower legs, causing an irresistible desire to move the leg in order to relieve the sensation; a leg may even involuntarily twitch or jump. The aetiology is uncertain, but it is strongly associated with pregnancy. Of 500 women interviewed at an antenatal clinic, 97 (19%) were diagnosed as having this syndrome (Goodman et al 1988), so it is important for the physiotherapist to be aware of it. The symptoms seem to be associated with fatigue, anxiety or stress.

Treatment

The following often give some relief:

- bed rest
- a period of reduced activity, e.g. giving up work.

The vast majority of women will be symptom-free soon after the birth of their baby. Reassurance and understanding, coupled with advice to rest more, will help to alleviate their worries.

UTERINE LIGAMENT PAIN

The 'remodelling' undergone by the skeletal ligaments and collagenous connective tissue is thought to affect the uterine suspensory ligaments. They are also under considerable stretch from the rapidly growing uterus. The sudden, sharp stabs of lower abdominal pain or the constant dull aches, often unilateral, in the iliac fossa are not only distressing, but can make the woman wonder if she is in labour. It is often helpful to explain that the uterus is 'tethered' to the pelvis like a tent, or a hot-air balloon, and that the worrying 'cramps' are not significant and are not damaging the baby.

Treatment

The following may help:

- warmth or cold
- massaging or stroking, over the site of the pain.

PAIN FROM ABDOMINAL ADHESIONS

Abdominal or pelvic pain in the pregnant woman may be a result of tension on, or subsequent stretching of, abdominal adhesions from previous surgical interventions. The symptoms may also be linked to pelvic inflammatory disease. Stress related to problems of conception (fertility surgery), which may have led to a lowering of the pain threshold when the long-awaited pregnancy is finally achieved, may be a contributory factor.

Treatment

This includes:

- emotional and physical support
- repeated explanation and reassurance
- warmth
- abdominal support
- TENS.

The physiotherapist is reminded to take careful note of current research with regard to use of interventional modalities.

FIBROIDS

These benign tumours tend to hypertrophy during pregnancy, when they can give rise to pain as a result of red degeneration. Sometimes they are actually visible and palpable through the abdominal wall. Following the birth of the baby, and as part of the process of involution, a decrease in size can be expected.

Treatment

This includes:

- reassurance that nothing untoward is occurring
- TENS as pain relief.

The physiotherapist is reminded to take careful note of current research with regard to use of interventional modalities.

FATIGUE

The tiredness so often experienced in the first trimester is usually less noticeable in the second, but becomes increasingly severe towards 'term' as weight increases and mobility becomes more of a problem.

Treatment

This includes:

- acceptance by the woman, her partner and her employer that there will need to be a reduction of 'normal' daily activity
- daily, lunch-time rest is *essential*
- weekends should be used wisely; the temptation to complete, at any cost, tasks such as redecoration before the birth of the baby should be resisted.

INSOMNIA AND NIGHTMARES

Many women experience a disturbance in their 'sleep pattern' as their pregnancies progress. Discomfort, visits to the toilet, cramp, heartburn and anxiety are just some of the 'culprits'. Vivid, and sometimes frightening, dreams are also common especially in the final trimester. These will all have an effect upon daytime functioning. Although a 'normal' occurrence, it can be frustrating, and can be seen as a 'dress rehearsal' for the broken nights of motherhood ahead.

Treatment

This includes:

- advice on positioning and support – pillows, bean bags, etc
- the use of relaxation techniques
- suggesting that, instead of tossing and turning, the woman gets out of bed, eats something light, has a *warm* drink, then goes back and practises a relaxation technique in a comfortable, well-supported position.

PRURITUS

Distressing skin irritation sometimes presents during the third trimester. The aetiology is uncertain.

Treatment

This includes:

- discontinuing the use of perfumed soaps, talcs and bath oils
- taking cold baths
- applying calamine lotion
- wearing light cotton clothes.

If not successful, the woman should be encouraged to consult her doctor.

HEARTBURN

This is a particular 'nuisance' to any woman experiencing the symptoms. It is a direct consequence of the 'relaxing' effect of pregnancy hormones on the smooth muscle of the cardiac sphincter at the base of the oesophagus. The reflux of acid stomach juices into the oesophagus actually burns its mucosa, and this problem is increased by the upward pressure of the growing uterus. The physiotherapist working in women's health is often asked what can be 'done' about it, though this is not strictly within her remit.

Treatment

Give advice to:

- eat 'little and often'
- avoid all foods that increase symptoms
- raise the head of the bed; extra pillows can give night-time relief
- consult the general practitioner/midwife to have suitable antacids prescribed (free during pregnancy in the UK).

MORNING SICKNESS

Nausea and vomiting are perhaps the most troublesome of all the symptoms during the first trimester, though not necessarily restricted to the morning! The raised level of HCG at this stage has been suggested as the cause, and it is often more severe in multiple pregnancies.

Treatment

This includes:

- acupressure (De Aloysio & Penacchioni 1992) between the flexor carpi radialis and palmaris longus, at the wrist
- acupressure 'bands' may be effective
- TENS (Kahn 1988) – 120 Hz 150 m/s to the web space between thumb and forefinger on the right arm
- eating ginger, e.g. biscuits, especially before rising, and crystallised ginger.

URINARY FREQUENCY

During the first trimester, when the still anteverted growing uterus presses against the bladder, and again in the final trimester when bladder compression between the abdominal wall and the much enlarged uterus prevents normal volumes of urine being comfortably contained, frequency of micturition is a common and often annoying problem. Nocturia in the first trimester is often a sign of pregnancy to many women who are unused to having to empty their bladder at night. Additionally, the increased volume of urine produced during pregnancy is partly responsible for frequency.

Urge and stress incontinence

This troublesome and embarrassing symptom can present during pregnancy, particularly in the third trimester. It is a condition that should be discussed regularly by the physiotherapist. Very few people have the courage to volunteer that they are experiencing bladder leakage. It can be reassuring for them to realise that they are not alone. For most women it will be a transitory problem, but for some it can continue after the birth of their baby and it can be treated. Persistence should be referred postnatally.

Treatment

This includes:

- pelvic floor muscle (PFM) exercises
- PFM contraction before, and during, coughing, sneezing or lifting.

References

Abramson D, Roberts S M, Wilson P D 1934 Relaxation of the pelvic joints in pregnancy. Surgical Gynaecology and Obstetrics 58:595–613.

Berg G, Hammer M, Möller-Neilsen J et al 1988 Low back pain during pregnancy. Obstetrics and Gynaecology 71:71–75.

Brayshaw E 2002 Pregnancy-associated osteoporosis. Journal of the Association of Chartered Physiotherapists in Women's Health 91:3–9.

Bullock J, Jull G H, Bulloock M I 1987 The relationship of low back pain to postural changes during pregnancy. Australian Journal of Physiotherapy 33:10–17.

Calguneri C, Bird H, Wright V 1982 Changes in joint laxity occurring during pregnancy. Annals of Rheumatic Disease 41:126–128.

Coxhead C E, Inshipp H, Mead T W et al 1981 Multicentre trial of physiotherapy in the management of sciatica symptoms. Lancet i:1065.

De Aloysio D, Penacchioni P 1992 Morning sickness control early in pregnancy by Neiguan pressure. Obstetrics and Gynaecology 80:852–854.

Don Tigny R L 1985 Function and pathomechanics of the sacroiliac joint. Physical Therapy 65:35–44.

Dunne F, Walters B, Marshall T, Heath D A 1993 Pregnancy-associated osteoporosis. Clinical Endocrinology 39:487–490.

Ekman-Ordeberg G, Salgeback S, Ordeberg G 1987 Carpal tunnel syndrome in pregnancy. Acta Obstetrica et Gynecologica Scandinavica 66:233–235.

Fast A 1999 Low back pain in pregnancy. Physical Medicine and Rehabilitation: State of the Art Review 12(3):509–519.

Fisher A P, Hanna M 1987 Transcutaneous electrical nerve stimulation in meralgia paraesthetica of pregnancy. British Journal Obstetrics and Gynaecology 94:603–605.

Fraser D 1976 Postpartum backache; a preventable condition? Canadian Family Physician 22:1434–1436.

Fry D, Hay-Smith J, Hough J et al 1997 Symphysis pubis dysfunction guidelines. Physiotherapy 83:41–42.

Funk J L, Shoback M, Genant K H, 1995 Transient osteoporosis of the hip in pregnancy: natural history of changes in bone mineral density. Clinical Endocrinology 43:373–382.

Golightly R 1982 Pelvic arthropathy in pregnancy and the puerperium. Physiotherapy 68:216–220.

Goodman J D S, Brodie C, Ayida G A 1988 Restless leg syndrome in pregnancy. British Medical Journal 297:1101–1102.

Gould J S, Wissinger H A 1978 Carpal tunnel syndrome in pregnancy. Southern Medical Journal 71:144–149.

Grieve G P 1981 Common vertebral joint problems. Edinburgh, Churchill Livingstone, p 398.

Gruber H E, Gutteridge D H, Baylink D J 1984 Osteoporosis associated with pregnancy and lactation: bone biopsy and skeletal features in three patients. Metabolic Bone Disease and Related Research 5:159–165.

Hall D C, Kaufman D A 1987 Effects of aerobic and strength conditioning on pregnancy outcomes. American Journal of Obstetrics and Gynecology 11:1199–1203.

Heckman J, Sassard R 1994 Musculoskeletal considerations in pregnancy. Journal of Bone and Joint Surgery 76A(11):1720–1730.

Hilde G, Hagen K B, Jamtvedt G et al 2002 Advice to stay active as a single treatment for low back pain and sciatica (Cochrane Review). In: The Cochrane Library, Issue 4. Update Software, Oxford.

Khan J 1988 Electrical modalities in obstetrics and gynaecology. In: Wilder E (ed) Obstetric and gynaecologic physical therapy. Churchill Livingstone, New York, p 113–129.

Laros R K 1991 Physiology of normal pregnancy. In Wilson J R, Carrington H R (eds) Obstetrics and Gynaecology. Mosby Year Book, St Louis, p 242.

MacLennan A H, MacLennan S C, Norwegian Association for Women with Pelvic Girdle Relaxation 1997 Symptom-giving pelvic girdle relaxation of pregnancy, postnatal pelvic joint syndrome and developmental dysplasia of the hip. Acta Obstetrica et Gynecologica Scandinavica, 76:760–764.

Mantle M J, Greenwood R M, Currey H L F 1977 Backache in pregnancy. Rheumatic Rehabilitation 16:95–110.

Mantle M J, Holmes J, Currey H L F 1981 Backache in pregnancy. II: Prophylactic influence of backache classes. Rheumatic Rehabilitation 20:227–232.

Melvin J L, Brunett C N, Johnsson E W 1969 Median nerve conduction in pregnancy. Archives of Physical Medicine 50:75–80.

Norén L, Östgaard S, Johansson G, Östgaard H C 2002 Lumbar back and posterior pelvic pain during pregnancy: a 3-year follow-up. European Spine Journal 11(3):267–271.

Nwuga V E B 1982 Pregnancy and back pain among upper-class Nigerian women. Australian Journal of Physiotherapy 28(4):8–11.

Östgaard H C, Andersson G B 1991 Previous back pain and risk of developing back pain in a future pregnancy. Spine 16:432–436.

Östgaard H C, Zetherstrom G, Roos-Hansson E et al 1994 Reduction of back and posterior pelvic pain in pregnancy. Spine 19:894–900.

Padua L, Padua R, Bondi R et al 2002 Patient-oriented assessment of back pain in pregnancy. European Spine Journal 11(3):272–275.

Reid L R, Wattie D J, Evans M C et al 1992 Post-pregnancy osteoporosis associated with hypercalcaemia. Clinical Endocrinology 37:298–303.

Sandler S E 1996 The management of low back pain in pregnancy. Manual Therapy 1(4):178–185.

Schemmer D, White P G, Friedman L 1995 Radiology of the paraglenoid sulcus. Skeletal Radiology 24(3):205–209.

Sims-Williams H, Jayson M V, Young S M S et al 1978 Controlled trial of mobilisation and manipulation for patients with low back pain in general practice. British Medical Journal 2:1338.

Smith R, Stevenson J C, Winearls C J et al 1985 Osteoporosis in pregnancy. Lancet i:1178–1180.

Smith R, Athanasou N A, Ostlere S J et al 1995 Pregnancy-associated osteoporosis. Quarterly Journal of Medicine 88:865–878.

Tulder M W van, Malmivaara A, Esmail R et al 2002 Exercise therapy for low back pain (Cochrane review). In: The Cochrane Library, Issue 4. Update Software, Oxford.

Voitk A E, Mueller J C, Faringer D E et al 1983 Carpal tunnel syndrome in pregnancy. Canadian Medical Journal 128:277–282.

Young G, Jewell D 2002 Interventions for preventing and treating pelvic and back pain in pregnancy, Cochrane Database Systemic Review (1):CD1139. Update Software, Oxford.

Further reading

Carlstedt-Duke B, Gustavsson P 2002 Pregnancy and work environment. Practical guidelines for risk assessment. Lakartidningen 10;99(1–2):34–38.

Grieve E 1980 The biomechanical characterisation of sacroiliac joint motion. MSc Thesis, University of Strathclyde.

Grieve G P 1976 The sacroiliac joint. Physiotherapy 62:384–400.

Lee D 1996 Instability of the sacroiliac joint and the consequences to gait. Journal of Manual and Manipulation Therapy 4:22–29.

Vleeming A, Mooney V, Dorman T et al (eds) 1997 Movement, stability and low back pain. The essential role of the pelvis. Churchill Livingstone, Edinburgh.

Watkins Y 1998 Current concepts in dynamic stabilization of the spine and pelvis: their relevance to obstetrics. Journal of the Association of Chartered Physiotherapists in Women's Health 83:16–26.

Wilder E (ed) 1988 Obstetric and gynecologic physical therapy. Churchill Livingstone, Edinburgh.

Useful websites

At work, and pregnant   www.hse.gov.uk.

Leaflets

ACPWH

Fit for Pregnancy (antenatal), *Fit for Birth*, *Fit for Motherhood* (postnatal), *The Mitchell Method of Simple Relaxation* (revised). Obtainable from Ralph Allen Press, 22 Milk Street, Bath BA1 1UT, Tel: 01225 461888.

Symphysis Pubis Dysfunction. Obtainable from Professional Affairs, CSP, 14 Bedford Row, London WC1R 4ED, Tel: 020 7306 666.

Chapter **6**

Preparation for labour

Sue Barton

CHAPTER CONTENTS

Introduction 165
Preparation 166
Relaxation 167
Breathing 170
Positions in labour 177
Massage in labour 180

Other coping strategies 184
Pain relief in labour 184
The third stage of labour 196
Birth plans 197
Variations in labour 198
The puerperium 199

INTRODUCTION

The process of preparing for labour is unique to each individual woman. No two women will experience the same process of labour and no one woman will experience two labour processes that are the same. The factors contributing to the experience are both physical and psychological and in combination result in the uniqueness (Holdcroft 1996). Therefore the preparation *must* be 'individual'. Each woman will have different hopes, fears and aims for her labour. The process of labour is an immense physical and emotional experience. Some will want to handle it with as little intervention as possible. Others will want to take advantage of all the technology available to them, in order to 'move' speedily and painlessly through the event. It is essential that health professionals do not impose their own opinions of the process on the client. They may well believe that the 'right' way to cope with labour is for a woman to use her own resources without resorting to analgesia, and that breastfeeding is the only way to feed a baby. The woman, however, may wish to prebook epidural anaesthesia, and may find the mere thought of breastfeeding repulsive. It is inappropriate to generalise, but surveys have shown that middle class women are more likely to demand a natural childbirth, whereas working class women do not have an issue with this; they tend to see childbirth as a means to an end and want it to be as comfortable, painless and safe as possible (McIntosh 1989, Nielson 1983).

It is essential that anyone preparing a woman for the process of labour is 'up to date' with the current practice locally, as well as with current national 'trends'. Physiotherapists must familiarise themselves, on a regular basis, with obstetric and midwifery developments, but also be aware of trends that may be affecting the woman and her partner. If particular 'modes' of delivery (e.g. water births) are being shown as 'positive' ways to deliver, then maternity units will make them available to the woman to enable 'free choice'. The physiotherapist must therefore be 'aware'. The role of the 'birth partner' at the labour process is constantly changing: from not present, to pressure to attend, to freedom of choice. It is not just the pregnant woman that the physiotherapist should be including in the preparation. There needs to be an awareness of the partner's role, and needs. Today, if it is their choice to attend, they are welcomed as part of the team, and the emotional and physical support they give is acknowledged by health professionals as well as by labouring women. What started as a demand from articulate middle class women in the late l950s and early 1960s, when women were often left unattended for many hours in the first stage of labour, has evolved into accepted practice.

The use of procedures such as routine 'breaking the waters', routine episiotomy, and forceps versus ventouse intervention have all been challenged, and discussion often follows in the media. Women will expect the health professional to be able to answer their questions knowledgeably and scientifically. The physiotherapist *must*, as part of her continuing development, prepare herself for every eventuality in order to fulfil the needs of the woman preparing for the labour process.

Labour, an 'inevitable' continuation of pregnancy, leading to parenthood and a totally new lifestyle, is a physical and emotional marathon. In some cultures it is considered to be a natural physiological occurrence whereas in others its importance is such that it must be prepared and even 'trained' for. Preparation, at whatever level, enables control, increases confidence, and provides coping strategies. There is a natural anxiety, in all women, about the unknown entity of the labour process and their ability to 'cope'.

PREPARATION

Preparation for childbirth will not alter the fact that labour, for the majority of women, is painful, but it can modify women's perception and interpretation of the process. Providing women with the 'tools' to counteract the 'problems' will increase their confidence, and that of the birth partner. This 'tool kit' of *coping skills*, non-invasive and without deleterious side-effects, can make the difference between confidence and fear, satisfaction and disappointment. Childbirth has become safer for mother and baby and the expected outcome is for both mother and baby to be in good health. Attention has therefore turned towards making it a physically and psychologically rewarding experience for all involved.

Women's expectations vary. Some set themselves goals that may be unrealistic and unattainable: labour without pain relief, with an intact perineum, the ultimate experience, the high 'spot' in their lives, pinnacle of achievement. There are many who do not have their 'hoped-for' pattern of labour. The psychological effect that this can have on the woman can be devastating: failure, disappointment, or guilt that may have far-reaching effects upon the early period as a mother. The health professional 'inputting' into the preparation for labour must accommodate for all eventualities with the aim of achieving a positive outcome for all.

EDUCATION

Education must prepare women appropriately; there will be a variety of approaches in their geographical area, and they need awareness of the unit in which they will deliver. The session should be as realistic as possible, 'delivering' the facts in an appropriate way relative to the group. Equipping the woman with knowledge and skills that will enable her to plan her labour is essential. Encourage the mother-to-be to put her wishes in writing. Most hospitals today follow a birth plan (see p. 197). Any specific requests should also be communicated, in advance, to senior personnel. Where a women's health physiotherapist feels strongly about the inadvisability of a labour ward procedure, it is the *professional's* duty to discuss it with midwives and doctors (e.g. a birthing position with a woman suffering the symptoms of symphysis pubis divarification). It is essential that the physiotherapist is able to support her concerns with research evidence.

Educational content should include:

- an introduction to the labour suite
- an introduction to pain relief available
- physiology of labour
- coping skills
- relaxation
- breathing awareness
- positions in labour
- massage.

RELAXATION

The approach to labour today is an active one, with a positive attitude towards coping with pain and stress. The muscular, wave-like, activity of the uterus is involuntary and therefore something over which the woman has no physical control.

TECHNIQUES

The use of relaxation techniques, as part of a coping strategy, has evolved over the years. Grantly Dick Read, one of the pioneers in this field, advocated the use of relaxation as a means of breaking the vicious cycle of pain–fear–tension (Dick-Read 1942) and began teaching it as early as 1933.

Randall (1953) has a chapter in her book *Fearless Childbirth* called 'Relaxation Makes you Fit and Fearless'. She suggested that there were two reasons for teaching relaxation to use in labour:

1. To prevent the mother becoming unduly tired, thereby causing nervous 'fatigue'
2. To help the mother control her thoughts and feelings or emotions.

Heardman (1951) said that by giving a positive idea to the mind the disturbing and worrying thoughts would be displaced. Rhythm is a mental release, and the natural breathing rhythm is incorporated in her scheme of progressive relaxation. These three authors used the 'tense–relax' technique of relaxation. Jacobson (1938), also used a tense–release approach that activates both antagonists and agonists maximally. This approach is often used where rest is prescribed, the maximal contraction gaining maximal release. Concerns with regard to use of this approach during labour might be:

- the initiation of cramp
- risks of hyperventilation
- it has been known to induce anxiety/anger
- it can exacerbate pain, especially back pain.

The Mitchell method

Since 1963 the Mitchell method of physiological relaxation has been widely used by physiotherapists in women's health. This method is widely practised as a stress-relieving strategy, and therefore a useful 'tool' during labour. Mitchell suggested that a woman should practise the approach, prelabour, whilst experiencing Braxton Hicks contractions. She claimed that the approach was successful in conserving the mother's energy during the first stage ready for the 'hardest work she will ever do'. Mitchell's method (1987) activates only antagonists, and moderately; therefore there are not the same concerns as with Jacobson if using during labour. Movements, once learnt, are performed in such a way that 'trigger' areas are put into positions of ease and comfort in a matter of seconds.

Dissociation and unblocking

Noble (1996) says that relaxation is more than rest or stillness; it involves recognising and releasing excess tension – whatever the cause. The passive relaxation practised in pregnancy should be replaced by an alert, but 'non-striving', state of relaxation in labour. She describes a sequence of 'dissociation' – selective relaxation which develops the body's ability to maintain a state of general release when one part of it (the uterus) is working hard. In 1983 Noble wrote that 'relaxation is the key to awareness and energy' (Noble 1983). 'Unblocking' the muscular system and breathing freely can be a blissful release when tension has developed. She points to the fact that women who have found ways to release tension in labour experience contractions that are very different to those felt by women without this 'safety valve' – the contractions are said to be almost pleasurable.

Touch relaxation

Kitzinger (1987) discusses the concept of 'touch relaxation', where a woman relaxes towards the touch of her partner. However many women cannot bear to be touched during labour contractions, it can also increase tension if inappropriately applied or, if the person administering it is tense, this may be relayed through to the woman.

Whatever the approach chosen for use during labour it is essential that it 'fits' the woman's needs. It is not advantageous to induce sleep when the woman is required to be alert and prepare for second stage, but sleep may conserve energy if there is a delay in progression.

Relaxation techniques can be learnt by anyone, can be applied to all aspects of daily living, there are no drugs involved, no strenuous exercise and there is no cost: it sounds too good to be true. In order for the approach to be successful, according to Madders (1998), there must be an understanding of the principles, practice and confidence. Relaxation techniques have not only been shown to have a positive effect upon the coping mechanism during labour; Janke's work (1999) showed that daily relaxation therapy has a positive effect upon preterm labour outcomes.

ASSESSMENT

So far as the physiotherapist is concerned, there must be an assessment of appropriateness of the approach used in order that it be advantageous to the woman. Payne (1995) describes relaxation as: an effective way of coping with stress and the disorders it causes, helping to avoid unnecessary fatigue and as aiding in recovery, raising the pain threshold, and improving physical skills and performance. These effects are all highly relevant during labour.

The physiotherapist should be as aware as she possibly can be of any emotional 'situation' that may be heightened by a relaxed 'state', be prepared to 'handle' an emotional, or physical, outburst, and know to whom or how to refer on if need be. It is important to raise this issue with the woman – that she may have a heightened awareness and she may feel distressed, and that this can be a normal reaction, but that it would be advantageous for the physiotherapist to be aware of 'situations' (in confidence) so that she can assist with 'coping' strategies (e.g. a previous traumatic pregnancy).

TEACHING TECHNIQUES

When teaching relaxation techniques consider the following:

- *enablement* – by choice of approach; reduced tension, ease and comfort, coping with the stress and pain of labour
- *understanding* – reasons behind the approach, the basic principles, and their effects
- *beware* – conflicting effects as a result of using a combination of techniques
- *the 'whole'* – combination of different coping strategies, (positioning, breathing, massage, etc.); relaxation alone is not generally enough to cope with the intensity of the 'wave'

- *flexibility* – venue, positioning, noise, pillows and blankets for comfort, etc. … to enable the woman to be successful in whatever situation prevails
- *practice* – to enable learning to take place, it should not be hurried, and should form part of daily life – practice in the clinic, with an unruly toddler, when unable to sleep, etc., leads to confidence in the approach therefore it is more successful when used in labour
- *motivation* – 'breeds' success; feedback – encouragement, praise
- *confidence* – physiotherapist, and mother-to-be; the freedom to change position if not at ease
- *long term* – once acquired, a skill for 'life'
- *safety* – the 'emotional reaction'; recovery must be slow and gradual; inhale, stretch. Return to standing must be staged: lying to side lying, to prone kneeling, to kneeling (with support), to standing. Discussion should take place with regard to the 'experience'.

With experience, the physiotherapist will learn to recognise a state of relaxation; the position of the body, the rate of respiration, eyes open or closed, fidgety 'state', and the overall look of comfort, are all clues which point to the success or failure of the method being used. Relaxation is classified as one of the main reasons (along with breathing) for women attending antenatal classes, therefore achievement is the 'goal'.

IMAGERY

This approach should come with a health warning. It is essential that physiotherapists are fully aware of the potentially 'major' emotional response that the woman might have. Imagery has the power to initiate an emotional reaction linked with a prior occurrence in people's lives.

A person's thoughts and emotions can produce powerful effects on their physiology, and imagery is a way of harnessing these thoughts to complement physical relaxation. Vivid personal thoughts can aid the process of relaxation. If it has the power to do this then it also has the power to do the exact opposite and perhaps trigger a negative experience.

The suggestions should be made while people are relaxing. They are instructed to imagine they are somewhere that makes them happy, somewhere they feel safe, doing things that they enjoy … wherever and whatever that might be. Examples can be given for those that might be finding it difficult, for example imagining a spring meadow, birds singing, walking with friends, or lying on a beach, watching the clouds moving, thinking of good times.

BREATHING

Breathing, a *normal*, involuntary process, continues at different rates and depths proportional to function. It can, however, also be a voluntary activity – consciously controlled and manipulated. Noble (1981) draws attention to the many physiological adjustments that occur in the respiratory and cardiovascular systems during pregnancy. Alveolar ventilation, tidal volume, cardiac output and blood volume are all increased. The whole system is 'perfectly' designed to enable adequate exchange of maternal and foetal blood gases. It is difficult, she says, to understand the justification for altering something as fundamental as normal breathing, especially during the increased metabolic demands that occur in labour. Yet, over the years, this is precisely what some authorities have recommended: 'controlled' respiration, with both the rate and depth consciously altered. In some cases breathing techniques are even dictated by a labour coach. Historically, different authors have suggested different ways of using breathing during labour.

THE EFFECTS OF ALTERATION OF 'BREATHING PATTERN'

Breathing is primarily controlled by carbon dioxide levels via the brain stem. Rises in carbon dioxide levels are not tolerated and are followed by *hyperventilation* to wash out the excess and restore normal levels. *Hypocapnia* (a low level of carbon dioxide) is tolerated, however, and results from voluntary or involuntary hyperventilation. Rises in oxygen levels are tolerated, but not falls. Carbon dioxide is acid; low levels will cause respiratory alkalosis (raised pH) leading to a decrease in calcium ionisation, which can affect nerve conductivity (Table 6.1).

The symptoms of hyperventilation can be relieved and the condition reversed if the mother breathes into her cupped hands or a paper bag, thus replacing carbon dioxide.

Theoretically, maternal hyperventilation could affect the *foetus* in two ways:

1. Low maternal carbon dioxide levels lead to reduced uterine blood flow (caused by lowered blood pressure and uterine vasoconstriction).
2. Haemoglobin 'hangs on' to oxygen when the blood is alkalotic; this reduces the amount of oxygen available to the foetus in the placenta.

However, it has not been shown that hyperventilation, which probably occurs physiologically in all labouring women, actually affects the normal, uncompromised foetus. Maternal apnoea (sometimes prolonged) follows periods of hyperventilation. It is this that may possibly affect the foetus. As the carbon dioxide level falls the oxygen level rises; neither of these states stimulate the brain to continue respiration. Until the carbon dioxide level rises again, the message 'breathe' will not be given – it is this apnoeic episode that could add to distress in the compromised foetus.

Table 6.1   Effects of hyperventilation

Signs and symptoms	Cause
Dizziness, 'wooziness', eventual unconsciousness	Cerebral hypoxia due to constriction of cerebral vessels and reduced blood pressure
Numbness and tingling in the lips and extremities; paraesthesia and muscle spasm	Changes in ionised calcium caused by alkalosis, which affects nerve conduction
Pallor, sweating, feelings of panic and anxiety	Possibly due to cerebral anoxia

It is advisable, therefore, for women to be encouraged to aim to return to their 'normal' level of breathing in order to redress the 'balance'. Talking will have a similar effect.

BREATHING FOR LABOUR

Breathing for labour (along with relaxation) is classified as one of the main reasons for attendance at antenatal classes. It can now be seen that teaching specific breathing patterns has a negative effect upon respiratory function, and may even produce negative symptoms.

Breathing *awareness* is, today, what the health professional should be aiming for in terms of breathing preparation for labour. This can be taught alongside relaxation with positive results.

Teaching techniques

A useful teaching approach is:

- Ask the women how many times they think they breathe out in 1 minute – responses will vary greatly.
- Ask them to count each outward breath made during a timed minute – again responses will vary greatly.

This will then reassure them with regard to the 'normal' range.

- Ask them to notice what happens when they breathe at rest – cool air can be felt entering the nostrils, warm air coming out.
- Ask them to focus on their own individual pattern of breathing: a breath in – momentary tidal pause – a breath out – and then a rest between breaths.
- Ask them to feel where movement takes place as they breathe; resting their fingers lightly on their 'babies', can they feel a rise and fall of the abdomen? Explain how slow, 'low', or 'deep', calm 'abdominal' breathing has a soothing, tension-releasing effect at times of stress.
- Tell the class to move their hands to the lower rib cage and ask what happens here as they breathe.

Mention that our bodies receive more oxygen when our breathing is slow and deep rather than fast and shallow, and this will be better for their babies in labour.

Once the slow, calm, easy breathing has been mastered it can be incorporated into relaxation practice. Explain how expiration can increase the depth of relaxation and relieve tension. When people are under stress, as well as adopting the 'tension' posture to a greater or lesser extent, they will tighten or pull in their abdominal muscles.

- Can they feel the ease and release gained from allowing the abdominal wall to swell and fall back instead?
- Ask them to practise calm, easy breathing when they relax at home and during stressful situations.

BREATHING AND CONTRACTIONS

Labour contractions may be painful, but it is essential to emphasise their positive, productive nature. Contractions are an 'absolute' certainly, they *will* happen. The course of each contraction will be identical.

There are three phases:

- *preparatory phase* – the time between contractions, the start of a new contraction, and the gradual build up
- *action phase* – the build up in strength and intensity, reaching a 'peak'
- *recovery phase* – receding from the peak, and recovering ready to prepare again for the next one.

These phases will form a complete and continuous cycle that culminates in the delivery. Each contraction is unique but will follow the same pattern. The woman can 'deal' with each contraction as an individual and then 'move on' to the next one, once recovered. Each contraction should be consciously welcomed as bringing the woman closer to her aim – the safe delivery of her baby.

The use of descriptive terms and phrases will help the woman to visualise what she may be about to experience. It is impossible to simulate a contraction.

Labour can be compared to the sea: usually calm and flat, with just the odd 'ripple' or 'wavelet' – Braxton Hicks contractions. As labour progresses, the sea gradually gets rougher; waves last longer, are higher and more demanding and they come closer together. The woman's aim is to let it happen, to ride the 'waves' produced by her working uterus; her breathing and relaxation, helped by positions of comfort and perhaps massage too, are surfboards or rowing boats taking her up, over the top, and down the other side. Each wave takes her nearer the shore and the birth of her baby.

It is helpful to draw diagrams of contractions, perhaps actual traces enlarged, to show the likely progress of labour (Gauge & Henderson 1992). Women should notice their 'trigger areas' of tension (jaw, shoulders, hands) and release these as they breathe slowly and comfortably up and over each contraction's peak. Some people find it helpful to say, in their head or out loud, 'relax', 'let go', or 'out' with expiration, linking it with the release of tension and relaxation. Every contraction should end with at least one deep breath in and then out – 'Hooray, I've done it, that's one less!'

First stage

Deep, slow, easy breathing – pausing between expiration and inspiration – may be all that some women use in the first stage. Most, however, will be unable to maintain this and a modification will be needed. Untrained women may either hold their breath or uncontrollably hyperventilate when contractions progressively become stronger and more painful. The respiratory response to exercise and effort is for breathing to become faster. This can be introduced as gentle 'feather' or 'candle' breathing. They could imagine that an ostrich feather or a candle is in front of their faces, and that they are very gently breathing in and out (this will probably be more comfortable through the mouth) so that the feather or candle flame would barely move on the outward breath. Each contraction will still start with the outward, relaxing, welcoming breath and continue with slow, deep, calm breathing; the lighter breaths will only be used at the contraction's summit. There should still be a momentary 'pause' between the outward and inward breath and respiration should be as slow and deep as is comfortable.

Transition stage

The end of the first stage (or transition) is a very special time for the labouring woman. The contractions are probably unremitting in strength and ferocity; the pain may well be intense. The woman may feel desperation, hopelessness, exhaustion, anger and perhaps irritation, and be aggravated by annoying symptoms such as limb shaking, nausea or belching. She will become withdrawn and find it difficult to articulate her needs. Occasionally she may feel the urge to bear down before full cervical dilatation is achieved. For a great many women this is the worst and most difficult time of all. Nothing seems to work; they are convinced labour will never end; their body cannot 'do it'; they want pethidine, an epidural, forceps or a caesarean delivery. For some women it is the point at which they decide that they have 'had enough', and attempt to go home. It is important to reassure women that this is a normal and positive response. They are signs that the second stage of labour is not far away. It is essential that vaginal assessment is carried out before pain relief is administered as it could delay imminent second stage if the cervix is almost fully dilated.

It is at this point in labour that hyperventilation, with its unpleasant side-effects, will be most noticeable, so thought must be given to not making the respiratory situation worse when suggesting 'coping' techniques. Various strategies have been recommended:

- SOS – 'sigh out softly' – gentle expiratory sighs, released at the peak of contractions.
- Sighing the breath out while saying 'hoo-hoo-hah' gently and slowly. Breathing in and out continues; only the 'hah' is a long expiration.
- Saying 'I won't push'; breathing in and out for the first two words, and giving a long sigh out for the word 'push'. This should also be gentle, and as slow as possible.
- 'Puff, puff, blow'; this should be a gentle panting interspersed with a sharp blow out, and is useful to overcome premature pushing urges.

Respiration during labour, particularly at this stage, will spontaneously become faster and more 'laboured'. It is therefore essential that women are warned about this possibility, and reminded of their coping strategies.

Many women worry about making a noise during labour. They should be encouraged to use their voices to express the difficulty they are having; the groans, moans and sighs will be those of effort, not necessarily pain. This can be likened to the explosive 'action' sounds of top class tennis players – expiration on effort. The suggestion has been made (Balaskas 1983) that making sounds stimulates the production of endorphins and alters the level of consciousness.

While it is impossible to enable women to experience a true 'dress rehearsal' in advance, a good teacher can talk them through a series of contractions, varying in length and severity, so that they can experiment with their coping strategies.

Following the effort of the transitional phase there is often a lull, a period of rest, when full dilatation is reached. Women used to be urged to begin pushing as soon as this happened. It is more usual today for pushing to be delayed until the foetal head has descended to the pelvic floor and the vertex is seen. The bearing-down urge is not usually experienced until the perineum begins to stretch; premature pushing can be unnecessarily exhausting and uses up the permitted time in labour wards that have a strict protocol in this respect.

Awareness of as many possible sensations as possible can only increase women's 'coping' with the labour process. These include:

- a feeling of 'fullness' in the rectum and anus (as if a large grapefruit is waiting to be expelled)
- a burning stretch of the perineal skin (two fingers in the mouth, pulling the lips out sideways, can mimic this) as it begins to bulge and distend
- the 'opening out' feeling in the sacroiliac, symphysis pubis and sacro-coccygeal joints, which can be frightening if they are not expected.

Stage two

Many women will be relieved with the start of the second stage that at long last there is something active that *they* can do; they may actually enjoy the wonderful feeling of working *with* the immensely powerful 'piston' that has developed within their body.

The pain of the first stage recedes and all becomes purposeful effort with stage two. Some women will be frightened of 'joining in'. They may fear that by pushing they will tear the perineum, cause themselves more pain, defaecate, or even harm their baby. For others the embarrassment of exposing this very private part of their body in that most threatening and vulnerable of postures (e.g. the lithotomy position) will be immensely inhibiting. Reassurance and the opportunity to voice their apprehensions antenatally, together with sympathetic and empathetic encouragement and support during labour, will go a long way towards helping women achieve normal delivery. It is difficult for some women to 'tune in' to their internal body sensations and to respond to these by pushing effectively. It must be mentioned during antenatal classes that several contractions may go by before the woman realises how to push her baby down and out. Each mother should be encouraged to work with her own internal expulsive urge, rather than have to push just because the cervix is fully dilated and the uterus contracting. The desire to bear down usually comes in waves, perhaps three or four 'emptying' urges per contraction, and she may not be able to push well until she actually experiences this. It is essential that she is in a position that is comfortable and feels right to her during this time, but also advantageous as far as effective expulsion is concerned (i.e. pushing 'down hill').

The length of time that a women is actively 'pushing' should be monitored and the physiotherapist must be aware of local procedures with regard to this phase so that she can communicate this accurately to the women she is preparing.

Prolonged 'pushing' will have the following physiological effects:

1. There is an initial large rise in blood pressure.
2. Venous compression in the chest and abdomen will increase intrathoracic and intra-abdominal pressure and therefore blood flow back to the heart is reduced.
3. A fall in cardiac output and blood pressure follows.
4. Dizziness results, the Valsalva manoeuvre is released, and cardiac output returns to normal.
5. Placental blood flow is reduced, which can be reflected in foetal heart decelerations.

Noble (1981) suggested that this sequence of events leads to pooling of blood in the pelvis and legs and could predispose a woman to varicosities. The tissues of the rectus sheath, linea alba and the pelvic floor will be unduly strained by artificially prolonged pushing. Caldeyro-Barcia (1979) has associated forced straining with an increased need for episiotomy as a result of there being insufficient time for the perineum to distend slowly and gradually.

The management of this phase of labour must be checked on a regular basis in order to avoid these potentially damaging events.

BREATHING AND 'PUSHING'

Breathing awareness can be used to facilitate pushing. The woman can be trained to breathe in, then slowly out on exertion (e.g. during defaecation) so that it will become instinctive to 'breathe' out as she pushes, and to maintain the push at the same time as she breathes in. Each push should last about 5 to 10 seconds, and each contraction may demand three to four pushes. The deep inhalation provides mother and foetus with a good supply of oxygen. Exhalation on exertion works with the muscular contraction of the uterus to best effect. It is absolutely essential that the push is 'felt' through the perineum.

Another option is to breathe in, and out, then in again and 'hold', for no more than 6 seconds, whilst 'pushing'.

At the end of the contraction, one or two deep breaths will redress the physiological balance, and initiate the relaxation/preparation phase for the next contraction. During this time movement is recommended, and 'mopping of the brow' will be welcomed.

The midwife will 'conduct deliveries on her own responsibility' (Midwives code of practice (Nursing and Midwifery Council 1998)), she will take the 'lead', for the delivery. It will be a combination of short pushes, longer pushes and a gentle sighing and panting – the best combination to enable the midwife to control the birth of the head and then the shoulders. With the mouth relaxed, the diaphragm moves rhythmically, thereby preventing an increase in intra-abdominal pressure. Awareness of these different approaches is vital to the effectiveness of the delivery and should be included in antenatal classes. Vocalisation is an integral part of the birthing process – women should expect to hear themselves making noises and *not* feel they must continually apologise for crying out.

The mother is likely to be also asked to push to assist with the delivery of the placenta.

POSITIONS IN LABOUR

The 'medicalisation' of childbirth saw the gradual immobilisation of women, culminating in their restriction to the delivery couch. Further hampered by intravenous drips and monitoring equipment, women have been prevented from following their instinctive internal body 'messages'. The way women moved about and the positions they adopted during the first stage of labour and then for the delivery of their babies have been historically and anthropologically recorded (Attwood 1976). Many authorities (Randall 1953, Smellie 1974, Vaughan 1951) have drawn attention to the positions women found comfortable and which seemed to facilitate progress. Although the expression 'active birth' is reasonably new – it was originally coined by Janet Balaskas, a yoga teacher and antenatal educator, in the late 1970s – its philosophy is old, and the exercises and postures Balaskas advocates (Balaskas 1983, Balaskas & Balaskas 1983) are all included in the early obstetric physiotherapy textbooks (Randall 1953).

There is now a wide range of research into the benefits or otherwise that can be gained from ambulation in labour, and into the help given by frequent changes of position and the adoption of forward-leaning postures (Calder 1982, Flynn & Kelly 1976, Lupe & Gross 1986, Poschl 1987, Roberts et al 1983, Russell 1982, Stewart & Calder 1984, Williams & Thom 1980). Although there is no consensus of opinion, one fact does repeatedly emerge: the comfort of the mother and her feeling of freedom and well-being are most important. All authorities recommend the encouragement of women who feel that ambulation and the use of different positions enable them to cope better with labour.

Normal, uninhibited labour is often a restless time; the mother will walk, squat, sit, stand, kneel and lie down, trying to find comfortable positions, 'listening to her body'. Passive confinement to the bed is rejected in the concept of 'active birth' – women want to use, and work actively with, their bodies; it is a return to the age-old customs of womankind since time immemorial.

Because of the anteversion of the uterus during first stage contractions, many women find that they instinctively need to lean forward on some sort of support; some like to rotate or rock their pelvis (Fig. 6.1). The different postures that women may like to use should be demonstrated and practised during antenatal classes, and their use at home encouraged; women should be able to move easily from one position to another and become used to those which may be uncomfortable or awkward at first (Fig. 6.2). Partners and carers should also be aware of these postures, because during labour it may be up to them to suggest alternatives; some women become so overwhelmed by what they are feeling that they become immobilised and frightened to move in case they make their pain

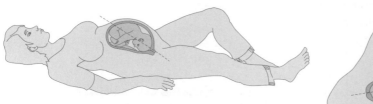

The supine position can reduce anteversion

The forward lean position facilitates anteversion. Many women feel most comfortable leaning forwards.

Figure 6.1 Anteversion of the uterus during first stage contraction.

worse. Roberts et al (1983) showed that it is actually the change from one position to another that stimulates efficient uterine activity.

Sometimes the cervix dilates unevenly, so that towards the end of the first stage of labour an anterior lip or rim remains between the presenting part and the pubis while the rest of the cervix is well drawn up. If this is the case the woman should be discouraged from pushing; lying on her side with the foot of the bed raised or adopting the prone kneel fall (pr.kn.fall) position can be helpful in this situation (Fig. 6.3).

Throughout history women have been depicted giving birth in many postures, but rarely recumbent. And yet the 'stranded beetle' position (sometimes with the additional 'benefit' of lithotomy stirrups) is how countless women may have been expected to give birth. There is no doubt that women have found it impossible to perform well in this posture; after all, defaecation is not normally carried out in the supine position, and birth is another form of body 'emptying'. It is hoped that, today, this posture would only be adopted in case of intervention. Russell (1982) demonstrated the increase in pelvic outlet size in the squatting posture, and any position that allows the pelvic joints to move freely during delivery must be preferable to those that restrict such activity. Gardosi et al (1989a) showed that the use of a 'birth cushion', which allowed the woman to adopt an upright 'supported squatting' posture, led to significantly fewer forceps deliveries and significantly shorter second stages. There were also fewer perineal but more labial tears. In a second paper Gardosi et al (1989b) reports that women who adopted upright positions (squatting, kneeling, sitting or standing) also had a higher rate of intact perineums and there was a reduction of forceps deliveries in the 'upright' group as compared with a 'semirecumbent' or 'lateral' group. What could be an important factor in the problem of pelvic floor muscle denervation was the fact that the mean duration of perineal distension before delivery, taken from the time when the head stopped receding between contractions, was shorter if the woman was kneeling than if she was semirecumbent. Once again, the comfort of each woman must be the prime consideration rather than the convenience of her carers during the second stage of labour; and it is also important that possible pushing and delivery positions be demonstrated and practised antenatally (Fig. 6.4).

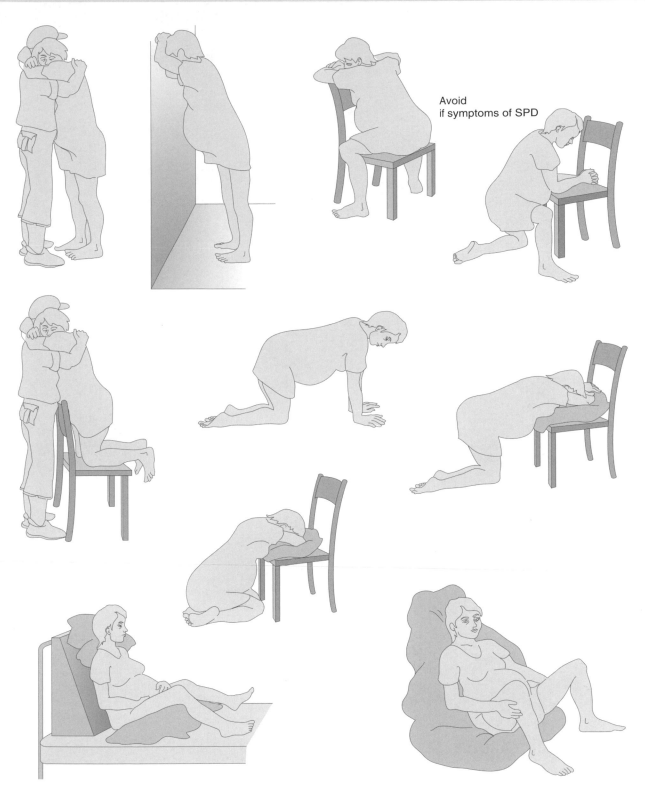

Avoid
if symptoms of SPD

Figure 6.2   Suggested positions of comfort for first stage labour.

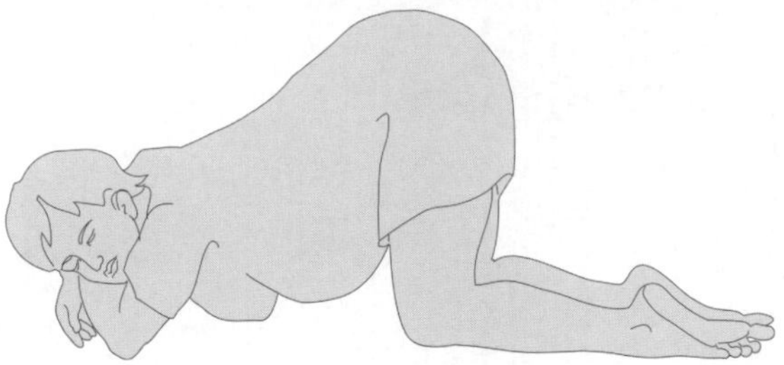

Figure 6.3 The prone kneel fall position may assist with the elimination of an anterior lip of the cervix.

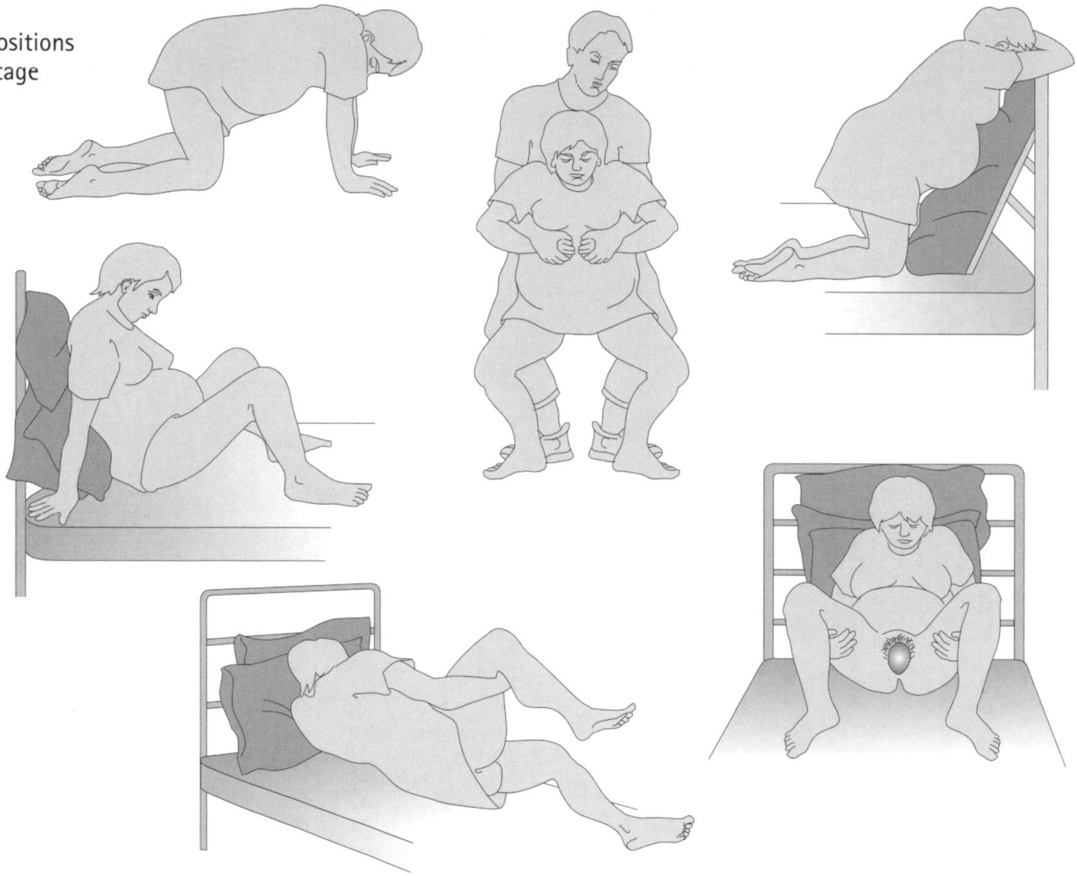

Figure 6.4 Suggested positions for second stage labour.

It is essential that labour partners and carers understand that the woman's head must *never* be 'forced' down on to her chest while she is pushing, whatever position she is using. Damage to the neck can easily occur leading to pain and inconvenience postnatally, making it difficult for the new mother to care for her baby.

MASSAGE IN LABOUR

Massage in labour is a very personal thing. Women who found the experience a positive one during pregnancy may find it aggravating during labour, and vice versa.

There have, as yet, been no controlled trials performed to determine the exact neurophysiological mechanisms by which massage moderates pain, but it is indisputable that 'rubbing' very often 'makes it better'. Before the advent of the use of anaesthesia during labour in the mid nineteenth century, midwives and labour supporters had little else to offer.

It is probable that the soothing sensory input from stroking, effleurage and kneading activates the 'gate-closing' mechanism at spinal level (Wells 1988). It may also be possible, by means of tissue manipulation (e.g. deep sacral kneading), to stimulate the release of endogenous opiates. In addition to its pain-relieving potential, massage demonstrates caring and non-verbal support and communication. This is particularly valuable when language barriers exist. It is most important that whoever is giving massage is sensitive to the changing needs of the woman, with regard to site, depth and technique, and uses advantageous well-supported positioning.

MASSAGE TO THE BACK

Back pain can be very demoralising, particularly when it is associated with a prolonged first stage of labour or where the foetus is in the occipitoposterior position. As shown in Figure 6.5, back pain in the first stage is experienced in the lumbosacral region, and it intensifies as labour progresses. Stationary kneading, either single handed or reinforced, applied slowly and deeply to the painful area is often helpful (Fig. 6.6). Elbows should be bent, and the masseur should use his, or her, own body weight combined with a gentle rotary movement to apply comfortable pressure, without fatigue, for a long period. Partners and midwives must be warned how easy it is to increase pain by overenthusiastic and vigorous application. Hands should be relaxed and moulded to the part. Uneven pressure, particularly with the heel of the hand, and straight arm application must be avoided especially over the bony sacroiliac region. Practice is essential both in antenatal classes and at home. Double-handed kneading, with loosely clenched fists, directly over the sacroiliac joints may be necessary as the pain becomes more severe (Fig. 6.7). Hand-held tennis balls can be a useful alternative where hands are small or become fatigued.

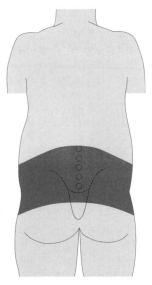

Figure 6.5 The site of possible back pain in first stage labour.

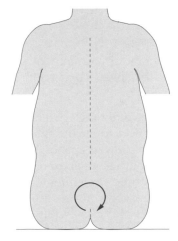

Figure 6.6 Deep, reinforced kneading to the painful area.

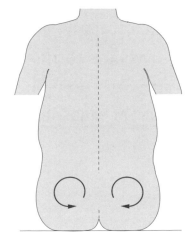

Figure 6.7 Double-handed kneading may be required if the pain becomes severe.

Figure 6.8 Effleurage and stroking for the relief of tension.

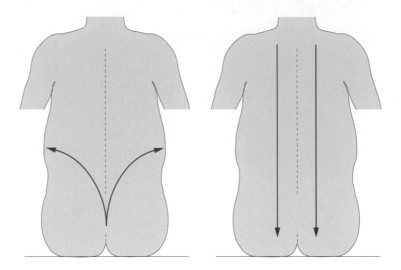

Effleurage from the sacrococcygeal area, up and over the iliac crests, will be even more soothing if a little oil is used to overcome the effects of sweating (Fig. 6.8). Slow, rhythmical longitudinal stroking, from occiput to coccyx, single or double handed, can relieve tension and facilitate relaxation. The strokes may be applied with the whole hands or the fingertips, actually over the spine or parallel to it. Pressure can become slightly deeper as the hands descend.

MASSAGE TO THE ABDOMEN

Pain is most commonly experienced over the lower half of the abdomen, particularly in the suprapubic region (Fig. 6.9). It is often described as nauseating. Deep massage will be totally unacceptable, but light finger-stroking or brushing from one anterior superior iliac spine to the other, passing under the bulge and over the pain, is often well received (Fig. 6.10). Another technique, best performed by the mother herself, is double-handed stroking ascending either side of the midline and across to the iliac crests (Fig. 6.11); this can be synchronised with easy breathing. Women often spontaneously and instinctively massage themselves; this should most certainly be encouraged and supplemented if it proves helpful.

MASSAGE TO THE LEGS

Occasionally labour pain may be perceived in the thighs, and cramp in the calf or foot may also occur; effleurage or kneading can relieve this.

PERINEAL MASSAGE

Some midwives will massage a mother's perineum in the second stage of labour in an effort to encourage stretching of the skin and muscle and thus prevent tearing or episiotomy. Grandmothers in some Eastern cultures also encourage their pregnant daughters or daughters-in-law to practise this simple stretching technique during pregnancy. The suggestion that it is possible to prepare the perineum for birth could be made during an antenatal class while discussing the second stage of labour, and how the mother can best help herself and her midwife to complete the delivery with an intact perineum.

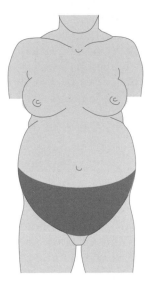

Figure 6.9 The lower half of the abdomen is the most common site for pain.

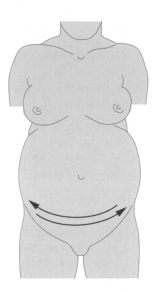

Figure 6.10 Lateral stroking, over the site of the pain, may give relief.

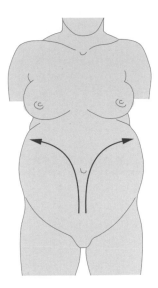

Figure 6.11 Double-handed kneading, self-administered and synchronised with breathing, may relieve pain.

This simple massage technique can be used by the woman herself leaning back in a well-supported position, or when squatting. Alternatively, some women may prefer their partner to do it for them. A natural oil (olive, wheatgerm, sunflower, etc.) can be used. Both index fingers or thumbs, or the index and middle fingers from one hand, are put about 5 cm into the vagina. A rhythmic 'U' or sling type movement, upwards along the sides of the vagina and with downward pressure, stretches the perineum from side to side. Maintaining a sideways stretch for a few seconds and gradually building up for 30–40 seconds can prepare the woman for the sort of sensation she can expect to feel as her baby's head begins to crown. As elasticity is improved it is suggested that three or four fingers could be used. As an alternative a kneading movement between index finger and thumb could be employed. If the woman contracts her pelvic floor during a perineal massage session she will realise how difficult it will be for her tissues to stretch if she 'holds back' while her baby's head is crowning. This may reinforce the idea of the need to relax the pelvic floor during delivery.

Avery & Van Arsdale (1987), two American nurse-midwives, evaluated the effect of perineal massage on 55 women (29 experimental and 26 controls). Massage began 6 weeks before the due date. In the experimental group 52% had an intact perineum or a first degree laceration; 48% had an episiotomy or a second, third or fourth degree tear, or both. In the control group, 24% had an intact perineum or first degree laceration, and 76% had an episiotomy or second, third or fourth degree tear, or both. When the episiotomy rate was examined, 38% of the experimental group and 65% of the control group had had an episiotomy. Third and fourth degree tears occurred only when an episiotomy was performed.

Some of the women in the trial experienced discomfort and discontinued the massage; they also felt it required a significant time commitment (5–10 minutes daily was suggested). However, many of the participants noticed a dramatic increase in perineal elasticity in the first 2 to 3 weeks of massage, which was maintained but not significantly increased if the massage was continued to term. No comment was made in this trial as to the strength of the pelvic floor muscles postnatally.

OTHER COPING STRATEGIES

Increasingly, maternity units are arranging for baths and showers to be available because it has been appreciated that some labouring women derive great benefit from them (Lenstrup et al 1987). Couples should be encouraged to bring tapes of favourite music which is relaxing and distracting. Television and games such as Scrabble or backgammon can be used to help pass the time.

The midwife can spend many hours in the delivery suite and can gain 'hands on' experience of the variety of labour sequences. The physiotherapist is not in that privileged position. It is therefore advisable for physiotherapists to study the labour reports in order that they are as prepared as they can be when teaching the 'mother-to-be'.

PAIN RELIEF IN LABOUR

Until the middle of the nineteenth century there were no really effective methods of anaesthesia, or analgesia, that eased labour pain. With the discovery of ether and chloroform, doctors were finally able to relieve the pain of the 'poor, suffering mother'. Many felt and some still feel that, as Sir James Young Simpson wrote in 1848, 'it is our duty as well as our privilege to use all legitimate means to mitigate and remove the physical sufferings of the mother during parturition' (Moir 1986).

The intensity of labour pain experienced varies from woman to woman, and from labour to labour in the same woman. The three P's: *power* (uterine contractions), *pelvis* (its shape and size) and *passenger* (the presentation and size of the baby), will all play a part in the length of labour and therefore the ability of a mother to manage without invasive analgesia. The level of anxiety experienced during pregnancy is also said to have a bearing on the analgesic needs of a labouring woman (Haddad & Morris 1985).

Wuitchik et al (1989) showed that the levels of pain and distress-related thoughts experienced during the latent phase of labour were predictive of the length of labour and obstetric outcome. Women registering high pain scores and distress-related thoughts during labour's latent phase had longer labours and were more likely to need instrumental delivery. Maternal distress during this time was also related to higher incidences of abnormal foetal heart-rate patterns and the need for neonatal assistance.

With the advent of reliable methods of contraception most pregnancies today will have been planned and the vast majority of babies will be wanted. Perhaps it is because of this that a sizeable proportion of women now express the desire to cope with labour 'on my own'. Many feel that labour, in spite of its pain, is the ultimate fulfilment of their femaleness, and they are prepared to suffer the pain of parturition, to deal with it as they might the pain of marathon running or mountaineering, in return for an enormous sense of achievement and self-fulfilment. Morgan et al (1982) showed that a completely painless labour is not always desirable for all mothers, and that analgesia is not the most important determinant of a satisfactory experience of childbirth. Reports of epidural anaesthesia (Billevicz-Driemel & Milne 1976, Crawford 1972) noted that some mothers felt 'deprived of the experience of childbirth' by perfect analgesia.

Many mothers regard the support of a sympathetic midwife as the most important factor in relieving their labour pain, and the presence of a *doula* (a lay female companion) during labour has been shown to shorten the interval, and therefore the pain, between the mother's admission and her baby's delivery (Sosa et al 1980). Melzack et al (1981) and Charles et al (1978) showed that antenatal preparation was related to lower levels of pain and higher levels of enjoyment during childbirth. Nevertheless, particularly in primiparous women, some form of analgesia will frequently be requested or be necessary, in addition to each mother's 'tool kit' of self-help techniques: positions of ease, mobility, body awareness and neuro-muscular control (relaxation), breathing, massage, distraction techniques, warm baths and showers, music, companionship and imaging. The following analgesic methods are in general use and should be discussed in antenatal classes. Although many women hope that they will manage to cope with labour without resorting to analgesia, it is important that they know what is available to relieve their labour pain and how it can help them, and also something about the side-effects they and their babies may experience.

TRANSCUTANEOUS ELECTRICAL NERVE STIMULATION (TENS)

TENS can be an additional tool that the women's health physiotherapist is able to offer to women in labour. Its non-invasive mode of action and absence of side-effects are very attractive to the woman hoping to cope with labour by relying on her own resources. TENS is a method of acute, or chronic, pain relief that is used widely throughout physiotherapy.

Johnson (1997) surveyed 17 896 women who hired Spembly Medical TENS units (PULSAR® TENS) which had a TENS and labour questionnaire enclosed. After labour 10 077 women returned completed questionnaires with their units (56.3%); of these 6733 were primiparas (73%), and the rest were multiparas or their parity was unknown. Forty per cent (4141) relied solely on the written instructions supplied with the unit and received no instruction from a health professional. Ninety-one per cent (9160) said they would use TENS again in labour. However, the fact that 7122 (71%) claimed excellent or good pain relief should be treated with caution as 6125 of these received additional analgesics. Johnson (1997) contends that TENS does have a role to play in the relief of pain in labour.

Carroll et al (1997) were more specific in a review of the use of TENS for labour pain. They stated: 'Randomised controlled trials provide no compelling evidence for TENS having any analgesic effect during labour. Weak positive effects in secondary (analgesic sparing) and tertiary (choosing TENS for future labours) outcomes may be due to inadequate blinding causing overestimation of treatment effects.' However, they go on to say that there will be a decreased need for additional analgesia if TENS is used. Crothers (1998) puts forward the theory that TENS is 'liked' by women, and is requested for subsequent labours, because they feel in control. It allows them to appreciate labour pain cognitively in a different way and thereby harness, to a deeper extent, the effects of endogenous opiate mechanisms. Pain perception is therefore more accurate, and therefore less of a threat. The control engendered allows the woman to 'cope' more efficiently and effectively.

If women find that TENS gives adequate pain relief during the latent phase of labour, this could possibly influence the length of labour, the mode of delivery and even the condition of the newborn infant. TENS may continue to be used if the mother opts to have additional help in the form of pethidine or Entonox. It may be helpful to retain TENS for post-delivery suturing, and it can also be useful for women experiencing severe after-pains in the early puerperium.

Modes of stimulation

TENS involves the transmission of electrical energy through the skin to the nervous system. Since it first became available in the mid 1960s, it has developed as a modality in its own right and is now more than just a model for the proof of the gate theory of pain (Melzack & Wall 1965). Two of the TENS parameters described by Walsh (1997) are used for labour. These are burst train TENS and brief intense TENS.

Burst Train TENS   This is characterised by low-frequency bursts (<4 Hz) of higher-frequency stimulation. This type of stimulation has the properties of both conventional TENS and acupuncture-like TENS. Conventional TENS has its effects by the stimulation of the Aδ and Aβ fibres to inhibit the C-fibre-mediated pain sensations presynaptically at spinal segmental level. Conventional TENS may take 5–10 minutes before pain relief is experienced. Acupuncture-like TENS will produce analgesia that is long lasting but may take about 30 minutes of stimulation before the effects are noted. This latency before onset of analgesia is due to the theorised mechanism of effect. It is thought that the stimulation affects the descending control mechanisms at both spinal and supraspinal levels by the production of opiate-mediated systems activated by the stimulation of Aδ nerve fibres.

Brief Intense TENS   This is characterised by a high frequency (>100 Hz), a long pulse duration (>150 μs) and the highest intensity that can be tolerated by the patient. It is best used for short periods of time (i.e. 10–15 minutes) owing to the fatigue generated in the nerves from this intense type of stimulation. The effect can be almost instantaneous owing to the localised blocking of nerve conduction.

These two modes of stimulation are used for the specific instance of labour because they suit the specific nature of labour pain. Labour pain consists of dull, aching period-type pains that are due to stretching of and pressure on the abdominal and pelvic viscera; these include the structure of the uterus, cervix, walls of the vagina and the pelvic floor muscles and fascia. Visceral pain is conducted to the spinal segment via C fibres and this type of pain is best ameliorated by the use of endorphin mechanisms and closing the pain gate. This is why burst train TENS is used all the time during labour. Brief intense TENS is also used as it acts quickly and has a strong counterirritant and nerve-blocking effect; this makes it suitable for the increased pain experienced during contractions (Crothers 1992).

Most TENS units that are used specifically for labour have these two types of stimulation. The burst train mode is the type of stimulation used all the time during labour and the brief intense mode is activated by the use of a press button mechanism when the woman experiences the beginnings of a contraction. The brief intense mode is then de-activated by pressing the same boost button so that the burst train mode is resumed.

Placement of the electrodes

The electrodes can be placed either over the relevant vertebral segments that receive nociceptive information from the painful areas or over the area that is giving pain. Bonica (1984) demonstrated that during the first stage of labour the pain information is transmitted to the dorsal horn of spinal segments T11–T12. Following 'intensity theory', the more intense the pain the more nociceptors are recruited to fire and eventually two additional segments are also transmitting pain information. Therefore, during the first stage, labour pain information, when pain is at its most intense, will be entering segments T10–L1. The information from the parasympathetic nerves and the pudendal nerve arrives at the spinal segments S2–S4. When choosing electrodes these will need to be long enough to cover these spinal segments. Each pair of electrodes will be placed on either side of the spinal column, one pair covering either side of the spinous processes of T10–L1 and the other pair covering either side of the spinous processes of S2–S4.

Some women feel considerable pain over the anterior aspects of the abdomen, especially during the late first stage. However, there is no research evidence to support or refute the safety of moving the sacral pair of electrodes to the abdomen.

Safety limits

There are only three papers that exist that were specifically designed to examine the effects on the foetus of the use of TENS as a method of pain relief during labour.

Bundsen & Klas (1982) suggested that the foetus was most at risk if:

- the electrodes were placed abdominally
- the woman was thin, having only 1 inch of abdominal fat
- the foetus was occipitoposterior.

They then tested the theory using an in-dwelling transducer in women's bladders, having estimated that at the time of delivery the 'at risk' position for the foetus would be 3 cm from the surface. They used both 60–80 Hz and 5 Hz frequencies and intensities of 20–40 mA, and they decided that the most important feature would be current density and suggested that this should not exceed 0.5 μA per mm^2 (hence the large electrodes that were used).

Bundsen et al (1982) tested these assertions on women during their labour and stated that 'no adverse effect upon the neonate by TENS is demonstrable by clinical laboratory or neurological examination of the infants after pain relief by TENS'.

The current density of the machines and electrodes in use in the department can be checked by dividing the average current output of the TENS unit by the area of the electrodes that are in contact with the skin (Low & Reed 2000).

Practical considerations in the use of TENS

Ideally women should be introduced to the TENS unit during a class with a health professional, preferably a physiotherapist. It should be clearly stated that:

- the unit should not be placed over the carotid sinus (the anterior neck)
- the unit should not be placed over the area where a pacemaker has been fitted
- the electrodes and the TENS unit should be removed before going into the bath or birthing pool
- the unit should only be used for the woman herself, and for her labour, unless she has been given instructions otherwise by a health professional

The placement of the electrodes, especially for the woman who is by herself at home, can be difficult. Practice before the 'event' is essential if the woman is to feel confident in the units' use. The following 'self-help' tips may be useful:

Spinal electrodes

- Locate the bottom of the bra strap.
- Place three fingers of the right hand below the level of the bra strap.
- Place the top of the electrode at this level to the right side of the spine, to roughly cover T10–L1.
- Repeat the process, for the other electrode of that pair, to attach it to the left side of the spine.

Sacral electrodes

- Locate the level of the iliac crest.
- Place three fingers of the right hand below this level.
- Place the top of the electrode at this level to the right side of the sacral area.
- Repeat the process, for the other electrode of that pair, to attach it to the left side of the sacral area.

Abdominal placement of the electrodes will be dictated by the site of pain and is usually not an issue until the woman is in the labour ward.

TENS units

There are a great variety of TENS units. The TENS unit should have a press release button (not press and hold) to enable switching to the brief intense mode. It should be described as an 'Obstetric TENS unit.' Units can be bought from the internet, or over the counter from many large retail stores, and can be hired without the involvement of any health professional. The woman will not necessarily have had any instruction in its use other than a written leaflet. If the unit is borrowed from a maternity unit, instruction will be given either 'one to one' or in the form of a 'special' TENS antenatal class. Instruction in use is strongly recommended.

Midwives and TENS

In June 1986 the UK Central Council (UKCC) accepted the recommendation of its Midwifery Committee that midwives should not, on their own responsibility, use TENS for the relief of pain in labour. However, they are allowed to use TENS under supervision provided that they have been instructed in its use in accordance with Rule 41(1) and (3) of the Nurses Midwives and Health Visitors (Midwives Amendment) Rule 1986. In many centres this is taken to mean that, within a 'blanket' referral from the consultants in charge of the obstetric unit, and with proper tuition and constant updating from women's health physiotherapists, midwives are able to use TENS in labour for those mothers who wish to use it as a form of analgesia.

ACUPUNCTURE

This ancient method of relieving pain is sometimes used in labour. Doctors, midwives and physiotherapists are all showing new interest in this field. Jackson (1988) describes general techniques and modern explanations for the pain-modulating effects of acupuncture, but although he suggests that it may be used for childbirth pain, he does not describe how this may be done. Skelton (1988) gives a comprehensive description of acupuncture techniques that have been successfully used in the treatment of labour pain, and suggests that this modality may be beneficially used. A randomised control trial by Ramnero et al (2002) concluded that acupuncture could be a good alternative, or complement, other forms of analgesia in labour, but no conclusion was drawn as to whether the effect was analgesic or relaxing.

HYPNOSIS

Anaesthetists, obstetricians and general practitioners have all described the use of hypnosis for the relief of labour pain, and also for the relief of tension and the promotion of relaxation in pregnancy. Women are usually treated individually, which is time consuming for the practitioner. Freeman et al (1986), in a randomised trial of hypnosis in labour, showed a trend for labour to be more satisfying for women who used hypnosis, although analgesic requirements were similar in hypnosis and control groups. Women who were good or moderate hypnotic subjects reported that hypnosis had been instrumental in reducing anxiety and helping them cope with labour.

HOMEOPATHY/ AROMOTHERAPY

Much work has been done in recent years looking at complementary therapies in the relief of pain in labour. In a review of clinical trials (Kleijnen et al 1991) of homeopathy, 77% yielded positive results and were therefore worthy of further research. In a trial conducted by Eid et al (1993), using Cauphyllum, average labour time was found to have been reduced by 90 minutes and the mother's emotional state was said to have been improved. Aromotherapy is a field that lends itself to physiotherapists, but it is *essential* that the therapist is fully trained in its use. It is potentially dangerous in 'untrained hands'. The reader is directed to Supper (1998).

WATER

Water births were first introduced in the UK in the 1980s and more than 200 hospitals (BBC press release 2002) now offer women the opportunity to labour or deliver, or both, in a birthing pool. The Health Committee (Maternity Services 1992) recommended that all hospitals 'make full provision, whenever possible for women to choose the position which they prefer for labour and birth and with the option of a birthing pool where it is practicable'. Balaskas & Gordon (1990) describe a labour in water as something which is shorter, easier and more comfortable. Physiotherapists are well aware of the positive mechanical and physiological effects of water, as well as the potential risks. Safety guidelines *must* be in place, and all parties must be fully aware of them before considering labouring or delivering in water. Clinical guidelines for a hospital water birth pool facility were revised in 1999 by Janet Balaskas and can be downloaded from the Active Birth Centre website (see Useful Addresses, p. 203). Balanced information to mothers is essential if they are to make an informed choice with regard to labouring or delivering in water. In the UK the Royal College of Obstetricians and Gynaecologists has published guidelines (RCOG 2001) on how to minimise the chances of complications. However, the American College of Obstetricians and Gynecologists has not endorsed the technique, quoting insufficient data to prove safety (BBC press release 2002).

ENTONOX

Various forms of inhalational analgesia have been available to women in labour in the past: 'gas' (nitrous oxide) and air, trichlorethylene (Trilene) and methoxyflurane (Penthrane) among them. They have mainly been superceded in the UK by Entonox, which is a mixture of 50% nitrous oxide with 50% oxygen. It is available in cylinders, but in many delivery suites will be piped in from a central source. Entonox is taken by the mother herself for each contraction, one at a time. It is not, nor should it be, administered by a midwife or labour companion. About 75% of labouring women use Entonox (Hobbs 2001).

Nitrous oxide is a weak anaesthetic, but has a good analgesic effect. Ideally women should be instructed in its use antenatally, with a quick revision in early labour. Deep breaths are essential to gain maximum effect, and 20 seconds of deep inhalation is necessary before the mother begins to feel the benefit. It is usually recommended that the woman starts using Entonox before a contraction or immediately it begins; 8 to 12 breaths may be all she needs to help her cope with it. Maximum analgesia will be reached after 45–60 seconds, and the effects wear off rapidly. The Entonox is usually administered via a plastic mouthpiece. A hissing noise will be heard if the apparatus is being used correctly.

Some women complain of nausea as a result of using Entonox, and some will find that the analgesia is insufficient or non-existent. Its use for long periods can also result in dehydration since breathing is through the mouth.

PETHIDINE

Pethidine is a synthetic opioid analgesic derived from morphine, and is the most common narcotic drug used in obstetric analgesia in the UK, although diamorphine is used in some centres. It is generally administered as an intramuscular injection in 100 mg doses, and is one of the drugs midwives may prescribe and give on their own responsibility to a woman in labour, to a maximum of 200 mg. Because the response to any drug is individual, and is related to body mass, 50 mg may be sufficient for some women, whereas others will need 150 mg. Self-administered controlled doses of intravenous pethidine via a pump have been found acceptable by some mothers. When the drug is administered parenterally it is recognised that there is unrestricted placental transfer from mother to foetus. As with other narcotic analgesics, side-effects can and do occur, and these are of particular concern during labour when the foetus must also be considered. However, pethidine is readily available in all maternity units and can help women relax when they become distressed by the intensity of their labour. Approximately 40% of labouring women use pethidine (Hobbs 2001).

Maternal side–effects

Pethidine can cause maternal nausea and sometimes vomiting; an antiemetic is often given simultaneously because of this. Other side-effects include drowsiness, distressing hallucinations and dysphoria, which can interfere with the mother's concentration on her own 'coping' techniques and affect her cooperation with her attendants. Pethidine is said to reduce the tone of the lower oesophageal sphincter and delay gastric emptying, which could have implications if a general anaesthetic has to be given. It could also give rise to hypotension and respiratory depression.

Foetal and neonatal side–effects

In common with other drugs, what affects the mother will also affect her baby, and although pethidine can be metabolised in the maternal liver and is eventually excreted from the mother's body, this may not be the case for the newborn infant. Because there will be a high concentration of pethidine and its metabolite norpethidine in the mother's bloodstream, the drugs will cross the placenta into the baby; in the first 2 to 3 hours following an injection, up to 70% of the dose plus some norpethidine will have accumulated in the foetus. Even at term the neonate's liver and kidneys are too immature to metabolise and excrete the drug effectively. After 3 hours, when the level of pethidine has fallen in the mother, the drug again crosses the placenta into the mother where it can be dealt with. Where labour is premature the problems are intensified. The preterm baby, being much smaller, will receive a proportionately larger dose of pethidine, and its more immature organs are even less able to deal with the drug.

Consequently, if the mother receives her dose of pethidine between 1 and 4 hours before the birth, it is possible (because pethidine will still be in the baby's bloodstream) that prolonged side-effects will be apparent in the neonate in addition to those observed in the foetus before delivery; foetal acidosis, a depressed foetal heart rate and a slower response to sound have all been reported. Respiratory depression in the neonate can occur following large or repeated doses; this can be reversed by the drug's antagonist naloxone, but, as naloxone has a shorter duration of action than pethidine, repeated doses may be required. Adverse neurobehavioural effects have been reported which are potentiated in the preterm infant; these include drowsiness (Richards & Bernal 1972) which can interfere with the early bonding process, and difficulties in establishing breastfeeding (Belsey et al 1981). Other, more subtle, side-effects have been observed, including the baby being less alert, more easily startled, less easily comforted, fretful and slower to respond to faces and sounds. It is easy to dismiss these changes as unimportant, but they could be distressing to new mothers who can lose confidence in themselves unless they have been warned in advance that they may need to persevere and devote more time to establishing breast-feeding and their new relationship.

It is advisable, therefore, for women to have pethidine at the times in their labour that can give them maximum help with least effect on their baby. More than 4 hours before delivery is said to be reasonably safe for the baby, who will then have low levels of pethidine in its bloodstream at birth – and, although it is difficult to predict exactly when a baby will be born, it is probably advisable for pethidine to be given following vaginal assessment in order to avoid severe neonatal side-effects.

Moir (1986) said that none of the narcotic analgesics provides complete pain relief to all labouring women when given in safe doses, and women must be prepared to feel some labour pain following an injection of pethidine.

EPIDURAL ANAESTHESIA

Continuous epidural (also known as extradural or peridural) anaesthesia is now widely used in the UK and may be available on demand in obstetric units that have full anaesthetic cover. As well as giving pain relief for labour, epidural anaesthesia may also be used for caesarean delivery. A full explanation is essential in antenatal classes for women who will have access to this form of pain control. Many 'young wives' tales' abound, and a great many women reject the idea of epidural anaesthesia without fully understanding its method of induction, the way it works, the different doses and how they can help themselves in the second stage of labour if they use it.

The benefits of epidural anaesthesia

- It may be administered as a single dose, as a continuous infusion, or as a client-controlled pump.
- Low-dose epidural, adding an opiate to reduce loss of mobility, if appropriate, is now available in some areas.

- The mother will be fully conscious, her mind unclouded by analgesia; she will be able to welcome her baby with an alert mind.
- The effects of bupivacaine on the baby are minimal compared with those of pethidine.
- Epidural anaesthesia may be helpful in cases of pre-eclamptic toxaemia and incoordinate uterine activity.
- Where a woman is exhausted from a long, painful labour, or is frightened and unable to tolerate her pain, an epidural anaesthetic can transform the experience for her and can reverse maternal and foetal acidosis.
- For a complicated delivery (i.e. twins, breech, forceps), epidural anaesthesia provides the obstetrician with the conditions needed for control and hence the safety of the baby. The mother has better pain relief than with a local nerve block, and general anaesthesia with its associated complications is avoided.
- Caesarean delivery can be carried out under epidural anaesthesia; the mother can be awake, and will escape the unpleasant after-effects of general anaesthesia and its dangers. An important plus is that the father can be present for the birth of his baby.

Technique

An intravenous infusion, usually Hartmann's solution, is always set up beforehand. The mother will either lie on her side, curled up as much as possible, or she may sit with her legs over the edge of the delivery table supported by her labour companion or a midwife. A small amount of local anaesthetic solution is injected into the surrounding skin at L2–L3 or L3–L4 prior to the insertion of a Tuohy needle. Some women may find the technique painful, whereas others do not seem to experience pain or discomfort. Pain is usually caused by difficulties, such as hitting bone. Relaxation, together with calm quiet breathing, can help fathers cope with what, for many, is a frightening ordeal. Once the Tuohy needle is inserted the anaesthetist moves it slowly from the resistance of the tough interspinous ligament into the epidural space. Before a dose of local anaesthetic (commonly bupivacaine, a 0.25% solution is often used) is injected, careful aspiration for blood or cerebrospinal fluid (CSF) is made. The presence of either of these could lead to complications, and the epidural would probably be resited at an adjacent intervertebral space. A fine plastic catheter is threaded through the needle and its tip positioned in the epidural space. The first dose will be given by the anaesthetist (the woman may notice a cold sensation in her back at first), and subsequent top-up doses will probably be given by a midwife. The effect of a good epidural anaesthetic should be to block the sensory nerves and eliminate pain, but leave motor power.

Side-effects and complications of epidural anaesthesia

1. There appears to be an increased rate of forceps delivery with its attendant maternal and foetal trauma. This could be due to three main factors:
   (a) There is normally a physiological increase in maternal oxytocin during the second stage of labour. This neuroendocrine response

is said to be due to stimulation of the pelvic stretch receptors by the descending foetus (Ferguson's reflex). However, where epidurals are used, Ferguson's reflex is abolished and uterine activity is measurably less, either because this oxytocic surge does not occur or because there is a drop in oxytocic output. Because of this an oxytocin infusion is often necessary to stimulate efficient expulsive contractions.

(b) The sensory blockade that eliminates labour pain also eliminates pelvic floor sensation, so the woman whose epidural is topped up will not appreciate the bearing-down reflex.

(c) Extensive epidural anaesthesia can lead to a relaxation and 'guttering' of the pelvic floor muscles, which may interfere with the rotation of the baby's head; additionally, the abdominal muscles may be affected.

The suggestion in antenatal classes that women consciously push in the second stage of labour as if they were trying to open their bowels can be helpful if an epidural has blocked sensation and also led to decreased motor power. It must be remembered, however, that the epidural may have been given *because* a forceps delivery was envisaged – it may not be correct to state dogmatically that forceps deliveries are always a direct result of a woman having had epidural anaesthesia.

2. Alongside the sensory blockade, the sympathetic nerves will also be affected. This leads to vasodilatation of blood vessels in the lower abdomen and the legs (which will be warm to the touch) and a consequent drop in blood pressure. This will be compounded if the mother is supine (although this should never happen), and could interfere with placental blood flow to the foetus. If this occurs the mother will be turned on her side; she may be given oxygen if there is foetal distress.

3. The mother's legs may feel 'heavy' and she may be unable to move them easily; walking will not be possible initially.

4. The mother sometimes feels dizzy, and shivering can be a nuisance.

5. Urinary retention may occur if the mother is unable to feel her bladder filling. She should try to micturate every 2 hours; a catheter will be passed if retention of urine becomes obvious. The mother *must* be encouraged to report any loss of sensation, or abnormality in micturition pattern. In some areas it is becoming standard practice to pass a catheter for women with retention, though this can be a contentious issue. The reader is directed to Maclean & Cardozo (2002) for further detail.

    It is recommended that physiotherapists be fully aware of ward protocol in their own area with regard to this issue.

6. Unblocked segments and unilateral blocks are common problems and can prove distressing for the woman who was hoping for total pain relief. They can sometimes be relieved by top-up doses in appropriate positions – but women should be warned antenatally that this may happen, also that it takes time to work.

7. The accidental puncture of the dura and consequent release of CSF can give rise to severe postpartum headache. In the past the mother was usually nursed flat for at least 24 hours and the intravenous drip of Hartmann's solution remained in place. In current practice, the drip may remain and the mother is encouraged to drink; she may not be required to remain supine. If the problem is prolonged and severe the anaesthetist may inject a 'blood patch' of the mother's own venous blood into the epidural space at the site of the damage. Women suffering from postepidural headache are usually distressed at their immobility and their inability to care for their baby and respond spontaneously and comfortably to its needs. They will need extra support and assistance, and the reassurance that the condition will resolve and that this initial problem will not interfere with the bonding process between them and their baby.

8. Many women complain of pain and tenderness postpartum at the epidural site, and for some this can be intolerable. The suggestion has been made that a tiny haematoma forms in the epidural space with consequent pressure on sensitive tissues, and women can be reassured if they are reminded that bruising often occurs around ordinary injection sites. The women's health physiotherapist can help alleviate this problem by offering a 'hot pack' or TENS, and suggesting that the mother rests in prone lying with appropriate pillows.

9. Total spinal anaesthesia can occur if the dose of local anaesthetic is accidentally injected into the subarachnoid space. This potentially fatal condition (severe hypotension and cessation of spontaneous respiration can occur very quickly) requires instant artificial respiration, the injection of vasopressor drugs and rapid fluid infusion. Rarely, spinal anaesthesia may follow a top-up.

10. Neurological complications may persist following epidural anaesthesia. Muscle weakness in a leg or foot, loss of sensation in an area of skin and paralysis occur.

11. Fusi et al (1989) have shown that women receiving epidural analgesia during labour are at increased risk of developing pyrexia. It is thought that this may be due to vascular and thermoregulatory modifications induced by epidural analgesia.

12. Bupivacaine, like other local analgesics, enters the maternal bloodstream from the epidural space, crosses the placenta and can be found in measurable (but clinically unimportant) concentrations in the foetal circulation within 10 minutes of injection (Caldwell et al 1977, Rosenblatt et al 1981). The neurobehavioural effects are clinically unimportant, unlike those of pethidine.

13. The issue of the possibility of long-term backache following epidural anaesthesia has been raised (MacArthur et al 1990), but later studies (MacArthur et al 1997, Russell et al 1996) show that there is no evidence to support *new* long-term backache. Previous reports may reflect high-dose epidurals, and stressed posture during labour.

Epidural anaesthesia for caesarean delivery

Epidural anaesthesia for caesarean delivery has become an increasingly safer and more popular option. The woman is conscious, and is therefore 'present' at the birth. Often her partner is able to be there too, which, psychologically, has great advantages in that the new family unit is together from the beginning.

When preparing women for an elective caesarean delivery, under epidural anaesthesia, it is important to mention that, because of the profound block required to achieve total analgesia, they may experience some side-effects. Hypotension can give rise to a feeling of faintness, shivering and vomiting can also be troublesome, and the mother may feel very cold.

Babies born by caesarean intervention do not expect to be delivered through the abdomen and it can come as a 'bit of a shock'. A paediatrician will be present at the operation to help the baby in whatever way necessary, for instance assisting in clearing mucus and liquor from the lungs, or giving some assistance to initiate breathing. It is important to warn women that, because of this, it may not be possible for them to hold the baby immediately after delivery but all being well they will be able to very soon.

Although epidural anaesthesia blocks pain, the woman must be made aware of the fact that she may feel sensations of pulling and tugging. One mother described her epidural caesarean delivery as being similar to having 'the washing-up done in my tummy'. It is also important, where possible, to prepare the father for this type of delivery.

Spinal anaesthesia is also used for caesarean delivery.

THE THIRD STAGE OF LABOUR

The third stage of labour has been called the most dangerous (Sleep 1989) because of the risk of maternal haemorrhage. It can be managed actively or passively, and it is important to prepare women antenatally for what is likely to happen and what may be expected of them. Couples are usually so overwhelmed by joy and excitement, and the wonder of actually seeing and touching their new baby, that this phase often passes by in a blur.

If the third stage is actively managed, a method in widespread use because it is said to reduce blood loss (Prendiville et al 1988), the mother will receive an injection of syntocinon and ergometrine as the anterior shoulder is delivered. She will be asked to lie back so that the midwife can palpate the uterine fundus, and the placenta will be delivered by continuous cord traction once it has separated from the wall of the uterus, which is achieved by strong uterine contractions (see p. 72).

Where passive physiological management is used to deliver the placenta, now considered a safe option if the mother has had a 'normal' delivery and accepted criteria are followed (Hobbs 2001), the mother will probably have to adopt an upright posture so that gravity and intra-abdominal pressure can play their part in helping the process. Once the midwife feels the strong uterine contraction that results in placental separation and its descent into the lower uterine segment, the mother will be asked to bear down in order to help push the placenta out.

If the baby sucks at the breast, oxytocin is produced, which stimulates contractions and a 'clamp-down' on the uterine blood vessels, thus aiding the physiological process. This is important because oxytocic drugs are not normally used when the third stage is passively managed. It is helpful for women to know that they may notice a gush of blood from the vagina as their baby suckles, a sign that the uterus is contracting well.

While the mother is made comfortable and has her perineum and vagina inspected for damage, the father can cuddle their new baby. This is often the time when parents want to talk about their experiences with the staff who cared for them in labour.

BIRTH PLANS

The birth plans which many hospitals now suggest their clients should prepare evolved from a reaction to the managerial approach of some obstetricians and midwives. The professionals thought that they 'knew best' when it came to childbirth. Women who felt that their needs and wishes would not be met by their carers wrote down their requests for the management of their labours and the care of their new baby. Because these early birth plans were sometimes written in an aggressive and demanding manner they were often met with hostility. But, as is often the case, the establishment began to realise that it was on the losing side in this confrontation, and hospitals began to produce their own formal printed plans for women to complete. This, of course, does make it seem as if women are being consulted and given choices, but in many cases, hospitals' ready-printed birth plans do nothing of the sort. They are often just a series of statements requiring a yes/no answer or a tick in the relevant box, and the kind of questions women are asked deal only with trivial, superficial matters. Furthermore, these birth plans are frequently handed out in antenatal clinics, without explanation, before women have started their course of antenatal classes – as early as 26–28 weeks. They will not yet have discovered what options are available to them. Kitzinger (1987) has written wisely of the special importance of birth plans where women do not know in advance who will be caring for them in labour, and also how they can help midwives and doctors understand what matters to each mother. She also mentions the anxiety some professionals feel when they are confronted by a birth plan that has been compiled by a well-informed woman. Articulate women and their partners tend to read widely and also attend the sort of antenatal class that questions interventionist obstetric practices. Some have very pronounced views on labour and how they hope their own experience will be managed.

Time should be devoted, during preparation for labour courses, to the consideration of birth plans and how they can be used to communicate to the caring staff not only each woman's feelings about her labour, but how she hopes necessary interventions such as caesarean delivery would be managed (e.g. epidural versus general anaesthesia), and also how she would like her baby to be handled after the birth. Within the birth plan should also be the mother's preferred choice of feeding. If birth plans are discussed within a class, women who find it difficult to express their feelings, needs and preferences can be helped by the encouragement of their fellows and the teacher. However, women and their partners must understand that, as obstetricians and midwives are responsible for the consequences of *their* decisions, so too are they.

While birth plans are particularly relevant for those women who have specific requests, very many expectant mothers will be happy to accept whatever their carers offer.

VARIATIONS IN LABOUR

It is important for awareness to be raised with regard to possible variations in the pattern of labour. The antenatal teacher must remain aware of changes in labour ward protocol and be able to give accurate, up-to-date information on the management of breech and multiple births, for example, and also guidance on the handling of such eventualities as occipitoposterior presentation. The following possibilities should be mentioned.

FIRST STAGE

The powers

Hypotonic contractions   Weak, infrequent hypotonic contractions with slow progress may necessitate oxytocin infusion.

Hypertonic contractions   Very powerful, frequent hypertonic contractions can lead to precipitate labour and delivery, and possible foetal distress. The mother should try to remain calm and relaxed, and will probably need to use lighter, quicker breathing.

Induction of labour   If the cervix is unripe, prostaglandins in one form or another will be administered. This may be followed by artificial rupture of the membranes (ARM) and intravenous oxytocin. Mothers must be warned that prostaglandins can give rise to unpleasant, 'colicky' contractions (TENS may be helpful), and that induced or accelerated contractions will be stronger, possibly more painful, and with shorter resting intervals than those of normal labour. In addition the woman may be immobilised by drips and monitoring equipment. She will need extra support and may require additional analgesia.

The passages

Cephalopelvic disproportion   The pelvis is too small for the foetus. Squatting may help overcome this in the second stage. (See p. 77.)

Cervical dystocia   There is failure of the cervix to dilate.

Placenta praevia   This can obstruct descent. (See p. 44.)

The passenger

Occipitoposterior presentations   These account for approximately 30% of labours. An aching, 'boring' backache will be apparent; it may persist between contractions. The first stage of labour can be long-drawn-out, with irregular contractions. The mother will be more comfortable in positions that take the weight of her uterus away from her back (e.g. prone kneeling);

between contractions, pelvic rocking and circling may help alter pressure within the pelvis. Deep back massage or pressure, heat or ice packs and resting in a warm bath may relieve discomfort. The foetus may rotate or be delivered face to pubes. An epidural anaesthetic may be necessary.

Breech birth Labour may be no different to a vertex presentation, but is likely to be actively managed with epidural anaesthetic in most hospitals. Pelvimetry and an ultrasound scan at 38 weeks will attempt to identify women whose babies will need delivery by elective caesarean section.

Malpositions or malpresentation These may be associated with an obstruction, such as disproportion or placenta praevia. (See pp. 75 and 43.)

SECOND STAGE

Episiotomy The possibility of this being used must be discussed antenatally.

Ventouse delivery This is the method of choice for assisted delivery as there is thought to be less risk of damage to mother and baby. A cap, attached to a suction pump, is fitted on to the baby's head whilst in the birth canal, and held in place by suction. Women should be shown the lithotomy position in antenatal classes.

Forceps delivery Most forceps deliveries today will be 'lift-out' procedures. It sometimes helps to describe the use of forceps as a 'shoe-horn', helping a baby out of a tight fit.

Caesarean delivery Women must be prepared for this eventuality; the reasons for both elective and emergency operations should be described. It is most important that women know how they may feel postoperatively, and how they can best help themselves in the immediate postpartum period.

THIRD STAGE

Lacerations and tears These must be mentioned, also the role of pelvic floor exercises in the relief of postpartum discomfort.

Retained placenta Although this is uncommon, women should be aware of its possible occurrence. A regional block or short general anaesthetic may be necessary to remove the placenta.

THE PUERPERIUM

By far the highest proportion of deliveries are 'natural', 'normal', happy events. There are, unfortunately, times when 'abnormal' events occur.

LOSS OF A BABY

Tragedies can and do occur. Little can be done to prepare a couple for coping with their baby's illness or death, yet the possibility of such a trauma occurring should be mentioned, and discussed if necessary, in antenatal classes.

MISCARRIAGE

Miscarriage is the spontaneous termination of a recognised pregnancy before 24 weeks. Although most miscarriages will take place before physiotherapists meet their clients, some of the women coming to 'early bird' classes may suffer a miscarriage and others admitted to gynaecological or antenatal wards because of miscarriage may be known to them. The emotional consequences of miscarriage can be great, and it is important that parents are allowed to mourn the loss. Sympathetic support is essential, both in hospital and once the woman returns home. Remarks such as 'Never mind, you can always have another baby', or 'You've got a lovely family already' can be wounding and do nothing whatsoever to help ease the pain.

PREMATURE DELIVERY AND ILL BABIES

Premature babies are those born after the 24th week and before the 36th week of pregnancy. With intensive care, the majority of tiny, early infants now survive, though some may have a physical or mental defect as a result. Mothers-to-be are encouraged to visit the special care baby unit (SCBU), in a positive way, to familiarise themselves 'just in case'. Those who are hospitalised because of the risk of preterm birth are often acclimatised to the unit before the birth.

An unexpected admission to SCBU can be emotionally traumatic for the parents. This, today, is acknowledged and the parents are given support in every way possible. There may be the added stress to the mother in terms of guilt. She may well feel a failure, and she may also be frightened to bond with a baby who might not survive.

Women need immense empathetic support at this time and often turn to their physiotherapist, whom they may already know from antenatal classes, for reassurance. Almost certainly, the last thing they will have a mind for will be themselves. Many will have had an elective caesarean delivery to prevent damage to very undersized or ill babies, and they will have to cope with their own physical discomfort as well as their emotional distress and anxiety.

STILLBIRTH

This is not an easy subject, but one that must be raised at some stage antenatally. Occasionally a baby dies in utero (IUD) and the mother will have to cope with the knowledge that her baby, although still within her body, is dead; sometimes a baby will die during the course of labour. A stillborn baby is one born dead after 24 weeks. This catastrophic experience is something no parent believes will happen to them, and one which the extended family often find very difficult to cope with themselves.

Very great care is taken today to make sure that the parents' wishes are adhered to. A humane, therapeutic approach is recommended. Parents are encouraged to look at and hold their baby, and photographs are often taken to provide a memento of the baby. It is essential that the parents are given the time or are encouraged to allow the normal grieving process to take its natural course. Bourne & Lewis (1983) described some of the long-term problems that may follow the inability to grieve properly. These include mothering difficulties with subsequent babies, marital problems, severe disturbances at anniversaries, puerperal psychosis in the next pregnancy and fracturing of the doctor–patient relationship. It is indeed difficult to bring this subject up in antenatal classes; some women have a superstitious inability to think of such things, but it must be mentioned. A women's health physiotherapist who is in contact with bereaved parents postnatally must not be ashamed of sharing their grief with them.

COT DEATH

There can be very little that is worse than the discovery that the baby who was apparently healthy a short while ago is cold and dead in its cot or pram. There are many causes for cot death or sudden infant death syndrome (SIDS). This unthinkable eventuality does happen and, while the women's health physiotherapist may not be in contact with women when it does, the subject often arises in antenatal classes if a woman has experienced this, or a stillbirth, previously.

Professionals undoubtedly have difficulty coping with the distress experienced by parents whose babies are ill, and more particularly with the despair of those whose babies are stillborn, handicapped or have died. Junior staff may not have received guidance in dealing with the anguish such tragic events can cause, and may well avoid bereaved and suffering parents. Great care should be taken when talking to these women avoiding thoughtless remarks, but at the same time not avoiding or ignoring them. Parents often appreciate the opportunity to talk about their lost baby and the events leading to the death, and, although this can be upsetting for others, the knowledge that it helps those who are distressed makes the discomfort easier to bear.

There are courses available for professionals who may be involved in the care of those who have experienced a miscarriage, stillbirth, neonatal, or cot death, and women's health physiotherapists would be well advised to attend.

References

Attwood R J 1976 Parturitional posture and related birth behaviour. Acta Obstetrica et Gynecologica Scandinavica 57(suppl):5–25.

Avery M D, Van Arsdale L 1987 Perineal massage: effect on the incidence of episiotomy and laceration in a nulliparous population. Journal of Nurse–Midwifery 32:181–184.

Balaskas J 1983 Active birth. Unwin Paperbacks, London.

Balaskas J, Balaskas A 1983 New life. Sidgwick & Jackson, London.

Balaskas J, Gordon Y 1990 Water birth. Thorsons, London.

BBC 2002 press release – health. Water birth drowning risk. Aug 5, http://news.bbc.co.uk.

Belsey E M, Rosenblatt D B, Liebermann B A et al 1981 The influence of maternal analgesia on neonatal behaviour: I. Pethidine. British Journal of Obstetrics and Gynaecology 88:398–406.

Billevicz-Driemel A M, Mime M D 1976 Long term assessment of extradural analgesia for the relief of pain in labour. II Sense of 'deprivation' after extradural analgesia in labour: relevant or not? British Journal of Anaesthesia 48:139–144.

Bonica J J 1984 Labour pain. In: Wall P D, Melzack R (eds) 'Pain its nature and treatment. Churchill Livingstone, London, p 377–392.

Bourne S, Lewis E 1983 Letter. British Medical Journal 286:145.

Bundsen P, Klas E 1982 Pain relief in labour by transcutaneous nerve stimulation (safety aspects) Acta Obstetrica et Gynecologica Scandinavica 61:1–5.

Bundsen P, Ericson K, Petersen L E et al 1982 Pain relief in labour by transcutaneous electrical nerve stimulation – testing of a modified stimulation technique and evaluation of the neurological and biochemical condition of the newborn infant. Acta Obstetrica et Gynecologica Scandinavica 61:129–136.

Calder A A 1982 Posture during labour and delivery. Maternal and Child Health 7:475–485.

Caldeyro-Barcia R 1979 Physiological and psychological bases for the modern and humanised management of normal labour. In: Recent Progress in Perinatal Medicine and Prevention of Congenital Anomaly, Tokyo, Ministry of Health and Welfare, p 77–96.

Caldwell J, Moffatt J R, Smith R L et al 1977 Determination of bupivacaine in human fetal and neonatal blood samples by quantitative single ion monitoring. Biomedical Mass Spectrometry 4:322–325.

Carroll D, Tramer M, McQuay H et al 1997 Transcutaneous electrical nerve stimulation in labour: a systematic review. British Journal of Obstetrics and Gynaecology 104:169–175.

Charles A G, Norr K L, Block C R et al 1978 Obstetric and psychological effects of psychoprophylactic preparation for childbirth. American Journal of Obstetrics and Gynecology 131:44–52.

Crawford J S 1972 Lumbar epidural block in labour: a clinical analysis. British Journal of Anaesthesia 44:66–74.

Crothers E 1992 Labour pains: A study of pain control mechanisms during labour. DPhil thesis, University of Ulster at Jordanstown.

Crothers E 1998 TENS for Labour pain. Journal of the Association of Chartered Physiotherapists in Women's Health 83:6–10.

Dick-Read G D 1942 Childbirth without fear. Heinemann, Oxford.

Eid P, Felisi E, Sideri M 1993 Applicability of homeopathic caulophyllum thalictroides during labour. British Homeopathic Journal 82:224–248.

Flynn A, Kelly J 1976 Continuous foetal monitoring in the ambulant patient in labour. British Medical Journal 2:842–843.

Freeman R M, Macaulay A J, Eve L et al 1986 Randomised trial of self-hypnosis for analgesia in labour. British Medical Journal 292:657–658.

Fusi L, Steer P J, Maresh M J A et al 1989 Maternal pyrexia associated with the use of epidural analgesia in labour. Lancet i:1250–1252.

Gardosi J, Hutson N, B-Lynch C 1989a Randomised controlled trial of squatting in the second stage of labour. Lancet ii:74–77.

Gardosi J, Sylvester S, B-Lynch C 1989b Alternative positions in the second stage of labour: a randomised controlled trial. British Journal of Obstetrics and Gynaecology 96:1290–1296.

Gauge S M, Henderson C 1992 CTG made easy. Churchill Livingstone, New York.

Haddad P F, Morris N F 1985 Anxiety in pregnancy and its relation to use of oxytocin and analgesia in labour. Journal of Obstetrics and Gynaecology 6:77–81.

Heardman H 1951 Physiotherapy in obstetrics and gynaecology. E & S Livingstone, Edinburgh.

Hobbs L 2001 The best labour possible. Books for Midwives, Oxford.

Holdcroft A 1996 The physiology and psychology of labour pain: a review. Journal of the Association of Chartered Physiotherapists in Women's Health 78:22–24.

Jackson D A 1988 Acupuncture. In: Wells P E, Frampton V, Bowsher D (eds) Pain: management and control in physiotherapy. Heinemann, Oxford, p 71–88.

Jacobson E 1938 Progressive relaxation. University of Chicago Press, Chicago.

Janke J 1999 The effect of relaxation therapy on preterm labour outcomes. Journal of Obstetrics, Gynaecology and Neonatal Nursing 28(3):255–263.

Johnson M I 1997 Women's health: transcutaneous electrical nerve stimulation in pain management. British Journal of Midwifery 5(7):402–405.

Kitzinger S 1987 Freedom and choice in childbirth. Viking, London.

Kleijnin J, Knischild P, Riet G 1991 Clinical trials of homeopathy. British Medical Journal 302:316–323.

Lenstrup C, Schantz A, Berger A et al 1987 Warm tub during delivery. Acta Obstetrica et Gynecologica Scandinavica, 66:709–712.

Low J, Reed A 2000 Electrotherapy explained. Principles and practice, 3rd edn. Butterworth Heinemann, Oxford.

Lupe P J, Gross T L 1986 Maternal upright posture and mobility in labour – a review. Obstetrics and Gynecology 67:727–734.

MacArthur A J, MacArthur C, Weeks S K 1997 Is epidural anaesthesia in labor associated with chronic low back pain? A prospective cohort study. Anesthesia and Analgesia 85(5):1066–1070.

MacArthur C, Lewis M, Knox E G et al 1990 Epidural anaesthesia and long-term back ache after childbirth. British Medical Journal, 301:9–12.

McIntosh J 1989 Models of childbirth and social class: a study of 80 working-class primigravidae. In: Robinson S, Thomson A M (eds) Midwives, research and childbirth vol 1. Chapman & Hall, London, p 189–214.

MacLean A D, Cardozo L 2002 Incontinence in women. RCOG Press, London.

Madders J 1998 Stress and relaxation – self help techniques for everyone Macdonald Optima, London.

Maternity Services Health Committee Report 1992 Winterton N. House of Commons Health Committee second report. HMSO, London.

Melzack R, Wall P D 1965 Pain mechanisms: a new theory. Science 150:971–979.

Melzack R, Taenzer P, Feldman P et al 1981. Labour is still painful after prepared childbirth training. Canadian Medical Association Journal 125:357–363.

Mitchell L 1987 Simple relaxation. John Murray, London.

Moir D D 1986 Pain relief in labour – a handbook for midwives. Churchill Livingstone, Edinburgh.

Morgan B M, Bulpitt C J, Clifton P et al 1982 Analgesia and satisfaction in childbirth (The Queen Charlotte's 1000 mother survey). Lancet ii:808–810.

Nielson M K 1983 Working class women, middle class women and models of childbirth. Social Problems 30:284–297.

Noble E 1981 Controversies in maternal effort during labour and delivery, I. Nurse–Midwifery 26:13–22.

Noble E 1983 Childbirth with Insight. Houghton Muffin, Boston.

Noble E 1996 Essential exercises for the childbearing year. John Murray, London.

Nursing and Midwifery Council 1998 Midwives code of practice. Introduction: definition of a midwife, section 3. www.nmc-uk.org

Nurses Midwives and Health Visitors (Midwives Amendment) Rule 1986. HMSO, London.

Payne R A 1995 Relaxation techniques: a practical handbook for the health care professional. Churchill Livingstone, Edinburgh.

Poschl U 1987 The vertical birthing position of the Trobrianders, Papua New Guinea. Australian and New Zealand Journal of Obstetrics and Gynaecology 27:120–125.

Prendiville W T, Harding J E, Elbourne D et al 1988 The Bristol third stage trial: 'active' versus 'physiological' management of the third stage. British Medical Journal 297:1295–1300.

Ramnero A, Hanson U, Kihlgren M 2002 Acupuncture treatment during labour – a randomized control trial. British Journal of Obstetrics and Gynaecology 109(6):637–644.

Randall M 1953 Fearless childbirth. Churchill, London.

RCM (Royal College of Midwives) 1994 Midwives code of practice. RCM, London.

RCOG (Royal College of Obstetricians and Gynaecologists) 2001 Statement No 1. Duley L M M Birth in water. www.rcog.org.

Richards M P, Bernal J F 1972 An observational study of mother–infant interaction. In: Jones (ed) Ethological studies of child behaviour. Cambridge University Press, Cambridge, p 129–197.

Roberts J E, Mendez-Bauer C, Wodell D A 1983 The effects of maternal position on uterine contractility and efficiency. Birth, 10:243–249.

Rosenblatt D B, Belsey E M, Liebermann B A et al 1981 The influence of maternal analgesia on neonatal behaviour. II. Epidural bupivacaine. British Journal of Obstetrics and Gynaecology 88:407–413.

Russell J G B 1982 The rationale of primitive delivery positions. British Journal of Obstetrics and Gynaecology 89:712–715.

Russell R, Dundas R, Reynolds F 1996 Long term backache after childbirth: prospective search for causative factors. British Medical Journal 312(7059):1384–1388.

Skelton I 1988 Two non-pharmacological forms of pain relief in labour. 1 Acupuncture. In: McKenna J (ed) Obstetrics and gynaecology. International perspectives in physical therapy 3. Churchill Livingstone, Edinburgh, p 129–140.

Sleep J 1989 Physiology and management of the second stage of labour. In: Bennett V R, Brown L K (eds) Myles' textbook for midwives. Churchill Livingstone, Edinburgh.

Smellie W 1974 A treatise on the theory and practice of midwifery. A facsimile printing of the 1752 edition. Ballière Tindall, London.

Sosa R, Kennell J, Klaus M et al 1980 The effect of a supportive companion on perinatal problems, length of labour, and mother–infant interaction. New England Journal of Medicine 303:597–600.

Stewart P, Calder A A 1984 Posture in labour: patients' choice and its effect on performance. British Journal of Obstetrics and Gynaecology 91:1091–1095.

Supper J 1998 Aromatherapy. The pregnancy book. Amberwood.

Vaughan K 1951 Exercise before childbirth. Faber, London.

Walsh D 1997 TENS – clinical application and related theory. Churchill Livingstone, New York.

Wells P E 1988 Manipulative procedures. In: Wells P E, Frampton V, Bowsher D (eds) Pain: management and control in physiotherapy. Heinemann, Oxford. p 181–217.

Williams R M, Thom M H 1980 A study of the benefits and acceptability of ambulation in spontaneous labour. British Journal of Obstetrics and Gynaecology 87:122–126.

Wuitchik M, Bakal D, Lipshitz J 1989 The clinical significance of pain and cognitive activity in latent labour. Obstetrics and Gynecology 73:35–42.

Further reading

Alexander J, Levy V, Roth C (eds) 1997 Midwifery in practice: core topics 2. Macmillan, London.

Balaskas J 1989 New active birth. Unwin Hyman, London.

Maclean A D, Cardozo L 2002 Incontinence in women. RCOG Press, London.

Sweet B, Tinan D 1997 Mayes' midwifery, 2nd edn. Baillière Tindall, London.

Wall P D, Melzack R (eds) 1989 Textbook of pain. Churchill Livingstone, Edinburgh.

Useful addresses

Active Birth Centre
25 Bickerton Road, London N19 5JT
Websites: www.activebirthcentre.com; www.homebirth.org.uk/homebirthlinks2htm

Cot Death Society
4 West Mills Yard, Kennet Road, Newbury, Berkshire RG14 5LP
Websites: www.SIDS.org; www.cotdeathsociety.org.uk

Miscarriage Association
c/o Clayton Hospital, Wakefield, West Yorkshire WF1 3JS
Website: www.agob71.care4free.net

National Childbirth Trust
Alexandra House, Oldham Terrace, Acton, London W3 6NH
Website: www.nctpregnancyandbabycare.com

SANDS (Stillbirth & Neonatal Death Society)
28 Portland Place, London W1B 1LY
Website: www.uk-sands.org

Twins and Multiple Births Association (TAMBA)
41 Fortuna Way, Grimsby, South Humberside DW37 95J
Website: www.tamba.org.uk

Useful websites

www.csp.org.uk
www.interactivecsp.org.uk
www.rcm.org.uk

www.rcog.org.uk
www.nelh.nhs.uk
www.nice.org.uk

Chapter 7

The postnatal period

Sue Barton

CHAPTER CONTENTS

Introduction 205
Postpartum physical/mental condition 206
Postnatal care 208

Immediate postnatal problems 221
Long-term postnatal problems 240

INTRODUCTION

It is in this period that the new mother's body begins its period of recovery and its return to 'normal'. However, the normality following the birth of a first baby will not be identical to that of prepregnancy. It will be a new normality: that of a mature female body that has undergone the process of pregnancy and birth. The pregnancy process will have resulted in a gradual change of body shape and function. At 'term' the woman sees a ripely swollen abdomen, enlarged breasts, possibly oedema of the face, hands and legs, deposits of fat on her upper arms, hips, buttocks and thighs, and even, perhaps, stretch marks. Although in the first few postpartum hours she may be thrilled with the softness and relative flatness of her abdomen, once she is mobile and sees herself in a mirror she will be confronted with a different image: an empty, sagging and still enlarged abdomen, maybe with 'tripe-like' wrinkled skin. As she moves, talks and laughs she may become aware of an almost complete lack of abdominal muscle control. She may have undergone an episiotomy, or a tear, which may be made more painful by bruising and oedema of the perineum; she may have difficulty in initiating micturition, or may experience retention of urine; she may also experience leakage when the intra-abdominal pressure is raised by coughing, sneezing or laughing.

Her immediate postpartum emotional state may be 'labile', varying between euphoric exhilaration, with an inability to sleep, and disillusioned disappointment (maybe as the result of unexpected medical intervention, or disappointment over the baby's gender) accompanied by total exhaustion.

The new mother, who may also be experiencing her first stay in hospital, may gradually become overwhelmed by the new responsibility of a totally dependent individual (the baby), may be feeling intense fatigue and may present with a lowered pain threshold. The women's health physiotherapist must be aware of this and complaints of 'aches and pains' should be appropriately assessed. Minor discomforts which would almost certainly not 'normally' affect the woman will respond well to physical treatment, delivered with empathy and understanding.

POSTPARTUM PHYSICAL/MENTAL CONDITION

Muscles and ligaments

The body's ligaments and collagenous connective tissue will still be softer and more elastic than prepregnancy and it will take 4 to 5 months (Calguneri et al 1982) for full recovery to take place.

The abdominal muscles, which will have been stretched, are now elongated, and a separation between the two recti abdominis muscles (known as a diastasis or divarification) will almost certainly be apparent in any woman who was at 'term' prior to labour. This can vary between a small vertical gap 2–3 cm wide and 12–15 cm long to a space measuring 12–20 cm in width and extending nearly the whole length of the recti muscles (Fig. 7.1). As a result, the entire abdominal 'corset' will be weakened

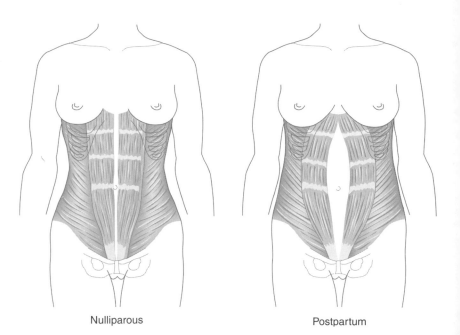

Figure 7.1   Diastasis recti abdominis.

Nulliparous

Postpartum

with very little apparent mechanical control. Those whose pregnancies necessitated prolonged inactivity, or those who habitually take very little exercise, will almost certainly find that their abdominal muscles are extremely weak. The combination of reduced mechanical control and increased elasticity of ligaments will render the back much more susceptible to injury. Those most at risk of developing a gross divarification are women with a narrow pelvis, those who carried large babies or who had a multiple birth, and multiparous women.

The pelvic floor will almost certainly be weaker than it was prior to the pregnancy. In addition to the stretching and trauma sustained during vaginal delivery, its muscles and connective tissue, will by the end of the 9 months have been partly responsible for continuously supporting as much as 6 kg of extra pelvic and abdominal weight (i.e. baby, uterus, placenta and liquor). The perineum itself will have been considerably stretched. It may also have been cut (episiotomy) or torn and then sutured, with resultant bruising and oedema. An additional trauma, and a cause of acute discomfort, may be the presence of haemorrhoids. The women's health physiotherapist should be aware that there may be neurological damage to the pelvic floor during the birthing process, resulting in temporary (days or weeks), longer-lasting (months) or permanent loss of sensation or muscle weakness, or both (Snooks et al 1984).

Oedema

Many women will complain of heavy, oedematous, aching legs, swollen feet and ankles in the immediate postpartum period that may not have been apparent before the baby was born. This may be unilateral or bilateral. The cause can only be speculated as probably prolonged pushing during labour, pelvic congestion, dysfunctional urinary tract, or the temperature on the postnatal ward.

Back pain

Back pain may not have been a symptom during pregnancy, but it frequently develops following the birth. The passage of the foetus through the pelvis, and the resultant stretching and movement of the lax joints, epidural anaesthesia, lithotomy position (especially if the legs were not placed and removed from the stirrups simultaneously), poor feeding or nappy-changing postures, tension and fatigue may all be causative factors.

Breasts

The breasts may become engorged, feel hot, full and painful (even up into the axilla where a 'tail' of breast tissue lies) when lactation begins on the 3rd or 4th postnatal day.

Psychological state

Psychologically a state of primary maternal preoccupation (Winnicot 1987) has been described; the mother's attention is fixed on her baby and she is often hypersensitive to every nuance of its behaviour. Her initial elation can change after a few days to a 'flattening' of her mood. She may well be more concerned with her baby than she is for herself. This could potentially be an issue for the physiotherapist attempting to achieve rehabilitative aims.

POSTNATAL CARE

ROUTINE CARE

The length of time before return to 'normal' activities has, over the years, become less and less, to the current expectation (if all has 'gone to plan') of a few days. The concern must be the wider picture (e.g. other children, a partner who works away, an elderly dependent relative, family support 200 miles away). Along with the reduction in the postnatal 'resting' period has come a much earlier discharge from care; the mother's return to home (if hospital delivery) may be within 6 hours following normal delivery, or up to 5 days if intervention has been necessary. The average discharge time is 24 to 72 hours, all being well.

There is a mandatory requirement for a midwife to attend the mother for the first 10 postpartum days as necessary; this can be extended to 28 days. The midwife will be concerned with the mother's well-being, the establishment of lactation, and the status of the baby. She will monitor the mother's vital signs, assess the mother's breasts, abdomen and perineum, check on the haemoglobin level at 24 hours postdelivery and repeat this at a later date as a preventative measure against anaemia.

If there are no complications the mother may not see a doctor during her hospital stay. The mother may need reassurance that this is 'normal' and that she would be referred to a doctor if it were found to be necessary.

ESTABLISHING BREASTFEEDING

The primary aim in the immediate postpartum period is the establishment of breastfeeding. For some women, and their babies, this is an instinctive activity. For others it will have to be 'learned', and for them to achieve it may require expert help, encouragement, support and advice from the midwife. Whenever, or however, the mother chooses to feed her baby it is essential that her positioning is not detrimental to her, physically. The baby must lie on its side facing the breast, not on its back with its head turned to the mother. Although it may be advantageous initially for the mother to lean forward so that the baby can be properly positioned on the breast, she should be encouraged to relax back on adequate support as soon as the baby is feeding well. A study by Ingram et al (2002) looked at a 'hands-off' (in terms of midwifery input) breastfeeding technique to see if it had any impact upon the success rate. They found it to be significant in empowering the mother and in improving breastfeeding rates.

Though not the province of the women's health physiotherapist, it can be useful to have some knowledge of the skills leading to successful feeding to avoid any conflicting advice. The nipple should be drawn into the baby's mouth against the hard palate, and the tongue should be underneath. To be properly 'fixed' on the breast the baby's mouth needs to be well open, with the chin resting on the breast and the lower lip curling down. The mother should not need to support her breast unless it is very heavy, in which case she can slip her hand underneath. Colostrum, and later milk, is drawn out by a wave of pressure from the baby's tongue on the lactiferous sinuses, and by a gentle, compressive milking action of the baby's lower jaw. This stimulates the 'let-down' or milk ejection reflex (oxytocin from the posterior pituitary causes the myoepithelial cells surrounding the alveoli to contract, thus releasing the milk). The response is highly individual: for some mothers it may give rise to sharp, needle-like pains in the breast, others may only feel a mild tingling sensation, and a proportion will feel nothing at all. This increase in oxytocin can also cause the characteristic 'after-pains' experienced by so many women during the early days of breastfeeding, as the uterus contracts in response to the variations in levels of the hormone. Deep breathing and conscious relaxation can help the mother cope with these discomforts.

The problems that may affect successful feeding are: engorgement, sore or cracked nipples, blocked ducts, and mastitis. The early days of breastfeeding can be the 'make or break' period for very many women trying to establish lactation. Good, consistent support from knowledgeable staff can help the mother overcome the early problems. Women's health physiotherapists, since they may be interacting with the woman at all stages of the puerperium, should remain informed with regard to protocols and regimens for breastfeeding so that they can support the woman as best as possible. By being aware, they are also able to 'refer on' appropriately should there be a need. It is essential to note that feeding 'takes priority' over any other activity. This can pose particular challenges to the physiotherapist who may be attempting to access the woman for treatment.

Pain management

The women's health physiotherapist must be alert to the pain of women who have experienced intervention deliveries, as this can often prevent the mother being relaxed and comfortable. A major role of the physiotherapist is to use her specialist knowledge, skills and experience to assist, in whatever way she can, for example with support, positioning, transcutaneous electrical nerve stimulation (TENS), ice, pulsed electromagnetic energy (PEME), pressure-relieving cushions, etc., to establish breastfeeding.

The postnatal check

It is traditional for a woman to be examined and assessed by a member of the obstetric team 6 weeks' postpartum. However, there is no good physiological reason for this timing apart from the fact that the uterus should have returned to its prepregnancy size by then, lochia should have ceased and any wounds healed. The negative side of this is if there are any problems they will already be well established.

The conscientious practitioner will also be interested in the mother's emotional state and how she and her family are adapting to, and coping with, the stress a new baby can bring, as well as her physical recovery. Women are extremely vulnerable postnatally; they have experienced a tremendous life change, and, particularly for primiparae, nothing will ever be quite the same for them again. Maintenance of links with support, in whatever form – groups, clinics, GP – are essential so that the woman does not feel abandoned. The women's health physiotherapist, is in an ideal position to reinforce issues and 'pick up' problems, at a postnatal reunion group.

The postnatal check should take the form of: assessing the mother's blood pressure, breasts, abdominal status, uterine involution and status of the cervix, performing a smear test, and discussing contraception and any problems that the woman may be experiencing. The women's health physiotherapist's knowledge, skills and experience are invaluable at this stage but it is unrealistic for her to expect to be present at all postnatal checks. Thus it is important that she ensures that those conducting the checks have the knowledge and skills to detect and refer for physiotherapy those women who may benefit. The physiotherapist will then be able to assess, treat and advise appropriately.

The women's health physiotherapist is not responsible for giving information and advice about contraception, but it is a subject that many women feel able to discuss in the friendly atmosphere of the antenatal or postnatal class. Misunderstandings, and 'young wives' tales', about this vitally important subject abound; physiotherapists, working with women of reproductive age, need access to up-to-date information about the methods, and their availability, that may be used to prevent conception in their area and need to be able to refer on.

It is essential that the physiotherapist make the important links with other health professionals in their area to, for example, learn from, know who to refer on to, acquire up-to-date leaflets, and invite to join postnatal group sessions. Time is 'well spent' with fellow professionals learning how they 'fit into' the wider picture. This time should not be seen as 'low' on the 'priority list', it should be an 'absolute' essential.

POSTNATAL PHYSIOTHERAPY

The role of the physiotherapist

The physiotherapist working in women's health, with her specialist skills, knowledge and treatment of neuromuscular–skeletal symptoms, ergonomics, rehabilitation and physiology of exercise, added to her knowledge and understanding of pregnancy, has an essential role to play in assessing, advising and treating women in the postnatal period. The physiotherapist is also ideally placed to encourage the new mother to discuss any concerns that she may have found difficult to discuss with other professionals (Brown & Lumley 1998).

The current trend is that of a shorter hospital stay. It is essential that the women's health physiotherapist deliver as effective a postnatal service as possible, taking into consideration the continuum from hospital to community. The approach and format will vary according to socioeconomic needs of the client group. Physiotherapists must be innovative in their approach, if they are to achieve their aims in today's ever-changing health-care structure. The principle aim should be to aid the body's recovery and encourage an interesting and safe exercise regimen (Livingstone 1998). Physiotherapists have to 'believe' in their role in order to justify their existence. Is there an evidence base supporting physiotherapy in postnatal care? We 'come up', yet again, with the issues around randomised controlled trials with this client group. A physiotherapist's strength is in 'core' skill and knowledge. The women's health physiotherapist's strength is in being able to use this in conjunction with specialist knowledge about this client group. An increasing number of postnatal units do not have a physiotherapy presence. Can this be justified? Can a leaflet replace the physiotherapist? Should all women be routinely seen by a physiotherapist? Is this cost effective? Should women be risk assessed? Who should do this? It is essential that all members of the 'team' are able to input their skills. Mørkved & Bø (2000) in their extensive work relating to pelvic floor muscle training clearly show, on many occasions, that only those women who had continued input from the physiotherapist beyond the puerperium were able to maintain muscle strength in a 1-year follow up. Östgaard & Anderson (1992) showed that 37% of women still had back pain 18 months postdelivery, thus reinforcing a true justification for physiotherapy intervention not only during, but beyond the pregnancy 'year'.

Suggestions for the physiotherapist's input include:

- the physiotherapist or midwife risk assesses the client from clear criteria formulated by the women's health physiotherapist
- group assessment/individual assessment is undertaken proportional to risk factors, e.g. medical, obstetric, social, etc.
- the physiotherapist or midwife implements the risk assessment following education (updated regularly) from the women's health physiotherapist
- a facility for referral is made available dependent upon risk assessment
- 'support' (not replacement) of all intervention is made available with literature.

Until we can fund having a 24-hour day or 7 days per week physiotherapy presence on the postnatal units, can we truly justify our existence on the unit? Should we be, therefore, redeploying some of our skills to other professionals, *or* should we be 'bidding' for more staff or hours? Unless physiotherapists are prepared to work the same hours as midwives there will have to be some rethinking of approaches.

Assessment

Ideally, the women's health physiotherapist should assess each new mother as soon as possible postdelivery, in order to determine her priority needs. It may be that another health professional can be equipped with the skills to perform a risk assessment, and the client, if necessary, be referred on to the physiotherapist for specialist assessment. Awareness of *needs*, proportional to mode of delivery, is essential. Thompson et al's (2002) study ($n = 1295$) showed for example, that:

Primiparas
- were more likely to report perineal pain, and sexual problems.

Caesarean births (when compared to unassisted vaginal deliveries)
- were more likely to suffer exhaustion and bowel problems
- reported less perineal pain and urinary incontinence
- were more likely to be readmitted.

Forceps and ventouse deliveries (when compared to unassisted vaginal deliveries)
- reported more perineal pain.

Symptoms to look out for/consider referral on (if non-physiotherapy assessment) include:

- diastasis recti abdominis
- inability to voluntarily contract the pelvic floor
- perineal pain or discomfort
- symphysis pubis pain or referred pain
- back pain or discomfort.

Individual versus group education

Immediate advice and initial exercise education is best given individually, and specific interventions, where needed, should be commenced as soon as possible.

In terms of cost effectiveness it may then be appropriate to continue intervention in a group. Individual suitability will be determined by assessment. The majority of new mothers enjoy the group approach, benefiting from the group interaction. The group approach is particularly useful in delivering the 'hidden curriculum' – the wealth of information and advice, over and above simple exercise instruction, which is particularly important for those women who did not attend antenatal classes.

Venue

The venue for the postnatal group can only be determined by what is available – within the ward, day room, or parent education room. Most women are happy to participate, but the physiotherapist must be sympathetic to the issues relating to the 'new mother', such as baby feeding, changing nappies, health concerns, waiting for the doctor, etc., and plan the group accordingly. If appropriate the baby can attend too. This provides an ideal opportunity to discuss functional activities, and their potential effect upon physical symptoms (e.g. baby feeding and nappy changing and their effect upon the neck and back). The benefits of group activity far outweigh the difficulties (sometimes) involved in getting a group together.

Exercise

The new mother should be encouraged to be mobile and therefore reduce the risk of circulatory and respiratory dysfunction. If she is confined to bed for a prolonged period of time then 'controlled', and deep breathing and 'vigorous' circulatory exercises should be encouraged.

Pelvic floor muscle exercises are valuable for their strengthening and pain-relieving properties. They will also speed healing by reducing oedema and encouraging good circulation. These exercises should be taught antenatally. Slow, progressive, controlled contractions along with fast, short, sharp contractions can be practised little and often. It will take all the physiotherapist's skill, and inventiveness to achieve compliance in this area. The mother may have an acutely painful perineum or several painful stitches and may be exceedingly reluctant to exercise these muscles. In order to gain compliance it is essential that the mother understand the benefits of performing the exercises. Three or four muscle contractions will begin to give relief by virtue of the pumping action on the local circulation. Finding the right starting position for the exercise will be the key to effectiveness (e.g. lean sitting increasing external proprioception anteriorally, sitting on a gymnastic ball, crook lying, standing, prone kneeling). A more efficient contraction may be obtained by contracting the transversus abdominis, before engaging the pelvic floor (Watkins 1998).

Two essential pieces of early advice to achieve physical relief and increase confidence are:

1. Contract the pelvic floor muscles (PFM) every time the intra-abdominal pressure increases, e.g. on coughing, sneezing or laughing.
2. Support sutures by applying pressure (hand) to the perineum using a sanitary pad or pad of soft toilet paper when defaecation is attempted, and until the perineal pain subsides.

For some women the memory of the postpartum perineal pain is more prominent than their memory of labour pain; it has been called the 'fourth stage of labour'!

The principles of muscle re-education should be followed when exercising the abdominal muscles, progressing from static (no joint movement), through to dynamic (joint movement). Commence at whichever starting position is appropriate for the individual, bearing comfort in mind, that is:

- side lying (s.ly.)
- prone lying (pr.ly.)
- crook lying (ck.ly.)
- sitting (sitt.)
- standing (st.).

The anterior abdominal wall should be drawn in on expiration, thereby increasing muscle tone.

Then progress through to static contraction *plus* active range of movement, that is:

- pelvic tilt
- flexion, in progressing ranges, of the lumbar spine.

It is important to include all muscles of the lumbar spine. Richardson et al (1998) describe the importance of the transversus abdominis and multifidus as stabilisers of the lumbar spine and these should therefore be acknowledged in an exercise regime. Looking (at the movement) and feeling (hand to abdomen) can increase facilitation of the contraction. It is important to emphasise that once the exercises have been learnt it is not necessary for them to be practised whilst lying down; they can be integrated into the daily routine, for instance whilst waiting for the kettle to boil. This increases compliance.

A static abdominal contraction followed by pelvic tilting, in crook lying, can aid the relief of 'after-pains' or backache. The speed of action can be varied from a slow 'hold' to a tilt/relax.

Rhythmical gluteal contractions may help ease the pain from haemorrhoids or bruising.

THE EARLY POSTNATAL CLASS

Setting up a class

Currently it is virtually impossible to set up a class within the hospital setting, but there is no reason why this could not be achieved in the community. The postnatal woman requires input from the physiotherapist, the expert in human function, in order to return to normal functioning and enabling her to 'manage' her 'new' life. The women's health physiotherapist will know her own 'patch' best and needs to determine the possibility of having a postnatal class in the community. An advice leaflet can greatly assist the scheme.

As with the 'setting up' of any class the client group should be taken into account. Are all individuals 'happy' with being in a group situation or are some likely to feel threatened? Appropriateness for inclusion should be assessed.

Teaching points

The arrangement of the group should enable all participants to: physically take part, interact with each other and the physiotherapist, see the physiotherapist for the non-physical aspects of the class, and be seen by the physiotherapist.

The starting position should minimise risk to participants, but enable participation. Participants may be sitting, standing or lying. The points to be covered in each position include:

Sitting

- *Well supported* back and comfortable perineum
- *Exercises* in sitting for posture, abdominals, pelvic floor muscles
- Regular reference to *daily activities* in sitting, e.g. feeding baby, in order to minimise symptoms.

Standing

- *Stable base of support* – leaning against something to increase stability, e.g. wall, back of chair
- *Appropriate footwear* – mules are *not* a good idea
- *Exercises* in standing for posture and abdominals; this can reduce the abdominal girth by up to 12 cm, especially if also standing tall; pelvic floor muscle exercises, trunk side flexion ('hiphitching').

Lying

- Pillows and wedges for *support* and exercise progression, plus mats (if there is no carpet) or rolls of disposable 'couch covering' paper (if there is carpet)
- *Teach* checking for separation of recti abdominis muscles
- *Raise awareness* regarding 'at risk' movements or exercises – strong side flexions and trunk rotations while lying should be omitted until the anterior abdominal wall is strong enough to allow these movements without shearing
- *Exercises* – abdominal muscle
  - abdominal muscle contraction, emphasis on transversus abdominis, increasing length of 'hold', with pelvic tilting, progressing to include active trunk movement, e.g. head raising and then head and shoulders raising
  - raise awareness regarding 'abdominal doming'

- posture, pelvic floor muscles
- all could be performed in the bath
- **NB** *Care must always be taken, with respect to starting position and exercises, with any woman experiencing symptoms of symphysis pubis dysfunction (SPD).*

Relaxation

If appropriate the class may be completed by a short period of relaxation. Relaxation techniques can be used successfully to reduce tension and maternal fatigue (Sapsford et al 1999). This element of the class should be included *only* if the physiotherapist has the appropriate knowledge and skills. It is *essential* that the women be 'risk assessed' as to their suitability for this element of the class. Relaxation therapy has the ability to enhance emotions and the physiotherapist must be absolutely sure that she has the skills to 'handle' an exacerbation of emotion, or know who or how to refer on to another professional if the situation arises. Relaxation therapy, in the wrong hands, is potentially dangerous.

The environment must allow for comfort of the participants – sufficient space for adequate pillow use, appropriate temperature, etc., and for it not to be a 'problem' if participants fall asleep. Simple relaxation suggestions linked with deep, calm, slow breathing will often result in some women falling asleep – this usefully demonstrates their intense fatigue and the importance of occasional power naps once they return home. The skill of relaxation also facilitates the 'let-down' reflex for breastfeeding (Sapsford et al 1999).

Educational principles

It is accepted that individuals learn:

- best from taking part, i.e. *doing* the exercise (if space, time, ability of the client allows); they are less likely to be afraid to do the exercises at home if they have 'tried' them under supervision
- next best from *watching* (if space, time, ability of the client does not allow participation); a demonstration of the exercise, with visual aids in the form of charts, diagrams, models, will increase the mothers' understanding of the purpose behind performing the exercises and therefore aid compliance
- least best from *listening* alone (last resort in terms of compliance)
- and all retain information better if there is a *combination* of the above and it is supported by *literature*.

Advice with regard to everyday functional activity such as baby bathing, lifting or carrying, cot or pram heights (Figs 4.4, 4.5, 7.2) etc. should be given by the expert – the physiotherapist. The physiotherapist has the knowledge and skills to teach the mother approaches that will minimise the effects on the musculoskeletal system. It is essential the women's health physiotherapist 'does her homework' – researches the 'in vogue' products on the market and is prepared with appropriate advice for the parents, for example on baby slings (Fig. 7.2) or car seats.

It is essential that the mothers be 'educated' not 'instructed' for the exercise programme or advice to be meaningful and lifelong.

Figure 7.2 Maintenance of good posture is essential at all times.

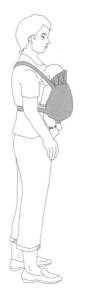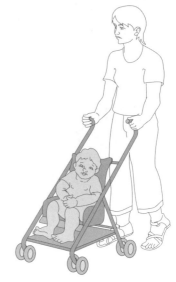

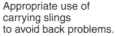

Appropriate use of
carrying slings
to avoid back problems.

Pram handles at the
correct height
to avoid back problems.

Teaching ergonomic principles

The new mother can experience cumulative physical trauma as a result of her new role. It is essential the women's health physiotherapist educate the mother in relation to ergonomic principles.

Sitting (sitt.)

- Thighs fully supported (at least ⅔) and horizontal – the sitting surface should *not* extend as far as the popliteal fossa to avoid potential impingement
- Feet flat on the floor, stable base of support, fully supported
- Weight evenly distributed over both buttocks – sitting on ischial tuberosities – 'sore' perineum/haemorrhoids may require 'cushioning'
- Sitting surface depressable to allow for pressure distribution
- Trunk fully supported maintaining natural spinal curves.

Standing (st.)

- Feet slightly apart, and angled (lateral rotation at the hips following 'true' line of femur) slightly (*not* like a ballerina!)
- Weight evenly distributed over both feet
- 'Soft' knees (*not* flexed, just 'off' full extension – do not 'lock' them back)
- Shoulders relaxed (*not* retracted or elevated)
- Arms held loosely at the side
- Maintain natural curves of the spine
- Head in line with trunk.

Lying (ly.)

- Fully supported (s.ly., pr.ly., ly.) with pillows – head, knees, low back, etc.
- Legs *not* crossed.

Figure 7.3 Suggested 'comfort' positions for feeding.

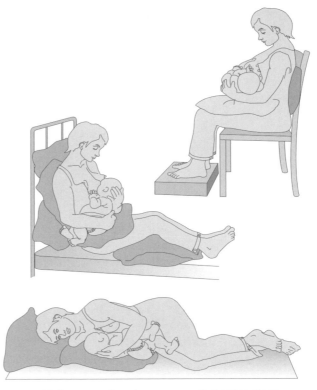

Mothers are strongly recommended not to sleep with baby in the bed

Kneeling (kn.)
- Avoid sustained, isometric trunk flexion, rotation
- Try to keep movement within the sagittal plane
- Perform activitites at an appropriate height surface

High. kn.
- Knees hip-width apart
- Knees directly under hips – maybe on a cushion
- Maintain natural spinal curves

Kn. sitt.
- Bilateral – maybe cushion to the back of the knees

½ Kn. sitt.
- Unilateral – sitting on one heel, other hip forward flexed with foot flat on the floor.

Feeding   The new mother may be feeding (Fig. 7.3) her baby eight or more times each day. However, what should be a happy, relaxed, shared time between mother and baby has the potential for resulting in *musculoskeletal symptoms* if she is positioned inappropriately. The women's health physiotherapist is the best person to teach the mother with regard to 'good' positioning, but the midwife is the person who is best able to reinforce this on a regular basis, so sharing of knowledge and skills between

Figure 7.4 Suggested positions for nappy changing, and maintaining good posture.

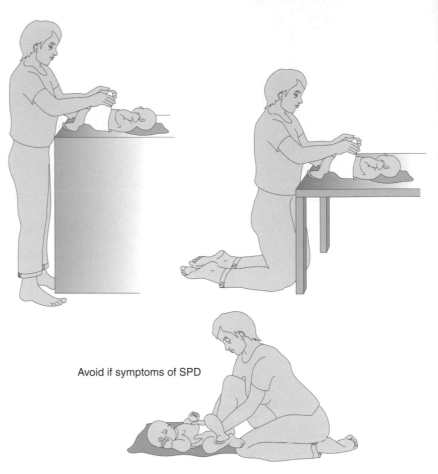

Avoid if symptoms of SPD

the professions is essential for the benefit of the mother. Whether the mother is breastfeeding or bottle feeding, and whether in sitting or lying, ergonomic principles must be followed to avoid musculoskeletal discomfort, or maybe even pain. She may be there for some time!

Nappy changing

Nappy changing (Fig. 7.4) is another activity that can result in incapacitating pain. A mother can change a nappy 10 times a day or more, and it is therefore considered a frequent activity. Frequent activities carry *musculoskeletal risk* if ergonomic principles are not followed. Positions that increase the risk to the mother should be avoided (e.g. st., knees extended, trunk flexed, and twisted). It is the role of the physiotherapist to teach not only the mother but other health professionals so that they are able to reinforce the principles. Many hospitals today insist that nappy changing is carried out in the baby's cot. The physiotherapist should be involved in the development of 'policies' that not only follow infection control guidelines, but also reduce the physical risk to the mother.

Suggested *positioning* for nappy changing could be:

• sitting (see ergonomic principles, p. 216) and changing on the lap
• standing (see ergonomic principles, p. 216) and changing on a surface of appropriate height (Fig. 7.4)

- kneeling (see ergonomic principles, p. 216) and changing on the floor (Fig. 7.4) or surface of appropriate height.

Bath time

Bath time should be 'fun' for all parties, but can be another source of *musculoskeletal problems.* Risk factors are as follows:

- Low baby bath on a stand resulting in the high-risk, isometric, trunk-flexed position
- A bath that requires filling, resulting in the carrying of water in jugs or buckets, and then the carrying of the bath full of water in order to empty it!

A variety of baby baths are now available to suit most requirements (e.g. those that can rest over an adult-sized bath so that the mother can kneel alongside). Other options could be to use a special washing-up bowl (non-slip) on the kitchen draining board, or the well-cleaned bathroom hand basin (if large enough).

If the mother has the knowledge of ergonomic principles she can hire or purchase something that is appropriate for her (and all others keen to bath the baby) thereby minimising the musculoskeletal risk.

Points to remember

- It is important that the women's health physiotherapist has a *belief* in what she is doing, has the ability to *motivate* and *encourage* the mother, and is, above all, *enthusiastic.*
- Many women will not want to exercise, and may have to be persuaded to participate.
- Do not burden new mothers with too many exercises – *prioritise* the essentials.
- Encourage *movement.* Reassure them that the stitches will not 'pop' if they move about.
- Although birth is usually a joyous experience, stillbirths, abnormal or ill babies and neonatal deaths do occur. These are difficult for all staff but, especially for the young and inexperienced. The women's health physiotherapist should establish the priorities and teach the mother exercises that are *appropriate.* She should not be afraid of *empathising* with parents in their anxieties or even joining them in their grief.

Postnatal 'home' exercises

To improve circulation during the first few weeks the new mother should try to have a daily *walk* with her baby in a sling or a pram: the change of scene will also benefit her emotionally. *Pelvic floor muscle exercises* can be done around the house. They should become routinely part of other activities. Reminders may be needed: post-it notes in obvious places – inside kitchen cupboards, by the phone, in the nursery.

Only when the recti muscles are closing satisfactorily can *abdominal exercise* be progressed to include side flexion and rotation exercises as well as 'curl-downs' (curling down halfway from crook sitting, holding briefly, and returning to the upright position), if the mother's perineum is not too painful.

Rest and relaxation are essential and should be continued on a regular basis whether it be in a chair, on the bed, or on the floor.

Postnatal exercise classes in the community

Individual *assessment* with regard to appropriateness for attendance at a postnatal class is essential. The 'status' of the mother's abdominal and pelvic floor muscles should be such that she is able to progress exercise activity. Perineal pain, stress incontinence and backache are the most common conditions that may still be giving problems. Ideally the women's health physiotherapists in the acute sector should *refer*, where necessary, to their colleagues in the community. In general, women wish to attend a postnatal exercise class because they have an issue with *body image*, i.e. abdomen, hips and thighs, or feel a need for *companionship* and *support*. The long-term benefits, hopefully, of attending a postnatal class, will also be an improvement in the 'bits' they cannot see (i.e. their pelvic floor and vagina). The 'hidden' agenda of the classes is the *group interaction* between women, all experiencing a particularly 'special' time in their lives, that can also be very daunting and stressful on occasions. Just being together and sharing can be a very worthwhile outcome.

The classes, if appropriate, should include exercises with the babies. The structure of the class should be *flexible*; for example if the women appear particularly tired then perhaps emphasis can be placed upon *relaxation*, whereas if they appear full of energy then there can be a concentration on *exercise*. Time should be 'built in' to the class to enable feeding, nappy changing, a drink and a chat. Useful topics can be brought into the '*chat*' so that it becomes semistructured and informative, for example: fatigue, depression, anxiety, loss of libido, support groups.

Return to sport and exercise

Even the athlete, dancer or dedicated sportswoman will have reduced the intensity and amount of exercise by the end of her pregnancy. After the postnatal period of recovery and gradual restoration of muscle strength, these women will be ready to return to their prepregnancy activity. Where the prepregnancy level of activity considerably decreased prior to delivery, a *gradual reintroduction* of sport and training schedules is essential. This is particularly important for the non-athletic woman who feels that she should be 'doing something' once her baby has settled down; she should be discouraged from joining a mass aerobics class at the local leisure centre, jogging long distances, or cycling many miles if she has not exercised for a long time. It is important that qualified instructors who understand the limitations of the postpregnancy woman supervise classes and activities – a communicative role here for the women's health physiotherapist. Swimming, an ideal activity for the fit and for those hoping to become fitter, may be resumed after the postnatal check.

Baby massage

In the same way that adults *enjoy*, and feel *relaxed* by, skilful massage, many babies respond with pleasure to simple stroking or kneading techniques. In the East and amongst many ethnic groups in this country, baby massage is practised regularly. In its simplest form, most mothers include a stroking movement when smoothing oil into their baby's skin following a bath or nappy change. A short baby massage session could enjoyably be included in a mother and baby exercise class or postnatal group; while massage is most successfully performed on the naked body (the room would have to be very warm in this case, and plenty of nappies available), it is perfectly possible to teach this form of massage where the baby is wearing a stretch, all-in-one suit. In some regions there are specific baby massage classes. Payne (1999) suggests that a baby massage class may in fact reduce the possibility of *postnatal depression*. Simple effleurage and stroking over the babies' backs, chests, abdomens, arms, legs, hands and feet can be taught, and practised by the group together. Mothers are probably most comfortable sitting on the floor with their backs supported by a wall, and baby lying across their lap. If baby starts to cry, for a feed or because of a wet nappy, and is therefore uncomfortable, the mother should feel sufficiently confident to halt the massage session. At home, mothers should be encouraged to massage their babies at appropriate times (i.e. when the baby is not hungry, and therefore likely to enjoy it). If baby is distressed despite having been fed, has a clean nappy and has been winded, a simple back and abdominal massage can sometimes soothe. Suitable oil can be used sparingly. The most important factor to remember is it should be enjoyed by both the baby and the masseur (mother, father, grandparent, friend), and that it should not become a chore. Experienced physiotherapists can easily adapt conventional massage strokes to their tiny clients.

Studies into sudden infant death syndrome (Gantley & Davies 1993) suggest that by increasing the 'sensory rich environment' its incidence may be reduced – another 'plus' for massage.

Mother and baby *postnatal exercise classes* in the community provide an excellent forum for introducing education on preventative health care, not only for the mother and her baby, but for all the family. This has the capacity to prevent, or alleviate, such 'problems' as backache, mild prolapse, stress incontinence and osteoporosis in later life. This education is of *great* importance and is an investment for their future.

IMMEDIATE POSTNATAL PROBLEMS

PERINEAL DYSFUNCTION/PAIN

Visible problems can include bruising, oedema, labial tears, haematoma, tight stitches, infection, breakdown of suturing and haemorrhoids. These may or may not cause varying degrees of pain. A vaginal haematoma will not be visible, but may, nevertheless, be intensely painful.

The physiotherapist has much skill, knowledge and experience in the treatment of pain, swelling, bruising, haematoma and infection. The women's health physiotherapist has in-depth knowledge of anatomy, physiology and human mechanics, and the changes that take place during and after pregnancy. Who better to treat these symptoms following a complete and thorough assessment?

The physiotherapist *must* always 'bear in mind' her treatment aims. For example, 'Physical' techniques might be used with the aim of promoting wound healing. The perineum is highly vascular and therefore ultrasound or PEME (megapulse) are unlikely to accelerate the process. Attempts to show objectively that ultrasound or PEME increase the rate of healing of the traumatised perineum have been inconclusive (Grant et al 1989). McLachlan (1998), however, suggests that pulsed shortwave will help to reduce swelling and inflammation. There are experienced women's health physiotherapists who will use these modalities, following a thorough assessment of the woman. The woman may be having great problems voiding owing to discomfort and fear and, by increasing the vascularity to the area even more by using 'physical' modalities, the therapist may 'speed' the physiological processes along just enough to avoid 'different' problems developing.

Treatment

Pelvic floor muscle exercises

One of the most physiologically sound self-help techniques for the relief of perineal pain must be the repeated contraction and relaxation of the voluntary component of the pelvic floor musculature. The resulting pumping action assists venous and lymphatic drainage and the removal of traumatic exudate, thus relieving stiffness and restoring function. It is also theoretically possible that the muscle activity triggers the 'pain-gating' mechanism and may also stimulate the production of endogenous opiates. Pain tends to be maximal with the first contraction and decreases with repetition as oedema disperses. It is essential that the woman is comfortable whilst performing the exercises. The appropriate position will be proportional to symptoms. Possible positions are: stride crook lying, prone lying, stride standing, or stride sitting.

Functional Activity

It is essential that the women find comfortable positions for feeding, relaxation and sleep, and they should be encouraged to experiment using pillows and pressure-relieving cushions. Pain relief can occur rapidly if positioning is appropriate.

Ice

The pain-relieving effect of cold therapy is well documented (Knight 1989, Lee & Warren 1978, Lehmann & DeLateur 1982, Palastanga 1988). Moore & James (1989) compared three topical analgesic agents in the treatment of post episiotomy pain (Epifoam, Hamamelis water and ice). All three agents were equally effective on the 1st day, although one-third of the women derived no benefit from any agent. Ice, however, gave better pain relief thereafter. It is an analgesic therapy which is readily available in hospital and at home, and is certainly the cheapest – a factor which must be taken into consideration in the current economic climate. The following are suitable techniques for the woman whose perineal pain is interfering with functional activities:

- Crushed ice, wrapped in damp disposable gauze or a disposable washcloth/surgical wipe, or put into a plastic bag (thus avoiding drips) and wrapped similarly, and applied to the affected area for 5–10 minutes (it should be remembered that plastic acts as an insulator and therefore effectiveness is reduced). Placing the ice in a 'split' damp sanitary towel is also an option. Ice packs specifically designed for the perineum are now available. The woman should be in a comfortable position, perhaps half-lying.

- Ice cube massage – an ice cube, held in a tissue, and used by the woman herself whilst in bed or whilst sitting over a toilet can give excellent pain relief.

The benefit of self-treatment is that it can be implemented when convenient, the woman knows the exact site of her pain, and can therefore gain most relief. The woman *must* always be warned of the dangers of using ice therapy, however, particularly since sensation may be diminished owing to 'birth trauma'. Ice packs or ice massage can be continued for as many days as they are helpful.

Warm baths and bidets   These are used principally to promote good hygiene. Although not strictly physiotherapeutic, most women experience relief of pain and a relaxed feeling of well-being following the traditional use of a warm bath. Women should be actively discouraged from staying in the bath too long, however, as traumatised skin quickly becomes 'soggy'. Warm water can also be poured over the perineum from a jug while the woman is sitting on the toilet. This eases the burning sensation some women experience when urinating, if they have sustained lacerations. The use of a bidet, as well as promoting hygiene, can also be soothing.

Ultrasound   Ultrasound has been shown to increase tissue temperature, which in turn leads to increased blood flow and increased repair (McMeehen 1994). It should be used in accordance with agreed local infection control procedures; each hospital should have a written protocol for its use and this should be checked on a regular basis.

Following assessment, treatment should commence as soon as possible after delivery and should continue twice daily until the woman is able to carry out functional activities without pain. The treatment is best given in the crook-lying or side-lying position as it is most important to be able to see the perineum and buttock area clearly. Using a cotton-wool swab and warm water, and swabbing from front to back, any lochia should be gently washed away. Using an appropriate cover, the ultrasound head is then applied through a coupling gel medium, and in accordance with local infection control guidelines. Normally pulsed ultrasound is used for its analgesic and exudates-removing properties, although it has been shown that the thermal and non-thermal effects of ultrasound are beneficial to all stages of tissue repair (Dyson 1987). For an initial treatment, a dosage of 3 MHz, 0.5 W/cm and 2 minutes per head-sized area of trauma was used by McIntosh (1988). It is thought unnecessary to increase the dosage if there is improvement in pain and decrease in swelling. Where the pain is too intense for direct contact a condom can be successfully used as a water bag – with couplant applied to the patient's skin, the bag and the treatment head. This also makes the application of ultrasound to haemorrhoids much more comfortable.

Pulsed electromagnetic energy

This technique is known variously as pulsed short-wave diathermy, pulsed high-frequency energy or pulsed electromagnetic energy (PEME). Both Bewley (1986) and Frank (1984) have described its pain-relieving and therapeutic effects for bruising, large haemorrhoids, extensive suturing, postcaesarean birth haematomas, and inflamed or infected wounds, in the early postnatal period. Its 'no touch' mode of operation must make it particularly suitable in the puerperium. The dosage usually used is mild; its exact parameter must depend on which machine is used. Acute conditions are said to respond well to a pulse width of 40–65 pulses with a repetition rate of 10–220 pulses per second (Low 1988), and it is suggested that treatment should be given at least twice a day, initially for 5 minutes and progressing to 20 minutes at a time. There is a variety of published opinions as to dosage and length of treatment; the women's health physiotherapist who is able to use this modality for postnatal problems will need to keep an open mind and be alert to newly published trials and their results.

GENITOURINARY DYSFUNCTION/PAIN

Incontinence

There is a close relationship between the pelvic organs, therefore an alteration in urinary and faecal control can occur following difficult forceps deliveries; even a normal birth can result in voiding problems. Thompson et al (2002), in a study of 1295 women, showed that bowel and bladder problems generally resolved between 8 and 24 weeks postpartum. Women who had caesarean births reported more bowel problems compared with those having unassisted vaginal deliveries, but reported less urinary problems. Fratton & Jacquetin (1999) suggest that the relationship between first childbirth and obstetric trauma is strong and may contribute to the development of stress incontinence (urinary and anal), and genital prolapse. Mørkved & Bø (2000) clearly show that physiotherapeutic input in the immediate postpartum period is effective in increasing pelvic floor muscle strength and reducing urge incontinence.

Faecal incontinence

In a study carried out on women who delivered vaginally between 1996 and 1997, Signorello et al (2000) showed that those women who experienced a midline episiotomy had a higher risk of faecal incontinence at 3 and 6 months postpartum compared with women with an intact perineum. Compared with spontaneous laceration, episiotomy tripled the risk of faecal incontinence at 3 months and 6 months. The effect of the episiotomy was independent of other influencing factors. It used to be thought that this highly embarrassing and distressing condition was only due to direct sphincter division or muscle stretching. However, research by Snooks et al (1985) suggests that this incontinence can result from damage to the innervation of the pelvic floor muscles during perineal descent in the second stage of labour. It is more common in women who have experienced difficult instrumental deliveries and in multiparae. Neuropraxia normally resolves by 2 months, but some women will be left with a long-term problem. Explanation, encouragement and pelvic floor muscle exercise instruction is the role of the women's health physiotherapist in the early treatment of a condition which most women are too ashamed to discuss. Rarely, a rectovaginal fistula following a fourth degree laceration may be the cause of apparent faecal incontinence. It is essential for the women's health physiotherapist to check whether a woman suffering from this condition is in fact able to initiate a pelvic floor contraction, and to follow her up if this is not the case (see Ch. 12).

Stress incontinence

Stress incontinence is a frequent early postpartum problem. It can be caused by distension and weakening of the pelvic floor musculature and connective tissue, and also by damage to their innervation (Allen et al 1990, Snooks et al 1985). Education with regard to structure and function is essential if the mother is to comply with a rehabilitation programme for her pelvic floor. Kegel (1951) suggested 200 contractions per day. It is more likely today to suggest that the mother contract her pelvic floor muscles a little and often, using both slow and fast contractions, whenever she can remember, aiming to increase the number, and length of hold, gradually. Counter-bracing these muscles whenever there is an increase in intra-abdominal pressure, as in coughing or nose blowing, can prevent leakage where the muscles are not strong enough. This knowledge will help increase confidence (see Ch. 11).

Constipation

Constipation is extremely common during the early puerperium and its cause is varied. It may be the result of weak abdominal muscles – a large diastasis recti abdominis would compound this, together with relaxation of the smooth intestinal muscles, the change from home to hospital diet (lack of fibre and fluid), iron medication, and the fear of increasing perineal pain or reopening the episiotomy wound or tears. As well as a full explanation of these causes (understanding a problem is often halfway to solving it), and their remedies, the suggestion that the perineum is supported with a pad of soft toilet paper during defaecation can be of great help. It should be impressed on the new mother that improving the strength of her abdominal muscles will help in relieving constipation. It is important that women realise that lifelong constipation can lead to the 'descending perineum' syndrome. Henry et al (1982) described this, and pointed out that repeated strain can lead to urinary stress incontinence and faecal incontinence (see Chs 11 and 12).

Urinary retention

It is most important that all health professionals involved in the care of the postpartum woman be fully aware of the problem a newly delivered woman may be experiencing in initiating and completing the act of micturition, and therefore showing symptoms of urine retention. There is some evidence to show that a single episode of bladder overdistension can produce chronic changes as a result of irreversible damage to the detrusor muscle (Toozs-Hobson & Cutner 2001). If retention of urine should occur, catheterisation can be necessary and the mother may need to have an indwelling catheter for several days.

Urinary retention can be caused by a prolonged second stage of labour, a large baby, instrumental delivery, or total/dense block from epidural. The urethra, being embedded in the anterior wall of the vagina, may be traumatised and unable to function normally. The mother may be too inhibited by pain, and fear, to allow voiding to commence. Apart from reassurance and simple explanation, the women's health physiotherapist can offer practical help with this worrying and uncomfortable situation. Frequent, gentle, pelvic floor contractions will reduce oedema and pain and give a feeling of normality. Controlled breathing with relaxation on expiration, while sitting on the toilet, may prove successful. Some women find that they are able to empty their bladder while sitting in a warm bath, or whilst having a warm shower.

Urgency

Sometimes postpartum urinary control can be affected by urgency, an increased feeling of needing to empty the bladder. This may result in being unable to reach the toilet before the bladder empties spontaneously. It is *essential* that symptoms are 'picked-up' early, and that urinary tract infection is eliminated. The important issue is 'is micturition "normal" for that woman?' Trauma to the nerve supply to the detrusor and the urethral sphincter mechanism, during labour or delivery, are possible causes. The initial suggestion from the women's health physiotherapist should be for frequent pelvic floor muscle exercises, and the mother's ability to perform this movement correctly must be checked. Contraction of the levator ani muscle directly inhibits the sacral micturition centre (McGuire 1979) and the voiding urge may be controlled.

Postpartum physiotherapy is *essential* in order to assess, treat and manage dysfunctions of the genitourinary tract.

MUSCULOSKELETAL DYSFUNCTION/PAIN

Diastasis recti abdominis

This is a common condition that varies in severity from woman to woman. It will mechanically interfere with the supportive and expulsive function of the abdominal wall unless it is recognised and treated. Noble (1980) and Boissonnault & Kotarinos (1988) both describe the condition, which can appear in pregnancy or be caused by bearing down in the second stage of labour. In some women gross diastasis will actually be visible when they try to sit up or lie down. A wide ridge of bulging tissue resembling a 'bowler hat', becomes apparent when the recti muscles are working actively against gravity, particularly when supine. The diastasis may simply extend a few centimetres above and below the umbilicus and only be 2–3 cm wide, it may only appear below the umbilicus, or it may involve the major part of the linea alba, extending from just below the xiphisternum to just above the symphysis pubis and can be as much as 20 cm in width. The size of the diastasis influences function and therefore postnatal care. It is therefore essential that all newly delivered mothers are assessed for diastasis. This can be performed by the physiotherapist or other health professionals provided the latter are skilled in the technique. The physiotherapist has a vital role to play in the education of other health professionals to enable reinforcement of rehabilitation principles in their absence.

Assessment technique

With the woman in crook lying (one pillow), the physiotherapist faces her and places the fingertips of one hand widthways on the abdomen, across the midline just below the umbilicus. The woman is asked to raise her head off the pillow and reach with her hands toward her feet. The medial edges of the two rectus abdominus muscles are then palpable and the distance between them is measurable in finger-widths. The length of any separation is also noted. The procedure is repeated palpating above the umbilicus. The woman is encouraged to assess herself, palpating with one hand reaching with the other. It is important to explain that the gap is not dangerous – nothing will fall out. However careful re-education to gain closure is crucial as the linea alba does not regenerate but strong muscles compensate for this and assist good functioning of the abdominal wall.

Re-education

It is important that there is a constant awareness of the abdomen, in all positions. Educate the woman with regard to structure of the abdominal wall and the changes that have taken place. It is now time for the elongated, separated, lax muscles to shorten, come closer together and tighten.

Technique

- *Abdominal retraction* – transversus abdominis; repeat frequently and integrate into all the activities of daily living
- *Pelvic tilting* – a dynamic progression, can be taught in ck.ly., s.ly., sitt. and st.; must be performed with full engagement of the abdominal muscles
- *Ck.ly. abdominal retraction* – pelvic tilt then head and shoulder raise; progress from pillow support to no support as muscle strength improves; if 'doming' occurs on the head raise the mother can apply external counter-pressure, and pulling medially, using crossed arms; at the point of doming 'hold', raise no further, and lower slowly.

Emphasis should be on isolation of the lower abdominal muscles. These are essential in order to maintain correct abdominal retraction. Lo et al (1999) advocate teaching transversus abdominis exercises along with pelvic tilting, postural correction and functional activity advice.

Watkins (1998) advocates that the primary emphasis should be on the recovery of endurance, in order to promote functional stability, rather than on dynamic work. Knowledge of the anatomical structure of the abdominal wall would suggest that, until diastasis recovery, strong rotational or side flexion activities should be avoided. Exercise should therefore be restricted to the sagittal plane.

It is essential that any woman who has an initial diastasis of more than 4 finger widths (6 cm) wide is reviewed at 6–8 weeks' postpartum in order to asssess her progress, and to update her exercise regimen. It is not advisable for a woman to begin another pregnancy before full recovery of the recti. In exceptional cases it may be helpful to suggest the temporary use of some form of abdominal support such as Tubigrip (double thickness), or 'support' underwear.

Back pain

Östgaard & Anderson (1992) in a study of 817 women found that 67% of women had back pain directly after delivery and that 37% still had it

18 months later. In comparing these figures with the general population they concluded that pregnancy was the cause of the back pain of the women studied. This view is also supported by Mørkved & Bø (2000). Back pain is a very common postnatal complaint and is not confined to women who experienced back pain during pregnancy. It can be coccygeal, lumbar, sacroiliac, thoracic or sometimes cervical in origin, and can seriously interfere with the quality of life of the new mother at this very important time. Analgesics and rest will not deal with the causative factors. Every woman complaining of postnatal back pain should have a thorough assessment and, where appropriate, active treatment from an appropriately qualified physiotherapist.

Low back pain

Low back pain may be relieved initially with a double-layered Tubigrip (sizes K or L) to support weak abdominal muscles. Resting in prone lying, well supported with pillows that allow a space for the enlarged breasts, is helpful for the mother. Ergonomic principles should be used in all functional activities. If the principles are followed then symptoms may abate. Specific mobilisation techniques for the sacroiliac, lumbar or lumbosacral regions may be appropriate.

Pain in the epidural site

It has been postulated that *pain in the epidural site* can be due to a tiny haematoma in the dura and epidural space. Heat, in the form of a hot pack, can be soothing, or alternatively an ice pack can be used. Appropriate warnings should be given about the use of both heat and ice.

Thoracic pain

Thoracic pain may be relieved by paying attention to postures during functional activity. Active exercises may give relief. Hot or ice packs may be effective.

Coccydynia

Coccydynia may be due to damaged ligaments, with or without displacement of the coccyx, or aggravation of a previous injury. Occasionally a coccyx may spontaneously fracture during the second stage of labour (Brunskill & Swain 1987). It can be a particularly painful and incapacitating condition in the early postpartum period, and can interfere with the mother–baby bonding process. It can also exist for a considerable length of time. Oral analgesia may be ineffective and functional activities become intolerable, particularly those in sitting positions. Active physiotherapeutic measures, such as ultrasound, ice or hot packs and TENS, can give relief. Martin (1998) suggests interferential therapy as an excellent form of anti-inflammatory and pain relief. Gentle mobilisations may also be helpful. In sitting, a cushion or pillows, arranged in such a way as to take pressure on the ischeal tuberosities and thighs, may assist comfort. Prone lying will be the most comfortable position, and frequent gluteal contractions are a self-help suggestion that may reduce initial pain. Until the pain subsides, it is essential that the mother receive all the support that is required, to enable her to function fully as a new mother.

Symphysis pubis pain

Pain in the region of the symphysis pubis is present in an ever-increasing proportion of postpartum women, and is under-recognised, suggests Fry et al (1997). Symphysiolysis or diastasis symphysis pubis may have occurred antenatally, or may follow a traumatic delivery. This joint separation, of either sudden or gradual onset, will give rise to varying degrees of pain from mild to moderate to severe and disabling. The pain distribution can be pubic, groin, inner thigh and suprapubic areas. It may be accompanied by sacroiliac joint pain or low back pain, or both, and it may be unilateral or bilateral. On occasions 'clicking' or 'grinding' may be audible and felt by the woman. The symptoms are aggravated by getting in or out of a car, walking, turning in bed, stairs, weight-bearing activities, hip abduction, and unilateral standing. (see Further Reading, p. 246.)

It is essential that the woman, and her family, fully understand her symptoms. Depending on the severity of pain, Fry et al (1997) advise 24–48 hours bed rest with analgesia and full assistance with baby care. Mobilisation will be gradual with walking aids if necessary. It is essential that weight-bearing stresses on the pelvis are minimised until symptoms resolve. Regaining functional spinal and pelvic stability is the main objective, with gradual progression in the re-education of applicable muscle groups. It is essential that the woman's pain level is 'managed' using whatever modalities are appropriate.

The women's health physiotherapist will have a great deal to offer by way of advice and treatment, for example:

- avoid non-essential weight bearing, abduction of the legs (getting out of a car, breaststroke), one-leg standing (sit down to get dressed), twisting and lifting
- teach functional activities to avoid aggravation (knees flexed and tightly adducted when moving in bed), exercise for dynamic stability (rotational control, adduction, transversus abdominis and pelvic floor muscles)
- discuss with other health professionals
- raise awareness of support groups
- encourage rest, accept help and support with baby
- ultrasound and ice may speed healing and absorption of oedema, and relieve pain
- warm baths may ease symptoms.

This condition has far-reaching effects and requires a multidisciplinary approach. The symptoms can have an effect upon 'bonding' with the baby and partner relationships, and pain-related depression can ensue (Wellock 2002). Protocols, therefore, must be put in place to assist with the management of this group of women.

'After–pains'

Many women experience postpartum lower abdominal pains – 'after-pains' – which are probably uterine in origin. Murray & Holdcroft (1989) showed that 50% of primiparous and 86% of multiparous women in a study complained of discomfort of a severity between menstrual and labour pain on the McGill pain questionnaire. Physiotherapy exercises relieved pain in 40% of the primiparous but only 16% of the multiparous women. Sleep, oral analgesics, a change in position and passing urine were also helpful. It is important that the woman *understands* where her pain is coming from. Practising the relaxation and breathing techniques used during labour may assist in its management. Where 'after-pains' are severe, TENS applied over the nerve roots innervating the uterus and perineum (T10–Ll and S2–S4) may be helpful.

CIRCULATORY DYSFUNCTION/PAIN

Varicose veins

Most women are pleasantly surprised by the appearance of their *varicose veins* after their babies are born, although some may experience pain along the length of the long saphenous vein. As a result, many do not appreciate the necessity for maintenance of circulatory leg care. There is an improvement in the severity of varicose veins following delivery, but, particularly in multiparae, once veins have become badly varicosed they will never recover completely.

Vigorous, and frequent, alternate dorsi and plantarflexion (at least 30 'pumps' at a time) will prevent stasis. Today's new mother is rarely confined to bed, but she is not as active as she would normally be. She will also be sitting feeding her baby for several long periods every day. Support tights or antiembolic stockings may be necessary for severe cases; advice about beneficial sitting positions with the legs raised, and the need to avoid crossing the legs, should be given. This should also be reinforced, and care taken to see that it is implemented.

Oedema

Although there is a massive diuresis following delivery, it can take several days (and even weeks) for the fluid retention of pregnancy to be reversed. Severely oedematous legs should be supported with antiembolic support stockings; the mother should rest with her legs in elevation. She should be encouraged to feed her baby with her legs raised, and vigorous foot and ankle exercises should be carried out half-hourly. Occasionally swelling of the feet and legs occurs for the first time after the baby is born, which can be upsetting and uncomfortable. Reassurance, explanation and encouragement from the women's health physiotherapist can turn what seems to be a major catastrophe into a transient inconvenience.

Superficial vein thrombosis

The mother may complain of tenderness over a palpable, superficial vein, and there may be redness of the overlying skin. This is often associated with varicose veins. The mother should be encouraged to remain mobile and to exercise her legs frequently. She may be more comfortable in support tights or antiembolic stockings until the condition subsides.

Deep vein thrombosis

With *deep vein thrombosis* (DVT) the mother will complain of pain and discomfort in her calf or thigh, and swelling may be present if the vein is occluded. Homans' sign (calf pain with ankle dorsiflexion and knee extension) may be positive. The main danger to the mother is the potential of a thromboembolism. Any woman showing signs should immediately be referred for medical intervention. Anticoagulant therapy and antiembolic stockings will be prescribed and, if the DVT is in the calf, mobility will be encouraged. The sufferer should avoid pressure on the back of her calf while feeding the baby, and all activities in sitting should be performed with the legs elevated. Vigorous foot and ankle movements should be performed on a regular basis, though these are no substitute for normal mobility. If the DVT is in the iliofemoral region, the woman may have to remain in bed until the swelling has subsided. The foot of the bed may be raised, or the legs supported in elevation. Exercises should be performed as a matter of great importance – foot exercises, quadriceps and gluteal muscle contractions and hip and knee flexion and extension can be valuable aids to circulation, if carried out vigorously until the mother is able to mobilise normally.

Pulmonary embolism

Pulmonary embolism, together with Mendelson's syndrome (inhalation of aspirated gastric contents while under general anaesthetic), constitute the two major causes of maternal mortality following delivery. In the case of a large embolus, death can occur within 15 minutes; with smaller emboli the symptoms can include dyspnoea, chest pain, pyrexia and malaise.

Haemorrhoids

Haemorrhoids are distended, and sometimes thrombosed, veins in the anal passage and can be a source of acute discomfort, and distress, in the immediate postpartum period. They may have been a problem antenatally, or may have appeared for the first time after the birth. Pushing in the second stage of labour can cause the veins to prolapse; on examination the swellings can resemble small to large bunches of grapes. The pain experienced by some newly delivered mothers is often described as excruciating.

Apart from doing the utmost to ensure the comfort of the woman while feeding, with a pressure-relieving cushion or strategically placed cushions, the women's health physiotherapist can use ultrasound (perhaps through a water-filled condom if the haemorrhoids are too tender to allow treatment in direct contact) and PEME, although Grant et al (1989) did not find that these therapies helped. Crushed ice packs also alleviate the pain and reduce the swelling. Frequent pelvic floor muscle contractions are probably the most helpful thing the mother can do as a self-help therapy, although resting in prone or side lying, or with the end of the bed raised may also be useful.

Steroid analgesic creams or foams are often prescribed, and if the haemorrhoids have prolapsed a gentle attempt may be made to replace them. The mother should be encouraged to drink plenty of fluid and have a fibre-rich diet in order to produce soft, bulky stools, thus reducing the pain caused by defaecation.

BREAST 'PROBLEMS'

Breast engorgement

Occasionally a woman may present with severe breast engorgement in the early puerperium, which is so acute that expression of milk using a breast pump or even by hand is too painful. Ultrasound, to the periphery of the breast initially and then moving the treatment head towards the nipple (Semmler 1982), warm compresses or crushed ice packs may be considered to relieve pain and encourage the milk to flow. PEME, as it is a non-contact treatment, might be less painful. These treatments have also been used to treat mastitis (see p. 243).

Sore and cracked nipples

The symptoms of sore and cracked nipples often lead to many new mothers abandoning breastfeeding in the immediate postpartum period. It has been suggested that the symptoms are directly related to the position of the baby on the breast. Sore or cracked nipples are not due to the mother's colouring, nor the 'toughness' of her skin, nor to the shape of her nipple. The position of the baby – facing the mother's body, with neck slightly extended, mouth well open with the lower lip curled down, and the nipple extending as far back as the soft palate (RCM 2003) – is all-important. If the baby is correctly attached, there should be no friction of the tongue, or gum on the nipple and no movement of the breast tissue in and out of the baby's mouth. Thus the baby's sucking will not traumatise the nipple and there will be no soreness. The women's health physiotherapist will advise a fully supported position for feeding, but it may be necessary for the mother to lean forward initially in order to obtain the most favourable position of her breast for the baby to 'latch-on' to and then feed successfully. If the mother is lying back in bed or on a chair, the naturally pointed shape of the breast is flattened and the baby is unable to take the nipple to the back of the throat. Experimentation may be necessary before the best feeding position for the individual mother and baby is found, and the situation will need constant review as the baby grows. The women's health physiotherapist will not be directly involved in the active treatment of sore nipples, but should be aware of the pain and discomfort that the woman is experiencing as it may have an impact on her recovery. The women's health physiotherapist should also make herself aware of current, local policies with regard to treatment and management of the 'problem', so that she is fully informed with regard to the mother's status.

The importance of technique cannot be emphasised enough and the midwife may spend many hours assisting the new mother to achieve what is 'right' for her and her baby. The women's health physiotherapist must be aware of the potential risk to the midwife in this situation. 'At risk' postures can be held for long periods of time and education in this 'scenario' is the role of the physiotherapist in order to maintain the 'team' effectively and efficiently.

FATIGUE

Fatigue is a 'normal' symptom, but can be 'overwhelming' in the early days, especially if the new baby is demanding and there are other small children. It is a frequent complaint by new mothers in the puerperium and is undoubtedly the result of an interruption in the usual sleep pattern, together with the constant daytime demands of a new baby. It can be exhausting physically and emotionally to very many women. This intense fatigue may not manifest itself immediately. The new mother is usually 'running' on an adrenaline (epinephrine) high for the first 2 or 3 days. Mothers who have had a long or difficult labour will probably react with immediate exhaustion. It is impossible to prepare women for the level of tiredness, but it is essential to raise their awareness, and confirm that it is a 'normal' occurrence that should be 'dealt' with by resting or sleeping as and when necessary. Help and support with household and family duties is therefore essential. It is very difficult for house-proud women, especially if they have previously combined managing a home with a full-time job, to accept that vacuuming, dusting and washing the paintwork does *not* have to be done daily. It is easy to become obsessive about housework. The new mother, however independent she is normally, should try to accept every offer of help (this is *not* an admission of failure). Frequent visitors should be discouraged unless they are prepared to be helpful, for example doing the washing up, the ironing, or delivering the shopping.

The main points of advice to give to the new mother are:

- Rest and sleep while the baby sleeps – household duties are *not* a priority.
- Ask the partner or a friend to take the baby for a long walk so that the mother can 'catch up' on sleep – *not* 'catch up' on household duties.
- Go to bed, if possible, after the early evening feed, and sleep until the baby wakes for the next feed. An understanding partner could bring the baby to her – she can breastfeed in bed – and then he can change and settle the child whilst she goes back to sleep. If the baby is bottle-fed they can share the task.
- prioritise household duties … accept offers of help.

Women who are used to being 'in charge' of their lives often find the first few weeks of life with a new baby (particularly if it is their first), totally exhausting. Society has acknowledged this fact with the introduction of paternity leave and extended maternity leave. It is important to reinforce suggestions for managing postnatal fatigue.

There will be an emotional, as well as a physical, aspect to the fatigue, and it is important for stress-coping strategies to be discussed. Even a simple thing like breast feeding lying down instead of sitting in a chair can be helpful, although falling is dangerous (see Fig. 7.3).

PSYCHOLOGICAL SYMPTOMS

Symptoms of *postnatal depression (PND) and anxiety* are ones that the woman herself may not recognise, but can be readily identified by family or health professional. Realising that the woman is not alone in her situation; suggestions for more rest, time on her own, daily outings with the baby in adult company, the occasional evening out with the partner (perhaps a friend or relative could babysit) are all self-help therapies. The midwife and the heath visitor can be a source of great support; then if the situation does not resolve, the general practitioner should be consulted, with possible referral to a psychiatrist to help the woman regain her mental health.

The emotional and psychiatric illnesses that can arise in normal, healthy women who have recently given birth are only now being recognised as separate pathological entities. Significantly, PND was omitted from the British and American classifications of disease which appeared in 1984. Until a few years ago psychiatrists believed that women were suffering from other recognised disorders such as schizophrenia, mania or depression. Now, however, it is accepted that not only is childbirth a mighty precipitating factor in those who are genetically and constitutionally predisposed to mental illness, but that childbirth frequently brings its own mental conditions as well. Psychiatrists are very much clearer about *what* happens than *why*, and many feel that the powers of prevention are puny (Cox 1986).

Abraham et al (2001) suggest that there is an association with body weight or shape concerns. They suggest a correlation between disordered eating patterns before and during pregnancy and postnatal problems. For some women pregnancy is the 'trigger' to obesity (Linne et al 2002). An increase in weight is an essential component of pregnancy, but for some women this becomes longer term. This may also have an effect upon mental 'state'.

The three common manifestations of postnatal depressive illness vary in their time of onset and in their degrees of severity.

The 'maternity', 'baby' or 'third day' blues

These occur in the first 2 to 3 weeks after delivery. The depression often follows a latent period of about 3 to 4 days, and is usually mild and transitory, but can be more intense. The mother is weepy, anxious and perhaps agitated. Maximum tearfulness and depression occur on the 5th postpartum day (Kendall et al 1981). A sore perineum, uncomfortable breasts, and fatigue from broken nights and endless visitors often aggravate the condition. A woman's sense of success or failure about her labour, delivery and baby, as well as thoughtless comments from hospital staff, can be triggering factors too.

The mother's response to her baby may not have been what she had expected; perhaps the automatic surge of love did not materialise, and the sudden realisation of the never-ending responsibility for the small, new life can be overwhelming. The fact that friends, relations and hospital staff seem more interested in the baby than in her, and her situation (being in hospital perhaps for the first time in her life, with strange food, bed and people), add to her sense of isolation, and maybe her guilt that she is not enjoying her baby. Any or all of these can play a part in the 'blues', which are experienced by as many as 80% of newly delivered mothers. Research suggests that about 25% of mothers experiencing severe postnatal 'blues' will go on to develop PND (Cox 1986).

Puerperal psychosis

Puerperal psychosis is a much more severe illness. The mother may seem to lose contact with reality, have delusions, hallucinations or extreme mood swings and behave abnormally. She can suffer from intense agitation and anxiety; insomnia and very early waking are also signs of this catastrophic illness.

Suicidal and infanticidal thoughts may also occur and, in its worst form, puerperal psychosis may require hospitalisation – ideally in a special mother and baby unit. There is a very high likelihood of its recurrence following future pregnancies.

Postnatal depression

Postnatal depression may also begin in the early postpartum period, but it can start, or become obvious, much later too. It presents in a variety of ways, and with varying degrees of severity. The mother may feel sad and depressed; she may worry constantly about herself and her baby, feel unable to cope and have a sense of futility and hopelessness. She may be tired to the point of exhaustion, but may be unable to sleep. She will probably suffer from a loss of libido and may have a delayed return of menstruation. Physical symptoms such as ankle swelling, loss of hair and a non-dietary weight gain may also be present. In very severe PND the mother may feel suicidal or may be frightened that she will harm her baby.

Although depressive illness is the most common, none of them is restricted to women in the affluent societies, and several authorities have described similar conditions in African women (Cox 1979, Ebie 1972, Oxley & Wing 1979).

There is still considerable conflict of ideas as to the aetiology of these disruptive illnesses. Hormonal, neuroendocrine and even social factors are all said to play a part. Recognition of PND and its treatment is imperative for the well-being of mother, baby and family. The size of the problem can be appreciated if, based on an annual birth rate of around 700 000 births in the UK, it is realised that 50–80% of women will have the 'blues' – that is 350 000 to 550 000 women; 10% (70 000) will go on to suffer from varying degrees of PND, and about two to three women in every 1000 will suffer from puerperal psychosis. That constitutes a great deal of unhappiness in new mothers and their families.

Every member of the caring team has a responsibility to watch for signs of any of these disorders occurring in women in the early postnatal days, and also in the weeks and months which follow once they have returned home. The women's health physiotherapist, who may have come into contact with a woman antenatally, and on the postnatal ward, and who may continue to see her at subsequent mother and baby exercise classes, may be the one member of the team who has known the mother continuously, and will therefore be most able to recognise any changes and alert the mother's health visitor and general practitioner (see Scottish Intercollegiate Guidelines Network (SIGN) 2002).

Sexual problems

The all-consuming role of new motherhood, and the fatigue with which it is accompanied, often result in a complete loss of libido. This can be made worse if the woman is still experiencing perineal or vaginal discomfort and is frightened that intercourse will prove painful. A partner who is demanding and lacking in consideration may add to her 'problem' and instill a sense of guilt – particularly if they had a good sex life before pregnancy. Reassurance that eventually she should regain her interest in sex, suggestions for the use of a lubricant where soreness is a problem, and alternative positions if she is fearful that the 'missionary' posture will be too painful, may all help. Self-referral for further help via the general practitioner or family planning clinic may be necessary for some couples. Some women and their partners will worry about what has happened to the vagina and pelvic floor muscles ('too tight' and 'too loose', 'not the same as before') – group discussions and laughter can ease what, to some people, is an intolerable situation.

AFTER–EFFECTS OF INSTRUMENTAL INTERVENTION

It is sometimes necessary for *instrumental intervention* (forceps or ventouse vacuum extraction) to assist with delivery. These techniques are generally accompanied by a substantial episiotomy and frequently by postpartum bruising and oedema. Assisted deliveries have been shown to be followed by a higher incidence of pelvic floor muscle denervation than normal vaginal or caesarean section deliveries (Snooks et al 1985). For some women a transient neuropraxia results in temporary numbness and muscle weakness, but for many the memory of their postforceps delivery pain is worse than that of labour. The consequent frustration felt by new mothers while they are learning to care for their baby handicapped by constant, throbbing discomfort, can mar what should be a happy time, and may delay the mother–baby attachment with subsequent feelings of guilt and disappointment.

It is important to make sure that adequate analgesia is available and that the woman has sufficient aids such as pillows, a pressure relieving cushion and a footstool, to ensure maximum comfort while feeding.

It is vital for active therapy aimed at reducing pain to be started as soon as possible. The physiotherapeutic techniques offered will depend on what is available in each maternity unit; ice and pelvic floor contractions cost nothing, however, and certainly reduce pain and swelling. The mother should be encouraged to exercise her pelvic floor muscles constantly. She should move her feet and legs freely and walk about, but should avoid prolonged sitting or standing. One of the most helpful suggestions is for her to rest in the prone position well supported by pillows. This is particularly useful if, in addition to oedema and bruising, the woman also has engorged haemorrhoids.

Whatever other modalities (ultrasound, PEME) are used, it is the duty of the women's health physiotherapist to review regularly the relevant infection control procedures and to ensure that no organisms are transmitted from patient to patient, or from patient to physiotherapist or vice versa.

If the woman is still in pain when she goes home, she can continue with treatment herself using ice, pelvic floor muscle contractions and brief warm baths, to assist resolution. It is important for the women's health physiotherapist to check, and record, whether a woman is able to perform a voluntary contraction of her pelvic floor muscles before she leaves hospital. Any woman who cannot achieve a pelvic floor muscle contraction should be referred to a women's health physiotherapist, to check whether the difficulty has been overcome. Any suspected problems should be reported to the obstetrician, or general practitioner.

CAESAREAN SECTION

Caesarean births are forever on the increase. Between 1997/8 and 2000/01 the caesarean rate has increased from 18.2% to 21.5%. In 2000/01 more than half of these were emergencies (DoH 2002). The national level was estimated at 14% in 1993 (Savage 1996). Medical reasons for this type of intervention suggest a level of 6–8% and, even in a high-risk area, it can be possible to achieve a rate of 9% (Savage 1996). In some areas the 'maternal request' rate is as high as 48% (Lowden & Chippington-Derrick 2002).

Although it is considered a comparatively risk-free procedure, it is a surgical procedure and not without problems for anaesthetists, obstetricians, midwives, physiotherapists and, most importantly, for the woman herself. It is the *only major abdominal operation* where there is little opportunity for an uninterrupted convalescence, and a new career (being a mother) commences within hours of surgery. The procedure can be carried out under general anaesthesia or epidural analgesia.

Danish research (Juul et al 1988) compared two groups of women who had undergone this operation, one with a general anaesthetic and one with epidural analgesia, for anaesthetic complications, postoperative morbidity and birth experience. The puerperal period was less complicated, there was quicker re-establishment of gastrointestinal function, and the women mobilised more quickly and were less tired following epidural analgesia. Eighty-six per cent of women would opt for an epidural in case of a repeat caesarean.

A further paper (Lie & Juul 1988) showed an interesting result with respect to breastfeeding following an epidural caesarean birth; these women breastfed significantly more frequently, and for a longer period after birth, than a similar group who had general anaesthesia.

The mother's reaction to this method of delivery will depend upon her own expectations and aspirations with regard to labour and birth. The relative issues are: planned/elective procedure or an emergency procedure during labour, conscious or unconscious, partner presence or absence; all are important factors in determining her degree of satisfaction. Postoperative status will be influenced by all these issues along with the woman's personal responses to surgery and pain. Women undergoing an elective procedure with epidural generally cope without difficulty, and will be readily mobile and able to care for their baby with minimal discomfort. Women undergoing the procedure following other previously failed interventions, may be in fear of moving, incapacitated by pain and able to care for their baby only minimally.

The physiotherapist's role

As well as routine postoperative measures designed to maintain good circulation and adequate respiratory function, the women's health physiotherapist must do her utmost to assist the woman to maintain function – cough, move, care for and feed her baby – as painlessly, effortlessly and as soon as possible. There is an increased risk of thromboembolism following caesarean birth (CEMD 2001); therefore prophylaxis is essential.

By virtue of the special physiology of pregnancy, and the fact that the timing of emergency intervention cannot be chosen, it is not uncommon for women postoperatively to have mild chest problems and secretions (they may have had the symptoms of a common cold at the time!). Coughing after any abdominal operative procedure is painful, but following a caesarean birth it can be complicated by the exceptionally 'slack' abdominal wall. Support is paramount, as is positioning. It is virtually impossible to cough comfortably and effectively in bed no matter what devices are used. The woman should be assisted to sit on the side of the bed with her feet supported on the floor or a stool. Her legs should be wide apart (but only if not experiencing SPD symptoms), a soft pillow should be clasped to her lower abdomen (to equalise internal pressure) and she should be encouraged to lean as far forward as possible. Coughing can be reduced to a minimum by using forced expiration or 'huffing' as an alternative or prelude.

Routine postnatal care is applicable to the postcaesarean woman, but must be introduced and progressed more slowly. Whilst immobile the priorities are the prevention of circulatory and respiratory dysfunction.

Exercises

Suggested exercises until mobile are:

1. ck.ly. – gentle pelvic tilting, principally gluteal muscles initiated
2. ck.ly. – gentle knee rolling from side to side (not with SPD)
3. ½ ck.ly. – hip hitching.

The exercises have the added benefit of facilitating the dispersal of 'wind' (which can be far more painful than the operation site itself!). Prolonged expiration, with abdominal contraction, may be effective.

Massage

Self-administered massage can have very positive results particularly if it follows abdominal exercise – vibrations/stroking over the 'wind' site, single or two-handed abdominal effleurage following the line of the colon (upwards on the right, transversely from right to left, and then downwards on the left) or in extreme cases, and if the woman can withstand it, double-handed kneading.

Feeding

Whatever abdominal incision has been performed, the mother will be 'guarding' the area, anxious that any external touch or pressure will be painful. She will be particularly anxious when feeding. The baby can be positioned in such a way as to allay her fears, For example tucking the baby's feet under her arm to avoid potential kicking, or positioning pillows to protect the wound (Fig. 7.5).

Wound healing

Some women may experience problems with wound healing. Those with pendulous abdomens, where loose flesh overhangs the wound, are particularly at risk. The skin may become unhealthily moist, providing a 'prime' site for the development of infection, thus delaying healing. These women should be risk assessed, and managed, in order to prevent infection at the wound site. Management should take the form of advice; encourage the woman to rest in extended positions that will expose the wound to the air, 'rearrange' superfluous flesh up and away from the wound for short periods, and consciously keep the area dry. PEME can be used, where infection is suspected, to relieve pain, improve local circulation and

Figure 7.5 Suggested breastfeeding positions for the mother who has delivered by caesarean.

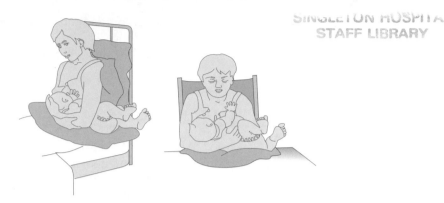

encourage speedy resolution without breakdown. Theoretically breakdown should not take place, but in any case it is essential to follow infection control procedures. Infections may be reduced by the use of prophylactic antibiotics with both elective and emergency caesarean deliveries, though have not been totally eradicated (Smaill & Hofmeyer 2002).

A postsurgery haematoma sometimes occurs, giving rise to considerable discomfort. It has been suggested that PEME (Golden et al 1981) or ultrasound may accelerate resolution but there is no research evidence.

Posture

Posture following caesarean intervention is likely to be one of protective flexion, complicated by weak abdominal muscles and possible backache. It is essential that the woman be encouraged to rediscover her prepregnancy posture. Success in achieving an upright posture will decrease pain and increase comfort, apart from making her look and feel more confident.

Postoperative pain

The majority of surgical procedures are followed by a period of convalescence. This is not the case following a caesarean birth since women have a responsibility to another, completely dependent, human being. Postoperative pain should not be such that it detracts from the woman being able to care for her baby. There is no reason today why this pain cannot be clinically controlled, either with medication or with physiotherapeutic modalities, to enable her to function comfortably.

MULTIPLE BIRTH

Mothers who have had a multiple birth, and who have had the joy of delivering more than one baby, will not only have very much weaker abdominal muscles, and possibly a larger diastasis recti abdominis, but they will also have less time to devote to themselves. Feeding demands will be greater, and they will be very tired. The women's health physiotherapist will need to introduce the idea of exercising a little and often, and should point out the importance of extra help at home and plentiful rest in the early postpartum period. Where possible these women should be seen in the community once they have adjusted to their new and demanding lifestyle, so that postnatal exercises can progress (or even commence if pressure at home has been too intense initially).

Parents coping with more than one baby at a time will appreciate the help, guidance and support they can receive from local branches of the Twins and Multiple Birth Association (TAMBA) (see Useful Addresses, p. 247).

LONG-TERM POSTNATAL PROBLEMS

Although the vast majority of postnatal aches, pains and problems resolve spontaneously after a few weeks, there are some that linger on (MacArthur et al 1991). There are also those that only become obvious once the new mother resumes her everyday routines; several months may pass before they become apparent. Awareness should be raised of these potentials antenatally, postnatally on the ward, or at the postnatal check, to avoid them being overlooked. It is reassuring for women to know that the 'team' (GP, physiotherapist) will continue to support her should the need arise.

PERINEAL/VAGINAL PAIN OR DISCOMFORT

For several weeks following the birth of a baby this can be a serious cause of anxiety, fatigue and even depression, as well as an obstacle to the resumption of sexual intercourse. Perineal pain can present up to 6 months postdelivery (Glazner et al 1995). The wound-healing rate varies from person to person, but no woman should be expected to cope with long-term perineal or vaginal pain. If no help is gained from 'self-help' techniques, such as warm baths, small disposable ice packs, the use of a pressure-relieving cushion or two pillows with a space between them, repeated pelvic floor muscle contractions or gentle self-massage with a bland vegetable oil (as long as the possibility of infection and a broken-down wound has been eliminated), then the mother must be encouraged to visit her GP in the first instance, with referral back to her obstetrician or gynaecologist as the next option. She should mention the continuing pain at the 6-week postnatal check and insist on a follow-up appointment. A rare source of postpartum discomfort and dyspareunia is the excessive formation of granulation tissue in the line of the episiotomy or tear (granuloma). Where this occurs it can be successfully treated by cautery. Painful scar tissue may also be helped by steroid injection. Ultrasound to external scar tissue may be useful in resolving pain which is not due to infection (Fieldhouse 1979, Hay-Smith & Mantle 1994). Clinical trials suggest that there is insufficient evidence as to the benefits or harms of using ultrasound (Hay-Smith 1999). However, those on the receiving end of the intervention are more likely to report improvement than those receiving a placebo. The trials reviewed by Hay-Smith (1999) suggest that there is little to support ultrasound, or PEME, but she suggests that at present there is insufficient evidence either way.

DYSPAREUNIA

Painful intercourse is possibly the most distressing long-term sequel to childbirth. Because fear of pain can prevent resumption of intercourse, simple advice as to the use of a lubricant, or a different position so that pressure is not an additional problem, may be all that is needed; ultrasound can also be helpful (Hay-Smith & Mantle 1994). The mother experiencing these symptoms must, however, be encouraged to seek a second opinion if her general practitioner and gynaecologist are not able to assist in the resolution of her problem; genito-urinary medicine and family planning clinics or psychosexual counselling services are often good sources of help.

INCONTINENCE

Stress incontinence

It has been shown that there is a dramatic drop in the strength of the pelvic floor muscles measured at 6 weeks' postpartum, compared with prepregnancy, and a slight, possibly physiological, recovery to levels still well below those prepregnancy by 12 weeks (Dougherty et al 1989). Stress incontinence (see Ch. 11) is probably the condition most readily accepted as a 'women's lot' by sufferers of all ages and parity. Mothers, and grandmothers, of recently delivered women often say that bladder leakage is a 'normal' consequence of childbirth, they have suffered from it themselves since their families were born, and nothing can be done about it other than surgery, so it has to be lived with. Researchers have demonstrated, however, that stress incontinence can be alleviated by a rigorous programme of PFM exercises (Berghmans et al 1998). Dougherty et al (1989) showed a dramatic improvement in pelvic floor strength and endurance following their programme of 6 weeks' intensive exercise with or without vaginal resistance. Too many women practise PFM exercises intermittently ('when I think of it'), too infrequently ('ten times after breakfast') or not at all ('I haven't got time').

Before embarking on a further programme of rehabilitative exercise, it is of prime importance for a full assessment to be made of each woman's PFM, including a vaginal examination; in addition a urine test to eliminate infection may be appropriate. Some women are unable to produce a PFM contraction, or are unable to maintain it for more than 3 seconds at best. The possibility of pelvic floor denervation must be considered. The experienced women's health physiotherapist should be able to grade the strength of the muscle contraction digitally.

Routines of PFM exercises must be tailored to each individual, and assessed and revised regularly. Progression should include the number of repetitions and the length of the 'hold'. The woman should be encouraged to exercise whenever she feeds her baby, and to counter-brace her pelvic floor on coughing, sneezing, laughing, blowing her nose, etc. If frequency and urgency are also problems, a strong pelvic floor contraction should be used to inhibit detrusor activity (McGuire 1979). If a woman is unable to produce a reasonable PFM contraction, electrical stimulation is an additional method of treatment which may be useful (see p. 375). It is vitally important that each woman knows, on her discharge from hospital, that she has an 'open door' to her women's health physiotherapist should urinary problems fail to resolve. A protocol should be in place to facilitate this. Where these are long lasting, a full urodynamic assessment will be necessary.

Faecal incontinence

Faecal incontinence does not, fortunately, affect as many women as urinary stress incontinence, though it is an intensely humiliating and embarrassing problem (see Ch. 12).

BACK PAIN

The physiological ligamentous changes during pregnancy take up to 6 months to reverse. Changes in bone density of the lumbar spine (but not of the radius) have been reported following 6 months' lactation (Hayslip et al 1989) caused by the lower levels of oestrogen. It seems probable that this loss is reversed when breast feeding ceases, although this may take some months. All these contribute to the symptoms of backache, therefore good back care and posture are essential. A great many women, of all ages, feel that their backache was a direct result of childbearing and its aftermath, whether this was in fact the true cause or not. MacArthur et al (1990) suggested that there may be a correlation between epidural analgesia and long-term backache. However Howell et al (2002), following a randomised study ($n = 369$) of long-term outcome, found no causal link between epidural analgesia during labour and low back pain. The postnatal class, with the women's health physiotherapist, is an ideal forum for discussion about the possible causes of back pain and the ways and means by which it may be prevented and relieved – yet another justification for the role of the physiotherapist.

DIASTASIS RECTI ABDOMINIS

The size of this intermuscular gap will reduce in most women as physical recovery from pregnancy and labour takes place; however, it may not disappear altogether without a careful exercise programme. It is most important for the correct mechanical function of the abdominal wall that the diastasis is eliminated. A great deal of encouragement may be necessary to stimulate women to keep exercising – those with multiple births will, understandably, have very little time or energy for themselves.

DIASTASIS SYMPHYSIS PUBIS

This incapacitating condition can persist beyond the puerperium. In most cases of pelvic 'relaxation' the symptoms clear spontaneously, or following the appropriate conservative treatment, during the weeks after delivery. However, morbidity may be weeks, months, or even years. It is hoped that early recognition and management of symptoms will reduce morbidity, although there is a tendency for recurrence in future pregnancies. For those whose symptoms are persistent it can become, understandably, a cause of depression and in turn anxiety for the partner and family, with resultant difficulties in relationships. The therapeutic aim to achieve spinopelvic stability is still paramount. If proving difficult to achieve conservatively, orthopaedic consultation may be necessary. Fixation of the symphysis pubis may be performed in cases of severe chronic instability (Rommens 1997). This condition, although noted by Hippocrates, has received serious attention only in the last few years. There is therefore a serious need for research into treatment modalities by physiotherapists (see Further Reading, p. 246).

CARPAL TUNNEL SYNDROME

If occurring during pregnancy this usually resolves shortly after delivery. It can, however, 'develop' in the puerperium and appears then to be closely associated with breastfeeding. Wand (1989) described a study of 27 women who developed carpal tunnel syndrome, on average, 3½ weeks following delivery. In three women who were bottle-feeding, the symptoms were mild and quickly resolved; the remaining four experienced painful paraesthesia, and 16 had such severe symptoms that their ability to care for their baby was affected. Complete resolution of the condition did not take place until breastfeeding had totally stopped; improvement began approximately 14 days following the beginning of weaning. Although this study shows the close association between the onset of symptoms and the establishment of lactation, and their disappearance following its cessation, the author did not offer any physiological reason for this. The suggestion therefore is that it is functionally related; maybe the breastfeeding technique is a contributable cause? Wrist splints, reassurance, diuretics, nonsteroidal anti-inflammatory drugs and steroid injections have been used to treat the condition with varying results. The women's health physiotherapist who encounters carpal tunnel syndrome in the postpartum period could use exercise, elevation, positioning, ultrasound or ice.

MASTITIS AND BREAST ABSCESSES

These may not present in the immediate postpartum period. Non-infective mastitis could arise if milk is not removed from the breast at the rate at which it is produced, or as a result of an obstruction (e.g. blocked duct, bruising following trauma or rough handling, or compression from fingers holding the breast, or a tight brassiere). Incorrect positioning of the baby could lead to ineffective breast emptying. Infection may occur externally, in the skin, and reach the inner tissue of the breast via damaged nipples. Unless mastitis is quickly treated, abscess formation requiring surgical incision and drainage can result. Apart from pain and redness or lumpiness in the breast, the woman may become pyrexial, develop a rigor and feel quite ill. Gentle massage towards the nipple to reduce lumpiness and encourage drainage can help relieve non-infective mastitis. Ultrasound has been used apparently beneficially in the treatment of these problems (Semmler 1982).

If surgery for a breast abscess is required, it is not thought necessary to abandon breastfeeding. It can be continued on the affected side so long as the position of the incision allows this. The baby may continue to feed normally on the unaffected side (RCM 2003).

HAIR LOSS

Hair is produced by hair follicles, which are epidermal structures. In the scalp the growing phase for hair (anagen) lasts for up to 3 years. The resting phase (telogen) lasts for a few weeks, after which the hair falls out. During pregnancy the number of hair follicles in telogen decreases and the woman's hair often seems thicker. After the baby is born, 3 to 4 months later the proportion of telogen follicles increases rapidly and there can be much hair loss, leading to thinning. In most women this will be temporary, and they will regain their scalp hair (Myatt 1988).

POSTNATAL DEPRESSION

For the 10% of all recently delivered women (Cox 1986) affected, the disturbing disorder of postnatal depression may not present until the baby is several weeks old. Symon et al (2002) found that at 8 months' postpartum, physical issues were a 'small' issue, but social and psychological issues were significant irrespective of age, parity or mode of delivery. Carers should watch for signs of its presence in any woman who expresses strong anxieties about herself or her baby, is sad and depressed, feels unable to cope, and is overwhelmingly tired yet suffers from sleep disturbances. The women's health physiotherapist is ideally placed to recognise this distressing condition, which can last for many months if not recognised and treated. Appropriate support in the community can decrease the prevalence of postpartum depression (Watt et al 2002). It is worth noting that depression can present in different ways: physical 'aches and pains' (somatisation) may in fact be a cry for help.

References

Abraham S, Taylor A, Conti J 2001 Postnatal depression, eating, exercise, and vomiting before and during pregnancy. International Journal of Eating Disorders 29(4):482–487.

Allen R E, Hosker G L, Smith A R et al 1990 Pelvic floor damage and childbirth: a neurophysiological study. British Journal of Obstetrics and Gynaecology 97:770–779.

Berghmans L C M, Hendriks H J M, Bø K et al 1998 Conservative treatment of stress urinary incontinence in women: a systematic review of randomized clinical trials. British Journal of Urology 82:181–191.

Bewley E L 1986 The megapulse trial at Bristol. Journal of the Association of Chartered Physiotherapists in Obstetrics and Gynaecology 58:16.

Boissonnault J S, Kotarinos R K 1988 Diastasis recti. In: Wilder E (ed.) Obstetric and Gynecologic Physical Therapy. Churchill Livingstone, Edinburgh, p 63–82.

Brown S, Lumley J 1998 Maternal health care after childbirth: results of an Australian population based survey British Journal of Obstetrics and Gynaecology 105(2):156–161.

Brunskill P J, Swain J W 1987 Spontaneous fracture of the coccygeal body during the second stage of labour. Journal of Obstetrics and Gynaecology 7:270–271.

Calguneri M, Bird H A, Wright V 1982 Changes in joint laxity during pregnancy. Annals of Rheumatic Disease 41:126–128.

CEMD (Confidential Enquiries into Maternal Deaths in the United Kingdom) 2001 Why mothers die 1997–1999. RCOG, London.

Cox J L 1979 Amakiro: a Ugandan puerperal psychosis? Social Psychiatry 14:49–52.

Cox J L 1986 Postnatal Depression. Churchill Livingstone, Edinburgh.

DoH (Department of Health) 2002 NHS maternity statistics, England. 1998–99 to 2000–01. Stationary Office, London.

Dougherty M C, Bishop K R, Abrams R M et al 1989 The effect of exercise on the circumvaginal muscles in postpartum women. Journal of Nurse-Midwifery 34:8–14.

Dyson M 1987 Mechanisms involved in therapeutic ultrasound. Physiotherapy 73(2):116–120.

Ebie J C 1972 Psychiatric illness in the puerperium among Nigerians. Tropical Geographical Medicine 24:253–256.

Fieldhouse C 1979 Ultrasound for relief of painful episiotomy scam. Physiotherapy 65:217.

Frank R 1984 Treatment of the perineum by pulsed electromagnetic energy. Journal of the Association of Chartered Physiotherapists in Obstetrics and Gynaecology 54:21–22.

Fratton B, Jacquetin B 1999 Pelvic and perineal sequelae of delivery. Review Prat 49:160–166.

Fry D, Hay-Smith J, Hough J et al 1997 Symphysis pubis dysfunction. Midwives 110(1314):172–173.

Gantley M, Davies D 1993 An anthropological perspective: ethnic variations in the incidence of SIDS. Professional Care of Mother and Child July/August:208–211.

Glazner C M A, Abdoula M, Stroud P et al 1995 Postnatal maternal morbidity. British Journal of Obstetrics and Gynaecology 102:282–287.

Golden J H, Broadbent N R G, Nancurrow J D, et al 1981 The effects of diapulse on the healing of wounds: double-blind randomised controlled trial in man. British Journal of Plastic Surgery 34:267–270.

Grant A, Sleep J, McIntosh J et al 1989 Ultrasound and pulsed electromagnetic energy treatment for perineal trauma. A randomised placebo-controlled trial. British Journal of Obstetrics and Gynaecology 96:434–439.

Hayslip C, Klein T A, Wray H L et al 1989 The effects of lactation on bone mineral content in healthy postpartum women. Obstetrics and Gynaecology 73:588–592.

Hay-Smith E J C 1999 Therapeutic ultrasound for postpartum perineal pain and dyspareunia. Journal of the Association of Chartered Physiotherapists in Women's Health 85:7–11.

Hay-Smith J, Mantle J 1994 Physiotherapy treatment of postnatal superficial dyspareunia. Journal of the Association of Chartered Physiotherapists in Obstetrics and Gynaecology 75:3–8.

Henry M M, Parks A G, Swash M 1982 The pelvic floor musculature in the descending perineum syndrome. British Journal of Surgery 69:470–472.

Howell C J, Lucking L, Dziedzic K et al 2002 Randomised study of long term outcome after epidural versus non-epidural analgesia during labour. British Medical Journal 325:357.

Ingram J, Johnson D, Greenwood R 2002 Breast feeding in Bristol: Teaching good positioning, and support from fathers and families. Midwifery 18(2):87–101.

Juul J, Lie B, Friberg Nielsen S 1988 Epidural analgesia vs. general anaesthesia for caesarean section. Acta Obstetrica et Gynecologica Scandinavica 67:203–206.

Kegel A H 1951 Physiologic therapy for urinary stress incontinence. Journal of the American Medical Association 146:915–917.

Kendall R E, McGuire R J, Connor Y et al 1981 Mood changes in the first three weeks after childbirth. Journal of Affective Disorders 3:317–326.

Knight K L 1989 Cryotherapy in sports injury management. In: Grisogono V. (ed) Sports injuries. Churchill Livingstone, Edinburgh, p 163–185.

Lee J M, Warren M P 1978 Cold therapy in rehabilitation. Bell & Ilyman, London.

Lehmann J F, DeLateur B J 1982 Cryotherapy. In: Lehmann J F (ed) Therapeutic heat and cold. Williams & Wilkins, Baltimore, p 562–602.

Lie B, Juul J 1988 Effect of epidural vs general anaesthesia on breastfeeding. Acta Obstetrica et Gynecologica Scandinavica 67:207–209.

Linne Y, Brakeling B, Rossner S 2002 Long-term weight development after pregnancy. Obesity Review 3(2):75–83.

Livingstone L 1998 Postnatal management. In: Sapsford R et al (eds) Women's health. A text book for physiotherapists. W B Saunders, London, p 220–246.

Lo T, Candido G, Janssen P 1999 Diastasis of the recti abdominis in pregnancy: risk factors and treatment. Physiotherapy (Canada) 51(1):32–44.

Low J L 1988 Shortwave diathermy, microwave, ultrasound and interferential therapy. In: Well P E, Frampton V, Bowsher D (eds) Pain: management and control in physiotherapy. Heinemann, Oxford, p 113–168.

Lowden G, Chippington-Derrick D, 2002 Caesarean section or vaginal birth – what difference does it make? AIMS Journal 14(1):1–5.

MacArthur C, Lewis W, Knox E G et al 1990 Epidural anaesthesia and long-term backache after childbirth. British Medical Journal 301:9–12.

MacArthur C, Lewis M, Knox E 1991 Health after childbirth. HMSO, London.

McGuire E 1979 Urethral sphincter mechanisms. Urology Clinics of North America 6:39–49.

McIntosh J 1988 Research in Reading into treatment of perineal trauma and late dyspareunia. Journal of the Association of Chartered Physiotherapists in Obstetrics and Gynaecology 62:17.

McLachlan Z 1998 Electrotherapy options for the perinatal period and beyond. In: Sapsford R, Bullock-Saxton J, Markwell S (eds) Women's health, a textbook for physiotherapists. London, W B Saunders, p 292–308.

McMeehan J 1994 Tissue temperature and blood flow – a research based overview of electrophysical modalities. Australian Journal of Physiotherapy, 40th Jubilee issue, p 49–55.

Martin D 1998 Interferential therapy. In: Kitchen S, Bazin S (eds) Clayton's electrotherapy. W B Saunders, London, p 306–315.

Moore W, James D K 1989 A random trial of three topical analgesic agents in the treatment of episiotomy pain following instrumental vaginal delivery. Journal of Obstetrics and Gynaecology 10:35–39.

Mørkved S, Bø K 2000 Effect of postpartum pelvic floor muscle training in prevention and treatment of urinary incontinence: a one-year follow up. British Journal of Obstetrics and Gynaecology 107:1022–1028.

Murray A, Holdcroft A 1989 Incidence and intensity of postpartum lower abdominal pain. British Medical Journal 187:1619.

Myatt A E 1988 Baldness. British Journal of Sexual Medicine Aug:260–262.

Noble E 1980 Essential exercises for the childbearing year, 2nd edn. John Murray, London.

Östgaard H, Anderson G 1992 Postpartum low back pain. Spine 17(1):53–55.

Oxley J, Wing J K 1979 Psychiatric disorders in two African villages. Archives of General Psychiatry 36:513–520.

Palastanga N P 1988 Heat and cold. In: Pain: management and control in physiotherapy. Heinemann, Oxford, p 176–179.

Payne J 1999 The benefits of baby massage in the prevention of postnatal depression. Journal of Association of Chartered Physiotherapists in Women's Health 84: 11–13.

RCM 2003 Successful breastfeeding. 3rd edn. RCM Press London.

Richardson C, Jull G, Hides J, Hodges P et al 1998 Therapeutic exercise for spinal segmental stabilization in low back pain: scientific basis and clinical approach. Churchill Livingstone, Edinburgh.

Rommens P M 1997 Internal fixation in postpartum symphysis pubis rupture: a report of three cases. Journal of Orthopaedic Trauma 11:273–276.

Sapsford R, Bullock-Saxton J, Markwell S 1999 Women's health. A textbook for physiotherapists. W B Saunders, London.

Savage W 1996 The Caesarean epidemic: a psychological problem? Journal of the Association of Chartered Physiotherapists in Women's Health 79:13–16.

Scottish Intercollegiate Guidelines Network (SIGN) 2002 Postnatal depression and puerperal psychosis: a national guideline (No 60). www.sign.ac.uk.

Semmler D M 1982 The use of ultrasound therapy in the treatment of breast engorgement. Australian

Physiotherapy Association. National Obstetrics and Gynaecology Journal, July.

Signorello L B, Harlow B L, Chekos A K et al 2000 Midline episiotomy and anal incontinence: retrospective cohort study. British Medical Journal 320:86–90.

Smaill F, Hofmeyer G 2002 Antibiotic prophylaxis for caesarean section. Cochrane Library. Update software, Oxford.

Snooks S J, Setchell M, Swash M et al 1984 Injury to innervation of the pelvic floor sphincter musculature in childbirth. Lancet, ii:546–550.

Snooks S J, Swash M, Henry M M et al 1985 Risk factors in childbirth causing damage to the pelvic floor innervation. British Journal of Surgery 72(suppl):515–517.

Symon A, MacDonald A, Ruta D 2002 Postnatal quality of life assessment: introducing the mother generated index. Birth 29(1):40–46.

Thompson J F, Roberts C L, Currie M et al 2002 Prevalence and persistence of health problems after childbirth: associations with parity and method of birth. Birth 29(2):83–94.

Toozs-Hobson P, Cutner A 2001 Pregnancy and childbirth. In: Cardozo L, Staskin D (eds) Textbook of female urology and urogynaecology. Isis Medical Media, London, p 486–487.

Wand J S 1989 The natural history of carpal tunnel syndrome in lactation. Journal of the Royal Society of Medicine 82:349–350.

Watkins Y 1998 Current concepts in dynamic stabilisation of the spine and pelvis: their relevance in obstetrics. Journal of the Association of Chartered Physiotherapists in Women's Health 83:16–26.

Watt S, Sword W, Krueger P et al 2002 A cross sectional study of early identification of postpartum depression: Implications for primary care providers. BMC Family Practice 113:5.

Wellock V 2002 The ever widening gap – symphysis pubis dysfunction. British Journal of Midwifery 10(6):348–353.

Winnicot D W 1987 Babies and their mothers. Addison-Wesley, New York, p 93.

Further Reading

Henchel D, Inch S 2000 Breast feeding: a guide for midwives, 2nd edn. Butterworth Heinemann, Oxford.

Linney J 1983 Multiple births: preparation – birth – managing afterwards. John Wiley, Chichester.

Livingstone L 1998 Women's health: a textbook for physiotherapists. W B Saunders, London.

MacLean A D, Cardozo L 2002 Incontinence in women. RCOG Press, London.

Nielsen C A, Sigsgaard J, Olsen M et al 1988 Trainability of the pelvic floor. Acta Obstetrica et Gynecologica Scandinavica 67:437–440.

Price F V 1990 Report to parents of triplets, quads and quins. Child Care and Development Group, University of Cambridge.

Price J 1988 Motherhood – what it does to your mind. Pandora, London.

Sweet B, Turan D (eds) 1997 Mayes' midwifery, 12th edn. Ballière Tindall, London.

Symphysis Pubis Dysfunction leaflet, published by ACPWH, obtainable from Professional Affairs, CSP, 14 Bedford Row, London WC1R 4ED.

Useful addresses

Association of Breastfeeding Mothers
PO Box 207, Bridgewater, Somerset TA6 7YT
Email abm@clara.net

PMS & PND Support
c/o University St, Belfast BT17 1HP
Email pmspndsupport@nthworld.com

British DSP Support Group
Room 2, Mount Hamel Place, Chapel Place, Ramsgate, Kent CT11 9RY
Website: www.spd-uk.org

CRY-SIS (Crying babies)
BM CRY-SIS, London WC1N 3XX
Website: www.our-space.co.uk/serene.htm

Episiotomy Support Group
232 Ifleld Road, West Green, Crawley, West Sussex RH11 7HY

Foundation for the Study of Infant Deaths
Artillery House, 11-19 Artillery Row, London SW1P 1RT
Website: www.sids.org.uk

La Leche League International (Breastfeeding)
BM 3424, London WC1N 3XX
Website: www.lalecheleague.org

Nippers (Premature babies)
Sam Segal Perinatal Unit, St Mary's Hospital, Praed Street, London W2 1NY
Website: www.tommys.org

National Childbirth Trust (NCT)
Alexandra House, Oldham Terrace, Acton,
London W3 6NH
Website: www.nct-online.org

Stillbirth and Neonatal Death Society (SANDS)
28 Portland Place, London, W1B 1LY
Website: www.uk-sands.org

The Child Bereavement Trust
Aston House, High Street, West Wycombe, Bucks HP14 3AG
Website: www.childbereavement.org.uk

Twins and Multiple Birth Association (TAMBA)
41 Fortuna Way, Grimsby, South Humberside, DW37 9SJ
Website: www.tamba.org.uk
Website: www.babyguide.co.uk/contacts

Chapter **8**

The climacteric

Pauline Walsh

CHAPTER CONTENTS

Introduction 249
Physical symptoms 251
Psychological and emotional symptoms 253

Sexuality in the climacteric 253
Postmenopausal problems 254

INTRODUCTION

The term *menopause* is used for the last menstrual flow experienced by a woman, and can be judged only retrospectively. The menopause occurs at some time between the ages of 45 and 55 years, with a mean of 50¾ years (Rymer & Morris 2000). Age at menopause is remarkably consistent worldwide, but there are variations with race, economic status and nutrition. For example, in India, on anecdotal grounds, menopause occurs about 3–5 years earlier (IMS 2002) than in Europe; women living at high altitudes tend to have an earlier menopause and cigarette smoking reduces menopausal age by almost 2 years (Spector 2002). Regardless of these factors, a few women experience a premature menopause before 40 years.

Menstruation may stop suddenly, or may be heralded by menstrual periods becoming more closely or more widely spaced. Alternatively a single menstruation, then two or three consecutive ones, may be missed, the flow may vary from cycle to cycle, or the flow may become progressively less with successive cycles. It is important for women to be able to discriminate between these normal variations and signs of disease. For example, bleeding that occurs more than 1 year after the menopause is known as postmenopausal bleeding, and may be indicative of pathology. Any such bleeding *must* be investigated. Prior to the actual menopause,

Figure 8.1 Terms used in relation to the climacteric.

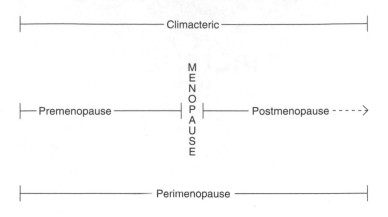

when periods are erratic, a woman may be referred to as being *premenopausal*, and following the menopause as *postmenopausal*. However, in popular usage the word 'menopause' is synonymous with the phrase 'the change of life', and is a broad concept including the unpleasant symptoms some women experience around this time – the *perimenopause*. More correctly, the interrelated anatomical and physiological changes that occur as a woman proceeds from her fertile to infertile years are termed the *climacteric* (Fig. 8.1). These changes occur because the ovaries become exhausted of viable follicles; they shrink and fail to produce oestrogens. The anterior pituitary gland is thus released from the cyclic inhibition of oestrogen and so continues to produce follicle-stimulating hormone (FSH) and luteinising hormone (LH). In most women some oestrogens continue to be produced in the suprarenal cortex, and by aromatisation of androgens (which are produced both in the ovaries and in the adrenal cortex) in fatty tissue. Thus heavier postmenopausal women have higher circulating levels of oestrogens (particularly oestrone) than slender women. Following the menopause there is a gradual atrophy of all the chief target organs for oestrogen. There is involution of the breast structure and a cessation of cyclic breast changes. The ovaries shrink, the uterus becomes smaller, the endometrium shows atrophic changes and becomes thinner, the cervix diminishes in size and its secretions decrease. There are atrophic changes of the vaginal wall with loss of elasticity and the fornices become shallower. There is a fall in the acidity of secretions within the vagina, making it more prone to infection. There is atrophy of the supporting structures to the genital tract and a predisposition to prolapse. The labia become flatter, and tend to gape, infection may occur (vulvitis), and pubic hair decreases. Atrophy of the epithelium of the bladder including the trigone and the urethra, and of the supporting connective tissue, may give rise to frequency, dysuria, stress and urge incontinence. These changes may predispose to infection, but may also present similar symptoms to an infection.

Approximately 10–15% of women pass through this stage in their life noticing very little difference either physically or mentally. They rejoice in the cessation of premenstrual tension and menstruation, and in their new sexual freedom with no need of contraception. However, there are others who experience moderate or severe physical and mental problems, and who are distressed by their loss of fertility. They experience some or all of the following: hot flushes, night sweats, vaginal soreness, dyspareunia, urinary disorders, dry skin, reduced concentration, loss of memory, inability to make decisions, anxiety, mood swings, irritability, tiredness and depression. Such unpleasant symptoms may begin premenopausally and can continue for several years after the menopause. Increasingly, doctors are administering hormone replacement therapy (HRT) through the worst of the unpredictable undulations in hormonal levels, with the option of gradually withdrawing therapy when body levels have stabilised. This usually prevents the worst of the symptoms, but some discomfort may be experienced when treatment stops.

Women who have a hysterectomy before their natural menopause but who retain at least one functioning ovary will cease to menstruate immediately but will not experience other menopausal symptoms until the ovaries naturally stop functioning. However, even with ovarian conservation, symptoms of oestrogen depletion are likely to become evident following hysterectomy (Khastgir & Studd 1998); the mechanism of this premature ovarian failure following hysterectomy is poorly understood, but it may be that circulation to the ovaries is compromised during surgery. If the ovaries are surgically removed or a woman has therapeutic irradiation of the pelvis she will experience an abrupt menopause, and severe climacteric symptoms may occur immediately and last for an indeterminate period. Since bilateral oophorectomy results in depletion not only of oestrogen, but also of endogenous androgens, women who undergo this procedure may become aware of a loss of confidence, energy, drive and libido, all of which are influenced by the presence of circulating testosterone.

PHYSICAL SYMPTOMS

HOT FLUSHES AND NIGHT SWEATS

Flushing and sweating occur, usually over the upper chest, neck and face. Sometimes this is triggered by a stressful situation, a hot drink or hot, spicy food; often, however, there is little or no apparent reason for these embarrassing and inconvenient events, which may happen occasionally or many times a day. The pulse rate rises and there may be palpitations. In addition (or alternatively) women may waken in the night soaked in perspiration, often needing to change their nightwear. These symptoms are known to be associated with low or falling levels of oestrogens in the blood, and may also be due to temporary rises in the levels of FSH and LH. They are certainly alleviated by HRT but may return as soon as it is stopped; for most women they will disappear, or diminish significantly, over time. The cause of this vasomotor instability is complex and unclear (Bachmann 2001) and severity varies widely between individuals.

VAGINAL SORENESS – ATROPHIC VAGINITIS

Vaginal and cervical secretions are decreased and become less acid; the vaginal lining becomes thin, dry and less elastic. As a result, the vagina becomes more prone to infection and vulnerable to soreness, irritation, burning and discharge. In addition there may be narrowing of the introitus and dyspareunia with consequent marital stress. These symptoms may respond well to the administration of oestrogen.

URINARY DISORDERS

Oestrogen receptors are present in the vagina, urethra, trigone and the pelvic floor (Hextall 2000). It is widely accepted that urogenital problems are associated with vaginal delivery (Wilson et al 1996), predisposing a woman to the development of urinary incontinence (stress and/or urge) or prolapse, or both. Toozs-Hobson (1998) suggests that vaginal delivery may not be the only culprit, but that pregnancy itself may have some causal significance. Although these disorders may develop at any time, symptoms commonly present, or are exacerbated, at menopause when declining ovarian function results in oestrogen depletion. Atrophy, inflammation and infection of the vagina may have secondary effects on the urethra and bladder. The vagina and urethra have a common embryological origin, both arising from the primitive urogenital sinus, and the presence of atrophic vaginitis suggests a concomitant urethritis. Oestrogen deficiency may have a role to play in atrophy of the trigone and associated supportive ligaments, and has been shown to result in a reduction in turgidity of the cells forming the urethra. These facts should be borne in mind if a woman complains of cystitis, urethritis, frequency, urgency and dysuria following the climacteric; this cluster of urogenital symptoms which presents postmenopausally is known as *urethral syndrome* (Gittes & Nakamura 1996, Wesselmann et al 1997). Oestrogen replacement may help to alleviate this problem.

DRY SKIN

The majority of age-related changes in the skin are secondary to chronic ultraviolet radiation exposure (Hawk 1998). There is also a reduction in epidermal cell turnover rate (up to 50% reduction by the age of 70), resulting in decreased ability of the skin to withstand and repair damage. Although oestrogen receptors are present in the skin, the precise mechanism by which, and the extent to which, this hormone is involved in preventing the pathophysiological changes of skin ageing is unclear. Maheux et al (1994) found that HRT administered to postmenopausal women resulted in increased dermal thickness, and a study by Pierard et al (1995) demonstrated improved dermal elasticity and deformability, and therefore a preventative effect on skin slackness. Some early work by Brincat et al (1987) found that the collagen content of skin was increased by 48% in women receiving HRT compared with those who were not. However, a more recent study, using oestrogen either alone or combined with a progestogen, failed to show a change in the amount of skin collagen or its rate of synthesis in postmenopausal women (Haapasaari et al 1997). Nevertheless it does appear that the decrease in oestrogen levels is partly responsible for the dryness, thinning and reduced elasticity of skin, and that use of HRT has been shown to improve some of these parameters (Bleiker & Graham-Brown 1999).

PSYCHOLOGICAL AND EMOTIONAL SYMPTOMS

Women blame the menopause for a great deal and complain of a variety of psychological and emotional difficulties. It is known that cholinergic neurons within the brain contain oestrogen receptors, and that a declining oestrogen level in postmenopausal women is likely to contribute to impaired cognitive performance and increased incidence of dementias (Genazzani et al 1998, Perry 1998). It is unsurprising that women report a general loss of well-being and diminished quality of life, since this sex steroid has a role to play in numerous physiological functions within the body. Many women experience an improvement in their psychological well-being after starting oestrogen therapy, although it should be noted that most double-blind placebo-controlled trials demonstrate a large placebo effect (Rees & Purdie 2002). It is worth considering, too, the other life stresses the average woman experiences through her late 40s and early 50s. For example, a mother's role has to change considerably as children go through teens and leave home, and the behaviour of some children causes huge stress; partners may seek other relationships, become ill or even die; redundancy or early retirement of self or partner alters status; and older relatives may need increasing time and support. These and other normal life events may well affect a climacteric woman. Gaining insight into the whole picture, understanding stress and having a selection of coping strategies may enable the woman to come to terms with these many, and sometimes very distressing, changes in her life – perhaps obviating the need for HRT.

SEXUALITY IN THE CLIMACTERIC

The consequences of the hormonal transition of menopause are declining levels of oestrogen and testosterone, the latter being associated with decreased sexual desire, sensitivity and response. The accompanying postmenopausal atrophic urogenital effects interfere mechanically with sexual comfort and pleasure, and disease and associated medications may also negatively affect sexuality (Gelfand 2000). However, some of these unpleasant symptoms may be alleviated by treatment and, psychologically, the loving support of an understanding partner may help to reduce a woman's anxiety, thereby increasing her pleasure.

Testosterone levels in the male begin to fall around the fourth decade, resulting in a decline in libido, physical performance and decreased sexual activity (Deck et al 2002). These symptoms are collectively accepted as the *andropause syndome* (Weidner et al 2001). Erectile dysfunction (ED) is defined as the inability to achieve and maintain a penile erection adequate for satisfactory sexual intercourse; this is a significant health problem, affecting approximately 150 million men worldwide (Kalsi et al 2002). Androgen deficiency is part of the normal male ageing process, but there are other independent factors which may contribute to ED, including radical pelvic surgery, diabetes, alcohol and smoking, certain medications for hypertension and depression, and performance anxiety.

Some couples, as they age, may find that the physical aspect of their relationship becomes less important and that they are happy to enjoy shared interests and companionship. Other couples remain sexually active into old age, each enjoying their physical relationship. However, many couples experience problems and, sadly, some men place the blame for their difficulties in sexual performance on their partner, further undermining her confidence. This is not an easy area to address, since a man may interpret any allusion to there being difficulties relating to *his* performance rather than to his partner's as an assault on his very manhood. If the lines of communication can be maintained, a woman, with understanding, sympathy and without attributing blame, may be able to persuade her partner to seek help, because treatment *is* available for many of the causes of male sexual dysfunction. The adoption of a healthier lifestyle may result in improvement: for example, reducing alcohol intake, giving up smoking, taking moderate exercise including PFM exercises (Dorey 2003), and perhaps learning relaxation techniques, which will help in reducing stress; a review of medication might be appropriate; and some couples are likely to benefit from relationship or psychosexual counselling. There is also available a range of medical options, including oral agents, surgery and a number of prosthetic devices (Kalsi et al 2002). If her partner refuses to seek help, as is often the case, a woman may need professional support; physiotherapists are good, non-judgmental listeners, but need to be aware of their limitations in this field, and of the sources of help that are available. (see Ch. 9 and Useful Addresses, p. 267).

POSTMENOPAUSAL PROBLEMS

The postmenopausal population has increased rapidly in the UK over recent years; better health and medical care has resulted in a life expectancy for women of approximately 80 years. With the menopause at around 50, a woman can now expect to spend more than one-third of her life in a state of oestrogen depletion.

Consequently, there is increasing interest in the effects on women over time of what has until recently been considered the normal and inevitable reduction in oestrogen levels. Some now call this an 'oestrogen deficiency', and there is much discussion of the desirability, efficacy and associated risks of long-term HRT (Stevenson & Whitehead 2002).

There are a number of notable sequelae of lowered oestrogen levels, some of which result in significant morbidity and mortality. The most critical known effect of oestrogen depletion is an acceleration of osteoporosis and subsequent fractures. Postmenopausal women are also at increased risk of cardiovascular disease (CVD), although the precise mechanisms governing its development and its relationship to falling oestrogen levels is complex and, at present, not well understood.

Long-term HRT has been shown to reduce bone loss and therefore prevent fractures (Cauley et al 1995, Iqbal 2000, PEPI Trial 1996, WHI 2002). Other benefits, too, have been identified: interim results from the

Women's Health Initiative (WHI) randomised controlled trial (RCT) support earlier observational studies, which have suggested fairly consistently that users of postmenopausal hormones may be at lower risk of colorectal cancer (Grodstein et al 1999), oestrogen replacement may protect against dental loss (Allen et al 2000) and assist in wound healing (Ashcroft et al 1997), and HRT may reduce the incidence of age-related macular degeneration (Smith et al 1997).

CARDIOVASCULAR DISEASE

Cardiovascular disease is the biggest killer of postmenopausal women in Western society. Following menopause, the incidence of CVD increases as oestrogen levels diminish; one in every two women who reaches the age of 50 will eventually die of heart disease or stroke (AHA 1997). Since the early 1980s, it has been generally accepted that postmenopausal oestrogen replacement confers protection against CVD, greatly reducing the risk (Mendelsohn & Karas 1999; Stampfer et al 1985). However, this postulation of significant cardiovascular protection has now been questioned (Burger & Teede 2001), and has been reinforced by interim results from the Women's Health Initiative RCT (WHI 2002). All previous evidence of benefits to the cardiovascular system by hormone replacement has been purely observational; the WHI trial of more than 16 600 postmenopausal women was designed to run for 8.5 years, with the objective of assessing the major health benefits and risks of the most commonly used combined hormone preparation (continuous combined oestrogen and progestogen) in the United States. One arm of the trial was halted early, at the 5-year point, since the number of cases of breast cancer had reached a prespecified safety limit, and no benefit to the cardiovascular system had been demonstrated. Although this is an important study, these results must be interpreted with caution: the findings apply only to this particular therapy regimen. There are many other replacement therapy regimes, using different oestrogens and progestogens in differing doses and with different routes of administration (a point acknowledged by the authors). Stevenson (2000) states that the metabolic effects of the many alternative therapy regimens are clearly different, and this is most likely to have an impact on their cardiovascular effects; it remains possible that transdermal estradiol (E_2) with progesterone, which more closely mimics the normal physiology and metabolism of endogenous sex hormones, may provide a different risk–benefit profile. The small increase in the number of patients with breast cancer accords with previous population studies, and overall mortality was not increased with therapy (Stevenson & Whitehead 2002). Within months of the halting of the WHI trial, another large prospective RCT (WISDOM 2002) was discontinued; its original aim was to recruit more than 20 000 women aged 50–69 from the UK, Australia and New Zealand, but early results suggested that, rather than a reduction in the incidence of coronary artery disease and strokes, there appeared to be an *increased* risk, albeit a small one. This trial used the same regimen as the WHI study, and therefore the same limitations apply. The effects of HRT on the cardiovascular system therefore warrant further investigation.

OSTEOPOROSIS

Osteoporosis is defined as 'a systemic skeletal disorder characterised by low bone mass and microarchitectural deterioration of bone tissue, with a consequent increase in bone fragility and susceptibility to fracture' (Consensus Development Conference 1993). Peak bone mass (PBM) is achieved late in the third decade or in the fourth decade. The greatest rate of bone loss, or reduction in bone mineral density, occurs in the first 3 years following menopause, when up to 15% of PBM may be lost, and lifetime loss may amount to 30–40% (Wark 1993). Bilateral oophorectomy, with sudden and complete cessation of ovarian oestrogen production, poses a particular threat to bone health.

There are three main factors involved in the development of osteoporosis: irreversible damage to the micro-architecture of bone, decreased bone mass and an increased tendency to fall. Bone is living tissue which undergoes constant remodelling, and it is this remodelling, or renewal, which gives bone its strength. Bone turnover is a balance of bone metabolism, whereby bone resorption (by osteoclasts) equals bone formation (by osteoblasts). Accelerated bone loss postmenopausally is associated with increased osteoclast activity: bone resorption occurs at a greater rate than bone formation and the balance between the two is disturbed, the net result being bone loss. Oestrogen receptors are present in osteoclasts (Ferguson 2000) and both oestrogen and androgen receptors have been found in osteoblasts (Kousteni et al 2001); this suggests that postmenopausal disruption of bone metabolism is, at least in part, hormonally mediated.

The axial skeleton is predominantly trabecular and the appendicular predominantly cortical bone. Trabecular bone is a honeycomb mesh of horizontal and vertical plates, which provide mechanical strength. Both trabecular and cortical bone are lost, there being greater loss of trabecular bone since it is more metabolically active and has a greater surface area. Bone loss is inevitable and is part of the normal ageing process, but the higher the peak bone mass (at age 30) the lower the risk of osteoporosis-related fractures in later life. Osteoporotic fractures are associated with significant morbidity and mortality; in the UK alone, it is estimated that there are more than 200 000 such fractures annually (Walker-Bone et al 2001), and the lifetime risk of fracture for a 50-year-old woman is 40% (Handy 2002). The most common sites for fracture are the proximal femur (in excess of 60 000 per annum), distal radius (50 000 per annum) and vertebral body (40 000 diagnosed per annum but many more go unrecognised). The incidence of osteoporotic fractures is increasing more than would be expected from the ageing of the population. This may reflect changing patterns of exercise or diet, or both, in recent decades (NOS 2002).

Osteoporosis is, to a great extent, a preventable disease, which until relatively recently has received little attention; the death rate from osteoporotic fractures at 14 000 per year, most of whom are women, rivals that of breast cancer, which causes 13 000 deaths annually. Following hip fracture, 25% will die within 6 months and 50% will lose their independence. Spinal involvement is likely to result in crush or wedge fractures of thoracic and lumbar vertebral bodies anteriorly, producing loss of height and, at their most extreme, the classic 'dowager's hump'. Spinal fractures are a source of significant pain and discomfort and, with increasing thoracic deformity, respiratory function may be compromised. Microfractures of the foot and ankle have been reported (Kaye 1998); these are often referred to as stress fractures, but are more correctly termed 'insufficiency' fractures in that they are produced when normal stress is applied to abnormal bone (Arendt 2000). These, too, are often undetected, causing significant pain and reducing mobility and independence. A fracture of the distal radius, which tends to occur in a woman's late 50s or early 60s, should sound an alert, as this may be the first sign of osteoporosis. Screening for the disease should be available for all such women, followed by the implementation of appropriate strategies (see below) for maintaining bone health and reducing, as far as possible, the risk of further fractures.

Prevention of osteoporosis

Box 8.1 shows the risk factors associated with osteoporosis. Prevention begins in childhood with the establishment of a healthy lifestyle, and the most significant aspects of this are diet (particularly calcium and vitamin D intake) and exercise. The bone mineral status of children aged 2–16

Box 8.1   Risk factors for osteoporosis (*indicates high risk)

- White or Asian ethnic group*
- Positive family history*
- Slim build/low BMI*
- Low peak bone mass (at age 30)*
- Early menopause or early oophorectomy*
- Elite athletes/excessive exercise, leading to secondary amenorrhoea
- Poor diet:
    - eating disorders
    - body fat composition of less than 17%
    - calcium and vitamin D deficiency
    - excessive or insufficient animal protein
    - high phosphate ingestion
- High caffeine intake
- High alcohol intake
- High intake of carbonated drinks
- Cigarette smoking
- Nulliparity
- Sedentary lifestyle
- Disorders affecting mineral metabolism
- Cushing's disease
- Rheumatoid arthritis; ankylosing spondylitis
- Corticosteroid treatment
- Long-term debilitating illness which results in decreased activity or immobilisation
- Very rarely, pregnancy

has been found to be positively associated with calcium intake (Chan 1994, Morris et al 1997). The health of bones is affected by the amount of stress placed on them; the pull of muscles and gravity which occurs during exercise makes bones stronger and heavier. In order to minimise the risk of osteoporosis later in life, it is important to build strong bones in adolescence and young adulthood. The lifestyle of today's children and adolescents is, in general, far less healthy than that of their parents and grandparents: often they travel by car rather than walking or cycling; leisure pursuits are more likely to include sedentary interests than physical activity; regular sport at school has, in many cases, disappeared from the timetable; indoor activities reduce exposure to sunlight, which is necessary for the production of vitamin D (without which calcium cannot be absorbed); and a diet of ready-meals and snacks high in fats, sugars and salt has replaced the healthier options which provide essential nutrients. Physiotherapists who work with women have an important health promotion role, educating them with regard to diet and exercise, not only for their children's sake but also for their own. It should be emphasised to women that a diet with adequate amounts of calcium and vitamin D, together with regular bone-loading exercise, should be followed for life in order both to attain optimal peak bone mass at age 30 and to reduce the rate of bone loss which commences early in the fourth decade and accelerates after the menopause. This lifestyle regimen should not prove to be too daunting a prospect for women; up to the menopause, daily the calcium requirement is 1000 mg, rising to 1500 mg postmenopausally (1 pint or 568 mL of skimmed, semi-skimmed or whole milk contains 700 mg of calcium, and hard cheese, white bread, yoghurt, sardines, broccoli and baked beans are also rich in this mineral). A *moderate* amount of UK sunshine will ensure sufficient production of vitamin D, and regular brisk walking or an appropriate exercise programme, or both (CSP/NOS 1999) will help to maintain bone density and muscle bulk. Additionally, at menopause, hormone replacement therapy or other pharmacological agents may be suggested for their role in reducing bone resorption.

Diagnosis of osteoporosis

At present, there is no mass screening of women for osteoporosis. It is offered only to those in the high-risk category (Box 8.1) or to women who would base their decision on whether or not to take HRT on a knowledge of their bone density. A low-trauma fracture is also an indication for screening and systematic evaluation. Bone densitometry, using a DEXA (dual energy X-ray absorptiometry) scanner measures bone mineral content at the hip and the lumbar spine, and compares it with that of healthy young adults and age-matched controls. Calcaneal ultrasound is another useful (and very much cheaper) option for assessing bone density. It should be noted, however, that the only way to assess fracture risk at a particular site is to screen that site; neither is bone density measurement a good predictor of fracture in the *individual*, but only in *populations*. What is clear is that the lower the bone mineral content, the higher the risk of fracture.

Treatment

The aim of treatment of established osteoporosis is to alleviate the patient's symptoms and to reduce the risk of further fractures. There are several drugs which may be used to prevent bone loss, and they can reduce significantly susceptibility to fracture. Other factors, too, should be considered: any secondary causes of osteoporosis should be treated, for example, endocrine disorders or rheumatological conditions. Assessment for dietary deficiencies is essential and, where relevant, review of corticosteroid use should be undertaken. The elderly, particularly those in institutions, may have little or no access to sunlight, and it may be appropriate for vitamin D, which is necessary for calcium absorption, to be administered by injection to this section of the population.

Pain relief may be provided by analgesic drugs, but physical measures such as a lumbar support and TENS may be helpful; referral for hydrotherapy or to a pain clinic may be indicated. If a foot or ankle insufficiency fracture is present, rest, decreased activity and mechanical support are likely to result in successful union.

Reduction of fracture risk

Kannus et al (2000) have found that patients who are wearing hip protectors at the time of a fall reduce their risk of hip fracture by 80%. However, these have not proved popular with patients, since the size of the pads creates a bulging appearance to both hips. Research is under way to develop materials which have similar shock-absorbing properties but are less bulky in size (Dubey et al 1998).

Falls are a particular problem in the elderly; with ageing comes vestibular impairment and loss of the righting reflex, so that the demands of a changing environment cannot be met – for example, a slippery or uneven surface (Hobeika 1999). Eyesight also deteriorates and avoiding obstacles becomes more difficult. If urinary urgency is present, trying to reach appropriate facilities quickly may precipitate a fall (Brown et al 2000, Canadian Consensus Conference 2000). There may be articular changes owing to a decrease in collagen content of ligaments and articular soft tissues (Whitehead & Godfree 1992); an overall reduction in muscle mass, with a decrease in both strength and endurance of muscle tissue, results in an increased risk of falling. Eastell & Lambert (2002) suggest that a lack of dietary protein contributes both to impaired bone mineral conservation and an increased propensity to fall. Sleep patterns and response to medication (e.g. sedatives) are altered in ageing, and these factors, together with an increase in nocturia, significantly increase the risk of falls at night (Martin et al 1999). It may be necessary to supply an appropriate walking aid, and it is important to ensure, as far as possible, that an elderly person is in a safe environment in which the risk of falling is minimised.

Exercise

Exercise has a vital role to play in the prevention and the management of osteoporosis; during recent years, researchers have looked at different exercise regimens and their effect both on prevention of falls and on bone mass. It is suggested that women who experience frequent vasomotor symptoms run a greater risk of balance disturbances, and therefore an increased tendency to fall, than do women without symptoms (Ekblad et al 2000).

Province et al (1995) state that there are documented benefits from having the mode of exercise incorporate movement for balance and flexibility, both of which are major factors in fall prevention. Weight-bearing exercise is popularly cited as the most valuable type of exercise for maintaining, and perhaps increasing bone mineral, and this mode of exercise certainly has a place. It is more appropriate, however, to refer to *bone-loading* exercise, which may not necessarily be weight bearing. Low repetitions with resistance (loading) are more effective than high repetitions with minimal or low loading. Kerr et al (1996) state that exercise effects on bone mass in postmenopausal women are site specific and load dependent.

The Chartered Society of Physiotherapy, in conjunction with the National Osteoporosis Society, has produced a comprehensive document (CSP/NOS 1999) on the management of osteoporosis, and consultation with this document is required in order to make informed clinical decisions. Exercise must be tailored to the individual, taking into account bone mineral status, and these guidelines recommend in detail the management of three distinct target groups who are at different stages of the disease. New research shows HRT is associated with an increased risk of incident and fatal breast cancer (Beral 2003).

Pharmacological management

There is now a wide range of drugs which are licensed for the prevention and treatment of osteoporosis. Initial assessment of the patient includes a review of diet, and if there is deficiency of calcium or vitamin D, or both, supplementation will be required.

Hormone replacement therapy

There is strong evidence that long-term HRT is effective in reducing bone turnover by inhibiting osteoclast activity (Delmas et al 2000, Peel 2002, WHI 2002) and, unless there are contraindications to its use, it is the treatment of choice (Iqbal 2000). In addition to its bone-sparing effects, there are other well-documented benefits mentioned previously, which may enhance a postmenopausal woman's quality of life. However, HRT is not without certain risks: there is an increased incidence (although not mortality) of breast cancer with duration of use, with a relative risk (RR) of more than 2 after 10 years' therapy (Magnusson et al 1999), and the incidence of venous thromboembolism is increased from 1 in 10 000 to 3 in 10 000 (Hulley et al 1998). Although the following regimen is no longer prescribed, unopposed oestrogen in a non-hysterectomised woman increases the risk of endometrial carcinoma, and even with the addition of a cyclical progestogen this risk is not reduced to unity; only with continuous combined oestrogen and progestogen (CCEP) is the endometrium fully protected. Recent studies have examined the association between oestrogen and ovarian cancer and there are suggestions that there may be a link (Lacey et al 2002). The issue remains unresolved, however, and requires further examination.

It is vital that the decision on whether or not a woman should take HRT be made on an individual basis; each woman should be assessed, informed, and allowed time to ask questions; *her* particular risk–benefit profile should be explained fully to her, and her preferences taken into account. There are many women for whom oestrogen replacement is appropriate; equally, there are some for whom it may be contraindicated (for e.g. a previous breast cancer or history of thromboembolism), some for whom there are no indications for its use, and others who simply do not wish to embark on this particular therapy. If HRT is contraindicated but bone protection deemed to be necessary, there are other agents available which will inhibit osteoclast activity and reduce bone turnover.

The administration of hormone replacement therapy   There is a large variety of ways in which HRT may be administered, and the dosage, type of preparation and route of administration should be tailored to the individual. It is not always possible to find the perfect regimen immediately, and it may be necessary to alter one or more of the parameters in the early months. Women will need support and encouragement at this time; side-effects, which are usually temporary, should be explained and reassurance given.

Oral administration   Tablets are taken daily. In a hysterectomised woman, unopposed oestrogen is appropriate; where there is an intact uterus, or where a women has undergone an endometrial ablative technique (in which it cannot be assumed that all the endometrial tissue has been removed even if amenorrhoea has been achieved), a progestogen should be added for at least 12 days of the cycle in order to prevent endometrial hyperplasia with its predisposition to malignancy. This regimen is referred to as a 'sequential preparation'; it will produce a monthly withdrawal bleed, which may be acceptable to a woman in her 50s, but is likely to be less so to a woman in her 60s and beyond. CCEP, where both hormones are taken continuously, will produce an atrophic endometrium within a number of months, for most women, and this 'no bleed' regimen is understandably popular, particularly in the ageing woman. The disadvantage of the oral route is the first pass effects on the liver and the consequent dominance of estrone (rather than estradiol, which predominates premenopausally) as the circulating oestrogen.

Implant   An oestrogen implant may be introduced into the abdominal cavity during hysterectomy. The gynaecologist may include a testosterone implant, particularly if bilateral oophorectomy is performed simultaneously, and the woman has complained of symptoms of androgen depletion (loss of confidence, energy, drive and libido). Alternatively, implants may be inserted subcutaneously under the skin of the abdomen. There is slow release of hormone over a period of 5–6 months. Implants are a highly effective method of mimicking the physiological and metabolic effects of endogenous hormones, but there are disadvantages to this mode of delivery. Firstly, once the implant is in the abdominal cavity, it is impossible to remove it should there be an indication to do so (although this is very rare). Secondly, a small proportion of women will experience decreasing effectiveness (tachyphylaxis): and will request further implants at ever-shortening intervals because they feel that oestrogen levels have fallen and symptoms are returning when, in fact, levels of plasma estradiol are still high, sometimes at a supraphysiological level. Tachyphylaxis precludes the insertion of further implants and an alternative route of administration should be sought.

If an implant is used in a non-hysterectomised woman, it is important that cyclical progestogen be added. A gynaecologist will continue to 'challenge' the endometrium with progestogen for many months after the final implant, since the residual effects of oestrogen on the uterus may last for up to 2 years; the aim is to ensure that there is no evidence of hyperplasia.

Transdermal   Oestrogen (and progestogen if indicated) may be delivered via a patch which is applied to an area of skin below the waist (buttock, thigh or abdominal wall). A matrix patch contains the hormone within the adhesive, while a reservoir patch delivers it via an alcohol medium. Both produce a slow release of hormone over 3–4 days, at which point a new patch is applied. Seven-day delivery patches are also available, either as an E_2-only matrix patch or a sequential E_2/progestogen delivery system. This route has the advantage of avoiding the first pass effects on the liver and gut, so the dominant circulating oestrogen is estradiol (E_2). The reservoir patch may produce some skin irritation, so it is wise to choose a different site for each new patch application.

The alternative transdermal route is by daily application of a gel, usually to the upper arm; at present, only E_2 is delivered in the form of a gel.

Topical (vaginal)   Oestrogen (often estriol) cream may be inserted into the vagina with an applicator, the dose ranging from application once nightly to once weekly, depending on the condition of the tissues. Alternatively, a vaginal ring may be inserted; this will provide slow-release estradiol over a 3-month period. Topical application may be very effective where there is atrophic vaginitis or urethritis and the presence of urogenital symptoms, since a preparation applied vaginally will be readily absorbed by the urethra. However, it should be borne in mind that, although there is unlikely to be any systemic effect from a topical application of oestrogen, this delivery system should be used for only a limited period in a non-hysterectomised woman: if the vaginal route of administration is continued, the uterus must be challenged with progestogen to ensure that there has been no significant proliferative effect on the endometrium. Alternatively, endometrial thickness may be measured by transvaginal ultrasound and it is generally accepted that up to 5 mm is within the normal range; if the endometrium is of a thickness any greater than this, tissue biopsy is indicated. It should be noted that topical application is appropriate only for the treatment of urogenital complaints due to oestrogen deficiency.

Nasal spray   Estradiol may be delivered via a daily application of nasal spray, from where it is absorbed rapidly. If the nose is blocked, for example during a cold, the spray may be used between the gum and the cheek; in these circumstances, the dose must be doubled.

Progestogen administration   Progestogen delivery by the oral route and by transdermal patch has been discussed. It is also formulated as a vaginal gel, or may be introduced directly into the uterus as a slow-release coil which remains in situ for up to 5 years. The uterine coil is not yet well established as an HRT preparation in the UK (although it is in other Western countries); it would therefore be prescribed only under the care of a gynaecologist, when first line progestogen preparations have proved to be unsuitable but endometrial protection is required. Other progesterone preparations are available but are not currently licensed for HRT.

Non–HRT drug therapies   All drug therapies which are recommended for the treatment of osteo-porosis (including HRT) are antiresorptive, that is, they produce a decrease in activation frequency of new remodelling sites by inhibiting osteoclast activity. This allows infilling of the remodelling space, which is reflected in a small increase in measured bone mineral density of 5–10% over the first 2 years of treatment (Wasnich & Miller 2000).

Bisphosphonates   This group of drugs includes etidronate, alendronate and risedronate; the latter two appear to be the more effective at reducing fracture risk (Black et al 1996, Harris et al 1999). They are characterised by highly selective localisation and retention in bone, but unfortunately demonstrate poor intestinal absorption. For this reason, they must be taken during fasting, making compliance difficult for some patients. Alendronate has recently become available in a once-weekly dose, which should prove to be a more acceptable option. Bisphosphonates are now the first choice of treatment for women unable or unwilling to take HRT.

Selective oestrogen receptor modulators (SERMS)   Raloxifene is a recent and second generation SERM (the first being tamoxifen). Its advantage is that it is tissue specific: it has an oestrogen-agonist effect on bone and the serum lipid profile, but an oestrogen-antagonist effect on breast and endometrial tissue. Although it was not a primary end-point in the trials, results demonstrated an unexpected 70% decrease in breast cancer incidence. Prospective RCTs to examine this apparent reduction in risk of breast cancer need to be undertaken. Although raloxifene reduces the risk of vertebral fractures, it does not appear to have the same benefi-cial effect on non-vertebral fractures; neither does it prevent the psycho-logical or vasomotor symptoms of menopause. In fact, it may worsen the latter, so it is not an appropriate choice of therapy for women who are still experiencing climacteric symptoms.

Tibolone   This is a synthetic steroid with oestrogenic, progestogenic and androgenic effects; it is licensed for osteoporosis prevention and may be used to treat the vasomotor, psychological and libido problems of the cli-macteric. It is not appropriate for the perimenopausal woman, in whom it may cause breakthrough bleeding, but for a woman who is at least 1 year past menopause it is an effective non-bleed regimen.

Calcitonin   Calcitonin is a polypeptide hormone, which, although not as effective in its antiresorptive action as other agents, has been shown to reduce vertebral fracture risk (Kanis & McCloskey 1999). It may be administered as a nasal spray or subcutaneously, but its use is limited by unpleasant side-effects (nausea, diarrhoea, flushing). However, it does have analgesic properties, which make it a useful short-term therapy in patients with an acutely painful vertebral fracture.

Other non–oestrogen–based treatments   There are several other drugs which are available but are, at present, less frequently used for preven-tion and treatment of osteoporosis. *Parathyroid hormone* (PTH), in combin-ation with HRT, may be used in the initial treatment of women who present with severe osteoporosis, although its precise mode of action in preventing bone resorption is unclear. It is suggested that, as understanding of PTH's interaction with the skeleton increases, this hormone is likely to be a major advance in the field (Cosman et al 2001). Another drug into which further research is needed is *calcitriol*; this is the active metabolite of vitamin D and increases intestinal absorption of calcium. It reduces fracture risk at both the spine and the hip.

The efficacy of *fluoride* has been, and remains, controversial; it is the only regimen which has a marked anabolic effect on bone, rather than being antiresorptive. However, while there is no doubt that it increases bone mineral density, there has been no corresponding reduction in fracture incidence from its use; it is hypothesised that, although there is an increase in bone mineral content, the mineral is of a poorer quality, which may lead to a higher rather than lower risk of fracture (Haguenauer et al 2000). The use of fluoride for the treatment of osteoporosis is currently not recommended.

One further line of research is the effect of *statins* on bone health; these are licensed as lipid-lowering agents, but new data suggest that they may also reduce the risk of osteoporotic fractures (Herrington & Potvin Klein 2001). This intriguing finding is in need of further study in RCTs.

For the sake of completeness, and because women increasingly are requesting information, it is important to mention the role of *phytooestrogens* (those which are derived from plants); soy has attracted the most interest and some trials have suggested a positive, albeit moderate, effect. However, the methodology of a number of these studies is questioned, and it is concluded that, although popular, these remedies have not been demonstrated to be effective in treating menopausal symptoms. The results are, however, sufficiently encouraging to warrant further research (Ernst 2002).

The role of the physiotherapist in health promotion must not be underestimated. Every opportunity should be taken to make women aware of how they can help to protect themselves and their children from problems which may not occur until decades later, but which nevertheless can have a devastating effect on quality of life as ageing progresses. With the incidence of osteoporosis rising exponentially, most women's health physiotherapists will come into contact with sufferers, and need to have an understanding of the pathophysiology involved and the interventions which are available. A knowledge of the many changes which occur naturally during the climacteric, and continue throughout the postmenopausal years, will enable the physiotherapist to deal sensitively with a woman at what is perhaps one of the most difficult periods of her life.

References

AHA (American Heart Association) 1997 Heart and stroke statistical update. AHA, Dallas TX.

Allen I E, Monroe M, Connelly J et al 2000 Effect of postmenopausal hormone replacement therapy on dental outcomes. Management Care Interface 13:93–99.

Arendt E A 2000 Stress fractures and the female athlete. Clinical Orthopaedics and Related Research 372:131–138.

Ashcroft G S, Dodsworth J, Boxley E V et al 1997 Estrogen accelerates cutaneous wound healing associated with an increase in transforming growth factor-β-1(TGF- β1) levels. Natural Medicine 3:1209–1215.

Bachmann G 2001 Physiological aspects of natural and surgical menopause. Journal of Reproductive Medicine 46 (Suppl 3):307–315.

Beral V, Million Women Study Collaboration 2003 Breast cancer and hormone replacement therapy in the Million Women Study. Lancet 362(9382):419–429.

Black D M, Cummings S R, Karpf D B et al 1996 Randomised trial of effect of alendronate on risk of fracture in women with existing vertebral fractures. Fracture Intervention Trial Research Group. Lancet 348:1535–1541.

Bleiker T O, Graham-Brown R A C 1999 Skin ageing in women: pathophysiology and treatment. Journal of the British Menopause Society 5(3):111–115.

Brincat M, Moniz C F, Kabalan S et al 1987 Decline in skin collagen content and metacarpal index after the menopause and its prevention with sex hormone replacement. British Journal of Obstetrics and Gynaecology 94:126–129.

Brown J S, Vittinghoff E, Wyman J F et al 2000 Urinary incontinence: does it increase risks of falls and fractures? Journal of the American Geriatric Society 48(7):721–725; 847–848.

Burger H, Teede H 2001 Cardiovascular disease. Maturitas 40:1–3.

Canadian Consensus Conference on Urinary Incontinence 2000 Physiological changes associated with aging that may influence continence. Canadian Continence Society Publications, Edmonton, Alberta, Canada.

Cauley J A, Seeley D G, Ensrud K et al 1995 Estrogen therapy and fractures in older women. Study of Osteoporotic Fractures Research Group. Annals of Internal Medicine 122:9–16.

Chan G M 1994 Dietary calcium and bone mineral status of children and adolescents. American Journal of Diseases of Childhood 145:631.

Consensus Development Conference 1993 Diagnosis, prophylaxis and treatment of osteoporosis. American Journal of Medicine 94:646–650.

Cosman F, Nieves J, Woelfert L et al 2001 Parathyroid hormone added to established hormone therapy: effects on vertebral fracture and maintenance of bone mass after parathyroid hormone withdrawal. Journal of Bone Mineral Research 16:925–931.

CSP/NOS 1999 Physiotherapy guidelines for the management of osteoporosis. (Chartered Society of Physiotherapy and The National Osteoporosis Society) CSP/NOS, London.

Deck R, Kohlmann T, Jordan M 2002 Health-related quality of life in old age: preliminary report on the male perspective. Aging Male 5(2):87–97.

Delmas P D, Confavreux E, Garnero P et al 2000 A combination of low doses of 17 beta-estradiol and norethisterone acetate prevents bone loss and normalizes bone turnover in postmenopausal women. Osteoporosis International 11:177–187.

Dorey G (ed) 2003 Pelvic floor exercises for erectile dysfunction. Whurr, London.

Dubey A, Koval K J, Zucherman J D 1998 Hip fracture prevention: A review. American Journal of Orthopedics 6:407–412.

Eastell R, Lambert H 2002 Strategies for health in the elderly. Proceedings of the Nutrition Society 61(2):173–180.

Ekblad S, Bergendahl A, Enler P et al 2000 Disturbances in postural balance are common in postmenopausal women with vasomotor symptoms. Climacteric 3(3):192–198.

Ernst E 2002 Herbalism and the menopause. Journal of the British Menopause Society 8(2):72–74.

Ferguson N 2000 Osteoporosis – prophylaxis and treatment. Hospital Pharmacist 7(3):69–71.

Gelfand M M 2000 Sexuality among older women. Journal of Women's Health and Gender Based Medicine 9 (Suppl 1):S15–20.

Genazzani A R, Bernadi F, Stomati M et al 1998 Sex steroids and the brain. Journal of the British Menopause Society 5(suppl 1):11–12.

Gittes F, Nakamura R 1996 Female urethral syndrome. A female prostatitis? Western Journal of Medicine 164:435–438.

Grodstein F, Newcomb P A, Stampfer M J 1999 Postmenopausal hormone therapy and the risk of colorectal cancer: a review and meta-analysis. American Journal of Medicine 106:574–582.

Haapasaari K M, Raudaskoski T, Kallioinen M et al 1997 Systemic therapy with estrogen or estrogen with progestin has no effect on skin collagen in postmenopausal women. Maturitas 27:153–162.

Haguenauer D, Welch V, Shea B et al 2000 Fluoride for the treatment of postmenopausal osteoporotic fractures: a meta-analysis. Osteoporosis International 11:727–738.

Handy M 2002 What is the evidence for once-weekly dosing of bisphosphonates? South Medical Journal 95:6.

Harris S T, Watts N B, Genant H K et al 1999 Effects of risedronate treatment on vertebral and nonvertebral fractures in women with postmenopausal osteoporosis: a randomized controlled trial. Vertebral Efficacy With Risedronate Therapy (VERT) Study Group. Journal of the American Medical Association 282:1344–1352.

Hawk J L M 1998 Cutaneous photobiology. In: Champion R H et al (eds), Textbook of Dermatology, 6th edn. Blackwell Science, Oxford, p 973–993.

Herrington D M, Potvin Klein K 2001 Statins, hormones and women: benefits and drawbacks for atherosclerosis and osteoporosis. Current Atherosclerosis Reports 3:35–42.

Hextall A 2000 Oestrogens and lower urinary tract function. Maturitas 36(2):83–92.

Hobeika C P 1999 Equilibrium and balance in the elderly. Ear, Nose and Throat Journal 78(8):558–562; 565–566.

Hulley S, Grady D, Bush T et al 1998 Randomized trial of estrogen plus progestin for secondary prevention of coronary heart disease in postmenopausal women. Heart and Estrogen/progestin Replacement Study (HERS) Research Group. Journal of the American Medical Association 280:605–613.

IMS (Indian Menopause Society) 2002 Panel report: Second national revised consensus and policy development summit on menopause. Indian Menopause Society Publishing, Hyderabad, India.

Iqbal M M 2000 Osteoporosis: epidemiology, diagnosis and treatment. Southern Medical Journal 93(1):2–18.

Kalsi J, Cellek S, Muneer A et al 2002 Current oral treatments for erectile dysfunction. Expert Opinion in Pharmacotherapeutics 3(11):1613–1629.

Kanis J A, McCloskey E V 1999 Effect of calcitonin on vertebral and other fractures. Quarterly Journal of Medicine 92:143–149.

Kannus P, Parkkari J, Niemi S et al 2000 Prevention of hip fracture in elderly people with use of a hip protector. New England Journal of Medicine 343:1506–1513.

Kaye R A 1998 Insufficiency stress fractures of the foot and ankle in postmenopausal women. Foot Ankle International 19(4):221–224.

Kerr D, Morton A, Dick I et al 1996 Exercise effects on bone mass are site-specific and load-dependent. Journal of Bone Mineral Research 11(2):218–225.

Khastgir G, Studd J 1998 Hysterectomy, ovarian failure and depression. Menopause 5(2):113–122.

Kousteni S, Bellido T, Plotkin L I et al 2001 Nongenotropic, sex non-specific signaling through the estrogen or androgen receptors: Dissociation from transcriptional activity. Cell 104:719–730.

Lacey J V, Mink P J, Lubin J et al 2002 Menopausal hormone replacement therapy and risk of ovarian cancer. Journal of the American Medical Association 288(3):334–341.

Magnusson C, Baron J A, Correia N et al 1999 Breast-cancer risk following long-term oestrogen and oestrogen-progestin replacement therapy. International Journal of Cancer 81:339–344.

Maheux R, Naud F, Rioux M et al 1994 A randomised, double-blind, placebo-controlled study on the effect of conjugated estrogens on skin thickness. American Journal of Obstetrics and Gynecology 170:642–643.

Martin J, Shochat T, Gehrman P R et al 1999 Sleep in the elderly. Respiratory Care Clinics of North America 5:461–472.

Mendelsohn M E, Karas R H 1999 The protective effects of oestrogen on the cardiovascular system. New England Journal of Medicine 340:1801–1811.

Morris F L, Naughton G A, Gibbs J L et al 1997 Prospective ten-month exercise intervention in premenarcheal girls: Positive effects on bone and lean mass. Journal of Bone Mineral Research 12:1453–1462.

NOS (National Osteoporosis Society) 2002 Introduction to osteoporosis – indications for bone densitometry. National Osteoporosis Society, p 5.

Peel N 2002 Treatment of postmenopausal osteoporosis: which agent at what age. Journal of the British Menopause Society 8(1):15–23.

PEPI 1996 Writing group for the PEPI trial. Effects of hormone therapy on bone mineral density: results from the Postmenopausal Estrogen/Progestin Interventions (PEPI) trial. Journal of the American Medical Assocation 275:1389–1396.

Perry E 1998 Alzheimer's disease, acetylcholine and oestrogen. Journal of the British Menopause Society 4(4):144–151.

Pierard G E, Letawe G, Dowlati A et al 1995 Effects of hormone replacement therapy for menopause on the mechanical properties of skin. Journal of the American Geriatric Society 43:662–665.

Province M A, Hadley E C, Hornbrook M C et al 1995 The effect of exercise on falls in elderly patients. A pre-planned meta-analysis of FICSIT trails. Frailty and injuries: cooperative state intervention techniques. Journal of the American Medical Association 273:1341–1347.

Rees M, Purdie W D (eds) 2002 Benefits and risks of hormone replacement therapy. Management of the menopause. BMS Publications, Marlow, p 45–46.

Rymer J, Morris E P 2000 Menopausal symptoms. British Medical Journal 321:1516–1519.

Smith W, Mitchell P, Wang J J 1997 Gender, oestrogen, hormone replacement and age-related macular degeneration: results from the Blue Mountains Eye Study. Australian and New Zealand Journal of Ophthalmology 25(suppl 1):S13–15.

Spector T 2002 Proceedings of the 10th World Congress on the Menopause. International Menopause Society, Berlin.

Stampfer M J, Willett W C, Colditz G A et al 1985 A prospective study of postmenopausal estrogen therapy and coronary heart disease. New England Journal of Medicine 313:1044–1049.

Stevenson J C 2000 Cardiovascular effects of estrogens. Journal of Steroid Biochemistry and Molecular Biology 74:387–393.

Stevenson J C, Whitehead M I 2002 Hormone replacement therapy: findings of Women's Health Initiative trial need not alarm users. British Medical Journal 325:113–114.

Toozs-Hobson P 1998 Pelvic floor ultrasonography: the current state of ultrasound imaging of the pelvic floor in relation to urogynaecology and childbirth. Journal of the Association of Chartered Physiotherapists in Women's Health 84:18–22.

Walker-Bone K, Pearson G, Cooper C 2001 Premenopausal risk factors for osteoporosis. Journal of the British Menopause Society 7(4):162–166.

Wark J D 1993 Osteoporosis: pathogenesis, diagnosis, prevention and management. Baillière's Clinical Endocrinology and Metabolism 7:151–181.

Wasnich R D, Miller P D 2000 Antifracture efficacy of antiresorptive agents are related to changes in bone density. Journal of Clinical Endocrinology and Metabolism 85:231–236.

Weidner, W, Altwein J, Hauck E et al 2001 Sexuality of the elderly. Urology International 66(4):181–184.

Wesselmann U, Burnett A, Heinberg L 1997 The urogenital and rectal pain syndromes. Pain 73:269–294.

WHI (Women's Health Initiative) 2002 Risks and benefits of estrogen plus progestin in healthy postmenopausal women: Principal results from the Women's Health Initiative Randomized Controlled Trial. Writing Group for the Women's Health Initiative Investigators. Journal of the American Medical Association 288(3):321–333.

Whitehead M, Godfree V (eds) 1992 Consequences of oestrogen deficiency. Hormone replacement therapy: your questions answered. Churchill Livingstone, Edinburgh, p 13–36.

Wilson P D, Herbison R M, Herbison G P 1996 Obstetric practice and the prevalence of urinary incontinence three months after delivery. British Journal of Obstetrics and Gynaecology 103:154–161.

WISDOM 2002 Women's international study of long duration oestrogen after menopause. Medical Research Council Expert Panel. WISDOM, London.

Further reading

Bain C, Lumsden M A, Sattat N et al 2003 The menopause in practice. Royal Society of Medicine Press, London.

Barlow D, Wren B 2003 Fast facts: menopause. Health Press/Plymbridge Distributors, Plymouth.

CSP/NOS (Chartered Society of Physiotherapists/National Osteoporosis Society) Physiotherapy guidelines for the management of osteoporosis. CSP London.

Henderson J E 2000 The osteoporosis primer. Cambridge University Press, Cambridge.

Lobo R 2000 Menopause: biology and pathobiology. Harcourt Brace, London.

Stewart D E, Robinson G E 1997 A clinician's guide to menopause. American Psychiatric Publishing, Arlington VA.

Woolf A 2002 The osteoporosis pocket book. Martin Dunitz, London.

Woolf A D, St John Dixon A 1998 Osteoporosis: a clinical guide, 2nd edn. Martin Dunitz, London.

Useful addresses

Amarant Trust
A charity for women going through the menopause
The Amarant Trust
Sycamore House, 5 Sycamore Street, London EC1Y 0SG

The Amarant Centre
Gainsborough Clinic, 80 Lambeth Road, London SE1 7PW
Menopause helpline tel 01293 413000
HRT helpline tel 09068 660620

Andropause Society
website: www.andropause.org.uk

British Menopause Society
4–6 Eton Place, Marlow, Bucks SL7 2QA
Tel 01628 890199; fax: 01628 474042
E-mail admin.bms@btconnect.com
Website: www.the-bms.org

Darsey Network (POF)
PO Box 392, High Wycombe, Bucks HP15 7SH
Website: www.darseynetwork.org.uk

Institute of Psychosexual Medicine
12 Chandos Street, Cavendish Square, London W1G 9DR
Tel 0207 580 0631
Website: www.ipm.org.uk

National Osteoporosis Society
Camerton, Bath BA2 0PJ
Tel 01761 471771; fax: 01761 471104; helpline 01761 472721
E-mail info@nos.org.uk
Website: www.nos.org.uk

Relate
Relationship counselling and psychosexual therapy
Helpline 0845 130 40 10
Website: http://www.relate.org.uk/contact_us.html

Chapter **9**

Common gynaecological conditions

Jeanette Haslam

CHAPTER CONTENTS

Introduction 269
Gynaecological health 269
Gynaecological disorders 271

Further gynaecological conditions of relevance
  to the physiotherapist 287
Sexuality 300

INTRODUCTION

Gynaecology is the study of diseases that are specific to women. It is a specialty that demands of the physiotherapist a particularly mature blend of attributes, which, when necessary, enable a woman to disclose confidently some of the most intimate and personal details of her life. In addition to sound theoretical knowledge and a high degree of clinical competence, the physiotherapist must always make time to listen, and be easily approachable, unshockable and non-judgmental.

GYNAECOLOGICAL HEALTH

It has been increasingly appreciated that some gynaecological conditions may be silent in progress, some simply debilitating, and others life threatening. Recent advances in the understanding of the early presentation and development of infections and malignant disease of the female reproductive organs and breasts has resulted in women in the UK being encouraged to avail themselves (once they are sexually active) of regular free screening by means of cervical cytology, and to learn to be breast aware by monthly systematic palpation preferably just after menstruation ends.

BREAST AWARENESS

Being breast aware means being aware of what is normal for yourself and being able to detect anything that is unusual. A practice nurse sometimes teaches breast awareness in the community-based well women clinics, where early detection and treatment of disease, prevention and health promotion are the chief objectives. However, it is acknowledged that the woman herself is best placed to detect changes in her own breast tissue. There are four stages of awareness often advocated. These are:

1. Observe any changes in appearance when standing in front of a mirror. (Look for any changes in the outline or size of the breasts, changes in the nipple position, shape or discharge, puckering or dimpling anywhere in the breasts, changes in skin texture, colour or a rash, constant pain in one part of the breast or axilla.)
2. Hands on hips, press down and tense the chest muscles; this will make changes easier to see.
3. With hands and arms raised above the head, observe particularly the upper tail of the breast towards the axilla.
4. Finally, palpate each breast in turn using the opposite hand spread flat, with the hand on the breast side placed behind the head. Using gentle pressure in a circular motion with the pads of the fingers, check the whole breast to detect any lump or thickening in the breast. This may be best done either lying flat on the bed or with a soapy hand in the bath or shower.

If any changes are observed, an appointment should be made with the GP for them to determine if a breast clinic appointment is necessary.

PHYSICAL CHECK-UPS

A visit to a women's health clinic is increasingly seen to be the ideal opportunity for a regular physical check, which may realistically include:

- measurement of blood pressure
- breast examination
- examination of perineum, vagina and cervix for signs of infection and prolapse, and cough test for stress incontinence
- cervical cytology
- bimanual pelvic examination, and test of pelvic floor muscle (PFM) strength
- urine test for infection, glucose, etc
- discussion of the woman's state of health and any problems she may be experiencing such as sexual problems.

Some well women clinics are extending this service with seminars on health matters, and exercise classes taken by physiotherapists to encourage fitness by improving mobility and strength and to try to delay osteoporosis; attention is also being given to weight control.

CERVICAL CYTOLOGY

All sexually active women are at risk of squamous cell carcinoma. It is recommended that a woman should have her first cervical smear at the age of 20 years with 3-yearly follow-up until the age of 65 years (Symonds & Symonds 1998). As a member of the well women or gynaecological team it is important for the specialist physiotherapist to know the classification of cervical cytology results. Results should be reported as agreed by the British Council for Cervical Cytology (Luesley 1997):

- *Negative* – a normal smear
- *Borderline nuclear abnormalities* – minor increase in the nuclear cytoplasmic ratio, but insufficient to be classed as dyskariotic
- *Mild dyskariosis* – abnormal, suggestive of, but not diagnostic of mild dysplasia (CIN 1)
- *Moderate dyskariosis* – abnormal, suggestive of, but not diagnostic of moderate dysplasia (CIN 2)
- *Severe dyskariosis* – abnormal, suggestive of, but not diagnostic of severe dysplasia (CIN 3)
- *Invasion* – abnormal, smear shows evidence of malignant fibre cells or necrotic debris
- *Koilocytosis* – cells suggestive of infection with human papillomavirus
- *Inadequate* – cellular content either insufficient or smear unsatisfactorily prepared to allow for cytological opinion.

Cervical cytology is not diagnostic but rather indicates when further investigation is necessary. If there are malignant or dyskariotic cells present, the woman should be referred for colposcopy. If there are borderline changes the smear should be repeated after 6 months and if the changes are persistent the patient should be referred for colposcopy.

Colposcopy (*colpos* = cervix or neck) involves the examination of the cervix with a binocular microscope. This will also enable biopsy of any abnormal epithelium and treatment of any intraepithelial neoplasia (Symonds & Symonds 1998).

GYNAECOLOGICAL DISORDERS

The most common disorders of the female genital tract can be classified as infections, cysts and new growths, or displacements and genital prolapse.

INFECTIONS

Full heed must be paid to infection control procedures with universal precautions being taken at all times. When intimately examining a woman, heed should always be paid to any visible abnormalities that may be infectious in nature. If any such lesions are observed it is wise to take medical advice before proceeding with a vaginal examination.

Vulva

Vulvitis

The continuous moist discharge from glands in the vulva supplemented by that from the uterus, vagina and cervix, together with traces of urine and faecal material, ensure that there is always a profusion of microorganisms in the perineal area. Infection may track up the vagina or may have tracted from it; thus vulvitis often becomes vulvovaginitis. It is suggested by some that the wearing of nylon tights, the habitual wearing of tight-fitting trousers by some women and increased sexual freedom have all contributed to maintaining the incidence of infections of the perineum and pelvic organs in women at a high level against the trend of many other infections. It is important to realise that pruritus vulvae, a severe and distressing irritation of some part of the perineum, is a common experience in women, but it is a symptom and not a condition in its own right. It requires careful investigation to determine the precise cause, which can be as diverse in nature as lichen planus, lichen sclerosus, psoriasis, intertrigo, incontinence, liver disease or Hodgkin's disease. Pruritus ani may be part of the same problem or have an individual cause such as threadworms. It is also worth remembering that the perineum may become sensitised to cosmetic or other chemical preparations causing an allergic dermatitis.

Gleeson (1995) quotes the following classification of vulval disorders (Ridley et al 1989), which has been adapted by the International Society for the Study of Vulvar Disease (SSVD):

Non-neoplastic disorders of the vulva

- Squamous cell hyperplasia
- Lichen sclerosis
- Other dermatoses

Vulval intraepithelial neoplasia (VIN)

- Squamous VIN
  - VIN I   mild dysplasia
  - VIN II   moderate dysplasia
  - VIN III   severe dysplasia and carcinoma in situ
- Non-squamous VIN
  - Paget's disease
  - melanoma in situ.

Infectious organisms

Infections of the vulva may be fungal, bacterial, viral or parasitic.

Fungal *Candida albicans* is frequently implicated in vulvitis in pregnancy, especially if the renal threshold for glucose becomes lowered. It is a yeast-like fungus, commonly called 'thrush', that flourishes in any warm, moist mucous surface in an acid environment, especially in the presence of glucose (Murray 1997). It is characterised by irritation, acute inflammation, rawness and a curdy, white discharge; the vagina is often also infected. The usual treatment is with Nystatin or Canestan vaginal pessaries or cream. Other factors that have been implicated in both the initial and recurrent disease are antibiotics, corticosteroids, immunosuppressive treatment, diabetes, orogenital contact and the presence of other sexually transmitted diseases (Adler 1990a). If a woman is having recurrent symptoms, her sexual partner should also be investigated for candadiasis and treated appropriately if it is present.

Bacterial *Staphylococcus* bacteria infect sebaceous glands and hair follicles on the perineum causing boils; gonorrhoea and syphilis are other infections that may affect this area.

Viral   *Human papilloma virus* (HPV) is the cause of common warts of the hands and feet as well as lesions of the genital area. As such it is one of the most commonly sexually transmitted viruses. They can be treated by cryotherapy or diathermy. They may be transient in nature but are potentially serious in nature as HPV type 16 and 18 are carcinogenic and others are reported to have a role in cervical carcinogenesis (Kjaer et al 2002). HPV-18 is the type most strongly associated with adenocarcinoma of the cervix (Woodman et al 2003). A Danish study followed up 10 758 cytologically normal women aged 20–29 years for development of cytological abnormalities (Kjaer et al 2002). It was found that infection with HPV at enrolment predicted future development of high-grade squamous intraepithelial lesions. Those women who were positive on repeated testing were at greatest risk of high-grade cervical neoplasia lesions.

Genital herpes is a sexually transmitted viral infection which has been linked with cervical cancer. Annual cervical cytology is recommended for all women with this condition. It is a serious problem in pregnancy, where it can cause abortion, and elective caesarean section may be indicated if the mother has active herpes at term; otherwise the foetus could become infected at delivery and subsequently die or suffer neurological damage (see p. 46).

Parasitic   Parasites such as lice can be transmitted from head hair to pubic hair and can cause perineal irritation. *Pediculosis pubis* may have symptoms of vulval irritation and is caused by infestation by the pubic louse.

Scabies is caused by a mite in which the female burrows into the upper layer of the skin; laying eggs and defaecating. They are transmitted by close but not necessarily sexual contact. They cause severe irritation and itching, especially at night-time (Adler 1990b).

Vagina

The *Bartholin's glands* are located on the posterior and lateral aspect of the vestibule of the vagina; the duct of each is narrow and easily becomes blocked. If this occurs mucoid secretions distend the gland, forming an often painless cyst. This may become infected forming an abscess, or an infection of the gland can occur independently of any duct narrowing; any such infection is excruciatingly painful. Cultures should be performed as *Gonorrhoea* may be a cause of Bartholin's abscess.

Gartner's ducts are found lateral to the vagina and may cause problems with dyspareunia if they become infected; they are usually treated by incision.

Vaginitis

The vagina can become infected by a variety of organisms similar to those found in the vulva, and 'vaginal discharge' is another symptom of which women often complain. Vaginitis may also be caused by sensitivity to spermicides, douches and perfumed sprays.

There is a normal cycle of changes in the amount and nature of secretions within and passed per vaginam associated with the menstrual cycle which has been described on page 31. Normally all secretions are transparent or white, so any change in colour, bleeding, or any unusual odour or quantity should be a cause for consultation.

Infectious organisms

Organisms that commonly cause infective vaginal discharge are:

- *Candida albicans* (see p. 272)
- *Trichomonas vaginalis*, a motile protozoan parasite causing vaginitis with a copious, malodorous (fishy smell), watery discharge and pruritis. It is usually sexually transmitted, has no serious effects but is often a marker for other sexually transmitted diseases especially chlamydia and gonorrhoea (Bradbeer 1997). Any sexual partner of a woman must also be treated.
- *Neisseria gonorrhoeae* is the causative organism of gonorrhoea. This may be asymptomatic or with a light discharge and can cause pelvic inflammatory disease. It can further affect the urethra, cervix, rectum and mouth. Transmission to a foetus at birth can cause neonatal conjunctivitis, which if it remains untreated can cause blindness (Murray 1997). It is a notifiable disease and is treated with penicillin; sexual partners should always be traced to be tested and treated if necessary.
- *Gardnerella vaginalis* is a genus of rod-shaped Gram negative bacteria that can be a cause of bacterial vaginitis. The discharge is thin, grey and foul smelling. Treatment is via appropriate medication, with sexual partners also requiring treatment (Govan et al 1993).
- *Chlamydia trachomatis* is an important cause of pelvic inflammatory disease. Gelatinous exudates are formed in the pouch of Douglas proceeding to multiple adhesions and tubal occlusion. It does not, however, produce a noticeable discharge. Vaginal organisms are transmitted sexually so, in treatment, partners must also be considered. Severe cases may present with cervicitis that looks like an infected erosion. It has also been suggested that *Chlamydia* may be an aetiological factor in cervical carcinoma (Govan et al 1993).

Cervix

Cervicitis

Erosions of the cervix are quite common; they can be infected but usually are not. Normally, columnar epithelium partly or completely lines the cervical canal and butts on to the stratified squamous epithelium which lines the vagina and covers the vaginal aspect of the cervix. Where there is an erosion, columnar epithelium appears to replace some of the cervical stratified epithelium. Erosions sometimes appear in pregnancy and in women taking oral contraceptives; they are rarely seen after the climacteric and improve when oral contraceptives are discontinued. This suggests a hormonal factor. Infections of the cervix are commonly caused by sexually transmitted organisms such as *Gonococcus* or *C. trachomatis*, and may follow trauma such as that which can occur at childbirth, abortion or as a result of operative procedures requiring dilatation of the cervix.

Acute cervicitis usually occurs associated with a generalised infection of the genital tract. There may be purulent discharge, low back pain, abdominal pain, dysuria and dyspareunia. The treatment depends on the organism causing the infection.

Chronic cervicitis is extremely common, often with minimal symptomology. However some women have more severe symptoms, such as acute cervicitis with occasional postcoital bleeding (Symonds & Symonds 1998).

Uterus

Endometritis

Infections of the uterus with resulting endometritis are less common than those of other areas of the genital tract by virtue of the protection afforded by the vagina and cervix – that is, the length of the vagina, the downward movement of secretions, the constriction formed by the cervix and the viscosity for much of the time of its secretions – and also by the cyclic shedding of the endometrium. However, infections do track upwards. It is possible that sperm can act as carriers, the tails of intrauterine devices have been implicated, and after delivery or abortion, the open placental site, the lochia or retained products of conception all potentially provide a superb culture medium. Any medical procedure that opens the cervix has the potential to introduce infection.

Fallopian tubes

Salpingitis

Infection of the fallopian tubes, which is often associated with infection of the ovary (salpingo-oophoritis), may result from ascending infection but can also occur following infection of the gut or other abdominal organs. Salpingitis may be acute or chronic and can be a cause of infertility (e.g. ectopic pregnancy) when scarring and adhesions block the tube, or damage muscle and cilia.

The principal organisms causing acute salpingitis are the sexually transmitted *N. gonorrhoeae* or *Chlamydia*. The symptoms can include low abdominal pain, purulent vaginal discharge, pyrexia, vomiting and diarrhoea; the signs can include tachycardia, signs of peritonitis and acute pain on pelvic examination (Symonds & Symonds 1998).

PELVIC INFLAMMATORY DISEASE

The close proximity of structures particularly within the true pelvis, and their interconnection via ligaments and peritoneum, means that infection is able to spread to involve other organs and produce what is known as pelvic inflammatory disease (PID). It is a combination of infection of the fallopian tubes, ovaries and peritoneum and may be a cause of ectopic pregnancies. In the UK a variety of bacteria can be responsible for PID, but *C. trachomatis* is the commonest cause, and *N. gonorrhoeae* and *Mycoplasma hominis* are frequent causes. Such infections may occur independently or concurrently, and are sexually transmitted. Since the United Kingdom Health Statistics (Office for National Statistics 2001) show that the annual number of new cases of *Chlamydia* continued to rise in the period 1991–1999 from 622.5 to 1077.3 per million women, it is probable that the number of cases of PID is also rising.

The infection causes inflammation, and the body's response in the highly vascular pelvic area is the production of adhesions (sometimes profuse) and scarring, which contort structures and glue or bind them to adjacent ones. In the acute phase women complain of pelvic or abdominal pain and of feeling thoroughly unwell; they may even be pyrexial. Sometimes there are difficulties in achieving an accurate clinical diagnosis owing to the problems in obtaining a sample from the infection site and because the accuracy of tests has been poor. Consequently the condition in many women becomes chronic and results in continuing ill health, persistent lower abdominal pain, serious internal damage and infertility. It adversely affects relationships and the ability to work successfully.

C. trachomatis is a Gram negative intracellular bacterium and is not detected, as *N. gonorrhoeae* can sometimes be, by routine microscopy. A special, time-consuming cell culture and staining test has been necessary to detect *Chlamydia*. However, quicker, simpler and more accurate tests are being developed; in some cases a specimen will need to be collected by laparoscopy. Chlamydial antigen is detected by a swab used to allow measurement of enzyme-linked immunoabsorbent assay (ELISA). If there is an equivocal result a cell culture will be done (Nash 1997). Many units now routinely test for *Chlamydia* prior to a termination or insertion of an intrauterine device.

N. gonorrhoeae usually responds to penicillin, but it is less well appreciated that *Chlamydia* does not; it is, however, usually sensitive to the tetracyclines. Several antimicrobials have also been shown to be effective in the treatment of *Chlamydia* infection. Sexual partners should be treated concurrently and sexual intercourse avoided until therapy is completed. Sometimes those women with a cervical smear showing 'inflammatory changes' have in fact got a *Chlamydia* infection; full bacterial and viral screening should be performed and the smear repeated after the cervical inflammation has been treated (Nash 1997).

Chronic PID does not run a predictable course. Some cases even resolve spontaneously. A broad-spectrum antibiotic is often given and surgery to remove the uterus, ovaries and fallopian tubes is often advocated (Govan et al 1993).

PHYSIOTHERAPY IN THE TREATMENT OF GYNAECOLOGICAL INFECTIONS

There is no role for physiotherapy in the acute phase of gynaecological infections. These must be promptly and properly diagnosed, and effectively treated with the correct pharmacotherapy. However, in the chronic phase, where the organism is resistant to antibiotics or when adhesions are causing pain, there may occasionally be a place for physiotherapeutic measures such as continuous or pulsed short-wave diathermy. The women's health physiotherapist can also offer coping strategies to deal with pain and stress, and advice on the promotion of good health.

ACQUIRED IMMUNE DEFICIENCY SYNDROME (AIDS)

AIDS is caused by a virus known as the human immunodeficiency virus (HIV). Infected persons carry the virus in body fluids, and may be fit and well for varying lengths of time. HIV is transmitted during intimate sexual contact, or through direct contact via mucous membrane or broken skin with infected blood or genital secretions from a carrier in any other circumstances. The virus can be transmitted to the foetus across the placenta and is present in the amniotic fluid of HIV carriers (see p. 46). The infection is diagnosed by the presence in blood samples of the appropriate antibodies. However, there is a time lag of months or years between acquiring the infection and developing antibodies. It is not yet known what determines if and when a carrier will develop the syndrome.

The latest figures obtainable from www.statistics.gov.uk show that there were 26 227 patients living in the UK who were seen for statutory medical HIV-related care in 2001. This included 877 mother-to-infant infections.

The women's health physiotherapist must heed universal precautions in all patients at all times; in this way they and their patients will not be put at risk. The Trust infection control officer should be consulted regularly to ensure that precautions are based on the latest information.

CYSTS AND NEW GROWTHS

Cysts

The term 'cyst' usually signifies a pathological fluid-filled sac bounded by a wall of cells. The fluid is often clear and colourless, and may be secreted by the cells lining the cyst or derived from the tissue fluid of the area. There are cysts peculiar to each organ, and these may be congenital or acquired. Congenital cysts occur in vestigial remnants of embryonic tissue; they are common in the genitourinary tract and the broad ligament is a frequent site. Acquired cysts may be caused by obstruction to the outflow of a duct and consequent retention of secretions (e.g. Bartholin's gland). Alternatively, distension cysts form in natural enclosed spaces; they are common in graafian follicles and corpora lutea.

Benign tumours

Benign tumours are formed by a mass of well-defined cells, which are still recognisably similar to the originating tissue, and the mass is encapsulated by a layer of normal cells so the tumour cells cannot escape. Benign tumours tend not to be troublesome and do not generally threaten life.

Malignant tumours

By contrast, the cells of malignant tumours show varying degrees of reversion to the embryonic unspecialised state, and look less like the original cells. They seem to lose control of cell division and divide repeatedly; they are less differentiated and lose the specialist function of their parent cell. They have no containing capsule and so invade surrounding tissue. Highly malignant cells lose the mature cell's adhesiveness to its neighbours, and regain the embryonic cell's ability to detach and migrate to form secondary deposits or metastases. They also have the ability to stimulate the growth of new blood capillaries around and within the growing cell mass, ensuring an adequate supply of nutrients. Thus malignant tumours tend to be life threatening until successfully treated.

Gynaecological cancers have been classified and clearly defined in stages by the International Federation of Gynaecology and Obstetrics (FIGO). The most recent definitions with the relevant papers are obtainable on www.figo.org.

Vulva

Vulvar cancer is classified in stages by FIGO (Beller et al 2001):

- *Stage 0* – carcinoma in situ and intraepithelial neoplasia grade III.
- *Stage i* – lesions ≤2 cm in size, confined to the vulva or perineum, with no modal metastasis
  - *1a* lesions ≤2 cm in size, confined to vulva or perineum and with stromal invasions ≤1.0 mm, no modal metastasis

○ *1b*   lesions ≤2 cm in size, confined to vulva or perineum and with stromal invasions >1.0 mm, no modal metastasis
- *Stage ii* – tumour confined to the vulva/perineum; >2 cm in greatest dimension, no nodal metastasis
- *Stage iii* – tumour of any size with adjacent spread to the lower urethra/vagina or anus, and/or unilateral lymph node metastasis
- *Stage iv* –
  ○ *iva*   tumour invades any of the following: upper urethra, bladder mucosa, rectal mucosa, pelvic bone and/or bilateral regional node metastases
  ○ *ivb*   any distant metastases including pelvic lymph nodes.

Both benign and malignant tumours occasionally arise on the vulva, particularly in postmenopausal women. Vulvar cancers may be primary, but where there are multiple foci they are commonly secondary growths as a result of lymphatic spread. Excision of the tumour or vulvectomy may be appropriate.

Bartholin's glands

In the sebaceous and Bartholin's glands of the perineal area, benign cysts can result from blockage of the ducts. They are of little significance unless they become large or infected. Cysts may be excised and the ducts opened (marsupialisation).

Vagina

Cysts, and benign and malignant tumours can occur; carcinoma of the vagina is rarely primary but most commonly spreads down from or via the cervix. It may then involve the rectum and other tissues and be very difficult to treat.

Uterus and cervix

Benign tumours

The most common benign tumour of the genital tract, found in 15–20% of women over 35 years of age, is the so-called *'fibroid'*, which grows on or within the wall of the uterus or cervix. In that it usually consists of unstriped muscle as well as fibrous tissue, the term 'fibromyoma' is more accurate. In the mature women, one or more fibroids of the uterus, with accompanying heavy menstrual bleeding (menorrhagia), are grounds for considering hysterectomy once childbearing is complete. In less severe cases myomectomy may be sufficient. Fibroids vary hugely in size and number and may develop on a pedicle, in which case the name *'polyp'* is more appropriate. They are uncommon in those under 20 years old but then are found most often in the nulliparous, possibly because they are causes of infertility and miscarriage. They occur three times more frequently in black women than in white women, although the reason for this is unknown.

In general fibroids grow slowly, and may atrophy following the menopause; they are prone to secondary degenerative changes such as hyaline degeneration, fatty degeneration and even calcification, all probably associated with gradual inadequacy of the blood supply to a particular fibroid. In pregnancy they tend to hypertrophy, may cause pain, and may be actually palpable and visible under the skin of the woman's distended abdominal wall in the third trimester. One particular type of degeneration – red degeneration – occurs most commonly in pregnancy, although it can occur at other times. This is the result of a rapidly renewed blood supply to a fibroid that has previously undergone some fatty degeneration, resulting in a degree of haemolysis and giving a local appearance of raw meat. The abdominal pain it causes can be alarming for the mother-to-be, but reassurance and palliative treatment only is required.

Malignant tumours   **Cervix**   Malignant tumours of the cervix most commonly arise in women between 45 and 55 years of age, but are apparently increasing among younger women. Almost all sufferers will have had sexual intercourse, but there is a more potentially significant correlation with those women who began to be sexually active very early and who have had several sexual partners. Once sexual activity has been commenced a woman must be encouraged to have regular cervical smears taken. Precancerous dysplasic changes in the cervical epithelium, if recognised, can be treated and the development of cancerous changes prevented.

Established carcinoma of the cervix is classified in stages by FIGO (Benedet et al 2001):

- *Stage 0* – malignancy suspected but not proven
- *Stage i* –
  - *ia*   tumour limited to the endometrium
  - *ib*   invasion to less than half of the myometrium
  - *ic*   invasion equal to or more than half of the myometrium
- *Stage ii* –
  - *iia*   endocervical glandular involvement only
  - *iib*   cervical stromal invasion
- *Stage iii* –
  - *iiia*   tumour invades the sertosa of the corpus uteri/adnexae and/or positive cytological findings
  - *iiib*   vaginal metastases
  - *iiic*   metastases to pelvic/para-aortic lymph nodes
- *Stage iv* –
  - *iva*   tumour invasion of bladder/bowel mucosa
  - *ivb*   distant metastases, including intra-abdominal metastases and/or inguinal lymph nodes.

In the UK about 4000 new cases of invasive cervical cancer are diagnosed each year. Cauterisation, cryosurgery and laser treatment effectively destroy tissue, and constitute conservative treatments suitable for women with early cervical changes (CIN 1). Cone biopsy may be used for CIN 2 and 3 (see p. 313).

The more serious stages of cervical carcinoma may be arrested and usually cured by radiotherapy or surgery, or a combination of the two. The surgery used is hysterectomy, extended where necessary. Surgery particularly for stage i cervical carcinoma may be preceded by treatment with radioactive isotopes aimed at destroying the malignant tissue and so avoiding spread of cells at surgery.

Uterus   Carcinoma of the uterine endometrium – that is of the uterine body (corpus) – is seen most commonly in women between 50 and 65 years of age, and does not have a coital correlation, as nearly 50% of the sufferers are nulliparous. The only constant symptom is irregular bleeding. Malignant changes begin in the glandular element of the endometrium. Spreading is less rapid than in cervical cancer, possibly because the myometrium forms some sort of containing barrier, but secondary growths may be found in the ovaries and liver. Treatment is again commonly a combination of radiotherapy and surgery.

Fallopian tubes

Despite being prone to infections, the fallopian tubes rarely support a primary carcinoma, although metastases or extensions of growths from the ovaries, uterus or gut do occur. Primary carcinoma is a relatively silent condition and therefore may either be found unexpectedly at surgery or not diagnosed until the condition is advanced.

Ovaries

There is a wide variety of possible cysts and benign or malignant tumours of the ovary. In some cases the menstrual cycle is disturbed and the patient may have pain, but often there is no obvious indication of the real cause.

Cysts

Follicular cysts are one of the most common types; most resolve spontaneously, while others can be surgically removed. Bleeding may occur into cysts, and if present for some time the altered blood will become tar-like, making the cyst look dark. Reports of surgery or laparoscopy may refer to 'chocolate' cysts. 'Oyster' ovaries indicate that the ovaries may appear enlarged, shiny and pearly; this is a sign of polycystic ovarian disease.

Cancer

Amongst women who die of cancer of the genital tract, ovarian cancer is the most common primary site, affecting about 4000 women per annum. The overall lifetime risk for developing ovarian cancer is 1 in 120 for the general female population. However, women with a first degree relative with a history of ovarian cancer before the age of 50 years have an increased risk at 1 in 40. If there are two affected first degree relatives this becomes a 1 in 3 risk. Both ovarian and endometrial cancer occur more often in families with breast or bowel cancer. Women in such families need to be particularly vigilant and avail themselves of any screening and family genetic counselling (Redman 1997). A major problem in early detection is that it is a silent cancer, often *without* symptoms until the tumour has extended into the peritoneum. In an attempt to combat this, voluntary ovarian screening by ultrasound and blood test is being offered in some centres. However unnecessary anxiety has been caused in some cases by false positive results, not least because with ultrasound scanning it is not easy to discriminate between benign and malignant structures.

The FIGO categorisation of ovarian cancer (Heintz et al 2001) is briefly as follows:

- *Stage i* – growth limited to the ovaries
- *Stage ii* – growth involving one or both ovaries with pelvic extension
- *Stage iii* – tumour involving one or both ovaries with histologically confirmed peritoneal implants outside the pelvis and/or positive retroperitoneal or inguinal nodes; superficial liver metastases equals stage iii; tumour is limited to the true pelvis, but with histologically proven malignant extension to small bowel or omentum
- *Stage iv* – growth involving one or both ovaries with distant metastases; if pleural effusion is present, there must be positive cytology to allot a case to stage iv; parenchymal liver metastasis equals stage iv.

Treatment consists of a combination of surgery, radiotherapy and chemotherapy.

Endometriosis

Endometriosis is a condition which, although not a cyst or a tumour, has certain aspects that make it an acceptable inclusion in this section. It is a disorder in which there is the presence of endometrium outside the endometrial cavity (Prentice 2001). Most pelvic endometrial deposits are found in the ovaries, peritoneum, uterosacral ligaments, pouch of Douglas and rectovaginal septum. Rarely there are extrapelvic deposits found in the umbilicus and diaphragm (Farquhar 2000). The tissue responds to the hormonal changes of the menstrual cycle, proliferates and may bleed at the appropriate point in that cycle. The bleeding causes inflammation, may be contained and fibrose, or track causing dense adhesions. The plaques grow, infiltrate and multiply, mimicking a malignancy. In severe cases, adhesions mesh the pelvic structures together; Llewellyn-Jones (1986) referred to such a pelvis as 'frozen'. Endometriomas are ovarian cysts of endometriosis. It has also been shown that there is a clear association between clear cell endometroid carcinomas and endometriosis (Stern et al 2001).

The prevalence ranges from 2 to 22% in the general female population, depending on the populations studied and the methodology used (Farquhar 2000). There is an increased risk in those females having an early menarche and late menopause. Oral contraception reduces the risk. There may be a disproportionate level of symptoms in comparison to the extent of the disease in the women's pelvis (Prentice 2001).

The presenting symptoms are variable, the most common being dysmenorrhoea. Other symptoms often presenting are: pelvic pain, lower abdominal pain, back pain, dyspareunia, dyschezia (pain on defecation), loin pain, pain on micturition, pain on exercise, fatigue, general malaise and sleep disturbance (Prentice 2001). As a result, patients are often referred to many different specialties prior to a gynaecological assessment. The women therefore become disheartened and often have the belief that nothing can be done for them. When there is more serious endometriosis it can be the cause of not only severe pain but also infertility. As a result of the pain, women often find that they need to take increasing amounts of time off work.

Whatever the cause, it has been estimated that 10 million women in the USA and 2 million women in Britain suffer with the condition.

Aetiology   The cause is unknown but there are several theories as to how this condition arises (see Further Reading, p. 306):

1. *The transportation theory.* In 1921 John Sampson (cited in Brentkopf & Bakoulis 1988) first used the term 'endometriosis'. He postulated that during menstruation there was reflux of endometrial debris and blood through the fallopian tubes and into the peritoneal cavity; endometrial cells could thus be deposited outside the uterus. In 1927 Halban (cited in Brentkopf & Bakoulis 1988) suggested instead that fragments of endometrium could be transported as emboli in veins and lymphatics.

2. *The metaplastic theory.* Meyer, (cited in Brentkopf & Bakoulis 1988) a contemporary of Sampson, suggested that repeated irritation (for example due to recurrent infection) might cause cells derived from the same embryological tissue as the endometrium to change and differentiate abnormally. A similar theory suggests that a chemical substance, perhaps environmentally derived, acts on cells outside the uterus causing them to be transformed into endometrial cells.

3. *Immune deficiency theory.* A further hypothesis is that women with endometriosis suffer from an immune deficiency such that the body does not reject and dispose of endometrial cells if they become displaced elsewhere in the body, as it would normally be expected to. The fact that endometriosis runs in families supports this theory.

Treatment

Pharmacological therapy   In primary care the first treatments to be considered should be non-steroidal anti-inflammatory drugs (NSAIDs) and the combined oral contraceptive (Prentice 2001). The NSAIDs have, however, the side-effect of possibly causing gastric irritation. Medical treatment may be hormonal, aimed at producing a pseudopregnancy or pseudomenopausal state of amenorrhoea. However some of the side-effects – bloating, fluid retention, breast tenderness, nausea, seborrhoea, acne, muscle cramps, weight gain and menopausal symptoms – are difficult to tolerate. Medical treatments have an 80–85% improvement rate for symptoms but the efficacy is dependent on the patient's ability to tolerate side-effects. It has, however, been claimed that many women are not treated adequately by laparoscopy because of the emphasis on medical management (Jones & Sutton 2002); they recommend that medical care should be used in primary care and then, only if unsuccessful, should patients be referred to a surgical unit.

Investigations   It is recommended that women presenting with pelvic pain, dyspareunia or dysmenorrhoea should have a transvaginal or abdominal ultrasound examination (Amso 2002).

Surgery   It is desirable to be referred to a unit where laparoscopic diagnosis and surgery can be carried out during the same operation. The laparoscopic surgery may be conservative, excisional or ablative, depending on the findings (Jones & Sutton 2002).

Hysterectomy and bilateral salpingo-oophrectomy may also be carried out for those with endometriosis if it is thought appropriate; however, use of hormone replacement therapy risks reactivating the disease. The Royal College of Obstetricians and Gynecologists (RCOG 2000) has also advocated the use of ablative surgery in the treatment of endometriosis. Women with endometriosis are encouraged to start their family as early as possible (Brentkopf & Bakoulis 1988). If there are problems of infertility associated with the endometriosis there should be a referral to a gynaecologist. There is evidence that surgery for endometriosis does not always assist conception in cases of infertility. A Canadian study of 348 women showed a benefit to fertility from surgical intervention (Marcoux et al 1997), but they found poor pregnancy outcomes in comparison to those receiving medical therapy. Also, an Italian study of 77 women found no benefit to fertility in the women who had a laparoscopic surgical intervention (Parazzini 1999).

More recently, lasers have been used to destroy endometrial implants and adhesions, and so can delay the progress of the condition. Surgery may also be used to remove adhesions thought to be causing pain, or to facilitate conception where adhesions have blocked or distorted the fallopian tubes.

Physiotherapy in the treatment of gynaecological cysts and new growths

Physiotherapy has no place in the actual treatment of cysts or new growths, but there are important prophylactic and therapeutic roles for the physiotherapist where chemotherapy or radiotherapy, involving bed rest, or surgery is undertaken. Patients will benefit from advice and assistance to optimise their physical and mental condition before as well as after such procedures. Appropriate physiotherapeutic modalities should be considered where pain is troublesome, but the value of pulsed short-wave diathermy or ultrasound (but not in the case of surgery) to assist in the softening and absorption of painful abdominal adhesions is unproven. However, the physiotherapist has much to contribute to the quality of life of those whose condition places heavy stresses on marital relationships and the ability to work, or who are terminally ill.

DISPLACEMENTS AND GENITAL PROLAPSE

The word 'prolapse' is from the latin *prolapsus*, meaning a slipping forth (Thakar & Stanton 2002). Therefore genital prolapse refers to a slipping of one of the pelvic organs into a displaced position. The woman may or may not be symptom free, depending on the severity of the displacement. Samuelsson et al (1999) reported that the symptomology and clinical findings may not correlate well. It has been reported that 20% of those on a waiting list for major gynaecological surgery are awaiting surgery for genital prolapse (Cardozo 1997).

The uterus is free to move according to the changing volumes of bladder and rectum. The cervix is directed backwards and the uterus is said to be 'anteverted'. Where the uterus is further bent forwards on itself, it is said to be 'anteflexed'. If, however, the cervix is found to be pointing forwards and the fundus of the uterus is directed backwards, the uterus is said to be 'retroverted', and where the uterus is then further bent backwards on itself it is said to be 'retroflexed'. Twenty per cent of normal women have retroversion of the uterus; infertility, backache and dyspareunia have been attributed to it. The uterus may be drawn or held in retroversion as a result of adhesions associated with endometriosis or pelvic inflammatory disease.

As described in Chapter 1, the pelvic organs are maintained and supported in position by a combination of fascia and ligaments, and indirectly by the pelvic floor and levator ani muscles. These vital supportive components are sometimes congenitally weak, or are weakened, elongated or actually damaged by childbirth. The factors at childbirth leading to genitourinary prolapse are: large babies, long labours, assisted delivery and poor postnatal exercise regimens (Jackson & Smith 1997). The same authors also cite connective tissue disease, hysterectomy, obesity, chronic respiratory disease and pelvic masses as other possible causes. Constipation is also considered to be a contributory factor to uterovaginal prolapse (Spence-Jones et al 1994). Prolapse most commonly occurs in women who have borne children, although it can occur in the nulliparous. It has been estimated that 50% of parous women have some prolapse; however, only 10–20% seek treatment for their condition (Beck 1983, cited in Glowacki & Wall 2002). There is also an increased risk of prolapse with age (Olsen et al 1997).

Following hysterectomy the vagina may be susceptible to prolapse owing to a decrease in the support of the vaginal vault (Jackson & Smith 1997). This can be due to the unsuccessful attachment of the incised uterosacral and transverse cervical ligaments for the conservation of the vagina. Figures 9.1 and 9.2 (p. 285, 286) illustrate the most common types of displacement and prolapse encountered by the physiotherapist, together with a rough guide as to how they may present at perineal examination. The symptoms are variable but patients may complain of a lump, a dragging sensation, 'something coming down' or a feeling of heaviness when they are standing, and as a progressive sensation through the day. It is 'not there' when the patient is lying down. There may be complaint of backache but it is not often caused by the prolapse. Sexual intercourse may be affected by difficulty in penetration, dyspareunia (see p. 296) or lack of satisfaction on the part of one or both partners. Displacement of the bladder (cystocoele) (Fig. 9.1a) does not always affect continence but some patients complain of frequency and urgency of micturition, and of stress incontinence, which may be anything from very mild to severe. A rectocoele (Fig. 9.1b) and an enterocoele may result in difficulty in defaecation, constipation and haemorrhoids. If there is concurrent urinary incontinence it should be fully investigated before any surgery (Jackson & Smith 1997). Any form of prolapse may lead to coital problems as a result of altered vaginal sensation, and dyspareunia and/or vaginal flatus (Jackson & Smith 1997).

Hormone replacement therapy in the form of postmenopausal oestrogen supplementation may be recommended to increase the skin collagen content, but its efficacy in preventing genitourinary prolapse is unproven (Jackson & Smith 1997).

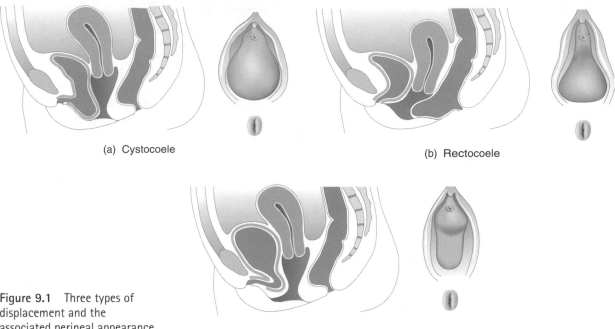

(a) Cystocoele

(b) Rectocoele

(c) Urethrocoele

Figure 9.1 Three types of displacement and the associated perineal appearance.

Prolapse of the genital organs can be described as occurring in the anterior, middle or posterior compartment.

1. Anterior compartment

Cystocoele (Fig. 9.1a)

Weakness of the pubocervical fascia allows the bladder to displace downwards and backwards against the anterior wall of the vagina. If this is slack it will protrude. In more severe cases a pouch is formed in the bladder which holds residual urine. Patients complain of frequency and incomplete emptying of the bladder, which predisposes to infection; they may also have stress incontinence. A cystocoele may occur in the absence of uterine descent; but where there is uterine descent it will be accompanied by some degree of cystocoele because of the intimate fascial connections between the bladder base and the cervix.

Urethrocoele (Fig. 9.1c)

The urethra alone, being closely attached to the anterior wall of the vagina, may sag backwards and downwards when it receives insufficient support from the vagina or surrounding fascia; it may also kink. It is the least common form of genital prolapse (Thakar & Stanton 2002).

Cystourethrocoele

A combination of a cystocoele and urethrocoele is the most common type of prolapse (Thakar & Stanton 2002). Cystourethrocoele may be associated with urinary stress incontinence, and urinary retention or recurrent urinary tract infection, or both (Jackson & Smith 1997).

2. Middle compartment

Enterocoele

A descent of the vaginal vault frees the upper part of the posterior vaginal wall to drop, bulge and protrude, allowing an extended pouch of Douglas to be herniated; it may contain small bowel and omentum. Thus an enterocoele usually accompanies a uterine prolapse.

Uterine prolapse

When lack of adequate support allows the uterus to descend, it causes the vaginal vault to descend also and the vagina to invert. Such a prolapse will be associated with a cystocoele and enterocoele (see above). Traditionally three degrees of uterine prolapse (Fig. 9.2) are used in clinical description:

First degree   The cervix remains within the vagina.

Second degree   A descent of the cervix to the introitus, which may protrude further on straining, with the possibility of damage, infection and ulceration.

Third degree or procidentia   The entire uterus descends outside the introitus of the body, causing total inversion of the vagina. A procidentia is almost inevitably associated with a cystocoele and an enterocoele.

However, it is now recommended that gynaecologists should use the parameters for measuring pelvic organ prolapse as described by Bump et al (1996) and agreed by the International Continence Society. This method uses anatomical reference points defined in terms of vaginal wall segments. There are six defined points located in the anterior, superior

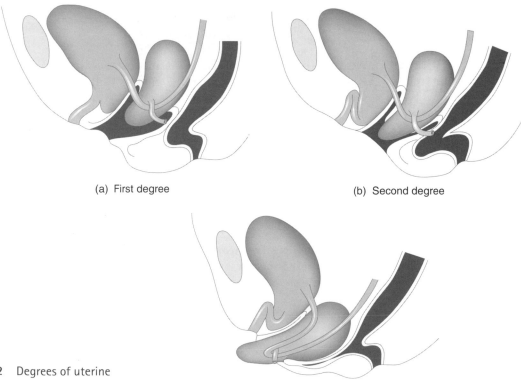

(a) First degree

(b) Second degree

(c) Third degree

Figure 9.2   Degrees of uterine prolapse.

and posterior vagina that are located in reference to the hymenal ring and measurements taken.

Uterine prolapse is associated with backache and difficulty in using tampons; procidentia may lead to ulceration (Jackson & Smith 1997).

3. Posterior compartment

Rectocoele (Fig. 9.1b)

Prolapse of the rectum forwards against the lower part of the posterior wall of the vagina is almost always associated with damage to the perineal body and consequent loss of the support it provides. Inadequate or ineffective suturing of episiotomies and perineal tears associated with childbirth, or lack of appreciation of the damage sustained, may contribute to this condition. Rectocoele is not necessarily associated with uterine prolapse because the rectum is not directly connected to the cervix. A rectocoele may lead to constipation and dyschezia (Jackson & Smith 1997). Faeces often 'pocket' in the rectocoele; women often report using perineal splinting or post-vaginal-wall pressure in order to empty their bowels fully.

Physiotherapy in the treatment of genital displacements and prolapse

Although not yet proven, it is believed that better education of women prior to childbirth with active pelvic floor muscle education will help in the prevention or delay of prolapse and its symptomology. Appropriate management in labour should also reduce the obstetric risk factors. Most patients with mild prolapse will benefit from physiotherapy directed at strengthening the pelvic floor muscles (see Chs 11, 12); this was recommended by both Jackson & Smith (1997) and Thakar & Stanton (2002). A physiotherapist should also consider giving attention to chest and other infections, obesity, constipation and the woman's workload. Considering the cost – both human and financial – and the inherent risks associated with surgery, it makes good sense for all patients to be offered an intensive 6–8-week period of specialist physiotherapeutic treatment before surgery is mooted or once they are placed on the surgical waiting list. In any case, surgery will be delayed whenever practicable until childbearing is complete; physiotherapy or a pessary may help to tide a woman over until then. For the more resistant cases, surgery in the form of a repair or hysterectomy will eventually be required (see p. 309); however long-term results for prolapse surgery are uncertain (Jackson & Smith 1997). It would seem sensible to teach all women appropriate pelvic floor muscle exercises prior to any prolapse surgery, in association with being taught 'the knack' (Miller et al 1998) and being given advice on appropriate moving and handling techniques. It is also advisable to teach defaecation technique (see p. 387) to any women presenting with prolapse, particularly if they are suffering with constipation.

FURTHER GYNAECOLOGICAL CONDITIONS OF RELEVANCE TO THE PHYSIOTHERAPIST

DISORDERS ASSOCIATED WITH MENSTRUATION

For most women, the onset of menstrual flow is a regular and reasonably predictable event, and the length of the menstrual cycle is individual and constant – usually somewhere between 27 and 32 days. However, there can be few women who do not, at some stage in their lives apart from pregnancy, experience irregularities or discomfort, or both, associated with their menstruation. The regularity of periods may change, and bleeding from the uterus may be delayed (*oligomenorrhoea*), more frequent (*polymenorrhoea*) or simply unpredictable, as is common in the menopause. The amount of menstrual flow may alter to be continuous or excessive (*menorrhagia*), or scant (*hypomenorrhoea*). A woman who experiences intermenstrual or postcoital bleeding should, however, always be investigated as it can be a sign of endometrial or cervical cancer (O'Brien & Doyle 1997).

'Menorrhagia' is a term used for excessive menstrual flow from the uterus. Bleeding may also arise from other organs in the tract (e.g. the vagina) and from other tracts (e.g. the urinary tract), and occasionally patients confuse these with menstruation. Not surprisingly it has been shown that women vary hugely in what they construe as abnormal and worthy of consultation, and reports of symptoms can be unreliable. Chimbira et al (1980) investigated 92 women complaining of menorrhagia (defined as heavy bleeding although the periods were regular), and found no correlation between the patients' subjective assessment of blood loss and the objectively measured menstrual blood loss. Once reported, such symptoms of change in pattern are worthy of investigation in many cases, to exclude organic disease.

The menarche

Menarche is the onset of menstruation, with a median age of 13 years in Britain; this has recently been confirmed by a study of 1166 girls from ten British towns (Whincup et al 2001). However the same study showed that almost one in eight girls reaches menarche whilst still at primary school. An early menarche tends to be followed by a late menopause, whereas a late menarche is often followed by an early menopause (Lewis & Chamberlain 1990). A girl's first cycles are often irregular and are usually painless, but may be anovular with the follicles failing to mature adequately and perhaps with prolonged bleeding.

Primary amenorrhoea

If a girl is developing secondary sexual characteristics, but has amenorrhoea, there is no cause for concern. If she has no secondary sexual characteristics developing at 14, or is still not menstruating by the age of 16 years regardless of sexual characteristics, the condition should be considered pathological; this is termed *primary amenhorrhoea* and it is believed by some that investigations should take place (Tindall et al 1991). However, others believe that if sexual characteristics are present then further investigation or management is not necessary, other than reassurance that normally developed girls will commence menstruation by the age of 18 years (O'Brien & Doyle 1997). Steele (1997) also states that the age that investigations take place should also depend on the family history and the level of anxiety shown by the girl and her parents.

Secondary amenorrhoea

'Secondary amenorrhoea' is strictly defined as the absence of menstruation for 6 months in those women who have previously menstruated (Steele 1997). Stress, emotional upset and regular strenuous exercise

(Beals & Manore 2002) are all known to cause the missing of one or more expected menstrual periods. Amenorrhoea or infrequent periods may also occur with serious illness, starvation (e.g. anorexia nervosa, where amenorrhoea may occur before excess weight loss is obvious) and gross obesity. Other possible causes of secondary amenorrhoea include: pregnancy and breastfeeding, polycystic ovary syndrome (PCOS), premature ovarian failure, pituitary tumour, Asherman's syndrome (uterine adhesions), radiotherapy and chemotherapy (Steele 1997). If the menstrual pattern is irregular but menstruation still present it is known as *oligomenhoroea*.

Dysmenorrhoea

The term 'dysmenorrhoea' comes from the Greek meaning 'difficult monthly flow' and it is used to describe pain associated with menstruation. The condition may be primary or secondary. It has also been shown in a small study of 18 women that those with dysmenorrhoea have symptoms of high nocturnal body temperatures and disturbed sleep throughout the menstrual cycle (Baker et al 1999).

Primary or spasmodic dysmenorrhoea

This is the more common type; there is no apparent structural abnormality or pathology. It is related to the increased production and release of endometrial prostaglandins resulting in increased and abnormal uterine activity (Pickrell 1997). The pain is felt over the lower abdomen and sacral region in the first hours of a period, and may be colicky. When pain is very severe, nausea, vomiting, headache, abdominal distension, irritability and even diarrhoea may be experienced. Pain decreases with increasing blood loss. Self-management is often by over-the-counter medication such as ibuprofen (Fraser & McCarron 1987). Medical management consists of reassurance and either prostaglandin synthetase inhibitors at the onset of menstruation or suppression of ovulation with oral contraceptives (Pickrell 1997).

Secondary or congestive dysmenorrhoea

This is associated with some structural abnormality or pathology (e.g. a fibroid, endometriosis or infection). The pain, which may be unilateral or bilateral, begins 3 days before menstruation and is relieved or temporarily exacerbated as bleeding commences. It may increase with activity.

The physiotherapist must assess every referral with care. Primary dysmenorrhoea may be managed using pain-coping strategies such as relaxation, breathing awareness, acupuncture, transcutaneous electrical nerve stimulation (TENS) and distraction techniques. A recent Cochrane review (Proctor et al 2003) reviewed the use of TENS for primary dysmenorrhoea; it concluded that high frequency TENS was found to be useful by a number of small trials. However, there was insufficient evidence to determine the effectiveness of low-frequency TENS. It also found from one methodologically sound study that there appears to be a benefit from the use of acupuncture in reducing dysmenorrhoea (Helms 1987). Where the patient's occupation and lifestyle are predominantly sedentary (as is often the case), or fitness is in question, guidance as to ways of wisely increasing physical activity may be helpful as exercise is known to produce endogenous endorphins, which have natural pain-relieving properties.

'Breakthrough bleeding'

This phrase describes intermenstrual bleeding; it is usually associated with the use of contraceptive pills. After checking that the pills are being taken correctly, the doctor may need to increase the progesterone dosage or change the preparation. Some women also experience this after having an intrauterine device (IUD) fitted. However if the woman is not on the contraceptive pill or has had an IUD recently fitted any intermenstrual bleeding should be investigated as it may be due to a carcinoma of the endometrium (Tindall et al 1991).

Premenstrual tension

Premenstrual tension (PMT) is more common in women over 30 years of age than in younger women; it is a diagnosis used to describe irritability, depression, lumbar backache, tenderness and enlargement of breasts, abdominal pain and distension, water retention, weight gain and insomnia associated with the menstrual cycle. In a sample of 1045 menstruating women from the UK, USA and France, up to 80% experienced mood and physical symptoms associated with their menstrual cycle; however, only 25% had ever sought treatment (Hylan et al 1999). Some or all of these symptoms commence up to 10 days prior to menstruation, and usually recede quickly once the menstrual flow has commenced. There is evidence in some women that their cognitive ability decreases and that they are more aggressive and accident prone at this time, which is relevant for those with demanding and responsible employment. There have been several legal cases where PMT has been used in defence.

The retention of fluid is thought by some to be due to a relative lack of ovarian progesterone, but there is also an increased output of antidiuretic hormone (ADH) by the posterior pituitary gland. There may also be reduced serotonin levels leading to mood swings; selective serotonin reuptake inhibitors (SSRI) may be an effective treatment.

Progesterone and progestegons have often been used in the management of the syndrome, but a recent systematic review concluded that the evidence does not support this treatment (Wyatt et al 2001). Another recent German study of 170 women suggests that the dry extract of agnus castor fruit is an effective and well-tolerated treatment for the relief of symptoms (Schellenberg 2001). Many women also consider that gamma linolenic acid, in the form of evening primrose oil, starflower oil or borage seed oil, is beneficial. There are contradictory studies regarding their efficacy, but as there are no reports of side-effects in their use, it may be worthwhile considering them (Andrew 1997).

The women's health physiotherapist has a role in helping women to understand the condition and to consider ways of adjusting the stress levels being placed on the body, both generally and at particular times. The Mitchell method of relaxation should be taught as fatigue and stress exaggerate the condition (see p. 111) (ACPWH 2002). Some women also find it helpful to consume small, frequent meals of complex carbohydrates, fruits and vegetables. Limiting salt intake can be helpful in avoiding fluid retention, and avoiding caffeine may help towards decreasing cyclic breast pain.

Dysfunctional uterine bleeding/menorrhagia

'Dysfunctional uterine bleeding' (DUB) is a term to describe abnormal uterine bleeding not due to organic disease of the genital tract. It is one of the most frequently encountered conditions in gynaecology, can occur at any age and is not one disease but a category of diseases (Dewhurst 1981). It is thought by some to be due to endocrine dysfunction. For example, girl infants may menstruate in the first weeks of life, probably as a result of no longer receiving placental oestrogens. All cases must be thoroughly investigated and if necessary reinvestigated; for example, anaemia may be the cause or the effect of menorrhagia, and malignant disease may become unmasked. Unfortunately there is evidence that many doctors do not necessarily prescribe what is believed to be the most effective first line treatment: tranexamic acid (Prentice 1999). Menstrual loss is reduced by about a half when taking tranexamic acid, and by one-third with NSAIDs; both are taken during menstruation. Progestogens have been found to be ineffective when given in the luteal phase of the cycle; they may be effective if taken for 21 days of the cycle but have unpleasant side-effects (Lethaby et al 1999). Other medical treatments may be combined oral contraceptives, or the levonorgestrel-releasing intrauterine system (Mirena). Appropriate medical treatment may be able to avoid the need for surgery. A physiotherapist's role may simply be to encourage a further consultation or second opinion.

BACKACHE AND ABDOMINAL PAIN

Women with gynaecological conditions frequently assume that this is also the source of their back pain. This is not always so, and much needless additional suffering could be avoided by appropriate physiotherapeutic assessment and care. However, back and abdominal pain, particularly chronic pain of gradual onset, may have a direct gynaecological origin (Fig. 9.3), and certainly gynaecological pain may coexist with pain from the back and is a late symptom of malignant disease.

The physiotherapist can be an invaluable member of the gynaecological team in helping to analyse the cause, particularly of back pain,

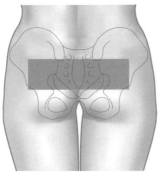
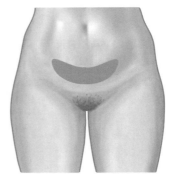

Figure 9.3 Zones of gynaecological pain.

(a) Posterior   (b) Anterior

and treating it where appropriate. Where pain cannot be cured but must be endured, TENS may be helpful.

Acute lower abdominal pain

Acute lower abdominal pain may be a sign of many conditions including an ectopic pregnancy in someone who is in the early stages of pregnancy, or a torsion, haemorrhage or rupture of an ovarian cyst. Any new abdominal acute pain should be immediately referred for medical advice.

Over the abdomen, true gynaecological pain rarely extends above the anterior superior iliac spines; when of uterine origin it may radiate to the anterior aspect of the thighs. Pain may be exacerbated by abdominal pressure over the site of the lesion. Posteriorly, it is usually located over the upper half of the sacrum and may extend laterally to the glutei. When involving lymphatic nodes around the sacral plexus, cervical cancer may cause pain radiating down the back of the legs. Backache associated with uterine prolapse is relieved by lying down; it becomes more severe on prolonged standing and as the day progresses.

Chronic lower abdominal pain with pelvic congestion

Beard et al (1984) suggested a cause for pelvic pain in women of reproductive age with no obvious somatic pathology; dilated veins and vascular congestion in the broad ligaments and ovarian plexuses were apparent in 91% of the women in this study. When examining the clinical features in women with pelvic pain and congestion, which was demonstrable on pelvic venography, the following results were found (Beard et al 1988):

- The women were more often multiparous.
- The pain was dull and aching with sharp exacerbations.
- Pain was commonly on one side of the abdomen, but could also occur on the other side.
- The pain was made worse by postural changes and walking.
- Congestive dysmenorrhoea, deep dyspareunia and postcoital ache were common.
- Evidence of significant emotional disturbance was present in 60%.

Alleviating factors were lying down, analgesics, local heat application and relaxation.

POLYCYSTIC OVARIAN SYNDROME

This syndrome is associated with menstrual disturbance and is the most common form of anovulatory infertility (Frank 1995). Women with this condition may also suffer with hirsutism, acne, obesity, increased testosterone activity, and elevated LH concentrations. It is thought that the underlying disorder is one of insulin resistance, with the hyperinsulinaemia stimulating excess ovarian androgen production (Hopkinson et al 1998). It is believed that insulin-sensitising agents such as metformin can play a major role in its treatment (Hopkinson et al 1998).

Women with this condition may become very anxious regarding infertility; the women's health physiotherapist may have a role to play in teaching stress control by relaxation techniques.

INFERTILITY

There have been increasing referrals for fertility investigations in recent years. This rise may be due to increased media exposure of the subject, but what is certain is that women are increasingly delaying childbirth until their thirties, and this practice has doubled in the last 25 years (Office for National Statistics 1997). Of those having regular intercourse without contraception, 90% of fertile couples should achieve a pregnancy within a year and this rises to 95% after 2 years. Therefore some people have low normal fertility rather than subfertility (Cahill & Wardle 2002). There are many causes of subfertility including sperm dysfunction, ovulation disorder and fallopian tube damage. The causes of these problems are many and varied and some couples may have more than one reason for their subfertility. Increasing age of the women reduces the women's fertility further and hence reduces the likelihood of treatment success.

Primary infertility is that occurring in women that have never conceived. If there has been a previous pregnancy it is termed as *secondary infertility*. A previous full term conception has been found to give a greater chance of conception either naturally or after treatment.

A couple should pursue early referral to a specialist infertility clinic if they have been attempting conception for more than 3 years, or the woman is over 38 years, has had serum *Chlamydia* antibody titre or has FSH concentrations or LH concentrations in the early follicular phase causing concern. Other possible reasons would be if the partner's sperm count, motility or appearance was causing concern (Cahill & Wardle 2002).

Women's health physiotherapists may encounter these patients only during or after a resultant pregnancy. They should be cognisant of the extra anxieties and concerns that these couples may have. Those that have had fertility problems may be more questioning of all that is offered to them and care must be taken to allay any of the very real anxieties that they may have. Physiotherapy should be directed appropriately towards any presenting condition.

PREMATURE OVARIAN FAILURE (POF), ALSO KNOWN AS PREMATURE MENOPAUSE

This distressing condition cannot be prevented or cured but can be treated and managed. The ovarian failure occurs some time between the menarche and the age of 40 years. The incidence is approximately 1% of women, rising to 8–10% when including gynaecological surgery, chemotherapy and radiotherapy (Farrell 2002). POF can be of different levels of severity and can not only result in infertility but also have the long-term consequences of a woman being at increased risk of osteoporosis and heart disease. The possible causes are many: gonadal dysgenesis, genetic associations, autoimmune disease, viral oophritis, or iatrogenic or idiopathic causes. Some causes are more rare than others, many falling into the idiopathic group.

This group of women often reports high levels of depression and stress and low levels of self-esteem and life satisfaction (Liao et al 2000). Those women that have POF as a sequellae of chemotherapy or radiotherapy may need effective crisis intervention (Pasquali 2002). It may be advisable to have a bone density scan as a baseline for future reference and practice breast awareness. The women's health physiotherapist must be aware of the possible psychological problems associated with the condition.

PSYCHOSEXUAL PROBLEMS

The women's health physiotherapist must be prepared for clients to want to discuss their sexual difficulties. Sometimes women may be directly referred suffering from dyspareunia, but frequently the subject will arise following surgery, or during treatment for various forms of incontinence and weak pelvic floor muscles, and of course during pregnancy or following childbirth.

Although sex and sexuality are more openly discussed today, most people have great difficulty in exposing their very personal sexual problems to outsiders. The physiotherapist must respect the woman's wanting to confide in her, provide a non-judgmental listening ear and, if unable to help directly, should know of further sources of psychosexual counselling in the area. A questionnaire sent to health professionals (doctors, nurses, physiotherapists and occupational therapists) revealed a lack of training; there were 813 respondents who believed that sexual issues needed to be addressed and discussed in the health service (Haboubi & Lincoln 2003). However, they felt that they were poorly trained, ill prepared and rarely had such discussions. The therapists in particular had less training, lower comfort levels and less willingness to talk about sexual issues than doctors and nurses; this needs to be addressed.

Aetiology

Female sexual dysfunction is caused by many variables. Hawton (1985) mentions three causal categories:

1. *Predisposing factors*, which include experiences early in life
2. *Precipitants*, which are events or experiences associated with the initial appearance of a dysfunction
3. *Maintaining factors*, which explain why a dysfunction persists.

Broadly, sexual problems can be classified as those that are physical and are caused by physical illness, trauma during surgery and drugs, and those that have a psychological origin. Obviously physical and psychological causes will interact closely, one with the other. Sexual dysfunction is a direct cause of disharmony and stress in relationships and leads to great personal anguish; female sexuality is frequently affected by life events such as pregnancy, birth, illness and the climacteric, all of which will be encountered by physiotherapists working with women.

Various authors (Gillan & Brindley 1979, Kegel 1952, Kline-Graber & Graber 1975; Masters & Johnson 1966) have drawn attention to the role played by the pelvic floor musculature, and particularly the bulbospongiosus, ischiocavernosus and the most medial fibres of the levator ani muscles, in the achievement of female orgasm. Kegel (1952) reported that weak pelvic floor muscles were accompanied by complaints of sexual dissatisfaction, and Graber & Kline-Graber (1979) have reported that orgasmic women had better circumvaginal musculature (pelvic floor muscles) based on clinical assessment and perineometer readings. Stimulation of the pelvic floor muscles using a vaginal electrode to treat urinary incontinence in women has produced increased coital satisfaction (Scott & Hsuch 1979). Shafik (2000) reviewed the role of the levator ani muscles in evacuation, sexual performance and pelvic floor disorders. He states that, during intercourse, the vaginal distension by the penis causes the vaginolevator and vaginopuborectalis reflexes with a resultant levator ani muscle contraction. The levator ani muscles also contract in response to stimulation of the clitoris or cervix uteri via the clitoromotor and cervicomotor reflexes.

All these findings have interesting implications for physiotherapists involved in pelvic floor muscle re-education; it could be that improving the strength of their pelvic floor muscles would help anorgasmic women.

Psychological causes play a large part in female sexual dysfunction (Masters & Johnson 1970), but disease and the oral contraceptive pill may also reduce libido. Dyspareunia can certainly inhibit sexual arousal; its causes are varied (see p. 296) and should always be properly investigated and treated.

General sexual dysfunction

There is a decrease in libido, leading to a lack of erotic feelings and reduced vasocongestion in the arousal phase; vaginal lubrication and expansion will not occur.

A lack of desire is often secondary to stress, fatigue, depression, physical illness, drugs, other sexual dysfunctions or relationship difficulties (Watson 1990). Testosterone production is shared between the ovaries and adrenal gland. If there has been surgery or chemotherapy affecting these there may be a loss of sexual desire (Butcher 1999a). There are also many drugs and other health problems that can affect sexual desire.

Orgasmic dysfunction

Although erotic sensations and vasocongestion may occur, orgasm is not experienced. This may be primary (orgasm has never been achieved) or secondary (having experienced orgasm previously, a woman is no longer able to reach a climax). Anorgasmia can be defined as an involuntary inhibition of the orgasmic reflex (Butcher 1999b). It becomes a problem only if the woman regards it to be one (Selby 1997). The media has sometimes made women have unreasonable expectations; 'normality' can range from those women who never or rarely experience orgasm to those who claim to have multiple orgasms. Treatment may start with the woman but continues with her and her partner; it is aimed at the 'holding back' that the woman may feel. Sexual therapists can further treat those women who are concerned by encouraging the use of 'superstimulation' using aids and by reassurance (Watson 1990).

Vaginismus

Vaginismus is an involuntary spasm of the pubococcygeal and associated muscles around the lower third of the vagina (Butcher 1999b); it may completely prevent penetration or make it very painful. If there is attempted penetration there may also be spasm of the adductors and abdomen. It can be a primary condition response caused by fear of penetration, in a woman who has never experienced vaginal peneration.

Secondary vaginismus is when there has been vaginal penetration without a problem in the past; it may be secondary to a traumatic experience such as childbirth or sexual abuse. Rarely there may be a physical cause, and dyspareunia, for whatever reason, may play a part in the aetiology of this distressing condition. There is a great spectrum of vaginismus, from woman who are happy to have anything but penetrative activity, even achieving orgasm, to those in whom the symptoms are so severe that it can lead to a general avoidance of any sexual or even affectionate touching (Butcher 1999b). Ultimately this can lead to pain, fear, humiliation and frustration, leading on to inadequacy and feelings of abandonment.

Women suffering from this condition will have difficulty in attending for any cervical smear or gynaecological assessment and be unable to use tampons. Treatment is often initiated using cognitive behavioural treatment programmes (Butcher 1999a). It commences with careful explanation of the nature of the problem followed by appropriate graded exercise whilst learning to gain control and relax the pelvic floor muscles. Training dilators may then be introduced in gradually graded sizes and ultimately partners are encouraged to participate in the therapy (Watson 1990). Treatment can succeed only if the woman manages to have what she perceives as 'ownership of her own vagina'.

The women's health physiotherapist must always be aware of a woman's body language when she attends for any therapy. Informed consent is always essential before any examination or treatment commences. Even if a woman gives consent to vaginal examination, any signs that she is unhappy to continue, such as legs adducted or disordered breathing, must be considered a sign for the examination to stop. Further conversation may elicit the cause of the unhappiness; it may be that the woman suffers from vaginismus. If so, it may need a great deal more therapy than merely being physically instructed in the use of dilators; unless the physiotherapist has received appropriate training it is wise to refer the woman for appropriate therapy.

Dyspareunia

Dyspareunia is defined as a recurrent genital pain with sexual activity. It may be further divided into primary dyspareunia, if intercourse has always been painful; and secondary dyspareunia, if it occurs after a period of pain-free sexual intercourse (Butcher 1999b). It is a distressing symptom and can lead to problems and conflict within a relationship. It is usually a description of pain with penetrative sexual activity but may also occur with genital stimulation. It may be described as being superficial or deep, and can be due to infection or allergy, trauma (such as episiotomy or perineal and vaginal tears accompanying childbirth or gynaecological surgery), postmenopausal changes, congenital defects, neoplasms, abuse or poor sexual technique. Recurrent sexual pain can become part of a cycle of pain in which fear leads to avoidance, a lack of arousal, failure to achieve orgasm and loss of desire; ultimately this leads to total avoidance and difficulties within the relationship (Butcher 1999b).

Superficial dyspareunia

There are many causes of superficial (at or around the vaginal entrance) dyspareunia:

1. Vaginal and vulval infections with such organisms as *Candida albicans, Trichomonas vaginalis* or herpes simplex; Bartholin's gland infections or infected cysts
2. Damage sustained during childbirth – a tear or episiotomy – or gynaecological surgery sometimes leaves scar tissue which can be acutely uncomfortable during intercourse, particularly that involving the posterior wall (Haase & Skibsted 1988); Spencer et al (1986) has shown that women repaired with glycerol-impregnated chromic catgut following childbirth were more likely to have perineal pain at 10 days and to suffer dyspareunia at 3 months than those who were sutured with untreated chromic catgut; Grant et al (1989) in a follow-up study of the original affected women reported that 3 years later, persistent dyspareunia was still being experienced by a significant number of women. It is surmised that the perineal tissues reacted differently to the glycerol-impregnated catgut, possibly by increased fibrosis; Grant suggested that there is no place for the use of this material in the repair of perineal wounds
3. Menopausal changes due to oestrogen deficiency giving rise to atrophic vaginitis or narrowing of the introitus and the vagina
4. Urethritis or a urethral caruncle
5. Congenital conditions such as rigid hymen or vaginal stenosis, or a vaginal septum
6. Inadequate genital lubrication – perhaps due to ineffective sexual arousal or psychological factors; this can be a problem following childbirth, surgery or the menopause, when fear of pain can inhibit the natural increase of vaginal and vulval secretions
7. Irritants such as spermicides or latex
8. Radiotherapy (radiation vaginitis)
9. Sexual trauma, abuse.

Deep dyspareunia

Deep dyspareunia is often described as pain as a result of pelvic thrusting during sexual intercourse (Butcher 1999b). It is often associated with pelvic pathology such as:

1. Acute or chronic pelvic inflammatory disease
2. Endometriosis
3. Ectopic pregnancy
4. Retroverted uterus, prolapse of the bladder, uterus or rectum, prolapse of the ovaries into the pouch of Douglas, or broad ligament tear
5. Postoperative scarring following vaginal repair or, occasionally, a high vaginal tear
6. Constipation
7. Neoplasm and its accompanying secondary infection
8. Gynaecological, pelvic or abdominal surgery
9. Postoperative adhesions
10. Fibroids

11. Irritable bowel syndrome
12. Urinary tract infections
13. Ovarian cysts.

Treatment

Treatment must always be directed first at any possible physical cause. Cognitive behavioural programmes may also be used in which the woman learns about her condition, and gradually feels that she has gained control over her vagina and sexual activity (Butcher 1999b).

Increasingly physiotherapists are being asked to treat patients complaining of dyspareunia, particularly postpartum. Usually the patient has had an episiotomy or a considerable tear needing suture following a recent delivery; occasionally this wound has become infected and broken down. A raised and sensitive scar may be palpable in some cases; in others there is nothing obvious. Obstetricians sometimes offer to excise such a scar and resuture, with a 50/50 expectation of improvement. Understandably women are reluctant to accept further trauma at such low odds. If the introitus has apparently been sutured 'too tightly', dilators may be suggested.

Physiotherapists are finding that they are able to treat many such patients very successfully using a combination of 'tender loving care', listening, counselling, education, ultrasound to soften scar tissue, and the teaching of self-massage and pelvic floor muscle exercises. No scientific evaluation of these techniques has so far been undertaken but the gratitude of patients and their partners is significant.

There are a few patients who, after childbirth or pelvic surgery, will be found to have fantasies concerning their pelvic floor, fearing trauma and deformity that make intercourse impossible. Often all that is needed is examination and reassurance by someone empathetic whom they trust, for example the postnatal class or clinic midwife or physiotherapist, insight into the fact that childbirth or surgery may have caused minimal changes, and guidance to self-examination using a mirror.

VULVODYNIA

In 1983 the International Society for the Study of Vulvar Diseases (ISSVD) developed the term 'vulvodynia' for a chronic condition with symptoms of burning and sometimes stinging, irritation and rawness in the vulval area previously known as 'burning vulva syndrome' (McKay 1984). It is different to pruritis vulvae in that there is no desire to scratch. Vulvodynia includes several disorders resulting in chronic vulval pain: vulvar dermatosis, cyclic vulvovaginitis, vulvar vestibulitis, vulvar papillomatosis and essential vulvodynia (McKay 1989). Sexual problems are quite common in patients with vulval pain and a psychosexual referral may be appropriate after the medical part of the condition has been appropriately treated.

Dysaesthetic vulvodynia

This condition is thought to be an abnormal pain syndrome similar to postherpetic neuralgia. The pain may be in a larger area including the inner thighs and around the anus and urethra. The pain varies from being comparatively mild to such a severe pain that the woman may even have a problem sitting comfortably. However, there are often no visible signs. Treatment may be with tricyclic antidepressants, but unfortunately these may have the side-effects of tiredness, dry mouth, constipation and occasionally blurred vision. Vaginal lubricants may make intercourse easier; aqueous cream is recommended for improving general skin condition.

Chronic vulvodynia may have an acute onset such as with vaginal infection, or after a change in pattern of sexual activity, or there may be nothing specific recollected by the woman prior to its commencement (Wesselmann et al 1997).

Glazer (2000) reported on the long-term follow-up of patients who had been treated with surface electromyography-assisted pelvic floor muscle rehabilitation; 38 out of 43 patients reported that they had suffered no further vulvar pain since completion of treatment more than 3 years previously. Vulvodynia has also been successfully treated with acupuncture (Powell & Wojnarowska 1999).

Vulvar vestibulitis

This is a subgroup of those with vulvodynia in which the pain is usually felt in the vaginal introitus from below the clitoris to the fourchette on any degree of touch. The characteristics of vulvar vestibulitis have been described as: severe pain on vestibular touch, or attempted penetration, tenderness to pressure in the vestibule, and vestibular erythema (Friedrich 1987), although not all women have visible signs. The simple swab test for the condition consists of elicitation or exacerbation of a sharp burning pain on touching the vulvar vestibule with a moist cotton-wool swab.

Unfortunately symptoms are often wrongly diagnosed as being a monilial infection. Women suffering from the condition with inappropriate treatment can then suffer with isolation, fear and self-treatment (Nunns & Hamdy 1998). As a result of this the Vulval Pain Society was founded in 1996 to give unbiased accurate information on the subject (for contact details see Useful Addresses on p. 307).

Treatment

Medical treatment can involve local anaesthetic creams and gels, tricyclic antidepressants, psychosexual counselling and vaginal dilators.

Physiotherapy has been used for the condition, with some degree of success. Glazer et al (1995) demonstrated an 83% improvement rate with 17 out of 33 women reporting pain-free intercourse at 6 months follow up. The 'Glazer' protocol includes a prebaseline 1-minute rest, five fast PFM contractions with 10 seconds rest between each, five 10-second contractions with 10 seconds rest between each, a single endurance contraction of 60 seconds and a 1-minute rest postbaseline (Glazer 1997).

Shelley et al (2002) describe fully the aetiology, physiotherapy assessment and treatment of many types of pelvic pain. The treatment methods include posture, body mechanics, relaxation, biofeedback, stress management and manual therapies. The women's health physiotherapist is well placed to learn and utilise these methods of treatment.

SEXUALITY

IN PREGNANCY

The physical and psychological changes of pregnancy have an effect on sexual activity. It has been shown in a Canadian study of 139 pregnant women that 58% (99 out of 139) reported a decrease in sexual desire (Bartellas et al 2000). In the same study it was also shown that vaginal intercourse and sexual activity decreased throughout the pregnancy. However, 8 out of 139 women reported an increase in intercourse during pregnancy and 32 out of 139 no change. Surprisingly 49% of the women thought that sexual intercourse may harm the pregnancy but only 29% (of the 139) had discussed this with their doctor. Most of the women (76%) felt that the subject should be discussed. Apart from physical discomfort and anxiety about the foetus, medical advice may be a reason for a reduction in coitus, although such advice is usually given only if there is a risk of preterm labour, antepartum haemorrhage or premature rupture of membranes.

The women's health physiotherapist may be in the position, together with their midwifery and medical colleagues, to dispel the myths concerning intercourse during pregnancy, particularly stressing that sexual intercourse will not normally cause complications in pregnancy (Bartellas et al 2000). They may also be able to help women understand that a progressive decrease in desire for sexual activity is more often apparent in women than men and that a change in coital positions can make sexual intercourse more comfortable and pleasurable.

Postnatal sexual problems are common and health professionals ought to be prepared to educate patients antenatally, be able to recognise problems and be competent to deal with them sympathetically (Glazener 1997).

IN THE PUERPERIUM

Female sexuality is often adversely affected in the puerperium and there are probably multiple reasons for this, including perineal trauma, hormonal readjustments, fatigue and psychological causes including anxiety and depression. Perineal pain and dyspareunia are common; there is a general decrease in desire for and frequency of sexual intercourse (Klein et al 1994). In a study of 796 women by questionnaire 6 months postdelivery, there was a 61% (494) response rate (Barrett et al 2000). Interestingly, six women refused to participate as they felt that the questionnaire was too personal. It was found that 67% of the women reported less frequent intercourse, with variability in the quality of intercourse. Problems with pain, lack of vaginal lubrication and loss of sexual desire all increased in the first 3 months after delivery. Dyspareunia was particularly common (see p. 296). Over 80% of women in the study experienced at least one postnatal sexual problem. Glazener (1997) found that 53% of women found problems with intercourse in the first 8 weeks postdelivery and 49% in the subsequent year.

Extreme tiredness, anxiety and depression can all contribute to the problem and make a women feel even more guilty for not complying with the expected image of being healthy, happy and coping (Saurel-Cubizolles et al 2000).

Women's health physiotherapists should take nothing for granted when assessing a postnatal patient. They should question a woman sympathetically and be very aware that a vaginal examination may be of great concern to the woman. They must pick up any signals that the woman is unhappy or concerned about her sexuality; there may be both psychological and physical issues. Furthermore, their role is to listen and not necessarily give advice unless they have the appropriate skills (Fleming & Crowley 1995). However, they should have knowledge of the appropriate referral pathways within their own vicinity for appropriate counselling if necessary.

PREMENOPAUSAL WOMEN

The late forties is a time when many women are achieving much in their professional lives but also having to cope with children growing into young adults, elderly parents and their own bodies starting to show some signs of deterioration. However, in recent years women have become more interested in their own health and often attend health clubs and gymnasia; this in itself may bring further pressures on their time. There are also expectations of a healthy sexual life. It has been found that a sexual self-rating (SSR) scale is positively related to oestrogen levels and negatively related to follicle-stimulating hormone (FSH) levels in women aged 45–49 years (Garratt et al 1995). It was further found that women experiencing pain with sex and dryness of the vagina had significantly lower SSR. It may be that a woman attending a women's health physiotherapist for problems of a urinary or faecal nature may disclose that she is also having sexual problems. Although simple problems of lack of vaginal lubrication or positioning for intercourse can be addressed, care should be taken not to proffer other advice unless appropriate training has been undertaken.

IN THE CLIMACTERIC

There are several factors other than body chemistry that can influence sexual fulfilment at the time of the climacteric. These include satisfaction with a relationship, emotional stability and psychological well-being (Abernethy 1997). The hormonal changes at the climacteric can significantly affect and reduce sexual activity. The vaginal epithelium changes at this time, with the vaginal walls becoming thinner and less elastic. Women may experience atrophic vaginitis with problems of vaginal dryness, hot flushes, night sweats, mood changes, weight gain and possibly bladder problems, all of which can play a part in altering a woman's sexual activity. Also, the skin may become dryer, thinner, itchy and bruise more easily, hair may become more sparse and dry, facial hair may increase, and the breasts start to shrink and sag – none of which make a woman feel more desirable. Ageing has also been shown to lead to a reduction in sexual interest, orgasmic capacity and coital frequency (Hallstrom 1980). This report also showed that sexuality is affected by psychosocial as well as by biological factors; higher social class was significantly related to normal sexual activity.

Hormone replacement therapy (HRT) may assist with those having problems with vaginal dryness, loss of libido and dyspareunia; topical application of oestrogens may be appropriate therapy (see p. 262). There is also some evidence that testosterone can assist in increasing sexual desire and is given alongside the oestrogen therapy (Floter et al 2002). However, many women report that non-medical problems have more effect on their sex lives than the actual menopausal changes (Pennell report 1998).

IN OLDER AGE

Most women live one-third to one-half of their life after the menopause (Pennell report 1998). More people of both sexes are reaching their 70s, 80s and even 90s, and many are in very good health. Continued sexual activity and enjoyment will be possible for many. For some, neurological damage or physical disability, or both, may affect it, needing thought and care regarding appropriate positioning. Thus it is important that those caring for the elderly should never assume that regular intercourse has ceased, particularly when arranging accommodation.

It is logical to suppose that, for a woman, sexual activity with the increased blood supply of arousal and muscular contraction of orgasm can only be beneficial to the pelvic floor, and, by inference, to the maintenance of continence. This contention appears to be supported by unsolicited opinions which have been voiced to physiotherapists by recently widowed women who experience incontinence, suggesting that it is because they are not now having regular intercourse that they are 'getting weak underneath'. It has also been reported by many post-menopausal women attending for PFM re-education that the sexual satisfaction of both themselves and their partners has greatly improved with increased PFM activity.

A German study reported that elderly and old women are increasingly seeking a gynaecological consultation for sexual difficulties (Neises 2002). However, such consultations may be hindered by feelings of shame, fear and embarrassment. The women's health physiotherapist may be of assistance by being prepared to lend a listening ear to any such patient prior to her gynaecological appointment.

Physiotherapists who become interested in this field should approach the Association of Chartered Physiotherapists in Women's Health for information regarding psychosexual counselling courses that will admit physiotherapists.

THE PSYCHOLOGICAL AND EMOTIONAL IMPLICATIONS OF GYNAECOLOGICAL DISEASE

Gynaecological disease strikes at the core of a woman's psyche, sapping her physical, mental and spiritual health. The effects are often covert and low grade, undermining a woman to the point that, although she goes through the motions of living, she temporarily or permanently becomes a 'second class citizen'. In more severe cases she tires easily and may not be able to hold down a full-time job; she is often in pain and irritable; she may not want or even be able to leave the house at times, and becomes moody and depressed; her closest relationships are stressed and her fertility threatened. She finds it hard to talk about her problems and experiences rejection by most people unless they are fellow sufferers. The partners of such women also have grave problems, for however much they give to the relationship it is never enough. Such a couple's social life is probably restricted; and sexual relationships are fraught because they cause pain, are curtailed by bleeding and are certainly no source of pleasure and strength. The further psychological effects of gynaecological surgery and incontinence are discussed on p. 321. Those woman who already experience some other disability may find that the gynaecological disease is the 'final straw'. The psychological support given to such people has been largely deficient but the growth in recent years of self-help groups has been particularly noticeable in this field; a list of these will be found in the Useful Addresses at the end of this and the next two chapters.

SEXUALITY AND BODY IMAGE AFTER CANCER

Many people survive treatment for their malignancies. However, they can find that they have emotional and physical changes that can affect their sexuality and sexual functioning (Sundquist & Yee 2003).

Patients with gynaecological cancers may feel shame and unease when talking of their sexual problems (Neises 2002); however, 80% definitely want to be informed of the possible consequences of the disease and its treatment on their sexuality.

Breast surgery patients in particular may be concerned about their own body image. It is common for women to have difficulties with sex and intimacy after their diagnosis (Love 2000). This may be a fear that their partner will find them less attractive, a practical issue of discomfort in positioning for sexual activity or a loss of libido after a chemical menopause. Tamoxifen is prescribed for those women with an oestrogen positive tumour; this may itself cause menopausal symptoms. Lymphoedema can bring additional physical and psychological problems in both gynaecological and breast cancer.

The psychological distress can bring about hormonal changes causing more psychological distress. It has also been found that most of such issues were resolved by 1 year, but somewhat bleakly, that if they were not resolved by then, they were never resolved (Ganz et al 1998).

All health professionals, but in particular women's health physiotherapists, are in an ideal position to give time to women who may suffer with these unmentioned fears. Therapeutic interventions where appropriate, listening and close liaison with the nurse specialist and other members of the team can ensure that there is seamless care. Also to be considered is the provision of information concerning patient self-help groups; some appropriate addresses are at the end of this chapter (p. 306).

References

Abernethy K 1997 The menopause. In: Andrews G (ed) Women's sexual health. Baillière Tindall, London, p 336–364.

ACPWH 2002 Mitchell method of simple relaxation (revised). Ralph Allan Press, Bath.

Adler M W 1990a Vaginal discharge management. In: Adler M W (ed) ABC of sexually transmitted diseases, 2nd edn. BMJ Publications, London, p 13–16.

Adler M W 1990b Genital infestations. In: Adler M W (ed) ABC of sexually transmitted diseases, 2nd edn. BMJ Publications, London, p 43–45.

Amso N N 2002 Clinicians and patients should be aware of association between endometriosis and malignancies. British Medical Journal 324:115.

Andrew G 1997 Premenstrual syndrome. In: Andrews G (ed) Women's sexual health. Baillière Tindall, London, p 314–335.

Baker F C, Driver H S, Rogers G G et al 1999 High nocturnal body temperatures and disturbed sleep in women with primary dysmenorrhoea. American Journal of Physiology 277(Endocrinology and Metabolism 40):E1013–E1021.

Barrett G, Pendry E, Peacock J et al 2000 Women's sexual health after childbirth. British Journal of Obstetrics and Gynaecology 107(2):186–195.

Bartellas E, Crane J M G, Daley M et al 2000 Sexuality and sexual activity in pregnancy. British Journal of Obstetrics and Gynaecology 107:964–968.

Beals K A, Manore M M 2002 Disorders of the female athlete triad among collegiate athletes. International Journal of Sport Nutrition, Exercise and Metabolism 12(3):281–293.

Beard R W, Higliman J H, Pearce S et al 1984 Diagnosis of pelvic varicosities in women with chronic pelvic pain. Lancet ii:946–949.

Beard R W, Reginald P W, Wadsworth J 1988 Clinical features of women with chronic lower abdominal pain and pelvic congestion. British Journal of Obstetrics and Gynaecology 95: 153–161.

Beck R P 1983 Pelvic relaxational prolapse. In: Kase N G, Weingold A B (eds) Principles and practice of clinical gynecology. John Wiley, New York, p 677.

Beller U, Sideri M, Maisonneuve P et al 2001 Carcinoma of the vulva. Journal of Epimediology and Biostatistics 6(1):155–173.

Benedet J L, Odicino F, Maisonneuve P et al 2001 Carcinoma of the cervix uteri. Journal of Epidemiology and Biostatistics 6(1):5–14.

Bradbeer C 1997 Sexually transmitted diseases. In: Luesley D M (ed) Common conditions in gynaecology. Chapman & Hall Medical, London, p 98–111.

Brentkopf L, Bakoulis M 1988 Coping with endometriosis. Grapevine, Thorsons, Wellingborough, p 38–44.

Bump R C, Mattiasson A, Bø K et al 1996 The standardization of terminology of female pelvic organ prolapse and pelvis floor dysfunction. American Journal of Obstetrics and Gynecology 175:10–17.

Butcher J 1999a Female sexual problems 1: loss of desire – what about the fun? British Medical Journal 318:41–43.

Butcher J 1999b Female sexual problems 2: sexual pain and sexual fears. British Medical Journal 318:110–112.

Cahill D J, Wardle P G 2002 Management of infertility. British Medical Journal 325:28–32.

Cardozo L 1997 Prolapse. In: Cardozo L (ed) Urogynecology. Churchill Livingstone, London, p 321–349.

Chimbira T, Anderson A B M, Tumball A C 1980 Relationship between measured menstrual blood loss and patient's subjective assessment of loss, duration of bleeding, number of sanitary towels used, uterine weight and endometrial surface area. British Journal of Obstetrics and Gynaecology 87:603–609.

Dewhurst J 1981 Integrated obstetrics and gynaecology for postgraduates, 3rd edn. Blackwell, Oxford, p 565–566.

Farquhar C M 2000 Extracts from 'Clinical evidence': Endometriosis. British Medical Journal 320:1449–1452.

Farrell E 2002 Premature menopause. 'I feel like an alien'. Australian Family Physician 31(5):419–421.

Fleming C, Crowley T 1995 How to help patients talk about sex. Student British Medical Journal 3:9–11.

Floter A, Nathorst-Boos J, Carlstrom K et al 2002 Addition of testosterone to estrogen replacement therapy in oophrectomized women: effects on sexuality and well-being. Climacteric 5(4):357–365.

Frank S 1995 Polycystic ovary syndrome. New England Journal of Medicine 333:853–861.

Fraser I S, McCarron G 1987 Ibuprofen is a useful treatment for primary dysmenorrhoea. Australian and New Zealand Journal of Obstetrics and Gynaecology 27:244–247.

Friedrich E G 1987 Vulvar vestibulitis syndrome. Journal of Reproductive Medicine 32:110–114.

Ganz P A, Rowland J H, Desmond K et al 1998 Life after breast cancer: understanding women's health-related quality of life and sexual functioning. Journal of Clinical Oncology 16(2):501–514.

Garratt A M, Torgerson D J, Wyness J et al 1995 Measuring sexual functioning in premenopausal women. British Journal of Obstetrics and Gynaecology 102:311–316.

Gillan P, Brindley G D 1979 Vaginal and pelvic floor responses to sexual stimulation. Psychophysiology 16:471.

Glazener C M A 1997 Sexual function after childbirth: women's experiences, persistent morbidity and lack of professional recognition. British Journal of Obstetrics and Gynaecology 104:330–335.

Glazer H I 1997 11 Vulvovaginal pain disorders. In: Electromyography applications in urology and gynaecology. Biofeedback Foundation of Europe.

Glazer H I 2000 Dysesthetic vulvodynia. Long term follow up after treatment with surface electromyography assisted pelvic floor muscle rehabilitation. Journal of Reproductive Medicine 45(10):798–802.

Glazer H I, Rodke G, Swencionis C et al 1995 Treatment of vulvar vestibulitis syndrome with electromyographic biofeedback of the pelvic floor musculature. Journal of Reproductive Medicine 40:283–290.

Gleeson N C 1995 The management of vulval dystrophy. In: Bonnar J (ed) Recent advances in obstetrics and gynaecology 19. Churchill Livingstone, London, p 191–200.

Glowacki C A, Wall L L 2002 Pelvic organ prolapse. In: Laycock J, Haslam J (eds) Therapeutic management of incontinence and pelvic pain. Springer, London, p 193–207.

Govan A D T, McKay Hart D, Callander R 1993 Gynaecological infections. In: Govan A D T, McKay Hart D, Callander R (eds) Gynaecology illustrated, 4th edn. Churchill Livingstone, London, p 143–178.

Graber B, Kline-Graber G 1979 Female orgasm: the role of pubococcygeus muscle. Journal of Clinical Psychiatry 40: 348–351.

Grant A, Sleep J, Ashurst H et al 1989 Dyspareunia associated with the use of glycerol-impregnated catgut to repair perineal trauma. Report of a 3-year follow-up study. British Journal of Obstetrics and Gynaecology 96:741–743.

Haase P, Skibsted L 1988 Influence of operations for stress incontinence and/or genital descensus on sexual life. Acta Obstetrica et Gynecologica Scandinavica 67:659–661.

Haboubi N H, Lincoln N 2003 Views of health professionals on discussing sexual issues with patients. Disability Rehabilitation 25(6):291–296.

Hallstrom T 1980 Sexuality in the climacteric. Clinical Obstetrics and Gynaecology 4:227–239.

Hawton S 1985 Sex therapy, a practical guide. OUP, Oxford.

Heintz A P M, Odicino F, Maisonneuve P et al 2001 Carcinoma of the ovary. Journal of Epidemiology and Biostatistics 6(1):107–138.

Helms J M 1987 Acupuncture for the management of primary dysmenorrhea. Obstetrics and Gynecology 69(1):51–56.

Hopkinson Z E C, Sattar N, Fleming R et al 1998 Polycystic ovarian syndrome: the metabolic syndrome comes to gynaecology. British Medical Journal 317:329–332.

Hylan T R, Sundell K, Judge R 1999 The impact of premenstrual symptomology on functioning and treatment seeking behaviour: experiences from the United States, United Kingdom and France. Journal of Womens Health and Gender Based Medicine 8(8):1043–1052.

Jackson S, Smith P 1997 Fortnightly review: diagnosing and managing genitourinary prolapse. British Medical Journal 314:875–880.

Jones K D, Sutton C 2002 Emphasis on medical treatment is misleading. British Medical Journal 324:115.

Kegel A H 1952 Sexual functions of the pubococcygeus muscle. Western Journal of Surgery in Obstetrics and Gynecology 60:521.

Kjaer S K, van den Brule A J C, Paull G et al 2002 Type specific persistence of high risk human papillomavirus (HPV) as indicator of high grade cervical squamous intraepithelial lesions in young women: population based prospective follow up study. British Medical Journal 325:572–578.

Klein M C, Gauthier R J, Robbins J M et al 1994 Relationship of episiotomy to perineal trauma and morbidity, sexual dysfunction and pelvic floor relaxation. American Journal of Obstetrics and Gynecology 71:591–598.

Kline-Graber G, Graber B 1975 A guide to sexual satisfaction – woman's orgasm. Popular Library, New York, p 21–54.

Lethaby A, Irvine G, Cameron I 1999 Cyclical progestagens for heavy menstrual bleeding. In: Cochrane Collaboration. Cochrane Library. Issue 1. Update Software, Oxford.

Lewis T L T, Chamberlain G V P (eds) 1990 Gynaecology by ten teachers, 15th edn. Edward Arnold, London, p 29–33.

Liao K L, Wood N, Conway G S 2000 Premature menopause and psychological well-being. Journal of Psychosomatic Obstetrics and Gynaecology 21(3):167–174.

Llewellyn-Jones D 1986 Fundamentals of obstetrics and gynaecology, vol 2. Faber, London, p 198–224.

Love S 2000 Life after breast cancer. In: Dr Susan Love's breast book. Perseus Publishing, New York, p 517–540.

Luesley D M 1997 The abnormal cervical smear. In: Luesley D M (ed) Common conditions in gynaecology: a problem solving approach. Chapman & Hall Medical, London, p 154–175.

McKay M 1984 Burning vulva syndrome: report of the ISSVD task force. Journal of Reproductive Medicine 29:457.

McKay M 1989 Vulvodynia. A multifactorial problem. Archives of Dermatology 125:256–262.

Marcoux S, Maheux R, Berube S 1997 Surgery in infertile women with minimal or mild endometriosis. New England Journal of Medicine. 337:217–222.

Masters W H, Johnson V E 1966 Human sexual response. Little, Brown, Boston.

Masters W H, Johnson V E 1970 Human sexual inadequacy Churchill Livingstone, Edinburgh.

Miller J M, Ashton-Miller J A, DeLancey J O L 1998 A pelvic muscle pre contraction can reduce cough related urine loss in selected women with mild SUI. Journal of the American Geriatric Society 46:870–874.

Murray L 1997 Sexually transmitted diseases. In: Sweet B R (ed) Maye's midwifery, 12th Edn. Baillière Tindall, London, p 570–577.

Nash J 1997 Sexual health and sexually acquired infection. In: Andrews G (ed) Women's sexual health. Baillière Tindall, London, p 287–313.

Neises M 2002 Sexuality and sexual dysfunction in gynaecological psycho oncology. Onkologie 25(6):571–574.

Nunns D, Hamdy D 1998 Vulval pain society provides information on vulval symptoms. British Medical Journal 316:706.

O'Brien S, Doyle M 1997 Abnormal vaginal bleeding. In: Luesley D (ed) Common conditions in gynaecology: a problem solving approach. Chapman & Hall Medical, London, p 57–80.

Office for National Statistics 1997 Birth statistics for England and Wales 1997. Stationary Office, London, Series FMI no 26, p 59–62.

Office for National Statistics 2001 United Kingdom health statistics. The Stationery Office, London, p 29.

Olsen A L, Smith V J, Bergstrom J O et al 1997 Epidemiology of surgically managed pelvic organ prolapse and urinary incontinence. Obstetrics and Gynecology 89:501–506.

Parazzini F 1999 Ablation of lesions or no treatment in minimal–mild endometriosis in infertile women: a randomised trial. Human Reproduction 14:1332–1334.

Pasquali E A 2002 Premature menopause and self-concept disjunctions. A case for crisis management. Journal of Psychosocial Nursing and Mental Health Services 40(9):20–29.

Pennell Report on women's health 1998 The Pennell initiative, Health Service Management Unit, University of Manchester, Manchester M13 9PL.

Pickrell D 1997 Gynaecological emergencies. In: Luesley D (ed) Common conditions in gynaecology: a problem solving approach. Chapman & Hall Medical, London, p 33–56.

Powell J, Wojnarowska F 1999 Acupuncture for vulvodynia. Journal of the Royal Society of Medicine 92(11):579–581.

Prentice A 1999 Fortnightly review: medical management of menorrhagia. British Medical Journal 319:1343–1345.

Prentice A 2001 Regular review: endometriosis. British Medical Journal 323:93–95.

Proctor M L, Smith C A, Farquhar C M et al 2003 Transcutaneous electrical nerve stimulation and acupuncture for primary dysmenorrhoea (Cochrane Review). In: Cochrane Library, Issue 1. Update Software, Oxford.

Redman C 1997 Gynaecological cancers. In: Luesley D M ed Common conditions in gynaecology: a problem solving approach. Chapman & Hall Medical, London, p 176–193.

Ridley C M, Frankman O, Jones I S C et al 1989 New nomenclature in vulvar disease: International Society for the Study of Vulvar Disease. Human Pathology 20:495–496.

Royal College of Obstetricians and Gynaecologists 2000 The investigation and management of endometriosis. Guideline no 24. RCOG, London.

Samuelsson E C, Arne V, Tibblin G et al 1999 Signs of genital prolapse in a Swedish population of women 20–59 years of age and possible related factors. American Journal of Obstetrics and Gynecology 180:299–305.

Saurel-Cubizolles M J, Romito P, Lelong N et al 2000 Women's health after childbirth: a longitudinal study in France and Italy. British Journal of Obstetrics and Gynaecology 107:1202–1209.

Schellenberg R for the study group 2001 Treatment for the premenstrual syndrome with agnus castor fruit extract: prospective, randomised, placebo controlled trial. British Medical Journal 322:134–137.

Scott R S, Hsuch G S C 1979 A clinical study of the effects of galvanic muscle stimulation in urinary stress incontinence and sexual dysfunction. American Journal of Obstetrics and Gynecology 135:663.

Selby J 1997 Psychosexual and emotional care. In: Andrews G (ed) Women's sexual health. Baillière Tindall, London, p 41–65.

Shafik A 2000 The role of levator ani muscle in evacuation, sexual performance and pelvic floor disorders. International Urogynecology Journal 11:361–366.

Shelley B, Knight S, King P et al 2002 Pelvic pain. In: Laycock J, Haslam J (eds) Therapeutic management of incontinence and pelvic pain, Springer, London, p 157–189.

Spence-Jones C, Kamm M, Henry M et al 1994 Bowel dysfunction: a pathogenic factor in utero-vaginal prolapse and urinary stress incontinence. British Journal of Obstetrics and Gynaecology 101:147–152.

Spencer J A, Grant A, Elbourne D et al 1986. A randomised comparison of glycerol-impregnated chromic catgut with untreated chromic catgut for the repair of perineal trauma. British Journal of Obstetrics and Gynaecology 93:426–430.

Steele J 1997 Common gynaecological problems. In: Andrew G (ed) Women's sexual health. Baillière Tindall, London, p 390–420.

Stern R C, Dash R, Bentley R C et al 2001 Malignancy in endometriosis: frequency and comparison of ovarian and extra ovarian types. International Journal of Gynecological Pathology 29:133–139.

Sundquist K, Yee L 2003 Sexuality and body image after cancer. Australian Family Physician. 32(1–2):19–23.

Symonds E M, Symonds I M 1998 Genital tract infections. In: Symonds E M, Symonds I M (eds) Essential obstetrics and gynaecology, 3rd edn. Churchill Livingstone, London, p 243–251.

Thakar R, Stanton S 2002 Regular review: management of genital prolapse. British Medical Journal 324:1258–1262.

Tindall V R, Oates S, Rimmer S et al (eds) 1991 Illustrated textbook of gynaecology. Gower, London, p 39–44.

Watson C 1990 Psychosexual counselling. In: Rymer J, Davis G, Rodin A et al (eds) Preparation and revision for the DRCOG. Churchill Livingstone, London, p 343–349.

Wesselmann U, Burnett A L, Heinberg L J 1997 The urogenital and rectal pain syndromes. Pain 73:269–294.

Whincup P H, Gilg J A, Odoki K et al 2001 Age of menarche in contemporary British teenagers: survey of girls born between 1982 and 1986. British Medical Journal 322:1095–1096.

Woodman C B, Collins S, Rollason T P et al 2003 Human papilloma virus type 18 and rapidly progressing cervical intraepithelial neoplasia. Lancet 361(9351):40–43.

Wyatt K, Dimmock P, Jomnes P et al 2001 Efficacy of progesterone and progestogens in management of premenstrual syndrome: systematic review. British Medical Journal 323:1–8.

Further reading

Andrews G (ed) 1997 Women's sexual health. Baillière Tindall, London.

Campbell S, Monga A (eds) 2000 Gynaecology by ten teachers, 17th edn. Edward Arnold, London.

Govan A D T, McKay Hart D, Callander R (eds) 1993 Gynaecology illustrated, 4th edn. Churchill Livingstone, London.

Laycock J, Haslam J (eds) 2002 Therapeutic management of incontinence and pelvic pain, Springer, London, p 157–189.

Luesley D M (ed) 1997 Common conditions in gynaecology: a problem solving approach. Chapman & Hall Medical, London.

Sampson J A 1927 Peritoneal endometriosis due to the menstrual dissemination of endometrial tissue into the peritoneal cavity. American Journal of Obstetrics and Gynecology 143:422–469.

Symonds E M, Symonds I M 1998 Essential obstetrics and gynaecology, 3rd edn. Churchill Livingstone, London.

Useful addresses

Anorexics Anonymous
45a Castelnau, Barnes, London SW13
Tel 020 8748 3994

Association of Chartered Physiotherapists in Obstetrics and Gynaecology
c/o CSP, 14 Bedford Row, London WC1R 4ED
Website: www.womensphysio.com

Breast Cancer Care
Kiln House, 210 New Kings Rd, London SW6 4NZ
Website: www.breastcancercare.org.uk

Cancerbacup
3 Bath Place, Rivington Ts, London EC2A 3DR
Website: www.cancerbacup.org.uk

Daisy Network (POF)
PO Box 392, High Wycombe, Bucks HP 15 7SH
Website: www.daisynetwork.org.uk

Eating Disorders Association
103 Prince of Wales Rd, Norwich NR1 1OW
Adult helpline 0845 634 1414
Youthline 0845 634 7650
Website: www.edauk.com

Herpes Viruses Association
41 North Road, London N7
Website: www.herpes.org.uk

MacMillan Cancer Relief
89 Albert Embankment, London SE1 7UQ
Website: www.macmillan.org.uk

National Endometriosis Society UK
50 Westminster Palace Gardens, Artillery Row, London
    SW15 1RL
Helpline 0808 808 2227
Website: www.endo.org.uk

Vulval Pain Society
PO Box 514, Slough, Berkshire SL1 2BP
Website: www.vul-pain.dircon.co.uk

Women's Nationwide Cancer Control Campaign
Suna House, 128–130 Curtain Rd, London EC2A 3AQ
Website: www.wncc.org.uk

Women's Reproductive Rights Information Centre
52–54 Featherstone Street, London EC1 8RT
Helpline 0845 125 5254
Website: www.womenshealthlondon.org.uk

Chapter **10**

Gynaecological surgery

Teresa Cook

CHAPTER CONTENTS

Introduction   309
Gynaecological excision surgery   309
Pelvic radiotherapy   314
Gynaecological repair surgery   314
Surgical treatment of stress incontinence   317

Definitions of other useful terms and
   procedures   320
Physiotherapy care of patients undergoing
   gynaecological surgery   321

INTRODUCTION

The women's health physiotherapist is a member of a multidisciplinary team looking after women requiring gynaecological surgery. To achieve an effective service, it is important that all members of the team are fully aware of the contribution that each can make to the holistic care of such women. The physiotherapist's principle role is concerned with pre- and postoperative care, but should include any relevant advice, treatment or referral judged appropriate to promote the health of each individual patient in the short and long term. The preoperative condition of patients admitted for gynaecological surgery will vary from the relatively healthy woman, who may have been waiting to be admitted for surgery for some time, to the severely ill. The physiotherapy needs of these women will similarly vary; therefore a thorough assessment of individual needs, as far as possible in advance of the surgery, is essential.

GYNAECOLOGICAL EXCISION SURGERY

HYSTERECTOMY

Hysterectomy is the surgical removal of the uterus, first successfully performed in 1853. Originally an operation of last resort, hysterectomy is currently performed for a variety of conditions. These include uncontrollable postpartum haemorrhage, malignant growths and a range of benign conditions such as dysfunctional uterine bleeding (DUB), fibroids, endometriosis, and prolapse. The operation is still considered to be major surgery, although the usual length of postoperative hospital stay is now between 3 and 6 days.

Information received from the Department of Health (DoH 2003) confirms that the number of hysterectomies performed in England increased through the early 1990s to a high of 69 396 in 1995–1996. Since then there has been a progressive decline, to 51 858 in 1999–2000, indicating that women are being offered treatment options other than surgery. Several alternative treatments are available for benign conditions: endometrial resection/ablation, oral/intrauterine progestogens, oral contraceptives and synthetic steroids (danazol) may be offered to women with DUB; myomectomy is an alternative for women with uterine fibroids; oral contraceptives, other hormonal treatments or laparoscopic resection may be suggested as treatment for endometriosis; vaginal pessaries are an alternative for women with uterine prolapse.

Through increasing media awareness and use of the Internet, women are finding it easier to access information about surgery, its risks, possible complications and the alternatives. This allows them to question recommendations for the management of their symptoms. For benign conditions, hysterectomy should obviously be considered as an option only for women whose childbearing is complete.

Hysterectomy may be carried out by either the abdominal or the vaginal route. During 1998–1999, 79% of hysterectomies performed in England used an abdominal approach, with 21% using the vaginal approach (DoH 2003). The route selected will be dependent on the reason for surgery and the size of the uterus and should be explained fully to the woman prior to surgery (DoH 2001). For malignant conditions the abdominal route is preferred to allow for proper assessment of adjacent tissue.

Abdominal hysterectomy

The abdominal route allows inspection of all the other pelvic organs and surrounding tissue. For this reason it is used for carcinoma, but would also be used to remove a large fibroid uterus or if there is restricted uterine mobility. Full pelvic clearance (exenteration) can only be performed by the abdominal route. Commonly a total abdominal hysterectomy (TAH) is performed which removes the complete uterus, including the cervix. It can be combined with the removal of one or both fallopian tubes (salpingectomy) and/or ovaries (oophorectomy) (see p. 313).

Procedure   The abdomen is opened via a Pfannenstiel (bikini-line) incision. This consists of a transverse incision through the skin and subcutaneous tissue. A further transverse incision is made through the anterior rectus sheath and linea alba, followed by dissection to separate the sheath from the rectus muscle. The peritoneum is identified between the bellies of the rectus muscle and a vertical, midline incision is made through both the peritoneum and transversalis fascia. This division of the layers in different directions reduces the risk of both wound herniation and damage to the nerve/blood supply of the anterior abdominal wall.

Once the pelvic organs are exposed the fallopian tubes, ovarian ligament and round ligament are divided on either side, at the top of the broad ligament. The broad ligament is opened to expose the uterine vessels, which are then ligated and cut. The cervix is excised from the vagina, leaving as much vagina as possible, and from the transverse cervical and uterosacral ligaments. This allows the removal of the entire uterus. Care must be taken to avoid trauma to the ureters, which run forward below the uterine arteries adjacent to the cervix. The upper end of the vagina is closed and attached to the ligaments for support and the abdominal cavity is closed in layers.

Other types of abdominal hysterectomy

- *Wertheim's hysterectomy* – this is the operation of choice for cervical carcinoma. A longitudinal incision may be used. The procedure involves removal of the uterus, fallopian tubes, ovaries, most of the vagina, associated pelvic lymph nodes and connective tissue. There is particular risk to the blood supply to the ureters in this radical operation.

- *Subtotal hysterectomy* – this is the removal of the fundus and body of the uterus, but leaving the cervix, and may reduce postoperative complications. For example, it may be performed where there is a known diagnosis of overactive bladder or where the woman is concerned that removal of the cervix will reduce sexual function (Grimes 1999, van der Vaart et al 2002). It has been suggested that women have an increased risk of developing urge incontinence symptoms following hysterectomy. Where a diagnosis of overactive bladder has been confirmed preoperatively, some surgeons will opt to avoid aggravating these symptoms by performing a subtotal hysterectomy. This procedure requires less bladder mobilisation and therefore less disruption to bladder innervation. In the late 1990s there was a flurry of media activity relating to the effect of cervical resection on sexual function. Although the research is not robust, some women state the desire to keep their cervix for this reason. When this option is considered, the woman needs to be made aware that she will still be at risk of cervical carcinoma and that regular cervical smears will continue to be necessary. However, recent research (Thakar et al 2002) found no significant differences in outcome regarding bladder, bowel or sexual function between total and subtotal hysterectomy.

- *Total abdominal hysterectomy with bilateral salpingo-oophrectomy* – this is the removal of the uterus as well as both fallopian tubes and ovaries. If this procedure is undertaken in the premenopausal woman, she may be offered hormone replacement therapy (HRT).

Postoperative condition   A drain is usually inserted into the abdomen, near to the wound. This is left in place for 24–48 hours, depending on the amount of drainage. A urethral catheter is inserted and left on free drainage, again usually for 24–48 hours. Micturition should be monitored following removal of the catheter. An intravenous infusion (IVI) will be in place, usually for 24 hours, until bowel sounds are heard and drinking and eating resumes.

Risks and complications There is some evidence to suggest that, whilst hysterectomy may solve some problems, others may be generated. Urinary incontinence (particularly urge), vaginal vault prolapse, dyspareunia and depression have all been cited in the literature (Brown et al 2000, Hidlebaugh 2000, Milsom et al 1993, van der Vaart et al 2002). Brown et al (2000) advised that women should be counselled regarding the increased likelihood of incontinence in later life and Clarke et al (1995) recommended that women should be warned preoperatively about early transient (postoperative) symptoms. Advice and exercises given to a woman by a specialist physiotherapist whilst she is in hospital can mitigate these possible short- and long-term problems (see p. 326).

Vaginal hysterectomy

Providing that the condition of the uterus is non-malignant, a vaginal hysterectomy may be the preferred route, particularly in cases of uterine prolapse. It is easily combined with anterior or posterior colporrhaphy, should this be indicated (see p. 314).

Procedure Surgeons vary with regard to the exact technique they employ but the general principles of the procedure are described here. The cervix is drawn down and an incision is made in the anterior vaginal wall. This is extended to encircle the cervix to enable the uterus and cervix to be further drawn down and out. The transverse cervical and uterosacral ligaments are divided from the cervix and the uterine blood vessels are ligated and cut. Once the fallopian tubes, round ligaments and ovarian ligaments are tied and divided, as near to the uterus as possible, the uterus with the cervix can be removed. The uterine ends of the fallopian tubes (pedicles), round ligaments, transverse cervical and uterosacral ligaments are sewn together and to the vault of the vagina, which is then closed with sutures – sometimes incompletely to allow drainage. This gives support to the vaginal vault and the pouch of Douglas, hopefully preventing a subsequent enterocoele. Finally the vaginal wall is closed, leaving the vagina as a cul-de-sac.

Postoperative condition The vagina is packed with gauze to control bleeding; this is left in place for 24–48 hours. A urethral or suprapubic catheter is inserted and left on free drainage, again usually for 24–48 hours. Micturition may be difficult owing to general trauma and should be monitored following removal of the catheter. An IVI will be in place (as in abdominal hysterectomy, see p. 311).

Risks and complications As well as those already listed under abdominal hysterectomy (see above) the most likely complication is haematoma of the vaginal vault, which occurs in 25% of cases (Thomson et al 1998).

Laparoscopic assisted vaginal hysterectomy (LAVH)

This procedure uses a laparoscope to inspect the pelvic cavity and to assist in the vaginal removal of the uterus. The abdominal incisions are small and recovery is as for vaginal hysterectomy. A study by Meikle et al (1997) comparing TAH with LAVH found that for LAVH there were more bladder injuries and longer operative time, but shorter hospitalisation, less analgesia needed postoperatively, a quicker return to full activity and generally lower costs.

OOPHRECTOMY

Oophrectomy is the removal of an ovary and is usually performed via a Pfannenstiel incision. If performed for a malignant tumour a decision has to be made about whether to remove other structures (e.g. the uterus and fallopian tubes). Other indications include removal of a benign ovarian tumour, ovarian cysts or diseased ovarian tissue. It may, however, be possible to remove part of an ovary (wedge resection) or to aspirate a fluid-filled cyst. The size of the incision depends on the surgery required and the size of the diseased ovary.

OVARIAN CYSTECTOMY

This is the removal of benign cysts from the ovary. The cysts are shelled out of the ovary and the remaining ovarian tissue is repaired.

SALPINGECTOMY

Salpingectomy is the removal of a fallopian tube. It is unusual for this to be carried out as an isolated procedure but it may be undertaken for ectopic (tubal) pregnancy or where an encapsulated quantity of fluid (hydrosalpinx) or pus (pyosalpinx) has collected within the tube.

MYOMECTOMY

This is the removal of one or more fibroids from the uterine wall via a Pfannenstiel incision. The procedure may be performed for a woman who has not completed childbearing. The fibroids are shelled out and the resulting cavities are closed with stitches.

VULVECTOMY

Radical vulvectomy

Radical vulvectomy is an extensive operation performed for carcinoma of the vulva. It involves removal of all the vulval tissue down to the bone and fascia, together with the superficial and deep inguinal glands and the glands associated with the external iliac vessels. Subsequently many women will experience complications, which include wound infection or breakdown, lymphoedema, urinary incontinence and sexual dysfunction.

Simple vulvectomy

Simple vulvectomy is a less common operation and much less extensive than the radical version (see above). It involves removal of superficial tissues and may be performed for isolated vulval lesions or vulval irritation.

LARGE LOOP EXCISION OF THE TRANSFORMATION ZONE (LLETZ)

This procedure is used for suspicious lesions or very localised carcinoma (CIN 1 and 2) of the cervix, either as a diagnostic tool or for therapeutic purposes. It has largely taken the place of cone biopsy. It involves the removal, by electrocautery, of a loop of tissue from the transformation zone of the cervix (the area between the squamous and columnar epithelium). It is usually performed as an outpatient procedure using a colposcope.

PELVIC RADIOTHERAPY

Radiotherapy for gynaecological cancer may be used in conjunction with or as an alternative to surgery. It can be given externally or internally. External radiotherapy (external beam radiotherapy) uses an X-ray beam directed at the malignant area. Outpatient treatment sessions, planned in advance, are usually short, although considerable time is taken to set the machine accurately. Internal radiotherapy (brachytherapy) involves insertion of an X-ray-emitting applicator into the uterus or vagina. The device is inserted under general anaesthetic and may remain in place for up to 24 hours. During this time the woman needs to remain as still as possible.

Treatment may be given preoperatively to sterilise any microscopic disease at the margins of the planned operative site. Postoperative treatment would be planned once information from the biopsy specimen is available. It may be used to reduce recurrence or as palliative treatment.

With the recent investment and improvements in services for cancer treatment, women will often be under the care of an oncology nurse specialist who will liaise between the patient and the various members of the team. Although the number of physiotherapists working with these women is small, an opinion or assessment may be requested when specific problems are encountered, such as a woman with a pre-existing respiratory problem who will be required to lie still for brachytherapy treatment. It is useful therefore to have some knowledge of the proposed treatment and to liaise with other team members as required.

Physiotherapists may also be involved in the treatment of long-term side effects, such as urinary frequency, urgency and incontinence, altered bowel habit and sexual dysfunction caused by narrowing and shortening of the vagina and possibly the urethra (Berek & Hacker 2000).

GYNAECOLOGICAL REPAIR SURGERY

COLPORRHAPHY

Colporrhaphy is an operation to repair the vaginal wall. It aims to reconstitute the normal anatomy of the area where prolapse is present and will usually be performed once childbearing is complete. Many surgeons now encourage women to consider how descent of their vaginal wall affects their quality of life, rather than just offering repair where few symptoms exist. When considering this type of surgery, women need to be assessed and receive counselling regarding aspects of their lifestyle that may have exacerbated their symptoms. Where poor collagen type is a factor, then adaptation or avoidance of particular activities (e.g. heavy lifting, high-impact exercise and straining to defaecate) may be appropriate. Improving the pelvic floor muscle strength may provide extra support. Where symptoms are mild, women should be offered a trial of this conservative option before surgery is discussed.

Anterior colporrhaphy

This is a primary procedure for the treatment of cystocoele or urethrocoele (see p. 285). The repair may be reinforced by use of a mesh.

Procedure   Approached via the introitus, the cervix is drawn down and the anterior vaginal wall over the cystocoele is opened. The protrusion is mobilised, then obliterated and supported in a more normal position by tightening and suturing available fascia, such as the pubocervical ligaments and fascia over the bladder. The positions of the urethra and bladder, and the level of the bladder neck are reviewed to ensure that continence is favoured. Finally a longitudinal or diamond-shaped strip of the stretched vaginal wall is excised and the vagina closed. If the uterus is tending to prolapse as well, the operation may be combined with either a vaginal hysterectomy or a Manchester repair (see p. 316).

Postoperative condition   This is as for vaginal hysterectomy (see p. 312).

Risks and complications   A short-term reduction in urinary flow rate has been reported. There is also a risk of postoperative stress incontinence (Stanton et al 1982). This latent or masked stress incontinence will not always be a new problem but may become apparent only following anatomical correction of the prolapse. Recurrence of the prolapse is common; it has also been suggested that dissection of the vagina during surgery has a detrimental effect on the innervation of the pelvic floor (Zivkovic & Tamussino 1997). (See also posterior colporrhaphy.)

Posterior colporrhaphy

This procedure is used to repair the posterior vaginal wall where a rectocoele or enterocoele is significantly symptomatic.

Procedure   For a rectocoele, the posterior wall of the vagina is opened and the rectocoele obliterated and supported using the perirectal fascia and by approximating and suturing the medial edges of the levator ani muscles. A section of the stretched excess vaginal wall is excised and the vagina is closed as for an anterior colporrhaphy.

An enterocoele is repaired in a similar way, but the peritoneal sac of the enterocoele is excised and the uterosacral ligaments sutured together to give support.

Perineorrhaphy is the suturing of the perineum, for example following childbirth trauma.

Colpoperineorrhaphy is a combination of a posterior colporrhaphy and a perineorrhaphy.

Postoperative condition   This is as for vaginal hysterectomy (see p. 312).

Risks and complications   Posterior colporrhaphy is associated with a postoperative increase in bowel and sexual dysfunctions. These symptoms include impaired bowel emptying (constipation, incomplete emptying and the need to use rectal digitation or external support to defaecate) and vaginal tightness or pain resulting in dyspareunia (Kahn & Stanton 1997). Long-term complications include recurrence of the prolapse, which may require repeat surgery. Olsen et al (1997) reported a retrospective cohort study of 395 women undergoing surgical treatment for prolapse and incontinence. The incidence of repeat surgery in this study was 29%, with the time intervals between repeat procedures decreasing with each successive repair. There is also a strong association between faecal incontinence and a history of more than one posterior colporrhaphy (Kahn & Stanton 1997).

SACRAL COLPOPEXY OR TRANSVAGINAL SACROSPINOUS FIXATION

These operations are performed to correct posthysterectomy vaginal vault prolapse. This appears to be a more common complication following vaginal, rather than abdominal, hysterectomy. It may be treated by conservative methods (ring or shelf pessaries) or by surgery.

The sacral colpopexy uses an abdominal approach. A mesh or sling is attached between the presacral fascia (at the level of S2–S3) and the vaginal vault.

The transvaginal sacrospinous fixation involves incision of the vaginal vault and the placement of sutures between the vault and the medial portion of the sacrospinous ligaments.

Postoperative condition   A urethral catheter and IVI are inserted following both procedures. For sacral colpopexy a drain may be inserted near to the abdominal wound (see abdominal hysterectomy, p. 311).

Risks and complications   Both of these procedures are not without complication, which may include urinary symptoms, infection or recurrence of prolapse.

The use of posthysterectomy HRT may be of benefit in addressing the possibility of recurrence, particularly for women who have their surgery for prolapse and who may have collagen deficiency (Barrington & Edwards 2000).

MANCHESTER REPAIR

This repair may be offered to women who have uterine prolapse but who do not wish to have a hysterectomy. The procedure involves amputation of the cervix, which may be elongated, as well as anterior and posterior repair and shortening of the transverse cervical and uterosacral ligaments. Subsequent pregnancy, whilst not recommended, is not impossible although delivery would be by caesarean section.

SALPINGOSTOMY

Salpingostomy is the microsurgery used to repair a fallopian tube. It may be performed via a laparoscope or Pfannenstiel incision, possibly in cases of ectopic pregnancy where it has not been necessary to remove the whole tube.

GILLIAM'S VENTROSUSPENSION

This procedure is performed to correct a retroverted uterus. Usually performed via a laparoscope, the round ligaments are shortened in order to pull the uterine fundus forward. Although the presence of a retroverted uterus may be asymptomatic, the procedure may be considered if the patient reports deep dyspareunia.

SURGICAL TREATMENT OF STRESS INCONTINENCE

Urinary incontinence is a common problem which, although not life threatening, has considerable impact on the quality of life for sufferers. Options for the treatment of urodynamic stress incontinence (USI) are conservative (physiotherapeutic) or surgical. Physiotherapy assessment and management are dealt with, in detail, in Chapter 11. Physiotherapy, however, must also be mentioned here, as the National Institute for Clinical Excellence has recently recommended that surgical options be considered only when conservative management has failed (NICE 2003). Laycock et al (2001) and the Royal College of Physicians (RCP 1995) have also recognised the importance of physiotherapy as providing treatments which are relatively inexpensive, readily available, have few complications and do not compromise future surgery. The role of PFM exercises as initial treatment or as a preventative measure premenopausally is recommended in *Good Practice in Continence Services* (DoH 2000).

Surgery has been performed on women with stress incontinence (SI) for over a century. A variety of procedures have evolved over the years, with anterior colporrhaphy (p. 314) being popular until recently. A systematic review by Black & Downs (1996) of the effectiveness of surgery for stress incontinence suggested that colposuspension appeared to be more effective and more long lasting than anterior colporrhaphy or needle suspension. Following this, Hutchings & Black (2001) reported on a multicentre (18), multisurgeon (49), non-randomised trial of the same three types of surgery; while their results suggest 'the results of surgery for SI are not as good as reported in the textbooks', they do confirm colposuspension to be the most successful. Hutchings et al (1998) reported that good surgical outcomes are more likely if there is no urge incontinence, no or only mild comorbidity, no or only slight obesity, preoperative urodynamic investigations are conducted and the surgeon is a gynaecologist.

Recently there has been a major new development from Scandinavia in the treatment of USI: the tension-free vaginal tape (TVT), a minimal access technique. The number of TVT procedures performed in England has risen from 214 in the year 1998–1999 to 2706 in the year 2000–2001 and early results appear promising. An appraisal of the TVT procedure has recently been completed by NICE. This appraisal reviews the clinical and cost effectiveness of the TVT procedure, in comparison with other surgical interventions, for women with uncomplicated urodynamic stress incontinence in whom conservative management has failed (NICE 2003). TVT, as with other surgical procedures for stress incontinence, is unsuitable for women who may go on to have children; however, it may be a suitable procedure for women who are too frail or unfit to undergo colposuspension (NICE 2003).

Whilst colposuspension and TVT are the two commonest surgeries used for USI, the choice of one procedure over another must be discussed on an individual basis. In comparing the two procedures, an increase in intraoperative complications with TVT contrasts with an increase in post-operative complications following colposuspension (Ward & Hilton 2002).

The long-term results and complications following colposuspension are well documented (Alcalay et al 1995). The TVT procedure appears to have similar effectiveness to colposuspension although the advantages of a minimal access technique need to be considered against the disadvantage of the absence of long-term data. Ward & Hilton (2002) suggest that follow-up will be necessary to inform on the incidence of long-term complications such as prolapse and tape erosion. Preoperative urodynamics are generally advised, before either procedure, to obtain an accurate diagnosis of USI and to determine whether the bladder shows any signs of overactivity (Rufford & Cardozo 2001).

COLPOSUSPENSION

This operation is designed to lift the bladder neck so that when the intra-abdominal pressure is raised it will act as a compressive force around the upper portion of the urethra. This reinforces urethral closure pressure and counterbalances the pressure being exerted on the bladder.

Procedure   Through a Pfannenstiel incision, four or five sutures are used to attach the paravaginal and vaginal tissue on either side of the bladder neck and upper part of the urethra to the ileopectineal ligament. The result is elevation of the bladder neck.

Postoperative condition   A suprapubic catheter is inserted which is left in situ for 3–4 days postoperatively. The catheter is left on free drainage initially and then clamped to allow the patient to attempt normal voiding. The catheter is removed once this has been re-established.

Risks and complications   Voiding dysfunction, de novo detrusor instability and genitourinary prolapse are the most commonly reported problems (Chaliha & Stanton 1999, Smith et al 2002). Patients should be counselled preoperatively concerning possible voiding difficulties in the immediate postoperative period. Skilled surgical judgement is required to produce the appropriate degree of bladder neck lift, otherwise voiding difficulty may persist, requiring long-term intermittent self-catheterisation. Occasionally the operation fails to improve continence.

LAPAROSCOPIC COLPOSUSPENSION

Over 90 articles have been published on this procedure (Smith et al 2002), which is adapted from the open procedure already discussed. The laparoscopic technique requires more skill than the open procedure (Jarvis 2000). Intraoperative time is also increased although there is a more rapid postoperative recovery. The data, however, do not appear to support the use of this procedure and the advent of the TVT counteracts the main advantage of a speedier recovery.

Risks and complications   No significant differences in bladder function have been observed between the open and laparoscopic procedures; however, the laparoscopic procedure may be associated with more surgical complications (Moehrer et al 2002).

TENSION-FREE VAGINAL TAPE (TVT)

The TVT procedure is a minimal access technique performed under local, regional or general anaesthesia. The TVT device consists of a polypropylene mesh (40 cm long, 1 cm wide) covered by a plastic sheath and attached to a needle at each end.

Procedure A 1.5 cm vaginal incision is made over the mid-urethra and two small (0.5–1 cm) suprapubic incisions are made on either side of the midline, about 4–5 cm apart. The needles, each connected to an applicator handle, are passed paraurethrally penetrating the urogenital diaphragm and passing through the retropubic space to emerge through the appropriate abdominal incision. The bladder neck and urethra are kept away from the needles by use of a rigid catheter guide and a cystoscopy is performed to check that there has been no damage to the bladder. The tape forms a U-shape sling around the mid-urethra, laying flat against the posterior urethral surface. If local or regional anaesthesia is used the bladder is filled to 300 mL and the tape is adjusted so that little or no leakage of urine occurs on coughing. If a general anaesthetic is used and the patient is unable to cough, the surgeon tests leakage by applying pressure to the abdominal wall, again with the bladder filled to 300 mL. Once the surgeon is happy with the position of the tape, the plastic sheath is removed. The ends of the tape are cut and left unfixed – hence the term 'tension free'. Finally the vaginal and abdominal wounds are closed.

Postoperative care The catheter will either be removed in theatre or left in place for several hours following surgery. It is essential that voiding is monitored to check bladder emptying. Length of postoperative hospital stay varies between 1 and 3 days (NICE 2003).

Risks and complications Bladder perforation (4%), urinary retention and haemorrhage are the most common short-term complications. Obturator nerve injuries, bowel perforations and vascular injuries have also been reported but are rare (Bodelsson et al 2002, NICE 2003). There are few reports of longer-term complications although urinary retention and difficulties with micturition may require the tape to be cut or removed. Erosion of the tape into the urethra, bladder or vagina is a potential problem, but the limited data suggest that this is a rare occurrence. New-onset symptoms of urgency and detrusor overactivity have also been reported (NICE 2003). There are many research papers regarding the effectiveness of TVT, but no information has been published about the effect on pelvic floor muscle function and there is little available on the issue of further surgery. One paper, published on abdominal hysterectomy after insertion of TVT, reported that the presence of the tape 'appeared to have no bearing on the difficulty of the procedure' (Neale 2002).

ALTERNATIVE PROCEDURES

There are several alternatives to the above procedures. These include endoscopic bladder neck suspensions (needle suspensions, such as the Pereyra, Raz and Stamey procedures), paravaginal repairs (Kelly), the Marshall-Marchetti-Krantz procedure, sling procedures (Aldridge), peri-urethral- or transurethral-bulking agents (Contigen, Macroplastique), and artificial sphincters. All of these procedures have their own complications and success rates. It is accepted that the success rates of these procedures are lower than the success rates following both colposuspension and TVT. The above procedures are therefore not generally recommended as a first surgical option, although this depends on individual assessment of the woman preoperatively, taking into account clinical features, urodynamic results, general health and previous surgical history (Chaliha & Stanton 1999, Jarvis 2000, Smith et al 2002).

DEFINITIONS OF OTHER USEFUL TERMS AND PROCEDURES

Colposcopy   This is the examination of the vaginal aspect of the cervix using a colposcope – a low-powered microscope.

Dilatation and curettage (D & C)   The cervix is gently dilated and the uterine cavity is systematically scraped using a curette. This procedure may be performed for diagnostic purposes (e.g. in abnormal bleeding), or for pregnancy complications (e.g. abortion).

Endometrial ablation   This technique usually uses heat to destroy the endometrium. It may be performed using high-frequency microwaves (microwave endometrial ablation) or laser. Both techniques are performed under general anaesthetic with the heat source inserted into the uterus via the vagina. It is an alternative, less invasive option to hysterectomy for women with DUB.

Hysteroscopy   An endoscope is passed along the vagina and introduced into the uterus through the cervix. It is used as a diagnostic tool to inspect the inside of the uterus.

Laparoscopy   An endoscope is introduced via a small abdominal incision into the pelvic cavity. It is used to inspect the lower abdominal cavity for diagnostic purposes, for example for assessment of acute or chronic abdominal pain. It may also be used for surgical procedures (e.g. sterilisation, ectopic pregnancy or ovarian cystectomy) or to assist vaginal surgery (e.g. LAVH). Additional surgical instruments will be introduced through new incisions as required. The benefits of laparoscopic surgery include small incisions, reduced surgical trauma, less postoperative pain, shorter hospitalisation and increased recovery rate. Laparoscopic procedures, however, require a high level of skills. If used as an alternative to procedures which are traditionally performed via laparotomy, the length of the procedure may increase with a resulting increase in anaesthetic risk.

Laparotomy   Any abdominal incision through which the abdomen is inspected is known as a laparotomy. For gynaecological purposes this will usually be a bikini-line (Pfannenstiel) incision, although a surgeon may occasionally use a vertical incision.

Marsupialisation of Bartholin's cyst   This procedure involves incision of the blocked duct within the Bartholin's gland. This is then opened and the edges stitched to the surrounding tissue.

PHYSIOTHERAPY CARE OF PATIENTS UNDERGOING GYNAECOLOGICAL SURGERY

The amount of physiotherapy care required by these patients varies considerably, depending on the individual condition of the patient and the nature of the surgery. There has been a move towards a shorter stay in hospital over recent years and for minor surgery there is usually no indication for physiotherapy intervention. The physiotherapist, however, may be involved in the preparation of information leaflets for women undergoing minor surgery.

The physiotherapist will usually have direct contact with women undergoing major gynaecological surgery and must therefore be familiar with both the procedure and the patient. Physiotherapy staff need to be up to date with surgical techniques in order to be able to use clinical-reasoning skills to adapt any rehabilitation programme. They also need to be aware of any psychological effect that surgery may have.

PSYCHOLOGICAL ASPECTS OF GYNAECOLOGICAL SURGERY

The psychological effects of gynaecological surgery are many and varied. Although some surgery is performed as an emergency, most will be elective, so the amount of preparation time may vary from a few days to many months.

Psychological reactions may be very complex and may involve relationships with both the partner and family or friends. The indication for the surgery may be part of this process, although again each woman is likely to have a different reaction. For women who are undergoing surgery for symptoms affecting their quality of life, the operation may be a relief. This could be the case for women who are having surgery to correct a prolapse, however, they may also fear that they will be 'tied too tight' or that their urinary control will be affected. There are few data regarding psychological status following surgery for stress incontinence. Studies by Black et al (1997, 1998) suggest that a considerable number of women report a deterioration in mental health; this may reflect the failure rate of the surgery. For women undergoing hysterectomy for DUB, the prospect of resolving this permanently may be liberating, although it could also be seen as a loss of femininity and of the childbearing role. If surgery is for malignancy there will obviously be anxiety as to the eventual outcome, which will affect all those involved with the patient. It is widely documented that depression may follow hysterectomy and the use of support groups may be helpful. It has been suggested that some of these feelings may be due to a lack of oestrogen after oophrectomy; however depression is not confined to this group of women (Hysterectomy Association 2002). For women admitted with an ectopic pregnancy there is the psychological effect of pregnancy loss.

All of these issues may be relevant, although the requirements to be admitted to hospital and to undergo surgery are factors in their own right. The woman may be anxious about being in an unfamiliar environment or being away from home. She may have concerns about those left to cope without her, particularly if she has carer responsibilities. Preparation and information prior to admission all help to reduce these anxieties.

In discussing the psychological aspects it is important to consider the partner, who may have his or her own anxieties and be unable to provide support. It may be difficult to articulate these feelings, resulting in a feeling of helplessness. Postoperatively the situation is just as varied: some will feel relieved, others overwhelmed.

Whatever the reaction, it is often the physiotherapist who appears to have the empathy and time to spend listening, explaining and drawing out unexpressed fears.

PREOPERATIVE PHYSIOTHERAPY

To enable the physiotherapist to give the most effective care, at least one preoperative session should be arranged in a calm, unhurried environment. It will comprise of assessment, instruction, discussion and possibly treatment.

In many hospitals, women attend a pre-admission clerking clinic and the physiotherapist may be able to see the patient at this appointment with other members of the team. If this is not possible, most women are admitted the day before major surgery and the physiotherapist should see them at this time.

In many units this preoperative session will be carried out with a group of patients, although the women should be assessed prior to inclusion in the group. If treatment is indicated this would be undertaken on an individual basis. Preoperatively, patients are generally well motivated, keen to learn and cooperative. They welcome the opportunity to ask questions and share their fears; they also appreciate the positive use of the waiting time. If they have already attended an outpatient clerking clinic they may recognise some of their fellow patients; a group physiotherapy session may therefore facilitate peer support. It is obviously more cost effective to see patients together, although this rationale should not compromise patient care and consent must be sought from all patients prior to the session.

Assessment

The initial impression should be obtained from the medical notes. The main reason for this is to establish the physical state of the patient and the risk status with regard to complications. It is imperative that the proposed surgery and rationale are understood by the physiotherapist. As well as warning the physiotherapist about the possible mental state of the patient, this also helps to prepare for questions.

The following checklist may be useful:

- pre-existing medical conditions – respiratory problems, mobility problems, backache, circulatory problems, diabetes, constipation
- smoking – number per day, smoker's cough
- proposed surgery and indication
- continence status
- previous surgery or physiotherapy for the condition
- any other relevant information – carer responsibilities, previously expressed concerns.

Patients who are undergoing surgery for stress incontinence, or possibly prolapse, may have been referred for physiotherapy prior to being put on the waiting list or whilst awaiting admission. This may have prevented some of these women from needing surgery. If an operation is still favoured such women should have been given a preoperative programme and should be adequately prepared.

If surgery is planned in advance and there are known risk factors (e.g. chronic obstructive pulmonary disease, COPD), preoperative anaesthetic assessment may have taken place. It may even be possible for such patients to achieve an improvement in physical condition prior to surgery.

Instruction and preparation

Patients should have a basic understanding of the procedure, in order to appreciate the relevance of physiotherapy. They need to be aware that it is routine for them to see a physiotherapist and that the objective is to help them to help their own recovery. Care must be taken with use of language, so that the physiotherapist is understood and patients are clear as to what they need to do. It is well documented (Devine 1992) that preoperative advice or information helps to reduce anxiety and prevent complications. Any verbal information should be reinforced by supporting information such as leaflets, tapes or videos (Theis & Johnson 1995). Many units have developed their own literature but general information booklets are also available such as the booklet by Haslett & Jennings (2003).

The main objective of the preoperative session is to give advice and teach exercises which are appropriate for the first few postoperative days. In many units this will be the only contact with the physiotherapist until several days after surgery, when further advice and exercise progression for discharge and afterwards will be given. There are several aspects that need to be covered.

Respiratory system

General anaesthesia and pain can both compromise respiratory function. The number of women experiencing respiratory complications following major gynaecological surgery is low (Amirika & Evans 1979); however there are a number of factors that increase the risk of postoperative respiratory complications. These include pre-existing lung disease (COPD, asthma), smoking, reduced mobility and prolonged anaesthesia (Berek & Hacker 2000). The existence of any of these risks should be determined from the records. In order to reduce the risk it is advisable to educate the patient with regards to both respiratory function and early ambulation. Patients also need to be aware of the need to accept good pain control, although this in itself can compromise respiratory and bowel function.

Upper abdominal surgery is known to cause severe and prolonged alterations in pulmonary mechanics (Richardson & Sabanathan 1997). Although there is little research in relation to gynaecological procedures, it is recognised that opiates and sedatives can affect the natural 'sigh' mechanism. This mechanism maintains the patency of the smaller airways, reducing the functional residual capacity.

A preoperative advice session allows the physiotherapist to identify patients at risk of respiratory complications as well as to teach appropriate techniques to optimise respiratory function. These techniques include the active cycle of breathing technique (ACBT), with the use of a sniff at the end of inspiration to increase lung volume for at-risk patients. The use of forced expiratory technique (huffing) and supported coughing is advised for use only if retained secretions are present postoperatively. Coughing is likely to cause less pain if the patient supports the perineum or abdomen, depending on the surgical approach.

Smoking should be discussed, although there is little evidence that stopping or reducing smoking immediately prior to surgery is of benefit. Some women will be keen to stop and see their admission to hospital as the right time to do so. In the UK, smoking cessation is the target of a national campaign (DoH 1998). Many Trusts employ or have access to smoking cessation advisors. Some hospital staff may also have been through a programme to give them skills to help patients in this situation. Physiotherapists need to be familiar with their local services.

Circulatory system

There is a postoperative risk of deep vein thrombosis (DVT) and possibly pulmonary embolus. This is due to intraoperative pressure and trauma to the pelvic vasculature, as well as enhancement of the normal clotting mechanism caused by surgery and bleeding. Risk assessment, which is usually completed at the preadmission clerking clinic, will direct appropriate prophylactic measures. These may include antiembolitic stockings and antithrombolytic drugs (e.g. Fragmin).

Early ambulation helps to reduce these risks, although full-range plantar- and dorsiflexion of the ankle will also increase venous return in the calves. Stiffness and soreness of the legs and buttocks can be reduced by active hip and knee flexion and extension and by weight transference and pressure relief. Women will usually be encouraged to sit in a chair for a short while on the first postoperative day and will start to mobilise more fully on the second.

Bed mobility

Movement in bed postoperatively is encouraged. Many hospitals have 'minimal-lift' policies and patients will find it difficult to master new movement patterns introduced after their operation. Techniques should therefore be taught preoperatively and the patient given time to practise on a hospital bed. As well as reducing the strain on the staff, this helps the patient to be independent and in control. It will also help to prevent wound complications (dehiscence) caused by the patient struggling to move and markedly raising intra-abdominal pressure in the process.

Women should be shown supported resting positions such as half lying with a pillow under the thighs, and side lying with pillows between the knees and under the lower abdomen. They should also be taught how to move from lying to sitting (and vice versa) via side lying, to minimise any increase in intra-abdominal pressure. When moving up the bed, women should be encouraged to bend their knees and use their thigh muscles, by digging in with the heels and straightening the legs. The upper limbs support the trunk and the patient pushes down with them at the same time as the knees are straightened so that the buttocks lift up off the bed and back towards the pillows.

All physiotherapists should be familiar with the manual handling policy of their unit and be able to adapt bed mobility patterns for their patients. They should also be aware of suitable transfer aids (slide-sheets, turntables, etc.) for less mobile patients.

Pelvic floor muscle exercises

These exercises are important regardless of the surgical route used. For women undergoing vaginal hysterectomy or repair, the pelvic floor muscles (PFMs) are directly affected by surgery and need to be strengthened to provide maximal functional support. The role of the PFMs in the treatment of stress incontinence is well documented (Berghmans et al 1998). For women who are having anti-stress-incontinence procedures, exercises should be encouraged, to strengthen and support. It is well documented that hysterectomy may affect bladder and bowel function (see p. 312). Therefore pelvic floor muscle exercises (PFME) are also recommended following abdominal hysterectomy.

It is easier to learn PFM contractions prior to surgery. It is known that brief verbal instruction is not adequate for many women to achieve correct pelvic floor action (Bø et al 1988, Bump et al 1991). It is not usually appropriate for women to undergo vaginal assessment of their PFM function at this preoperative session. The physiotherapist must therefore use diagrams or models and provide sufficient detail when explaining the anatomy, function and contraction of the muscles. A combination of fast (phasic), slow maximal and submaximal (tonic) contractions should be encouraged, as well as the use of an anticipatory PFM contraction ('the knack') for activities causing any increase in intra-abdominal pressure (Miller et al 1996, Naylor 2002).

Abdominal muscle exercises

Whilst it is assumed that the abdominal muscles are directly affected by abdominal surgery, there is currently no evidence to support this. Following the clinical-reasoning process with regard to pain causing muscle inhibition, it seems appropriate for women to work these muscles in order to restore normal function following abdominal surgery.

Transversus abdominus contractions (submaximal) are believed to facilitate pelvic floor muscle activity and enhance core stability (Sapsford et al 2001). These exercises, which can be difficult to teach, should be taught in a position appropriate for the postoperative period (e.g. crook lying or standing). Pelvic tilting taught in crook lying works the oblique abdominal muscles but may also help to reduce wind pain. The same appears to be true of gentle trunk rotations, although, as yet, there is no research evidence to support this.

Gentle abdominal muscle exercises also help to facilitate trunk movement and early mobilisation, by reducing the fear of movement. Whilst it may be possible to teach these exercises in a group setting, they will need to be performed on a hospital bed and checked individually.

Posture and back care

Decreased mobility, poor positioning and lack of lumbar support may cause backache in the postoperative period. As well as the above abdominal muscle exercises and early mobilisation, patients should be advised to adopt supported positions, using appropriately placed pillows or lumbar rolls. This may also help to reduce neck pain and headaches.

Wind pain

This can be caused by stationary air in the gut due to reduced peristalsis following general anaesthetic. It is also thought to be caused by air in the peritoneal cavity, and this takes time to be absorbed. The resulting pain can be acute, within the abdomen or referred to the right shoulder, or both. Early ambulation, gentle abdominal muscle exercises and abdominal massage have all, anecdotally, been reported as helping to reduce this pain.

Patient discussion

Having discussed all of the above areas, the patient may still have concerns. It is important that anxiety levels are reduced as far as possible so, given sufficient time, the rapport built between the specialist physiotherapist and the patient should make raising of concerns easier. The matter can then be discussed and referral to another team member arranged if thought appropriate.

Treatment

Any treatment indicated by the preoperative assessment should be undertaken on an individual basis and may include adaptation of routine advice and exercises to a pre-existing condition, teaching additional respiratory techniques, or providing mobility aids to facilitate independence.

POSTOPERATIVE PHYSIOTHERAPY

The main objective of postoperative physiotherapy is that patients return to their normal function, or better, in an optimal timescale and without complication.

Early treatment

The immediate objectives are to achieve good respiratory and vascular function and early mobilisation. For most patients who have received a thorough preoperative preparation, these issues will not be a problem and no intervention will be required for the first day or two following surgery. Nursing staff should be familiar with the need for patients to perform breathing and circulatory exercises. They should also be able to facilitate appropriate transfers and mobilisation.

If no preoperative preparation has taken place, however, early assistance may be required. This can be a slow and time-consuming process, as patients may be affected by either anaesthetic or postoperative analgesia. They may not be receptive to an unfamiliar person or understand the rationale behind the new advice they are given.

For patients with known risk factors or early respiratory complications, assessment and appropriate treatment must be commenced as soon as possible.

Further progression

Pelvic floor muscle exercises

Ideally these will have been learnt preoperatively. PFME should be encouraged as soon as possible after surgery. Pain will cause muscle inhibition and so encouragement to take adequate analgesia, along with a delay in commencing exercises, is important if pain is a problem. Many physiotherapists believe that PFME should be delayed if a catheter is present in the urethra, although there is no evidence to prove any harmful effects (Haslam & Pomfret 2002). The PFME may be started if a supra-pubic catheter is in place, although abdominal discomfort around the catheter during cocontraction of the tranversus abdominus may again cause a delay in starting these exercises.

A combination of fast (phasic), slow maximal and submaximal (tonic) exercises are appropriate, with varying emphasis depending on the type of and rationale for surgery (Naylor 2002). If surgery has been performed for prolapse, submaximal contractions held for several seconds may help to increase the resting tone of the PFM and increase postural support. Following abdominal surgery, the exercises are used to enhance the function of the trunk stabilisers, by cocontraction of the transversus abdominus, and to reduce the possibility of urinary incontinence. Again, slow recruitment, submaximal holds are more important (Sapsford et al 2001).

The use of PFM 'bracing', known as 'the knack' (Miller et al 1996), is important following all gynaecological surgery. This contraction counteracts the increase in intra-abdominal pressure and both fast and slow maximal contractions are needed for this to be effective. This is particularly important for women after continence procedures.

Abdominal muscle exercises

Ideally these will have been taught preoperatively. The preoperative section gives information about the rationale for abdominal muscle exercises (see p. 325). The importance of pain causing muscle inhibition cannot be understated (see PFME, p. 326).

Transversus abdominus, pelvic-tilting and knee-rolling exercises in crook lying will help to reduce backache, stiffness and wind pain. They may be commenced as soon as pain allows, usually within the first few days. Care, however, must be taken when recommending any progression of abdominal muscle exercise as any increase in intra-abdominal pressure could put a strain on healing tissues.

The most important reason for performing abdominal muscle exercises is to improve the support provided by these muscles. In order to do this the local and global stabilisers need to be functioning well before further progression occurs.

Posture and back care

There is a tendency to adopt protective flexed postures following surgery. Abnormal postures require correction. The patient must be made aware of the problem and be encouraged to sit, stand and walk 'tall', using the transversus abdominus, the PFMs and lumbar support where appropriate. It is important that the woman understands how to take care of her back and this must be discussed prior to discharge.

Mobilisation

Early ambulation helps to prevent respiratory and vascular complications, as well as reducing backache, stiffness and wind pain. Women will often be sitting out of bed, for a short while, the day following surgery and will start to mobilise the following day. Initially this will be short walks, probably as far as the toilet or bathroom. Mobilisation is not solely the responsibility of the physiotherapist, but referral by other members of the team is appropriate if difficulties occur with individual patients. A gradual increase in mobilisation is essential prior to discharge.

Stairs are not usually a problem for women after gynaecological surgery. However, if there is concern about the woman's ability to climb the stairs at home following discharge, or if indicated for other reasons, then the physiotherapist can assess and advise.

Rest   This is as important as mobilisation. Too much activity will cause tiredness, which can delay recovery. Sleep and relaxation can be difficult to achieve on a busy ward; but adopting comfortable resting positions and discussing anxieties will help. For some patients, the teaching of relaxation techniques or a recommendation that they move to a quieter part of the ward may be beneficial.

Immediate postoperative complications

Chest infection

The patient will be given antibiotics. ACBT, huffing and supported coughing are recommended. Humidification and positioning, as well as ambulation, may help to improve expectoration.

DVT   Prophylactic care has been discussed in the preoperative section (see p. 324). Should a DVT occur then anticoagulant therapy will commence with instructions on mobility status.

Wound infection   As for chest infection, the patient will be given antibiotics. Any wound infection may reduce the exercise level, which will have a knock-on effect on recovery rate.

Voiding dysfunction   Routine postoperative nursing observations should pick up any problems with voiding, such as retention, urgency and frequency, although it is the responsibility of all members of the multidisciplinary team to monitor and act on any problems. Straining to void must be discouraged as this will increase the pressure on both the PFM and other healing structures. Infection of the urinary tract or bladder will be treated with antibiotics. The patient may report symptoms of urinary incontinence directly to the physiotherapist, particularly if the patient is aware of the role of physiotherapy from preoperative contact.

PREPARING TO LEAVE HOSPITAL

Patients should be adequately prepared for discharge home. The information they have been given verbally must be reinforced in written or audio format. This will allow them to refer to the advice once at home but it also allows the advice to be accessible to carers and other members of the family. Any carer demands on patients themselves should have been resolved whilst in hospital, if not before.

If patients have been seen preoperatively then some of the discharge advice may have been given at that stage. This would be appropriate if concerns regarding discharge are causing anxiety before surgery. All women must be seen at least once following their operation for advice on progression to their normal activity level and to prevent long-term complications or, in some cases, recurrence of the initial problem.

Discharge advice following uncomplicated major gynaecological surgery

- The first 1–2 weeks should be a continuation of hospital care. This means a combination of gentle mobilisation and rest, with someone to prepare meals and perform other household tasks.
- It is crucial that constipation is avoided. Straining at defaecation will increase the pressure on the PFM as well as other healing structures. Advice should be given regarding fibre and fluid intake as well as short-term laxative use if required. All women will benefit from being given advice on appropriate positioning and defaecation technique (Markwell & Sapsford 1995). (See p. 387.)
- After a few days, short walks outside can be introduced with a gradual progression in distance and speed as recovery occurs.
- After 1–2 weeks light household activity can be recommended, but prolonged standing should be avoided. Activity levels can gradually be increased so that slightly heavier jobs (e.g. light shopping and ironing) are undertaken by 4 weeks.
- Lifting more than 1 kg must be avoided for 4 weeks; after that a gradual increase is recommended but it will take at least 3 months to return to heavy lifting. It must be emphasised that the transversus abdominus and PFM should be braced during any lifting. If, despite this, breath holding or abdominal straining occur, the load is too heavy. It may be recommended that some women never return to their usual preoperative lifting level.
- Driving may be recommended at about 4–6 weeks; however, women should be advised to check their insurance cover. The main concerns are the ability to perform an emergency stop (and the effect this would have on healing tissues), general movement in the car and heavy steering. Women are well advised to try an emergency stop before driving on public roads; if they are hesitant to do so they should not drive.
- Encouragement should be given to continue the exercise programme with gradual progression.
- By 6 weeks, household activities such as vacuuming and laundry tasks may be recommended.
- Most units will arrange an outpatient review with a member of the consultant team at about 6 weeks. This is the earliest at which women are advised to return to work – the more active the job, the longer is required off work, with some women returning to work as long as 3 months after their operation.
- Some physiotherapists provide a postoperative class about 6 weeks after surgery. This can be used to reinforce information about PFME, defaecation technique, moving and handling, general back care and return to fitness.
- Sexual activity is recommended when comfortable, but most women wait until after their 6-week review appointment. Dyspareunia can be a complication of vaginal surgery, owing to physical or psychological problems, or both (see p. 296)
- General exercise is not recommended until at least 6 weeks. Ballistic activities and those causing large increases in intra-abdominal pressure are to be avoided initially and for some patients permanently. The progression of walking, swimming or water-based exercise is particularly beneficial.

LIFELONG ADVICE

The importance of maintaining good PFM function cannot be emphasised enough and women need to be aware that PFME should be as much of a habit as cleaning their teeth!

Although the recovery rate and routine are similar regardless of the surgical route, the rationale is different. For women with poor quality connective tissue who have undergone surgery for prolapse, the contributing lifestyle factors must be discussed so that they are able to reduce recurrence. This means the avoidance of constipation, heavy lifting, weight-bearing exercise and management of any aggravating respiratory conditions. It may also mean weight reduction, for which they may need advice and support. The body will be getting older over time and women need to be aware of the adverse role these factors can play, although this may require huge lifestyle changes. By educating patients, physiotherapists are able to empower patients to help themselves.

References

Alcalay M, Monga A, Stanton S 1995 Burch colposuspension: a 10–20 year follow up. British Journal of Obstetrics and Gynaecology 102:740–745.

Amirika H, Evans T N 1979 Ten year review of hysterectomies, trends, indications and risks. American Journal of Obstetrics 134:431–437.

Barrington J W, Edwards G 2000 Posthysterectomy vault prolapse. International Urogynecology Journal 11:241–245.

Berek J S, Hacker N F 2000 Practical gynecologic oncology, 3rd edn. Lippincott Williams & Wilkins, Philadelphia.

Berghmans L C M, Hendriks H J M, Bø K et al 1998 Conservative treatment of stress urinary incontinence in women: a systematic review of randomized controlled trials. British Journal of Urology 82:181–191.

Black N A, Downs S H 1996 The effectiveness of surgery for stress incontinence in women: a systematic review. British Journal of Urology 78(4):497–510.

Black N, Griffiths J, Pope C et al 1997 Impact of surgery for stress incontinence on morbidity: cohort study. British Medical Journal 315(7121):1493–1498.

Black N A, Bowling A, Griffiths J M et al 1998 Impact of surgery for stress incontinence on the social lives of women. British Journal of Obstetrics and Gynaecology 105(6):605–612.

Bø K, Larsen S, Oseid S et al 1988 Knowledge about and ability to correct pelvic floor muscle exercises in women with urinary stress incontinence. Neurourology and Urodynamics 7:261–262.

Bodelsson G, Henriksson L, Osser S et al 2002 Short term complications of the tension-free vaginal tape operation for stress urinary incontinence in women. British Journal of Obstetrics and Gynaecology 109:566–569.

Brown J S, Sawaya G, Thom D H et al 2000 Hysterectomy and urinary incontinence. Lancet 356:535–539.

Bump R C, Hurt W G, Fantl J A et al 1991 Assessment of Kegel pelvic muscle exercise performance after brief verbal instruction. American Journal of Obstetrics and Gynecology 165(2):322–329.

Chaliha C, Stanton S L 1999 Complications of surgery for genuine stress incontinence. British Journal of Obstetrics and Gynaecology 106:1238–1245.

Clarke A, Black N, Rowe P et al 1995 Indications for and outcome of total abdominal hysterectomy for benign disease: a prospective cohort study. British Journal of Obstetrics and Gynaecology 102(8):611–620.

Devine E C 1992 Effects of psychoeducational care for adult surgical patients: a meta-analysis of 191 studies. Patient Education and Counseling 19:129–142.

DoH (Department of Health) 1998 Smoking kills: a white paper on tobacco. DoH, London. Online. Available: http://www.doh.gov.uk/tobacco/smokexec.htm

DoH (Department of Health) 2000 Good practice in continence services. DoH, London. Online. Available: http://www.doh.gov.uk/continenceservices.htm

DoH (Department of Health) 2001 Good practice in consent implementation guide: consent to examination or treatment. DoH, London. Online. Available: http://www.doh.gov.uk/consent/

DoH (Department of Health) 2003 Hospital episode statistics. OPCS4, Codes for Hysterectomy Q07, Q08. Available: http://www.doh.gov.uk/hes/index.html

Grimes D A 1999 Role of the cervix in sexual response: evidence for and against. Clinical Obstetrics and Gynaecology 42(4):972–978.

Haslam J, Pomfret I 2002 Should pelvic floor muscle exercises be encouraged in people with an indwelling urethral catheter in situ? Journal of the Association of Chartered Physiotherapists in Women's Health 91:18–22.

Haslett S, Jennings M et al 2003 Hysterectomy, vaginal repair and surgery for stress incontinence, 5th edn. Beaconsfield Publications, Beaconsfield.

Hidlebaugh D A 2000 Cost and quality-of-life issues associated with different surgical therapies for the treatment of abnormal uterine bleeding. Obstetrics and Gynecology Clinics of North America 27(2):451–465.

Hutchings A, Black N A 2001 Surgery for stress incontinence: a non-randomised trial of colposuspension, needle suspension and anterior colporrhaphy. European Urology 9(4):375–382.

Hutchings A, Griffiths J, Black N A 1998 Surgery for stress incontinence: factors associated with a successful outcome. British Journal of Urology 82(5):634–641.

Hysterectomy Association 2002 Online. Available: http://www.hysterectomy-association.org.uk.

Jarvis G J 2000 Surgery for urinary incontinence. Ballière's Clinical Obstetrics and Gynaecology 14(2):315–334.

Kahn M A, Stanton S L 1997 Posterior colporrhaphy: its effects on bowel and sexual function. British Journal of Obstetrics and Gynaecology 104(1):82–86.

Laycock J, Standley A, Crothers E et al 2001 Clinical guidelines for the physiotherapy management of females aged 16–65 with stress urinary incontinence. Chartered Society of Physiotherapy, London, p 12–14.

Markwell S J, Sapsford R R 1995 Physiotherapy management of obstructed defaecation. Australian Journal of Physiotherapy 41:279–283.

Meikle S F, Nugent E W, Orleans M 1997 Complications and recovery from laparoscopy-assisted vaginal hysterectomy compared with abdominal and vaginal hysterectomy. Obstetrics and Gynecology 89(2):304–311.

Miller J M, Ashton-Miller J, DeLancey J O L 1996 The Knack: use of precisely timed pelvic muscle contraction can reduce leakage in stress urinary incontinence. Neurourology and Urodynamics 15:392–393.

Milsom I, Ekelund P, Molander U et al 1993 The influence of age, parity, oral contraception, hysterectomy and menopause on the prevalence of urinary incontinence in women. Journal of Urology 149(6):1459–1462.

Moehrer B, Ellis G, Carey M et al 2002 Laparoscopic colposuspension for urinary incontinence in women. Cochrane Database of Systematic Reviews. Update Software, Oxford. Online. Available: http://www.cochrane.org/cochrane/revabstr/ab002239.htm

Naylor D 2002 Which is the best way to exercise pelvic floor muscles? Journal of the Association of Chartered Physiotherapists in Women's Health 91:23–28.

Neale E J 2002 Abdominal hysterectomy after insertion of tension-free vaginal tape. British Journal of Obstetrics and Gynaecology 109:731–732.

NICE (National Institute for Clinical Excellence) 2003 Technology appraisal of tension-free vaginal tape for stress incontinence. Online. Available: http://www.nice.org.uk

Olsen A L, Smith V J, Bergstrom J O et al 1997 Epidemiology of surgically managed pelvic organ prolapse and urinary incontinence. Obstetrics and Gynecology 89(4):501–506.

RCP (Royal College of Physicians) 1995 Incontinence: causes, management and provision of services. RCP, London, p 1–5.

Richardson J, Sabanathan S 1997 Prevention of respiratory complications after abdominal surgery. Thorax 52(suppl 3):S35–S40.

Rufford J, Cardozo L 2001 The role of TVT in genuine stress incontinence. Reviews in Gynaecological Practice 1(1):7–11.

Sapsford R, Hodges P, Richardson C et al 2001 Co-activation of the abdominal and pelvic floor muscles during voluntary exercises. Neurourology and Urodynamics 20:31–42.

Smith T, Daneshgari F, Dmochowski R et al 2002 Surgical treatments of incontinence in women. In: Abrams P, Cardozo L, Khoury S et al (eds) Incontinence, Ch. 11. Health Publications, Plymouth, p 825–863.

Stanton S L, Hilton P, Norton C et al 1982 Clinical and urodynamic effects of anterior colporrhaphy and vaginal hysterectomy for prolapse with and without incontinence. British Journal of Obstetrics and Gynaecology 89(6):459–463.

Thakar R, Ayers S, Clarkson P et al 2002 Outcomes after total versus subtotal hysterectomy. New England Journal of Medicine 347(17):1318–1325.

Theis S L, Johnson J H 1995 Strategies for teaching patients: a meta-analysis. Clinical Nurse Specialist 9(2):100–105.

Thomson A J, Sproston A R, Farquharson R G 1998 Ultrasound detection of vault haematoma following vaginal hysterectomy. British Journal of Obstetrics and Gynaecology 105(2):211–215.

van der Vaart C H, van der Bom J G, de Leeuw J R J et al 2002 The contribution of hysterectomy to the occurrence of urge and stress urinary incontinence symptoms. British Journal of Obstetrics and Gynaecology 109:149–154.

Ward K, Hilton P 2002 Prospective multicentre randomised trial of tension-free vaginal tape and colposuspension as primary treatment for stress incontinence. British Medical Journal 325(7355):67–70.

Zivkovic F, Tamussino K 1997 Effects of vaginal surgery on the lower urinary tract. Current Opinion in Obstetrics and Gynaecology 9(5):329–331.

Further reading

Cardozo L, Staskin D (eds) 2002 Textbook of female urology and urogynaecology. Isis Medical Media, London.

Smith T, Daneshgari F, Dmochowski R et al 2002 Surgical treatments of incontinence in women. In: Abrams P, Cardozo L, Khoury S et al (eds) Incontinence, Ch. 11. Health Publications, Plymouth, p 825–863.

Useful addresses

Hysterectomy Association
Tel 0871 7811141
Website: www.hysterectomy-association.org.uk

Chapter **11**

Urinary function and dysfunction

Jill Mantle

CHAPTER CONTENTS

Introduction   333
Normal lower urinary tract function   336
Lower urinary tract dysfunction   342
Incontinence of urine   343
Voiding difficulties   348
Physiotherapy assessment methods   349

Urodynamic, radiological and electromyographical
    assessment   361
Understanding urinary dysfunction   364
Physiotherapy treatment   364
Management of persistent urinary
    incontinence   379

The terminology used in this chapter largely complies with the ICS Standardisation of terminology of lower urinary function (Abrams et al 2002a), which is published in full in Appendix 1 on p. 427. However, to assist readers in consulting literature published earlier than 2002, the 1988 version (Abrams et al 1988) is also included as Appendix 2 on p. 449.

INTRODUCTION

The term '*continence*' is used to describe the normal ability of a person to store urine and faeces temporarily, with conscious control over the time and place of micturition and defaecation. Continence of urine and faeces is fundamental to the sociological, psychological and physical well-being of an individual. Infants do not have such control, but develop the neurological maturity and form the habits necessary, usually by 3 or 4 years of age. In the adult there is considerable normal variation in the volume of urine and of faeces that is stored, and in the frequency of micturition and defaecation. A subtle combination of factors contribute to continence so that it is not only the condition and integrity of the specific organs involved and the immediate surrounding tissues that is important, together with the general health and well-being – both physical and mental – of the whole person, but also the environment. This includes privacy and cleanliness.

In addition, society places demands that voiding occurs at a time and in a place that is acceptable to the majority. For example, when out for a walk in the countryside, it is acceptable to empty one's bladder behind a hedge on the edge of a deserted field, but to do so behind a hoarding in a crowded street is not acceptable. If a person passes urine or faeces into clothing, in a bed or chair, on to the ground or into a receptacle not designated for the purpose the person is likely to be labelled as 'incontinent'.

'Incontinence' has been defined as the involuntary or inappropriate passing of urine or faeces, or both, that has an impact on social functioning or hygiene (DoH 2000). This definition applies only after early childhood. Incontinence of urine or faeces is a symptom or a sign with a cause, not a condition or a specific disease. It may be a temporary state associated with a transient cause (e.g. transient unconsciousness, infection, or drug side-effects), or it may be persistent resulting from longer-lasting or even permanent causes (e.g. trauma in childbirth, stroke). Incontinence is not life threatening, but it is humiliating, distressing, degrading and expensive (Hu 1990) for the sufferer. Where it persists, it can lead to isolation, depression, loss of self-esteem, and ill health, for example infections (Wyman et al 1990). The odour and damage to property it causes militate against proper social integration (Grimley et al 1993) and, especially for children and the elderly, can even result in the person being ostracised, abused and receiving insufficient care from unsympathetic or poorly informed carers. It has been suggested that incontinence is a major factor in sufferers and carers reaching crisis point with consequent referral to residential care (Continence Foundation 2000).

There is considerable individual variation in what each person classes as a 'continence problem'. Furthermore there are many sufferers who do not seek help because they are too embarrassed to consult their general practitioners or anyone else, and others who consider their state to be inevitable (Hampel et al 1997). Sufferers naturally oppose the 'incontinent' label – 'I'm *not* incontinent, I just leak sometimes!' Researchers have used a variety of parameters regarding amount lost and frequency of loss in their definitions of incontinence, which makes firm statements on prevalence unwise. However, the Royal College of Physicians (RCP 1995) produced a useful synthesis of the literature and the Continence Foundation (2000) expanded on this to produce a model to enable readers to produce an estimate of prevalence in their particular area, which is certainly a useful starting point when appraising services for sufferers in a locality. It is safe to say that in the UK, incontinence, both urinary and faecal, is more common in women than men and that it increases with parity and age (RCP 1995, Thomas et al 1980, 1984). Faecal incontinence is probably less common than urinary incontinence but there is no doubt that faecal incontinence is underreported for obvious reasons. Faecal incontinence is more often accompanied by urinary incontinence (double incontinence) than occurring alone. It is also safe to say that most sufferers would benefit from specialist assessment and active treatment and, where this is not successful, management measures prescribed by specialists (e.g. appliances, pads or home adaptations) would improve the person's quality of life.

The prospect for incontinence sufferers has greatly improved in recent years. Collaborative lobbying by individuals and organisations has raised awareness, culminating in 2000 with the publication of Government Guidelines entitled *Good Practice in Continence Services* (DoH 2000). Social mores are changing, allowing freer discussion and publicity about such matters. Women's magazines, 'soaps' and chat shows have played an important part, and the caring professions are working together with greater success to seek solutions tailored to individual sufferers. The International Continence Society (ICS), formed in 1971, has fostered much valuable exchange of knowledge and collaborative research, and has since become multidisciplinary. The ICS Standardisation of Terminology Committee has made an important contribution by setting standards in word usage and for investigations, facilitating a common language and comparisons of results between investigators.

Prevention of continence problems

Prevention has always been much better than cure – assuming that cure is even possible once a health problem has started. Continence is priceless and an unappreciated gift until it is lost. Much suffering could be avoided if individuals had in-depth understanding of how to promote their own continence. Repetitive coughing, smoking, frequent constipation, obesity, repeated heavy lifting and poorly controlled diabetes are just some of the factors that can lead to continence problems and over which an individual has some control (Hannestad et al 2003). A simple understanding of the workings of the tracts concerned, what is and is not normal, what to avoid and where to go for speedy advice would make a start in continence promotion. Following childbirth, it is important to regain prepregnancy strength of the pelvic floor muscles (PFMs) as far as humanly possible. As a prophylactic measure, every woman should be encouraged from a young age to make a regular habit of PFM contractions (Wall & Davidson 1992), and it is never too late to start!

Physiotherapists interact with large numbers of people in a wide range of contexts. Physiotherapists are good communicators and also have the knowledge and skills to make a substantial impact in this field of prevention. Continence status and continence promotion should be considered routinely for *all* patients, clients and carers. This imperative is not limited to physiotherapists working in obstetrics and gynaecology, although obstetrics in particular offers unique opportunities in prevention. For example, patients with hay fever, asthma, chronic chest conditions, back problems, stroke, multiple sclerosis, Parkinson's disease, Alzheimer's disease, hypertension and diabetes, those undergoing hip replacement, the elderly, the obese, those on crutches and those confined to a wheel chair are all at particular risk of developing bladder and bowel dysfunctions.

NORMAL LOWER URINARY TRACT FUNCTION

The basic anatomy of the lower urinary tract was described in Chapter 1 (see p. 18). Urine is produced continuously by the kidneys. It passes, via the ureters by means of peristalsis, from kidneys to the bladder in varying amounts – more during the day and less at night owing to the diurnal rhythm of antidiuretic hormone secretion. The bladder acts alternately as a storage organ and then as a pump to void urine in a cyclic fashion. The act of voiding urine is called *micturition* – hence the use of the term – 'the micturition cycle'.

THE MICTURITION CYCLE

The micturition cycle (Fig. 11.1) consists of two phases: bladder filling and bladder emptying. During the filling phase, the detrusor muscle is compliant and the detrusor pressure is usually less than $15\,\text{cm}\,H_2O$. At a volume of 150–200 mL the first mild desire to void is commonly felt. Normally this desire can be postponed, at least to allow for completion of the necessary preparations for voiding, although more often it is postponed for longer. Eventually, with increasing stored volume, the pressure within the bladder begins to rise and the sensation of fullness becomes more consciously apparent and persistent. A decision to void is taken, a socially acceptable site is found and necessary preparations are made. The levator ani and urethral sphincter muscles relax and then the detrusor muscle contracts. On completion of the void the levator ani and sphincter muscle contract and the detrusor muscle stops contracting and is ready to store again.

STORAGE OF URINE

The normal bladder's compliance accommodates and stores the incoming urine without a significant rise in pressure within the bladder, and without involuntary contractions of the detrusor even with provocation (e.g. a cough, change of position). The actual pressure in the bladder is the sum of intra-abdominal pressure on the bladder from outside and the

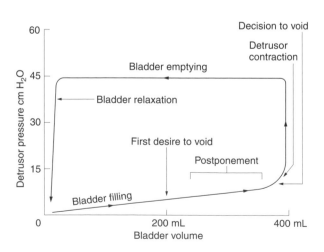

Figure 11.1 The micturition cycle.

pressure produced by the elasticity of the connective tissue and muscle of the bladder wall. Normally the intra-abdominal pressure on the bladder is counterbalanced by intra-abdominal pressure also compressing the proximal portion of the urethra above the pelvic floor. Thus the effective pressure in the bladder, in the storage (filling) phase, is produced by the bladder wall and is usually less than 15 cm H_2O. This elastic ability of the bladder to accommodate an increasing volume of fluid without a rise of pressure is called 'compliance', and is objectively measured in mL/cm H_2O using the following formula:

$$\text{Compliance volume} = \frac{\text{Volume change}}{\text{Change in detrusor pressure}}.$$

Reflux of urine up the ureters when the detrusor contracts is prevented by peristaltic waves of muscular contraction that pass down the walls of the ureters. Also, by their oblique entry into the bladder, which results in their closure when the detrusor muscle contracts (see p. 19), reflux is discouraged. Urine is prevented from leaving the stable bladder via the urethra by a considerable closure pressure, about 50–70 cm H_2O in pre-menopausal women and 40–50 cm H_2O for postmenopausal women (**NB** the figure for men is between 60 and 90 cm H_2O), to which the following factors contribute:

- the elastic connective tissue, including muscle fibres in the neck of the bladder and urethral wall, placed obliquely and longitudinally, closing the lumen of the urethra
- the turgidity of the cells of the walls and the blood supply
- the adhesive force of contact of the moist epithelial lining of the urethral walls
- the length of the urethra – 3–5 cm in women
- the steady contraction of the type 1 striated muscle of the external urethral sphincter (see p. 20)
- the support, occlusive compression and lift applied by the type 1 fibres and, when necessary, the type 2 fibres of the levator ani muscles
- the intra-abdominal pressure applied to the proximal portion of the urethra above the pelvic floor.

Eventually, as filling continues, the limit of distensibility of the bladder wall is reached and the pressure then begins to rise. The average daytime tolerable bladder capacity in women is between 350 and 500 mL; the first void of the day may be greatest and may be greater than 500 mL. Continence is maintained so long as the pressure within the bladder is lower than the closure pressure of the urethra. Even in a normal, healthy person there is a point, as bladder pressure rises, at which urethral pressure could be overwhelmed and leakage occur.

VOIDING OF URINE

Micturition is normally achieved by voluntary, cortically mediated relaxation of the external urethral sphincter and levator ani muscles, which is followed a few moments later by a detrusor contraction. In the absence of stressful environmental or other factors (e.g. urethral obstruction), the detrusor contraction, combined with the normal slight shortening and opening up of the relaxing urethra, empties the bladder in a continuous steady stream in a short time. As women have a short urethra (3–5 cm), the detrusor is not required to contract very strongly to complement gravity to achieve emptying; normally it should not be necessary to bear down to empty. The flow rate, that is, the volume of liquid in millilitres expelled via the urethra per second, has a strong dependency on the total voided volume (see Appendix 1 on p. 427) A normal flowmetry chart will show a smooth bell-shaped curve (Fig. 11.2) rising to a peak (maximal urine flow rate – MUFR) and falling back to zero. From such a trace, the average urine flow rate is calculated (AUFR). In women with no gynaecological problems the AUFR may vary between 5 and 15 mL/s for a voided volume of 100 mL and between 12 and 25 mL/s for 400 mL (Haylen et al 1989). After gynaecological surgery or for patients with urinary problems, the rates are often lower (Haylen et al 1990, 1999). (**NB** The median MUFR and AUFR for men are lower than for women, possibly owing to the resistance of a longer urethra.)

It is important that women have privacy, are relaxed and are seated to micturate. Lack of privacy may be stressful and result in sympathetic nerve discharges, which favour storage rather than voiding, and can even result in the person being unable to void. Moore et al (1991) showed crouching over the toilet reduced AUFR by 21% compared with sitting, and predisposed to incomplete emptying and thus higher residuals.

The detrusor muscle is able, by virtue of its intermeshed fibres, to reduce all dimensions of the bladder when it contracts. This, and the fact that the PFMs relax to facilitate voiding and so allow the bladder base to descend a little, results in the urethrovesical angle being lost, and the urethra and trigone become aligned. Contraction of the detrusor also opens up the bladder neck so that urine is funnelled into the relaxed urethra. When micturition is complete, the PFMs and urethral sphincter contract and the detrusor muscle relaxes ready for the next storage phase, and the

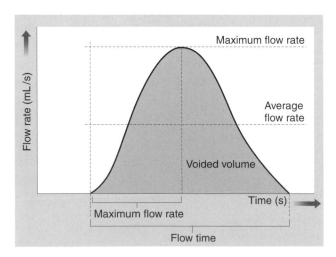

Figure 11.2 Urine flow rates.

bladder base returns to its higher position. Some women develop the habit of bearing down or contracting the abdominal muscles, or both, at the end of micturition in an attempt to squeeze out a final drop. Women in a hurry may bear down during voiding to try to increase the flow rate. Conversely many women are able to slow or even stop urine flow midstream by voluntarily contracting their PFMs strongly and then relaxing to restart the flow, for example to collect a midstream urine specimen. Voluntary contractions of the PFMs may also be used to encourage detrusor relaxation in order to defer micturition for short periods or overcome urgency, or both, utilising the perineodetrusor reflex (Mahony et al 1977). Several authors (Bø et al 1989, Bump et al 1991, Kegel 1948, Shepherd 1990) have claimed that about 30% of parous women have no innate ability to consciously contract their PFMs voluntarily; however, expert opinion suggests that most can be taught the skill.

THE NEUROLOGICAL CONTROL OF CONTINENCE

Continence is controlled neurologically at three levels – spinal, pontine and cerebral. Normally these harmoniously interact by means of a combination of somatic and autonomic pathways – chiefly parasympathetic (Fig. 11.3). Urine is stored and micturition initiated periodically, usually four to six times a day.

Storage

The bladder wall is richly supplied with stretch receptors whose discharge is proportional to the intramural tension. As the bladder begins to fill, parasympathetic afferent fibres convey this information via the pelvic nerves to sacral roots S2–S4, to the sacral micturition centre. From there the impulses ascend in the lateral spinothalamic tracts, and are then relayed back to the pons where there are areas capable of inhibiting or exciting the sacral micturition centre. In the early stages of bladder filling, detrusor muscle contraction is inhibited by descending inhibitory impulses to the sacral centre. As the volume of stored urine increases, so does the strength of the receptor discharges from the bladder wall. This causes them to be relayed higher to several areas of the cerebral cortex including the frontal lobe, so that the desire to void may be consciously perceived. Thus the cortex now becomes involved in detrusor inhibition and, if micturition is not to take place, it is usually possible to suppress the voiding urge to a subconscious level again and postpone bladder emptying. In addition, sympathetic afferent input via the hypogastric nerves (T11–L3) from the bladder wall, trigone and smooth muscle of the urethra is able to stimulate sympathetic efferent impulses to reduce the bladder's tendency to contract and to increase urethral pressure. This is probably the mechanism brought into play intuitively if the point of extreme bladder filling has been reached and a suitable site has yet to be found, and it can be complemented to advantage by conscious pelvic floor contraction (Hilton 1988). It is also the mechanism that makes it difficult to micturate in stressful circumstances.

Mahony et al (1977) described a series of storage and voiding reflexes. One of these, the perineodetrusor inhibitory reflex, is of particular

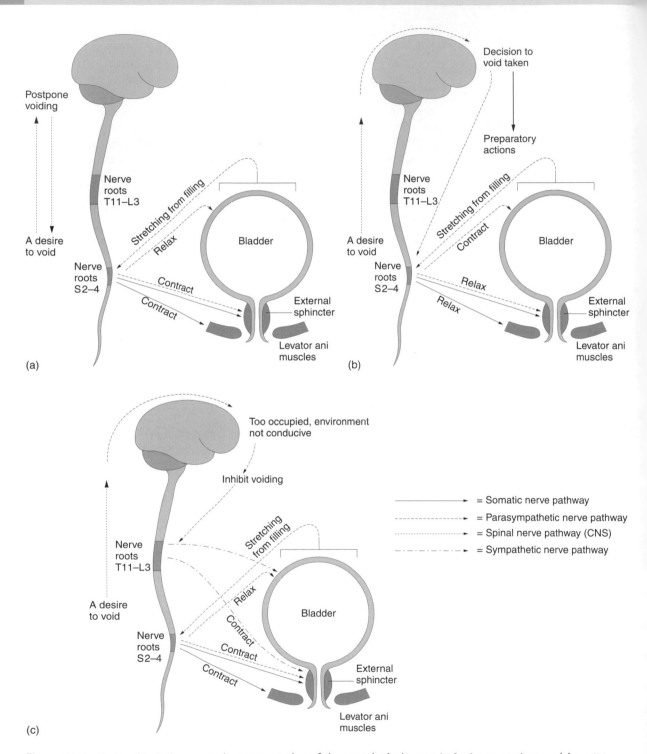

Figure 11.3 A simplified diagrammatic representation of the neurological control of urinary continence: (a) a mild desire to void; (b) decision to void; (c) desire to void but environment not conducive.

interest to physiotherapists, who have used the concept quite widely, including it in the treatment of detrusor overactivity incontinence. This reflex is said to be the means by which detrusor muscle contractility may be inhibited in response to increasing voluntary contraction of the PFMs.

Voiding

When the decision to micturate is taken, descending efferent impulses are released. In addition to initiating all the preparatory activity, these impulses cause inhibition of pudendal and pelvic nerve firing, so that the PFM and external uethral sphincter relax, and inhibition of sympathetic impulses, which, as suggested above, may have been reducing detrusor muscle contractility and increasing closure pressure of the bladder neck and urethra.

Then the cortex and the pontine centre suppress their inhibitory output to the sacral centre, and enhance excitory output to allow firing of the pelvic efferent parasympathetic nerves to cause the detrusor to contract. With suppression of any efferent sympathetic discharges, the detrusor muscle is free to contract and the sphincter to relax. The result is a marked fall in urethral closure pressure, followed by a rise in pressure in the bladder and urine flow. Once emptying is complete, impulses initiated by tension in the bladder wall are no longer produced and the whole sequence begins again.

A SUMMARY OF FACTORS WHICH FAVOUR NORMAL URINARY FUNCTIONING

- The bladder and urethra are structurally sound and healthy; damage or pathology, such as infection, will affect function.
- The nerve supply to the bladder, urethra, external sphincter and PFM is intact; conditions such as multiple sclerosis and diabetes, or childbearing, can cause disruption.
- The bladder is positioned and tethered so the neck is well supported and able to close, and the urethra is not kinked; the angle made by the urethra with the bladder may also be of some importance; childbearing can cause damage to supporting structures.
- The bladder is positioned and supported high enough in the abdominal cavity that intra-abdominal pressure is transmitted both to it and to the proximal portion of the urethra; the latter is referred to as the 'pinchcock' effect, and should result in continence being relatively unaffected by intra-abdominal pressure changes.
- Bladder size and capacity are normal.
- There are no pathological changes in surrounding structures (e.g. fibroids causing pressure on the bladder).
- The woman has the ability to move sufficiently quickly and freely to a socially acceptable site in order to void (e.g. such conditions as arthritis may make going upstairs to the toilet too painful to contemplate).
- The woman is able to adjust clothing and position herself for voiding unaided; anything that causes difficulty and delay (e.g. inappropriate clothing, mental confusion, heavy doors, or dependence on others) may dispose to 'accidents'.

- The woman does not suffer from faecal impaction, for this can cause urinary incontinence. An inappropriate diet, reduced fluid intake or inactivity can cause constipation.
- The woman is in good general physical health, alert, and free from confusion, depression or serious stress; she does not smoke and is not obese.
- There is a fluid intake of about 1½ litres per day, and avoidance of excess alcohol or caffeine (e.g. coffee, tea, cola, chocolate, Lucozade).

Though the maintenance of urinary continence is multifactorial, experience indicates that considerable damage or deterioration in these factors, or both, can occur without inevitable loss of continence.

LOWER URINARY TRACT DYSFUNCTION

The ICS Standardisation of terminology of lower urinary tract dysfunctions document (Abrams et al 2002a – Appendix 1) describes and defines lower urinary tract symptoms (LUTS), signs and syndromes in detail and the reader is advised to study it in depth. It divides LUTS into three main groups: storage, voiding and postmicturition symptoms. The patient with continence problems who seeks help from health professionals, most commonly comes complaining of symptoms. The ICS model is a very useful one for the physiotherapist to have in mind when listening to the patient.

Storage symptoms are experienced during the storage phase (e.g. abnormal bladder sensations, frequency, urgency and leakage of urine).

Voiding symptoms are experienced during the voiding phase, and include any description or deviation from a speedy and continuous flow of urine (e.g. a slow or intermittent stream, hesitancy at the start of micturition, terminal dribble).

Postmicturition symptoms are experienced immediately after micturition (e.g. a feeling of incomplete emptying, and postmicturition dribble).

There are also specific symptoms associated with sexual intercourse and pelvic organ prolapse, and a variety of pain syndromes experienced in the genitals and lower urinary tract with which the physiotherapist should be familiar.

Some useful definitions

- *Enuresis* means any involuntary loss of urine.
- *Nocturnal enuresis* is involuntary loss of urine during sleep.
- *Nocturia* is the complaint that the individual has to wake at night one or more times to void. Technically this term should be reserved for passing urine at night as a result of being roused from sleep by a strong desire to void. It is different from a habit of always waking at a certain time to void whether one needs to or not, and different from happening to wake up (or being woken) and deciding to void without real need.
- *Increased daytime frequency* (pollakisuria) is the complaint by patients who consider that they void too often during the day.

Stanton (1986) defined frequency as the passage of urine seven or more times during the day, or the need to wake more than twice at night to void.

- *Urgency* is the complaint of a compelling desire to pass urine which is difficult to defer.
- *A normal desire to void* is defined as the feeling that leads a person to pass urine at the next convenient moment, but voiding can be delayed if necessary.
- *The urinary voiding stream* may be described as slow, spitting or spraying, or intermittent (i.e. stops and starts).
- *Hesitancy* describes difficulty in initiating flow.
- *Dysuria* is pain on passing urine.
- *A postvoid residual* (PVR) is defined as the volume of urine left in the bladder at the end of micturition.

INCONTINENCE OF URINE

The main groups of patients referred to the physiotherapist are those with *storage* symptoms resulting in urine leakage. Incontinence of urine was defined by the ICS (Abrams et al 1988) as the involuntary loss of urine that is objectively demonstrable and is a social or hygienic problem. However, involuntary urinary leakage may be a symptom of which the patient complains or a sign seen on examination, which may be urethral or extraurethral leakage. In women, urinary leakage may need to be distinguished from sweating or vaginal discharge (Abrams et al 2002a).

COMMON TYPES OF URINARY INCONTINENCE

Extraurethral incontinence

Loss of urine through channels other than the urethra is called *extraurethral incontinence*. This may be due to congenital abnormality (e.g. an aberrant ureter draining into the vault of the vagina). Fistulae between the bladder or urethra and the vagina are most commonly the result of trauma at pelvic surgery such as hysterectomy, particularly where the pelvic anatomy has been distorted by disease such as endometriosis, infection or carcinoma. In the Developing World, childbirth is still a major cause of trauma resulting in fistulae (Wall 1999) (see pp. 88 and 94) and it is not yet unknown in the West. Management usually requires reconstructive surgery (Hilton 2001, 2002, Shah & Vakalopoulos 2002).

Detrusor overactivity incontinence

Detrusor overactivity may present as a symptom, a sign, and as a condition:

1. *The symptom*. The patient with detrusor overactivity complains of urge incontinence, which is involuntary leakage of urine accompanied by or immediately preceded by urgency, that is, a strong desire to void (Abrams 2002a). The amount lost is related to the intensity of the urgency and the amount of urine in the bladder.
2. *The sign*. Detrusor overactivity is confirmed as a sign and observed at urodynamic assessment as spontaneous or provoked detrusor contractions during the filling phase.

3. *The condition*. Detrusor overactivity may be further qualified as neurogenic, where there is a relevant neurological condition, or as idiopathic, when there is no known cause.

Changing terminology

The ICS (Abrams et al 2002a) has recommended that the terms 'motor and sensory urgency motor urge incontinence' and 'reflex incontinence' should no longer be used; also that 'detrusor instability' and 'detrusor hyperreflexia' respectively should be subsumed into the detrusor overactivity idiopathic and neurogenic categories respectively.

The urgency and possible incontinence resulting from detrusor overactivity has a variety of causes. It is naturally associated with frequency; it is the second most common cause of urinary incontinence in women in their middle years (McGrother et al 2001) and the most common cause in the elderly. The precise aetiology is not fully understood, but usually the unwanted detrusor activity can be demonstrated by means of cystometry.

Local pathology such as infections, malignancies, interstitial cystitis or stones leads to hypersensitivity of the receptors in the bladder wall, and sometimes the urethra. Thus, as the bladder fills, early and unwanted detrusor contractions are either produced spontaneously or provoked by activity. Cystitis is the most common example of this manifestation. The patient responds by voiding frequently in an effort to reduce leakage episodes, and this behaviour may even continue after the cause has been removed.

Neurogenic detrusor overactivity presents in a variety of forms. For example, there may be detrusor contraction and urethral relaxation in the absence of any perceived sensory desire to void, owing to neurological impairment. This condition is outside the scope of this book, but is essentially the result of an uninhibited sacral micturition centre and associated reflex arc. It is seen in paraplegics, and the bladder empties incompletely and without proper conscious control.

In patients experiencing urgency, with or without leakage, there may be apparently spontaneous detrusor contractions or contractions provoked by such common activities as walking or coughing. In the latter case any resulting leakage is sometimes confused with urodynamic stress incontinence until urodynamic assessment is made. Such contractions may indicate a neurological disorder such as multiple sclerosis. However, it is known that they may occur in the apparent absence of neuropathology, and may even be asymptomatic, in which case they are considered significant only if the patient complains of them. Where there is no known cause, a diagnosis of *idiopathic detrusor overactivity* would be appropriate.

Management is crucial, particularly in the elderly where urgency and detrusor overactivity incontinence predisposes to falls and fractures as people try to rush to the toilet (Brown et al 2000). It consists of removing the cause whenever possible and explaining the problem to the patient. This should be followed by pharmacotherapy to reduce detrusor activity, exercises to strengthen the PFM if necessary, and then teaching deferment techniques using repeated voluntary PFM contraction (VPFMC), and bladder training to regain confidence and to improve the ability to hold reasonable volumes of urine. In addition, continence-promoting advice may be helpful. The pharmacotherapy brings the possibility of side-effects (e.g. a dry mouth, constipation) and is poorly tolerated by some patients. An alternative therapy, which is successful in some cases, is continuous electrical stimulation with a pulse duration of 500 μs at 5–10 Hz applied daily for 20–30 minutes (see p. 376).

Urodynamic stress incontinence

The phrase 'stress incontinence' may be used to denote a symptom, a sign and a condition.

1. *The symptom.* The patient complains of incontinence on stress, that is, when the intra-abdominal pressure is raised by exertion or effort (e.g. sneezing, coughing or walking). This may be due to urodynamic stress incontinence, but could be entirely or partly due to detrusor contractions provoked by these activities – that is, detrusor overactivity.

2. *The sign.* An involuntary spurt, dribble or droplet of urine is observed to leave the urethra immediately on an increase in intra-abdominal pressure (e.g. when coughing). This test should be performed with a reasonable amount of urine in the bladder, and may need to be conducted standing up, rather than lying down. The patient may also be able to demonstrate how a particular activity such as jumping produces a leak.

3. *The condition.* Urodynamic stress incontinence (USI) is the name coined to denote the condition in which there is involuntary loss of urine when, in the absence of a detrusor contraction, the intravesical pressure (pressure in the bladder) exceeds the maximum urethral pressure. Essentially the detrusor activity is normal but the urethral closure mechanism is incompetent. There may be associated bladder neck hypermobility. Urodynamic assessment is the only reliable way of diagnosing this, and indeed urethral sphincter incompetence and detrusor overactivity frequently coexist.

Mixed urinary incontinence is the complaint of involuntary leakage associated with urgency and also with exertion, effort, sneezing or coughing.

USI is often associated with urgency and frequency. This may be due to a heightened awareness of any desire to void for fear of leakage. The woman will try to keep her bladder as empty as possible by repeated voiding, and it is possible that this might remove the normal healthy challenge to the muscular elements of the closure mechanism, possibly predisposing to atrophy and producing a vicious circle.

How the various factors comprising the urethra closure mechanism interact, and in what proportion, is not fully understood, nor is it known to what degree each may be compromised before USI occurs. Prolapse of the bladder and urethra, due to damage to supporting structures or associated with uterine descent, may be a cause, possibly due to loss of the pinchcock effect of the intra-abdominal pressure. Conversely prolapse, particularly if it substantially involves the anterior wall of the vagina, may favour continence by causing a kink in the urethra. Atrophy associated with reduced oestrogen and ageing presumably attacks the elastic and adhesive factors of the urethral wall. However, weakness and sagging of the pelvic floor are the factors on which physiotherapists have concentrated their attention. This weakness may result from any of the following:

- trauma to muscle or adjacent tissues (e.g. from abuse, surgery or childbirth)
- damage to the nerve supply to the sphincter or levator ani muscle (e.g. from surgery, stretching or tearing at childbirth)
- weakness from underuse (the patient may sit around all day, perhaps suffering from depression)
- stretching from overuse (e.g. repeated coughing, straining at the stool because of constipation, heavy lifting or obesity).

Management of USI begins with a thorough assessment, including the assessment of the precipitating factors, followed by a clear explanation of the problem to the patient. The treatment of chest infections or respiratory allergies, cessation of smoking, reduction in obesity, help with a heavy dependent relative, relief of constipation, treatment for depression, encouragement to activity and other general health- and continence-promoting advice may be enough to relieve symptoms. After that the options are conservative treatment or surgery according to the nature and severity of the condition, and to the preferences of doctor and patient. Regardless of which option is chosen, every woman should be encouraged to make a daily habit of VPFMCs. Where there is considerable prolapse with obvious bladder neck descent, surgery will probably be required, although it is not always successful and has its own morbidity (Black & Downs 1996) (see p. 309).

For conservative treatment to effect the urethral closure mechanism, it would seem logical that only patients who can voluntarily contract their PFMs and produce a reasonable closure between the two medial margins of the puborectalis muscle will benefit from an intense PFM rehabilitation. Where the PFMs are very weak or the patient is unable to produce a VPFMC, biofeedback with or without electrical stimulation should be offered (see p. 372). In addition this brings her into contact with the encouraging, supportive and motivating influence of the physiotherapist so that she does her PFM exercises more regularly. These and other modalities are described later in this chapter. Occasionally, a woman is found to leak only with a particular strenuous activity that she wishes to continue (e.g. sporting activities, dancing). Following all reasonable attempts to gain natural control, it is sometimes appropriate to consider the use of intravaginal devices (see p. 379).

Nocturnal enuresis

Nocturnal enuresis is urinary incontinence during sleep, or 'bed wetting' at an age when a person could be expected to be dry – usually agreed to be the developmental age of 5 years. It affects 15–20% of 5-year-old children and up to 2% of young adults (Glazener & Evans 2003). It must be differentiated from waking with urgency and failing to reach the toilet in time (i.e. detrusor overactivity incontinence). It is often associated with daytime leakage. The vast majority of children who suffer from nocturnal enuresis are dry by puberty but the condition causes great psychological suffering and social deprivation. The child has difficulties staying overnight with friends or going on school trips; it can cause stress between parents and the child, and even abuse (Warzak 1993). The condition requires specialist care and this is usually given by the continence advisor. Parents and sufferers should also be encouraged to seek help and advised to contact the Enuresis Resource and Information Centre (ERIC).

Management begins with a full assessment, possibly with cystometry to detect detrusor overactivity. The young patient and carer must understand the problem. It may be necessary to change diet to reduce caffeine intake, such as cola drinks and chocolate. Reward charts and scheduled awakening may be tried. Where it is thought that the child sleeps too deeply to be aware of the desire to void, various alarm systems can be used. Antidiuretic drugs may be prescribed, for example desmopressin, which can be administered as a nasal spray or orally (Glazener & Evans 2003). Specialised bedding products may reduce the need for changes in the night, and it is never a waste of time to teach PFM contractions, which may have some inhibitory effect on the detrusor muscle.

Giggle incontinence

Girls in particular go through a giggling phase around puberty, if not before. A few find this results in embarrassing leakage of urine. There is often a positive family history of this problem. It is thought that giggle incontinence is caused by detrusor overactivity induced by laughter (Chandra et al 2002).

Following careful assessment and elimination of pathology, treatment is as for detrusor overactivity; in severe cases this may include pharmocotherapy. Time is well spent explaining exactly why the leakage occurs and teaching PFM exercise and deferment techniques. Not only should the girl practise PFM exercise regularly to build up strength and endurance but she should be encouraged to develop the habit of contracting these muscles before and while giggling. Continence-promoting advice should include fluid intake and bowel habits (see p. 368).

Incontinence associated with sexual activity

The urethra and bladder lie in close proximity to the vagina; thus sexual activity can cause urinary symptoms and lower urinary tract dysfunction, and this in term may give rise to sexual problems. 'Honeymoon cystitis' or postcoital dysuria, with and without infection, is common in young women, and dysuria, urgency and urinary tract infections are noted by postmenopausal women following intercourse. Many women also have the urge to void urine during or immediately following coitus, and some experience actual leakage during intercourse on penetration or orgasm. Leakage on penetration is more commonly associated with USI, urgency, whereas detrusor overactivity as well as USI may be implicated with leakage at orgasm (see p. 294). Women who experience this distressing condition may be comforted by the realisation that they are not alone; Hilton (1988) found 24% of 324 sexually active women referred to a gynaecological clinic experienced incontinence – two-thirds on penetration and one-third on orgasm.

The women's health physiotherapist is often the first person in whom the patient confides the presence of this embarrassing problem, and, in view of the paucity of research, would be the ideal professional to research it further. Simple advice to empty the bladder prior to intercourse or to change the coital position may be helpful. Drug therapy may be prescribed to reduce detrusor overactivity. VPFMC to control leakage and inhibit the detrusor muscle may also be helpful to control urgency.

Functional incontinence

This section includes all cases where there is involuntary loss of urine resulting from a deficit in ability to perform toileting functions secondary to physical or mental limitations. This is a very important group for physiotherapists and highlights the need for *all* physiotherapists to consider the continence status of *all* patients and to have its promotion as an implicit objective in *all* rehabilitation across *all* specialties. Being dependent on others for toiletting is a recipe for disaster. It may well be that it is the women's health physiotherapist on whom rests the responsibility to raise the awareness of colleagues.

Only careful assessment will reveal the crux of the problem; physiotherapists, in collaboration with occupational therapists, will look first for evidence of insufficient mobility in strength and range of movement, and balance difficulties – in which case the solution will lie in improving these where possible, or arranging for the toilet to be more easily accessible (e.g. moving the toilet nearer, or the seat higher, or adding grab rails). Other types of obstacles include heavy difficult doors, insufficient turning space, complicated clothing and fear of falling. Each of these requires an individualised solution in collaboration with the continence advisor and the occupational therapist. Physiotherapists are particularly skilled at assisting carers to plan transfers and lifts.

In hospitals and care homes, it is crucial that toilets are clearly marked to overcome problems associated with poor sight and confusion. New patients/residents should be actually shown where the toilets are – several times if necessary. It is important that there are sufficient toilets to avoid queuing and that they are kept scrupulously clean. Many women dislike using toilets away from their own home and deferring voiding and defaecation will inevitably lead to accidents. More difficult is trying to facilitate, as far as possible, independent voiding for the confused and demented. Studying the relevant key mannerisms and natural habits of these individuals can lead to an individualised programme of *prompted voiding*. Alternatively *timed voiding*, for example being taken to the toilet every 2 hours or so, may be successful in some cases (see p. 377).

VOIDING DIFFICULTIES

Urine is stored in the bladder and may have difficulty in escaping. In simple cases this may be due to faecal impaction, to a large cystocoele kinking the urethra, to inhibition due to an unsuitable environment, or to the patient crouching over the toilet. More complex problems arise if either the nerve supply to the detrusor is impaired so it does not contract or does so too weakly; or the detrusor is so stretched by virtue of the volume of urine, caused by the urethra being obstructed, that it cannot contract effectively. Urethral dyssynergia, which occurs often with multiple sclerosis, is a condition in which the urethral musculature does not relax when the detrusor contracts for voiding. The result may be chronic urinary retention. Eventually the pressure in the bladder rises and overcomes the urethra closure pressure, and urine is passed in small amounts as a dribble or spurt, often on movement or effort, until the pressure in the bladder and the urethral closure pressure equate. This leaves a significant volume of residual urine, and the pressure then quickly builds up again.

This situation can arise from neurological damage affecting the pelvic innervation, for example diabetic neuropathy; some damage may result in detrusor atonia, for example spinal shock, or cauda equina lesions. Urethral obstruction in women may be caused by faecal impaction or acute infection in the urethra, or can result from fibrosis following, for example, bladder neck surgery or pelvic irradiation for carcinoma.

Assessment should first be by uroflowmetry to assess the flow rate, if any, and a bladder scan will give an indication of the volume of urine in the bladder following voiding. Management consists of removing the cause where possible. Faecal impaction can be relieved and followed by attention to diet and bowel training. Urethral obstruction due to urethral fibrosis may be improved by laser treatment or urethral stretching. Weak detrusor activity may sometimes be enhanced by drugs such as bethanechol chloride. In intractable neurological cases, clean intermittent self-catheterisation may be taught, or a suprapubic catheter implanted.

PHYSIOTHERAPY ASSESSMENT METHODS

The assessment appointment letter from the physiotherapist to the patient should be clear and give an outline of the structure and purpose of the initial session. The addition of a short, simple explanatory leaflet may be appropriate. Some patients feel disappointed that they have not immediately been offered surgery, and often have low expectations of physiotherapy. Many patients start with misconceptions, for example that 'pelvic floor muscle exercises' are exercises done on the floor, and this prospect may be unappealing! A 3–5-day frequency/volume chart and a 'Quality of Life Questionnaire' (QOLQ), with instructions on completion, may be enclosed with the appointment letter for the patient to complete before she attends. If as part of previous recent investigations the patient has kept such a chart or filled in a QOLQ, or both, it is usually unnecessary to repeat these at this stage.

If it is possible that a perineal and vaginal assessment will be offered at the first session then this must be clearly stated in the initial appointment letter and the patient invited to bring a friend or relative with her if she wishes. Many physiotherapists choose to delay offering such an assessment to the second attendance of the patient, giving time to build rapport and trust.

The patient with urinary problems should be interviewed and examined in a quiet, private room, in an unhurried manner and without

PHYSIOTHERAPY ASSESSMENT – URINARY DYSFUNCTION

Name: Age: DOB: Hospital No:

Address:

Tel' No: Home: Mobile: Work:

GP name/address:

Consultant name/address:

Last seen

Diagnosis

Patient's description of problem:

....

....

STORAGE SYMPTOMS	FREQUENCY OF LEAKAGE
Stress leakage	Never
Urgency	About 1 per week or less
Urge incontinence	2–3 per week.
Frequency	About once a day.
Nocturia	More than 1 per day
Nocturnal eneuresis	
Other	**QOL SCORE**

VOIDING SYMPTOMS	SEVERITY OF LEAKS
Hesitancy	None
Slow stream	A little amount
Intermittent stream	A moderate amount
Feeling of incomplete emptying	A large amount

Other symptoms e.g. pain, feeling of something coming down...........................

....

HISTORY OF PRESENT CONDITION

Onset date
Triggers for leakage
Type of pads
No. of pads used per day
Cystitis?

INVESTIGATIONS e.g. MSU, Urodynamics..

....

GYNAE. HISTORY	FREQUENCY/VOL
Menstruation/cycle	Frequency day/night
Menopause/yr/HRT	Average voided vol. per 24 hrs
Sexually active	Max. voided vol.
Dyspareunia	Min. voided vol.
Surgery	Average vol. drunk in 24 hrs
	Average vol. caffeine,
Other	Average leaks per 24 hrs
Occupation	
Hobbies, leisure activities	
	Height /weight/BMI:

OBSTETRIC HISTORY

Parity   Duration

Year	Type delivery	Wt	1st	2nd	3rd	Tear/Epis	PN exs?
1.							
2.							
3.							
4.							

Figure 11.4 Physiotherapy assessment form.

MEDICAL HISTORY

Other conditions (e.g. back pain problems, allergies, hayfever, asthma, chronic cough, diabetes, high BP, depression)...
....

Obesity
Smoking
Bowels – B/O per week......................................
Leakage wind/fluid/solid..

SURGICAL HISTORY

*

*

*

CURRENT MEDICATION

....
....

EXAMINATION – Informed consent Y/N

Dermatomes..
Myotomes...
Reflexes..
Abdominal examination...
....
Observation of perineum..
....
Effect of cough..

DIGITAL EXAMINATION

Vagina ....
....
Sensation/pain...
Anterior wall/grade..
Posterior wall/grade...

Pelvic floor muscle

Contraction – aware/not aware

Grade   L   R

Hold time
Repetitions
Fast repetitions
Reflex to cough
Co-contract with TA

Patient's priorities for improvement and comments:

Signature   **Date**

Figure 11.4   (Contd).

interruption. Figure 11.4 shows an outline assessment form which gives some guidance as to the principal information it will be useful to record.

HISTORY OF THE PATIENT'S CONDITION AND DETAIL OF PRESENT STATE

The initial priority is to gain insight into the problem as the patient perceives and experiences it, and the specific ways in which the condition is affecting her life. It is also important to note aspects of the person's life, past and present, which may have a bearing on the current situation (e.g. occupation, childbearing, or back problems). Where the patient has been referred from a consultant unit following full urodynamic testing, it should not be necessary, nor is it a cost-effective use of the physiotherapist's time, to submit the patient to yet another tedious rehearsal in minute detail of her full medical history. Nor should it be necessary for the patient to repeat assessments such as frequency/volume charts or questionnaires. Every effort should be made to encourage the health professionals concerned to keep joint records in a mutually beneficial form, and these and the patient's main notes must be available to the physiotherapist, ideally well before the first appointment. When the patient is referred directly by her general practitioner, or another health professional or has self-referred, the physiotherapist will wish to construct fuller documentation. Two things are worth remembering: first, that retrospective memory is notoriously inaccurate so, for example, detail regarding births of children should be treated with caution. Secondly, a patient's impression of such details as the volume and frequency of urinary leakage may be unreliable. The former should be checked against the written records if possible; the latter emphasises the importance of objective measurement of the present condition if this has not already been done.

It is also important to ascertain from the patient at this early stage what exactly needs to change and by how much for the patient to be satisfied with her condition.

URINALYSIS

Urinalysis uses reagent strips and is a simple cost-effective way of detecting a number of substances in urine such as sugar, blood, leucocytes, proteins, nitrites and ketones. The patient is asked for a specimen of urine and *within 1 hour* a reagent strip is dipped into it as per the instruction on the reagent strip container. Sections of the strip change colour according to abnormal content of the urine. The strip can then be read against the normal coding key on the strip container. If the result is positive a midstream urine sample should be sent for full laboratory testing.

Physiotherapists are strongly advised to seek official training in the reading of these strips and in judging smell, colour and degree of cloudiness of the urine (see Addison 2002).

FREQUENCY/VOLUME CHART (BLADDER DIARY)

This is an invaluable tool in assessment. The patient is asked to note the time of day and to measure the volume of urine voided each time she goes to the toilet. This is recorded on a special chart over a period of days decided with the patient or her carers, or both jointly (Fig. 11.5). Most conveniently the patient voids into a large measuring jug, which may have to be supplied to her. However, some people find this stressful. Patients are recommended, where possible, to place the jug between their thighs and sit on the toilet. Crouching over the lavatory, rather than sitting relaxed on the seat, can result in an abnormal, interrupted or incomplete micturition sequence (Moore et al 1991). Patients may prefer to place a small washing-up bowl into the toilet, micturate into it and then pour the urine into the jug. This collecting process can be very demanding;

Date:

I woke up at:

I went to sleep at:

Time	Record drinks taken (type and amount)	Record (✓) each time you use the toilet to pass urine	Tick when you changed a pad/pantyliner	Each time you leak urine, circle whether you were:	REMINDERS:
6 am				Almost Dry Damp Wet Soaked	
7 am				Almost Dry Damp Wet Soaked	1. Don't forget to record the time **you woke up** in the morning and the time you **went to sleep.**
8 am				Almost Dry Damp Wet Soaked	
9 am				Almost Dry Damp Wet Soaked	
10 am				Almost Dry Damp Wet Soaked	
11 am				Almost Dry Damp Wet Soaked	
Midday				Almost Dry Damp Wet Soaked	2. Don't forget to record what happened **overnight** when you get up in the morning.
1 pm				Almost Dry Damp Wet Soaked	
2 pm				Almost Dry Damp Wet Soaked	
3 pm				Almost Dry Damp Wet Soaked	3. Try and make a record of things just after they happen in case you forget them later on.
4 pm				Almost Dry Damp Wet Soaked	
5 pm				Almost Dry Damp Wet Soaked	
6 pm				Almost Dry Damp Wet Soaked	
7 pm				Almost Dry Damp Wet Soaked	4. Record things to the **nearest hour.**
8 pm				Almost Dry Damp Wet Soaked	
9 pm				Almost Dry Damp Wet Soaked	5. Record type and amount of **drinks taken** (e.g. 2 cups of tea, 1 mug of coffee, 1 can of coke, 1 glass of water/wine/juice, 2½ pints of beer)
10 pm				Almost Dry Damp Wet Soaked	
11 pm				Almost Dry Damp Wet Soaked	
Midnight				Almost Dry Damp Wet Soaked	
1 am				Almost Dry Damp Wet Soaked	
2 am				Almost Dry Damp Wet Soaked	6. Start a new sheet for each new day.
3 am				Almost Dry Damp Wet Soaked	
4 am				Almost Dry Damp Wet Soaked	
5 am				Almost Dry Damp Wet Soaked	

Figure 11.5   A 1-day frequency/volume chart for assessment. (Courtesy of Leicestershire MRC Incontinence Study.)

it may be too difficult to carry out in the workplace because of the need to have the measuring jug available. It requires agility and some dexterity, and consequently it is not suitable for all patients. However, it is a test physiotherapists can use and, for those patients who can cope, it is helpful to keep a record for several days, according to the exact information required. It is often helpful if this includes weekdays and a weekend, or days of paid employment and 'home' days. Where incontinence is associated with a particular part of the menstrual cycle, recording over a longer period may be necessary. In addition, on the same chart it is possible to record urinary accidents and the time, type and amount of drinks taken.

From the chart it is possible to determine:

- the actual frequency of micturition compared with the patient's subjective impression
- the precise degree of nocturia
- whether the patient has an altered diurnal voiding rhythm and is voiding more by night than by day
- the total and individual volumes being voided per 24 hours
- the incidence of urinary accidents; and possible causes or triggers
- the total volume and what is being drunk per 24 hours
- the volume of liquids being drunk containing caffeine.

A woman with normal control does not usually void more than six to eight times per 24 hours and does not wake from sleep more than once a night to void. Normal daytime volumes voided are 250–450 mL, with the first volume of the day often being the greatest and sometimes greater than 450 mL.

PAD TEST

The test approved by the ICS (Abrams et al 1988 see Appendix 2) takes 1 hour and comprises the following sequence:

1. The test is started without the patient voiding.
2. A preweighed absorbent perineal pad is put on and the timing begins. The patient is asked not to void until the end of the test.
3. The patient drinks 500 mL of sodium-free liquid (e.g. distilled water) within 15 minutes, then sits or rests to the end of the first half hour.
4. In the following half hour the patient walks around, climbs up and down one flight of stairs, and performs the following exercises: standing up from sitting (×10); coughing vigorously (×10); running on the spot for 1 minute; bending down to pick up a small object (×5); washing the hands under cold running water for 1 minute.

At the end of the hour the pad is removed and weighed; any difference from the starting pad weight constitutes fluid loss, and this is recorded. If the pad becomes saturated during the test then a second pad may be used. In this assessment, an increase of up to 1 g is considered normal to allow for possible sweating and vaginal discharge.

The critics of this test highlight its stressfulness and artificiality. Versi et al (1988) showed it to be unsatisfactory as a screening test; it gave a false negative result in 32% of 311 women presenting at a urodynamic clinic, almost two-thirds of whom were subsequently shown to have urodynamic stress incontinence. Physiotherapists using a 1-hour pad test as a quantitative monitor of response to treatment should note that patients with urodynamic stress incontinence may not have a positive result, and that the reproducibility of this pad test has been questioned (Harvey & Versi 2001, Jeyaseelan et al 1997, Jorgensen et al 1987). A better correlation has been found by filling the bladder with a fixed volume (e.g. 250 mL), extending the time to 90 minutes and using more provocative activities (Jorgensen et al 1987). Twenty-four-hour and 48-hour pad tests have been devised whereby the patient is supplied with and wears preweighed perineal pads continuously for 24 or 48 hours, removing them only to void or to change to a fresh pad. Discarded pads are placed directly into individual self-sealing plastic bags, and may be weighed immediately by the patient using a supplied spring balance or returned to the clinic. The patient may also be asked to keep a frequency/volume chart, and to record fluid intake and urinary accidents. Otherwise the patient continues with her normal activities. This test has some advantages over the 1-hour test in measuring the patient in more normal circumstances and over a long period. However, it is hugely demanding and entirely dependent on patient compliance and diligence for completeness and accuracy. Versi et al (1996) deduced the normal increase in pad weight to be less than 8 g for the 24-hour test and less than 15 g for the 48-hour test.

PAPER TOWEL TEST

This test is derived from a test used in research by Miller et al (1998). In standing, the patient holds a coloured paper towel against the perineum and coughs strongly three times. Any leakage is absorbed by the paper towel, which, where damp, changes colour. Alternatively, having removed lower underwear the patient stands astride the paper towel and coughs three times; any leakage falls on to the towel. Assessment of the amount of leakage can be measured by weighing or measuring the area of the dampness. This test has been criticised as being undignified for the patient. However, for those who do not leak whilst lying down, it can be a satisfying vindication of their complaint.

PERINEAL AND VAGINAL ASSESSMENT

The Royal College of Obstetricians and Gynaecologists (RCOG) has published guidelines for intimate examinations (RCOG 2002). The Association for Continence Advice (ACA) has produced comprehensive guidelines entitled *Examination and Assessment of the Female Pelvic Floor* (ACA 2003) which describe how to perform such an examination. The CSP information paper no. PA 19 entitled *Pelvic Floor and Vaginal Assessment* (CSP 1996) sets out the range of options for acquiring the skill, and the CSP information paper no. 19B entitled *Association of Chartered Physiotherapists in Women's Health (ACPWH) Guidelines for Tutors Teaching Pelvic Floor and Vaginal Assessment* (CSP 1998) offers advice to tutors. Physiotherapists are strongly advised to study all these guidelines *and* undertake specialist practical training in this intimate examination, from an expert. ACPWH has information on training sessions currently available. (See Useful Addresses on p. 382.)

The procedure in brief

The whole procedure must adhere to the locally agreed infection control policy. An explanation of the examination procedure and its purposes is given to the woman; this is first, to enable the physiotherapist to have an accurate knowledge of the condition of the perineum and vaginal and, second, to establish the condition and strength of the PFMs. It is important to check whether the patient has a known allergy to latex and it may be helpful to use a simple diagram or model of the pelvis and its contents to aid the patient's understanding of the procedure. The patient must be given the option of having a chaperone present during the examination, whether the person is brought by the patient or provided by the physiotherapist. Furthermore, the patient must be informed that she can opt out at any stage. If at any point in the procedure the physiotherapist becomes aware of even the slightest sign of emotional or physical discomfiture, the examination should be discontinued immediately.

The woman's informed consent to the examination must be obtained and documented (DoH 2001). She is then given privacy (and help if needed) to remove underwear and prepare herself on a couch in crook lying. The couch should have been covered with disposable paper with two pillows at the head. The patient is covered with a disposable paper sheet, and an absorbent pad may be placed under the buttocks. The physiotherapist talks through the examination, explaining what she is doing and simply reporting what she is finding. The perineum is observed first for skin condition, signs of infection, vaginal discharge, haemorrhoids, prolapse and evidence of episiotomy or previous surgery. The patient is asked to cough and strain; evidence of prolapse, ballooning of the perineum or any leakage of urine or faeces is noted.

Wearing gloves and using a lubricant, the physiotherapist then separates the labia; after further observation the index finger of the dominant hand is gently inserted into the vagina. The texture of the walls, evidence of prolapse, quality of sensation and any pain caused are noted. The physiotherapist curls her finger over the levator ani muscles and the woman is asked to contract the pelvic floor muscles as if to stop leakage or stop passing wind, or to grip the therapist's finger and prevent its withdrawal. The ability to contract or not is recorded, and where voluntary contraction is possible it is graded. With training and experience, judgements can be made concerning the texture and integrity of the muscle, scarring, the width between the two medial edges of the PFM, and degrees of prolapse. The presence of reflex contraction to cough, and coactivation of the PFMs by contraction of the transversus abdominis muscle, are tested. The sensation over the perineum and of the anal sphincter to touch, and the anal reflex may also be checked. The patient is assisted to get off the couch and replace clothing. The patient is then given a clear description of the findings and their implications for treatment.

Manual grading of the strength of a PFM contraction

The method of grading most commonly used in the UK was proposed by Laycock & Chiarelli in 1989. It is a six-point scale (0 = nil contraction, 1 = flicker, 2 = weak, 3 = moderate, 4 = good, 5 = strong) modelled on the Oxford scale. Laycock & Jerwood (2001) built on this by developing and validating the 'PERFECT' scheme whereby:

P = power – which is more correctly the 'strength' of the PFM determined on the six-point scale; both the left and right sides of the levator ani muscles are graded

E = endurance – i.e. the time measured in seconds (up to 10) that a maximum voluntary contraction (MVC) can be held before fatigue sets in

R = repetitions – i.e. the number of MVCs which can be performed (up to 10) interspersed with rests of 4 seconds

F = fast – i.e. the number of 1-second contractions (up to 10) performed, contracting/relaxing as quickly as possible, up to 10 or until fatigue sets in

ECT – i.e. 'every contraction timed' – to complete the acronym.

An intertester reliability test of digital vaginal assessment of the PFM (Jeyaseelan et al 2001) found that intertester reliability could not be assumed but, where physiotherapists had received adequate specialist training, it was good.

Thirteen ways of confirming a contraction of the PFM

These are:

1. vaginal examination by the physiotherapist
2. self-examination by the patient
3. hand on perineum by the physiotherapist
4. hand on perineum by the patient
5. observation of perineum by the physiotherapist
6. observation of perineum by the patient – using a mirror
7. perineometer
8. stop and start midstream – only occasionally for suitable patients
9. using the Neen Healthcare 'Educator' (see p. 359)
10. using a cone in the vagina and applying traction to the string while trying to grip the cone
11. asking the partner at intercourse
12. manometric and EMG biofeedback
13. transperineal or labial ultrasound.

BIOFEEDBACK

The ICS definition of 'biofeedback' is the technique by which information about a normally unconscious physiological process is presented to the patient or therapist, or both, as a visual, auditory or tactile signal. For the pelvic floor musculature, proprioceptive techniques of touch, stretch, pressure and verbal encouragement can all be used during digital assessment; cones provide similar possibilities. The following may also be available to the physiotherapist in assessment (see also Haslam 2002); before using any of these the patient's informed consent should be gained.

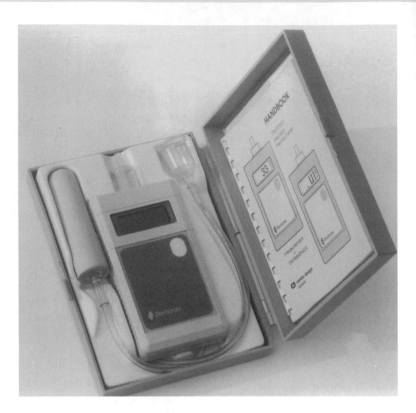

Figure 11.6 The Peritron. (Courtesy of Cardio Design, Australia; Neen Healthcare, UK.)

The perineometer

Perineometers record changes in activity in the region of the vagina. There are two types, one recording pressure changes, the other monitoring electromyographic activity (EMG). The most commonly used simple perineometer in the UK is the Peritron (Fig. 11.6). It is designed to record the changes in pressure produced by voluntary contraction of the PFMs. This is achieved by means of a vaginal pressure probe, which is usually covered for use with a condom; if necessary a little lubricant jelly is applied. Patients should be asked if they wish to introduce the probe themselves, and every care should be taken to maintain their dignity. The whole procedure must also adhere to the locally agreed infection control policy. The visual display is motivating for the patient providing she can produce a voluntary contraction, but if not, it is depressing to see nil being recorded. Great care must be taken if the results of use are to be treated as a monitor and compared over time. If physiotherapists try the equipment out on themselves they will appreciate how many confounding factors can effect the reading, such as the position of the probe, time of day, day of month, load in bowel, breath holding, position on couch, whether the head is supported or not, etc.

The Educator

Neen Healthcare UK has developed a simple device called the 'Educator' (Fig. 11.7), which is inserted into the vagina with the patient in crook half-lying. A voluntary contraction of the PFM will cause the indicator to

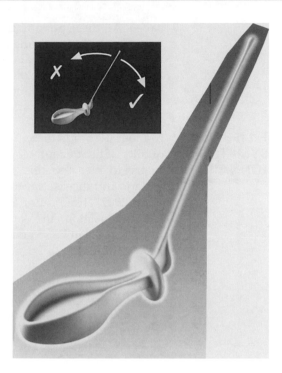

Figure 11.7 The Educator.
(Courtesy of Neen
Healthcare, UK.)

move downwards and is one way of confirming a contraction. An upward movement of the indicator indicates valsalva manoeuvre. Alternatively the Periform electrode can be used similarly, having first attached the indicator provided.

Computerised manometric and electromyographic equipment

There are complex clinic-based computerised manometric and electromyographic pieces of equipment which provide a visual display; some also have facilities for electrical stimulation.

For manometric equipment a vaginal pressure probe is used; for EMG equipment, two electrodes are mounted on a vaginal probe, for example the Periform produced by Neen Healthcare UK, or other surface electrodes may be used. In either case, signals are produced, relayed to a visual display unit (VDU) and seen by the patient and physiotherapist, often as a brightly coloured trace against a squared-graph background. The probe is introduced into the vagina with the woman in a comfortable supported crook half-lying position, but could equally well be used in standing. The whole procedure must adhere to the locally agreed infection control policy. Once the machine is switched on and adjusted, the woman is asked to contract the PFM. Signals from the activity of these muscles are shown in proportion to the strength and duration of the contraction. Templates can be chosen and screened of varying contraction intensity, duration and rest periods, for the patient to try to follow. These serve to motivate the patient not only to practise but also to work for longer, stronger contractions. The resulting traces can be printed out and saved. All these possibilities can be used in assessment, in treatment and as a means of monitoring a patient's progress.

There are smaller handheld devices which can be used in assessment although they are of doubtful reliability for monitoring. They are better suited to use during home treatment sessions as motivators.

QUALITY OF LIFE AND SYMPTOMS QUESTIONNAIRES

In the last decade there has been an increasing awareness of the affect on quality of life of continence problems, and an explosion of questionnaires to try to measure this. There are two main groups of questionnaire: generic and disease specific, and these are well documented by Donovan et al (2002). It is important to use validated questionnaires. The King's Health Questionnaire is commonly used; it is specific for urinary incontinence and can be scored (Donovan et al 2002, Kelleher et al 1997). It has been thoroughly tried and tested, and is now translated into several languages. However, it takes a patient about 30 minutes to complete and 10 minutes to score. In contrast, the new International Consultation on Incontinence Questionnaire (ICIQ), in its short form (ICIQSF), has been rigorously pruned down to just 6 questions and will take a patient only a few minutes, and is scored in moments! It will be found in full in Appendix 2 in the second edition of the documentation of the second Consultation of Incontinence (Abrams et al 2002b) This has been validated and the short completion time is an obvious plus point for physiotherapists. Work is in progress toward producing a modular ICIQ – modules of which may well be useful to physiotherapists in certain circumstances.

VISUAL ANALOGUE SCALE

A helpful measure of the severity of symptoms of incontinence as they affect the patient is the visual analogue scale (VAS). This technique has been used widely for pain measurement, and is useful in other fields. Such an approach makes due allowance for the variation in what individuals accept as normal or tolerable, and gives insight into the patient's perception of any problem. The patient is asked to place a cross at the appropriate point on a 10 cm line, one end of which is marked, for example, 'no leakage', 'no incontinence' or 'no problem', and at the other end 'always wet', 'totally incontinent' or 'massive problem'. Bø et al (1989) used a VAS before and after a course of treatment to measure ability to participate in a variety of social activities without leaking.

IMAGING – ULTRASOUND SCANNING OF THE BLADDER

Many obstetric units now own a small portable ultrasound scanner designed to scan the bladder and calculate the volume of urine in the bladder. This has obvious use postnatally where there is concern of acute retention. It can also be helpful to the physiotherapist with a patient who reports a feeling of incomplete emptying postmicturition. A postvoid residual of <100 mL may be considered within normal limits for symptom-free women.

It is possible to use ultrasonography to visualise the lower urinary and intestinal tracts including the bladder, urethra, external urethra sphincter, rectum and anus, PFMs and associated connective tissues (see reviews by Artibani et al 2002; Khullar 2001, 2002). Contraction of the PFM can be seen by the operator and the patient, and the amount it lifts cephalically can be observed. Damage to muscle and connective tissue is sometimes discernible. It has been used transvaginally with a vaginal probe, and transperineally or translabially with the probe held against the perineum or between the labia. The transvaginal approach has been largely discontinued because the probe distorts structures around the vagina.

So far the use of ultrasonography in this way has been chiefly confined to research and diagnostics. However, it is probable that as equipment becomes cheaper that it will become more widely available. This is a modality that will appeal to physiotherapists and one that, with appropriate training, could be useful in assessment and treatment. It can also be used to image the transversus abdominis muscles.

URODYNAMIC, RADIOLOGICAL AND ELECTROMYOGRAPHICAL ASSESSMENT

Most patients presenting with incontinence will be asked for a midstream specimen of urine, which is sent for laboratory testing. Urinary tract infection is commonly associated with dysfunction. Patients may have both lower urinary and upper renal tract infections. Midstream specimens are inappropriate for urethral infection because the urethra is first washed through; a perineal swab may be better. All urine specimens should be as fresh as possible for accurate microbiological investigation. Infection by *Chlamydia* will need a special test (see p. 276). However, more sophisticated methods of assessing some important aspects of the micturition cycle and the factors involved in maintenance of continence are now available, and have proved helpful in diagnosis, although they are all to some degree invasive. Physiotherapists treating patients with continence problems should endeavour to observe these.

CYSTOMETRY

This test (see reviews by Garnett & Abrams 2002; Hughes & Abrams 2001) determines the relationship between the volume of fluid and the pressure in the bladder, during both filling and voiding. Accurate technique is essential and the ICS Report on good urodynamic practice (Schafer et al 2002) is to be found at www.ics.org.uk.

Two catheters are introduced into the bladder, one to fill it, the other to record pressure – a combination of the intra-abdominal pressure and detrusor pressure. A third catheter is introduced into the rectum to record rectal pressure, which is generally the same as intra-abdominal pressure although muscle contraction of the rectal wall will be evident. This information is interpreted electronically and is available as two continuous graphic traces or on a VDU. The rectal or intra-abdominal pressure is automatically subtracted from the total bladder pressure, and the result, the intrinsic detrusor pressure, is available as a third trace. It is therefore possible to watch and have a permanent record of the detrusor pressure as the bladder is filled with warmed normal saline (or contrast medium if radiological video imaging is to be used). Any spontaneous detrusor contractions, or provoked contractions when the patient is asked to cough or change position, may suggest detrusor overactivity. As filling progresses the volume at which the first desire to void is perceived and noted – usually 150–200 mL. Filling continues and the volume is noted at which the patient reports a normal desire to void. Filling is stopped at the volume which the patient interprets as a strong desire to void. This gives evidence of bladder sensation and capacity, and the general trend of detrusor pressure is a measure of compliance – a steady low pressure is indicative of normal bladder compliance, and a rise of >15 cm H_2O is abnormal.

Up to this point in the test the patient usually lies flat or sits. Next the patient is tilted to the erect position, and if this provokes detrusor contraction it will be seen on the trace. Standing causes a general rise in pressure in both the bladder and rectum, but the detrusor pressure should remain as before. With radiological screening it is possible to see the outline and shape of the bladder for any hints of pathology, also the level of the bladder base and neck, and whether the neck and urethra are open or well closed. The patient is again asked to cough strongly several times, and both provoked detrusor contractions and evidence of sphincter incompetence in terms of leakage are noted. With video imaging (Herschorn 2001) it is possible, on coughing, to watch fluid being forced into the urethra and past an incompetent sphincter. The patient is then asked to commence voiding, and then to stop and restart midstream before completing voiding. The strength of detrusor contractions appears on the trace; the behaviour of the bladder neck, the rate of flow, the ability to stop or reduce flow, any effort needed to void and any residual urine can all be ascertained and visualised if necessary.

The emotional and physical stress placed on a patient by such a procedure must never be underestimated, and its artificiality must be remembered when considering the results. The test has its own morbidity in that occasionally patients develop urinary infections afterwards and its reliability is not 100%.

URETHRAL PRESSURE PROFILOMETRY

The pressure in the urethra may be measured in both the storage and voiding phases by means of a microtransducer mounted on the tip of a fine catheter (Garnett & Abrams 2002, Lose 2001, Versi 1990), or by a fluid-filled or gas-filled catheter attached to an external transducer. The catheter is drawn down the urethra from the bladder neck to the external meatus during the storage phase, with or without provocative stress (coughs), and the urethral closure pressure is measured at several points to give a urethral pressure profile (UPP). A trace is produced.

The procedure may be carried out during voiding (VUPP) to detect obstruction; in such cases it is necessary to measure the bladder pressure simultaneously.

UROFLOWMETRY

This is quite a reliable indicator of normal detrusor contraction and urethral relaxation. The patient is asked to void, in private, into a toilet in which a flow meter has been fitted. It is important that the patient sits to void. This device measures the quantity of fluid passed per unit of time. The necessary equipment can be easily transportable and could be available to physiotherapists.

DISTAL URETHRAL ELECTRIC CONDUCTANCE

The accurate detection of leakage of urine is obtained by inserting a short probe with two ring electrodes into the distal part of the urethra until the distal ring is 1.5 cm from the external urethral meatus. Passage of urine past the electrodes increases conductivity between them, and this can be recorded electronically (Peattie et al 1989).

ELECTROPHYSIO- LOGICAL TESTS

For some time it has been possible to record the electrical activity associated with resting and contracting muscles (see reviews by Fowler & Vodusek 2001, Fowler et al 2002, and Vodusek & Fowler 2001). Considerable research effort has been channelled into electrophysiological studies of the levator ani muscle – particularly the puborectalis and the external anal sphincter. This was because it became evident that childbirth could cause not only direct division of the anal sphincter (Sultan 2002) and stretching of the PFM, but also injury to the innervation (Snooks et al 1984). Single fibre density (FD) and pudendal nerve and perineal nerve terminal motor latencies (PNTML, PerNTML) have been measured (Snooks et al 1984, Swash 1985).

Electromyography

Single needle EMG has been used to examine the puborectalis and external anal sphincter. A fine EMG needle is inserted and the motor unit action potentials in the immediate vicinity of the needle can be recorded at rest and on contraction on an oscilloscope. In both these muscles, activity will be expected at rest as well as on contraction. Duration, amplitude and the number of phases of the action potentials of individual motor units can be measured. Normal muscle has a typical pattern of measurements (Swash 1985).

Single fibre density

A motor unit is comprised of an anterior horn cell and its myelinated axon, which divides into a number of terminal branches, each of which serves a single muscle fibre. When the axon or any of its branches are damaged, reinnervation of the bereft muscle fibres may occur by regeneration of the axon or by collateral sprouting of neighbouring healthy motor nerve axons. In the latter case the number of muscle fibres supplied by that motor unit is greater, and the FD is said to be increased. In addition, the motor unit activity recorded is of greater length and amplitude, and is polyphasic. The normal FD in the puborectalis and anal sphincter muscles is 1.5. It is calculated by taking 20 recordings during mild contraction in various parts of a muscle, counting the components making up the 20 individual motor unit action potentials, and taking the mean (Swash 1985).

Motor conduction tests

Pudendal nerve terminal motor latency

If a nerve is stimulated electrically, there is a delay before the muscle responds. The latency of response can be measured and is increased where a nerve passes through areas of localised injury or disease, for example the median nerve at the wrist in carpal tunnel syndrome, or where there is actual neuropathy. An intrarectal stimulating and recording device is introduced into the anus to stimulate the pudendal nerve and record the response of the external anal sphincter muscle. The latency of the response is measured and recorded on a graphic printout (Fowler & Vodusek 2001, Snooks et al 1984).

Perineal nerve terminal motor latency

This is a similar test using a catheter-mounted recording electrode in the urethra (Swash 1985).

Central motor conduction times

By stimulating the motor cortex it is possible to record a response from the pelvic floor. It has been found that patients with multiple sclerosis have longer cortical conduction times than healthy persons (Eardley et al 1991).

IMAGING

One of the most exciting developments in investigating urinary dysfunction is the increasing use of ultrasound imaging and, more recently, magnetic resonance imaging (MRI). (See reviews by Artibani et al (2002) and Khullar (2001, 2002).)

OTHER TESTS

Measurement of perineal descent

Perineal descent is recognised clinically by ballooning of the perineum during straining effort. This is measured using a graduated latex cylinder held against the anus which moves on a frame pressed against the ischial tuberosities (Kiff et al 1984). Using the tuberosities as a reference point, the position of the perineum can be measured at rest and on straining.

Cystourethroscopy or cystoscopy

This is an endoscopic investigation of the bladder and urethra to look for pathological lesions which could explain the signs and symptoms.

UNDERSTANDING URINARY DYSFUNCTION

Following collation of the full history and the results of appropriate tests, the physiotherapist must seek to understand the patient's condition and how the signs and symptoms are being produced (Table 11.1). Only then can the best treatment be selected.

PHYSIOTHERAPY TREATMENT

In the 1940s and 1950s, physiotherapists in some UK centres were regularly involved in the treatment of urinary incontinence. They used PFM exercise, often treating patients in groups, and electrical stimulation, which chiefly consisted of 'faradism'. Through the 1960s and 1970s,

Table 11.1 Causes of urinary dysfunction

Signs and symptoms	Explanations	Possible causes
Storage phase		
1. Frequent desire to void, small amounts of urine passed	Bladder or urethra is hypersensitive Neurological inhibition of the detrusor is reduced Bladder capacity is reduced Detrusor contracts spontaneously or is easily provoked, e.g. by cough, changing position, cold, water Learnt habit Woman is acutely anxious, afraid or stressed	Infection, inflammation or other pathology, e.g. fibroid, neurological disorders, alcohol, coffee, tea, cola intake
2. Frequent desire to void, normal volumes of urine passed	Pregnancy or recent childbirth Woman has drunk large amounts, or eaten water-filled food	
3. Urine leaks on physical effort	Urethral closure pressure is low Activity provoked detrusor contraction	
4. Uncontrollable urges to void, leaks	Detrusor overactivity Neuropathology Bladder inflamed Urethra, surrounding tissue and/or vagina traumatised	 Infection Recent childbirth
Voiding phase		
1. Passing urine takes a long time, flow is poor	Urethra is partially obstructed Detrusor is underactive Neurological disorder	Pressure from faeces in rectum, tumour, oedema, prolapse, inflammation, urethral kink, or stricture Drugs Detrusor sphincter dyssynergia
2. Woman has desire to void, is ready but cannot start	Stress or embarrassment or adverse environment causes sympathetic inhibition of voiding Neurological disorder Urethra is obstructed by a full bowel Acute urethritis with obstruction or pain inhibition	 Detrusor sphincter dyssynergia
3. Woman bears down to void	Habit See also (1)	
4. Urine dribbles after micturition completed (rare).	Urine collecting in introitus Urethrocele with 'kinked' urethra	
5. On standing up, patient feels there is still urine in the bladder at the completion of micturition and that she may pass more if she sits down again	Residual urine Haste – woman stopped micturition prematurely Bladder was so full that urine had pooled in ureters and was released when the detrusor relaxed	Uterine descent, cystocoele, urethrocoele
6. Woman has to press perineum to assist voiding	Cystocoele with part of bladder hanging below the level of bladder neck	

doctors increasingly turned to surgery as the treatment of choice for stress incontinence and to drug therapy for the alleviation of urge incontinence. Older surgical techniques were revised and new innovative approaches devised. In addition urodynamic and electrophysiological tests were developed or became more sophisticated, improving understanding of the patient's condition and accuracy of diagnosis.

In the last decade increasing attention has been drawn to overestimation of cure rates, some morbidity following surgery and of recurrence of relieved symptoms (Black & Downs 1996, Kjolhede & Ryden 1994). So once again urologists and gynaecologists are showing increasing interest in conservative therapies, to the point that expert opinion recommends that women with urodynamic stress incontinence should receive a trial of conservative treatment from a specialist physiotherapist before surgery is considered (Berghmans et al 1998, Bø 2002, DoH 2000, NICE 2003).

It is worth considering the implications for the affected woman of a choice between conservative therapy and surgery. There is a world of difference between passively undergoing an operation 'to be put right', and being expected to cooperate over a period of 3–6 months in a treatment that is repetitive and potentially boring, and demands a high degree of discipline, perseverance and self-motivation. Many women are simply unable or unwilling to give what it takes. Many more would be able and willing if they understood their condition, and the pros and cons of the options, and were given the benefit of working with a committed specialist physiotherapist. Whether surgical or conservative treatment is chosen, it is important for women to understand that a total cure of their incontinence may not be possible.

In terms of offering women physiotherapeutic treatment, there is an increasing sociological problem in the UK which makes it difficult for them to attend for treatment. First, most women under 60 have paid employment of some sort and, regardless of age, many have a substantial carer role (e.g. of grandchildren), often so that the next generation may undertake paid employment. Secondly, travel is becoming more time consuming, overcrowded and expensive; roads are congested and, for car drivers, parking is very limited. Third, there is concern particularly amongst older women about safety when going out alone. These aspects may account for non-attendance and certainly affect the amount of personalised attention that a physiotherapist is able to give to an individual. In addition there are the constraints placed by NHS management and the need to be cost effective. It is therefore of prime importance that treatment is well chosen and valued by the patient, that it is delivered on time and efficiently, and that attendances are kept to a minimum.

It is obviously desirable that patients be empowered to take responsibility, as far as possible, for their own treatment. PFM exercises are ideally suited to this and research supports this modality of therapy for patients with stress, urgency and mixed symptoms (Hay-Smith et al 2001). However, research has shown that patients comply better when they are supervised, with periodic monitoring and encouragement (Thow 1990/1). Over recent years, there has been a boom in the production of small biofeedback devices and battery-operated electrical stimulators that a patient with urinary dysfunctions might use at home. Ideally equipment designed for home use should have a facility to record how long and how often the equipment is actually used. Bidmead et al (2002) reported only 45% compliance in using a loaned electrical stimulator daily in addition to an intensive PFM exercise programme, and no significant benefit from its use compared with PFM exercises only for patients with urodynamic stress incontinence.

Physiotherapists who wish to consider the possibility of these types of home treatment should ask first who is to pay for the equipment; there may or may not be a NHS budget to cover it. Chiefly this is because the research evidence, particularly for the efficacy of electrical stimulation, is poor. If it is to be bought by the NHS and then loaned to patients, a very strict protocol needs to be in place, perhaps requiring a deposit; there is anecdotal evidence of failure to return such equipment. If patients are expected to buy their own device, criticism may be made that this is discriminatory. Also equipment that has been out on loan needs to be checked professionally (e.g. by the Medical Physics Department) and have a new battery fitted before it is loaned out again; this is an additional cost. There is also the matter of infection control to be considered.

GENERAL PRINCIPLES

All patients with a continence problem referred to a physiotherapist, following assessment, should receive assistance to clearly understand the nature of their problem and what they can do to help themselves. This will take time and will be facilitated by diagrams, models and good communication skills. Any other health problem which might be contributing to the continence dysfunction (e.g. back pain, chest infection or hay fever) or medications for other conditions such as high blood pressure should be considered and the patient referred where appropriate. Information regarding self-help should include individualised continence-promoting advice as to the amount of fluids consumed and what is drunk, bowel habits to avoid constipation and straining, the position for micturition and defaecation, lifting activities, and sport and leisure activities (see below). If no VPFMC is possible, every effort should be directed to facilitate that ability, including electrical stimulation.

ADDITIONAL TECHNIQUES

For patients with stress urinary incontinence

If no VPFMC is possible then biofeedback and electrical stimulation should be considered. If VPFMC is possible then patients should be taught 'the knack' (Miller et al 1998b) and encouraged to follow an intensive programme of daily exercise individually designed to increase the strength and endurance of their PFM (Hay-Smith et al 2001). This may be augmented with biofeedback (home or clinic based), electrical stimulation (home or clinic based), or cones. The objective of electrical stimulation is to produce PFM contractions. Commonly a pulse duration of $250\,\mu s$ with a frequency of 30–40 Hz, and an individualised duty cycle to match the patient's ability to contract the PFM, is recommended once or twice a day for 10–20 minutes. A vaginal electrode is used and the patient is encouraged to 'join in' with the stimulator. Occasionally it may be appropriate to consider an intravaginal or urethral device (see p. 379).

For patients with urgency or urge incontinence, or both

Assuming VPFMC is possible, patients should be taught deferment techniques such as 'the knack', series of repeated strong PFM contractions, distraction, or perineal pressure, and encouraged to desist from going 'to the loo just in case', to increase the period between voids. In addition, patients will probably be receiving pharmocotherapy. Some patients find the side-effects of medication too unpleasant to continue; others seem not to benefit at all. For these patients, it may be appropriate to offer a trial of electrical stimulation from a home stimulator. This should be set to deliver a current of 5–10 Hz in continuous mode with a 500 μs pulse duration. The objective of this is to try to inhibit the detrusor muscle and normalise reflex activity. The suggested treatment regimen would be once or twice a day for 20–30 minutes.

For patients with mixed symptoms

A combination of the above would be considered.

CONTINENCE-PROMOTING ADVICE

An adult should drink 1000–1500 mL per day, but consideration should be taken of diet because some people take in more fluid with their food than others (e.g. as soups, stews, citrus fruit, etc.). It has been suggested that a urine output of about 1500 mL is a better guide. Suffice to say that some people drink unnecessarily large volumes and others do not drink enough. Concentrated urine may irritate the bladder; drinking large volumes will cause frequency. Patients are generally advised to restrict their caffeine and alcohol intake, as both are diuretics and tend to heighten the activity of the detrusor muscle and reduced tension in the external urethral sphincter. Caffeine should be reduce gradually to avoid withdrawal symptoms such as headache. Although there is some controversy over the adverse effects of caffeine, the effect of limiting this produces a marked improvement for some patients. Hannestad et al (2003) reported a strong correlation between smoking, even when it had been discontinued, tea drinking and obesity and incontinence. Women should sit, not crouch to void and defaecate. Every effort should be made to avoid regular straining at stool and to use an optimal sitting position (see p. 388).

Responsibilities (for children, the elderly, or disabled) and occupations that involve heavy lifting and leisure activities that result in ballistic movements (e.g. netball, aerobics or weight training) need to be reviewed. Advice, equipment and training may be needed for carers straining daily to lift and handle family members in the home. As a general principle, if an activity causes leakage the patient should discontinue it and maybe with treatment it can be resumed later. Medication being taken for other health problems can also cause leakage, particularly diuretics and those for high blood pressure. Physiotherapists are advised to consult the British National Formulary. A change in the time of administration and use of alternative medication are worth considering.

TEACHING PFM CONTRACTIONS

The teaching of PFM contractions is one of the most difficult tasks required of the physiotherapist, probably because the muscles are not directly visible to either patient or therapist, and demonstration cannot be used. It requires a high level of skill particularly in communication, is time consuming, and uninterrupted privacy is essential.

Teaching points

Visualisation

A large, simple diagram or a model (or both) of the pelvis, pelvic organs and the levator ani muscles is helpful to show the three openings, and the lifting and gripping effect of the muscle action.

Language

Throughout the teaching session the language must be chosen specifically for each individual patient, employing words and images that are likely to be familiar and easily understood, for example asking the patient to simulate:

- stopping passing water/urine
- stopping passing/breaking wind
- stopping yourself 'blowing off'/farting
- stopping diarrhoea/shit/'poo'/'crap'
- stopping doing a 'pee'/'wee'
- stopping yourself 'having an accident'/'bursting'
- trying to stop yourself 'leaking'/'wetting your pants'
- gripping to stop a tampon falling out
- gripping your partner's penis/willy.

Starting position

PFM contractions can be performed in any position, but a useful initial position is sitting on a hard chair leaning forward with support from the forearms on the thighs, with knees and feet apart. It is a non-threatening, unexposed position and the patient is not required to undress. The perineum is against the chair seat so there is some perineal sensory stimulation as feedback, and a change of sensation is usually apparent over the pelvic outlet, particularly the anterior part, on contraction.

Example of instruction to a patient

Are you comfortable on that chair? Now can you sit like this, knees and feet apart? Lean forwards a little and support yourself with forearms on thighs. Can you feel your back passage near the chair seat? Think about the back passage, imagine you want to pass wind or empty your bowels; close shut your back passage as tightly as you can and try and pull it up toward your waist. Now let go. Try twice more. What can your feel? Try not to clench your buttocks at the same time or hold your breath! Now let's imagine you have a full bladder but there are no toilets available and you must wait! Squeeze shut your front passage tight and try to lift it away from the chair. Now let go. Try twice more. What do you feel? Be sure not to clench your buttocks, hold your breath or pull your tummy in strongly. (**NB** Noticeable cocontraction of the transversus abdominis muscles may occur with VPFMC.) Now think about your vagina/birth canal; pretend you have a tampon slipping out and are trying to grip it. What can you feel? Try twice more, then have a rest.

'Now let's try tightening, closing and lifting back passage, front passage and the vagina, all three together. What can you feel? Now let go. Try again and let go. Can you feel any lift?

Now try a cough; what happens to your pelvic floor? Yes, it goes down. Now pull up your pelvic floor 'up and in'; hold it tight and give another cough. Did it still go down against the chair seat? Tightening like that would be a good way of trying to stay dry when you cough or sneeze, or of helping you 'hold on' when you get the urge to pee.

Now try tightening and letting go quite quickly and count. See how many tightenings you can do before you feel the muscles getting tired. Well done! How many was that? Have a rest. Now tighten as strongly as you can and hold, and see how long you can hold before you feel the muscle just letting go despite you trying to keep holding. Have a rest and we'll try again and I'll time you to see how many seconds you can hold. Well done, that was X seconds. Have a rest and we will do that again, etc.

Duration and repetition of contractions

The patient is asked to perform long, strong contractions one after the other with a rest of about 4 seconds between, each held for as long as possible, to see how many contractions can be performed before serious fatigue sets in. The length of the hold and the number of repetitions are recorded. The patient is also asked to try repeating short, sharp quick contractions until fatigued and the preceived number is recorded.

Patients should be warned that there may be a little variation from day to day in performance, according to the time of day, and even the time of the month if they are premenopausal; but that overall, in the coming weeks, an increase in duration and in the number of contractions possible is the objective and is the expected reward for practising regularly. They can be reassured that the research evidence supports this form of treatment (Hay-Smith et al 2001, Wall & Davidson 1992, Wilson et al 2002). However, it will take time!

Changing the starting positions

The patient will probably find that PFM contractions performed in other positions (e.g. supine lying, crook lying and standing) will each 'feel' different. It is a useful exercise, having started in sitting, to experiment in the initial teaching session by going on to try contracting in other positions. Sometimes the patient reports more sensation or better quality contraction, or both. This illustrates the fact that contractions can be performed in virtually any position. It also gives a further opportunity for checking for contraction in the gluteal, hip adductor and abdominal muscles, and for whether the patient is holding her breath or bearing down. The patient should also understand that it is possible to exercise the PFM in a variety of situations: while queuing, telephoning, on the bus or train, watching television or waiting for the kettle to boil.

Confirmation of a PFM contraction

Some physiotherapists choose to teach PFM contractions in the way described above at the first attendance and then to send the patient away for a week 'to practise and get to know your pelvic floor'. A full vaginal and pelvic floor muscle assessment is offered at the second attendance. In the mean time the patient may be encouraged to feel her perineum when attempting to contract in bed or in the bath. For patients who refuse a vaginal examination there are other ways of confirming a contraction (see p. 357).

General advice

The patient is advised to contract her PFM before and during any of the events, which, for her, normally trigger leakage, for example when coughing, sneezing, laughing, nose blowing, lifting, running or jumping, or with a strong desire to void. This technique is called 'the knack' (Miller et al 1998a, b) or counter-bracing.

Number and content of practice sessions

In discussion with the patient, possibly at the second attendance, a plan of daily practice sessions is made. This must be realistic and attainable as well as being agreeable to the patient. Some people are best able to exercise 'a little and often' (hourly or half-hourly); others practise more reliably using two or three intensive sessions per day. The fact that the more exercise that is done the sooner results will be noticeable, and that even then it will take time, must be impressed on the patient. Olympic gold medals are not won by people who train occasionally! Some patients are helped to comply by keeping an exercise diary (Bø 1990).

The most advantageous programme of exercises to strengthen and improve the endurance of the PFM is not known and probably will vary from patient to patient. Women should be encouraged to do both sub-maximal holding contractions and fast, short maximal contractions. Bo et al (1989) showed improvement in patients with stress incontinence using 8–12 groups of contractions, each of which consisted of one contraction held for as long as possible followed by three or four short ones. This regimen was repeated three times each day and contractions were carried out in a variety of positions. The greatest improvement was found in those patients who also attended the clinic for practice sessions which included general exercise.

Further sessions, reassessment and progression

Each time the patient attends for treatment a verbal reassessment should be made. If good progress seems to be being made, a repeat digital examination is not usually necessary on each visit. If there is no improvement or if the patient is doubtful as to whether the right muscles are being used, a repeat examination should be offered. However if clinic-based biofeedback equipment is available, its use may serve two purposes – remotivating the patient and enabling the physiotherapist to reappraise the exercise programme.

As with all re-education, the patient needs regular encouragement to increase the length, intensity and number of repeat PFM contractions. A variety of positions should be used, working toward those in which leakage used to occur; PFM contractions will be more difficult in some positions (e.g. squatting). Once a satisfactory routine of simple daily PFM contractions has been established, it may be appropriate to teach transversus abdominis muscle contractions in four-point kneeling, sitting and standing to try to encourage coactivation with the pelvic floor (Jones et al 2002, Sapsford 2001). It is a contraction that lends itself to combination with activities of daily living (e.g. walking).

If the patient has evidence of back pain or core instability, or both, this should be addressed. As the woman regains reliable continence, other activities designed to develop physical fitness should be suggested, such as walking, swimming or dancing. Women must appreciate that the best hope for maintaining improvement is to continue with their programme.

Attendance for treatment

It has been suspected for many years by physiotherapists that most patients start with great enthusiasm and complete the assigned number of contractions for the first few days; but if they are left to follow the programme uncoached or monitored the daily number of contractions drops in most cases rather than increases. Research by Thow (1990/1) seems to support this, and others (Bø et al 1989, Wilson et al 1987) have shown that patients who are sent away to practise at home on their own, experience less improvement than those who attend the physiotherapy department regularly. In response to an open question in a survey concerning physiotherapeutic services for stress incontinence (Mantle & Versi 1989), physiotherapists strongly indicated that they considered the patient's motivation to be critical to outcome; yet it is difficult to maintain motivation alone. Could it be that the apparent benefit sometimes seen from the addition of regular clinic-based biofeedback or electrical muscle stimulation (or both) to the treatment regimen has more to do with the recharging of the patient's determination to persevere with the exercises than anything else?

To derive the maximum improvement possible from a programme of PFM exercises, it will need to be continued for 3 to 6 months. The woman should be seen by the physiotherapist after no more than a week for a thorough check and further instruction if necessary. Initially appointments should be frequent to provide regular reinforcement and encouragement. Thereafter they can be more widely spaced in order to develop the woman's independence and responsibility for her own therapy. Group treatment sessions can be very cost effective for the therapist as well as therapeutic and pleasant for women. A friendly telephone call periodically can be very supportive and is a valuable method of maintaining contact with women who are unable to make regular visits to their physiotherapist.

BIOFEEDBACK

Biofeedback equipment is of two types: for clinic use and home use. Biofeedback may be used in assessment (see p. 357), in treatment as a challenge and motivator and, with great care, as an audit tool (see also Haslam 2002). It is time consuming so in treatment a judgement needs to be made by the physiotherapist and the patient as to its cost benefits, and this may vary through an episode of treatment. A systematic review (Berghmans et al 1998) could find no added benefit from biofeedback over PFM exercises alone. However, a further meta-analysis (Weatherall 1999) disputed this, and many physiotherapists claim to find it highly motivating for some patients.

Manometry

Manometric devices are used with a vaginal pressure probe and give biofeedback by means of a manometer or a visual display. Where units of measurement of pressure change are given, centimetres of water (cm H_2O)

are usually used, but because there are so many possible variables the results are not transferable from one piece of equipment to another, or from one patient to another. Even with the same patient and with the same equipment, every effort must be made to control the variables (see also p. 358).

Computerised manometric equipment

The display from such equipment is shown on a VDU screen and in preparing the patient it is essential for both physiotherapist and patient to see it. The patient is usually positioned initially in well-supported half-lying with the head supported. If measurements are going to be used comparatively, then detail must be recorded of the exact position of back-rest and pillows. A vaginal probe is used in accordance with local infection control policies. The deflated probe is introduced into the vagina to a predetermined depth and then pressures are normalised to the baseline. Using a blank screen, the patient is then asked to perform a VPFMC and the result is visualised. It may be wise to allow the patient practice (warm-up) time before recording the reading. The patient is then asked to perform a suitable series of held contractions and a series of fast, short contractions appropriate to her ability. This may be repeated or screens can be changed and templates used to add further degrees of difficulty – mental as well as physical. Records may be kept for future comparison.

Perineometer

In 1948 Kegel described a pneumatic device which he used to measure pressure within the vagina and to motivate women to practise PFM exercises. A compressible air-filled rubber portion (sensor) was inserted into the vagina by the woman and attached by rubber tubing to a manometer. The woman then contracted her pelvic floor several times and noted the highest reading on the dial and the length of time for which she could hold a contraction.

The Peritron (Cardio Design, Australia; Neen Healthcare, UK), described under Assessment (see p. 358), is currently available and can be used for motivation. It is essential that the procedure used adheres to the locally agreed infection control policy; usually a condom is used over the probe and in some centres each patient has her own probe. Expert supervision is needed to ensure that the intra-abdominal pressure is not being measured rather than the result of PFM activity, and as many factors as possible should be held constant at each use.

Handheld devices

Manometric handheld devices have been produced for home use but there are cost implications for either the NHS or the patient. It is important to be sure of benefit before suggesting use. Such gadgets tend to be seven-day wonders!

Electromyography

Computerised electromyographic equipment

This equipment is designed to pick up the bioelectrical activity and show it on a screen. It can be used to observe PFM activity. Usually a vaginal electrode is used but this must be comfortable for the patient; the Periform is popular because its ellipsoid shape helps it to stay in place even if it is decided to record activity in standing, walking or jumping. However, occasionally there is a patient with a scarred and narrowed vagina, the presence of which should have been noted at assessment, who will need a different type of electrode.

The same concerns apply to this equipment as to computerised manometers regarding infection control, controlling for variables, time usage and cost benefit.

Other

Vaginal cones

In the rehabilitation of muscle, resistance in the form of weights has long been used to increase strength and endurance. Attempts to find a means of applying graded resistance to the PFM led to the development and marketing of vaginal cones in 1988. The theory underpinning cone usage is that there is increased reflex activity of the PFM to support and retain the cone against gravity, and to counteract downward slippage. Over the years companies have manufactured these in sets of five to nine small, progressively weighted cylinders, ranging from 10 to 100 g or as a set of weights which fit into a single cone. Each cone is about the size and shape of a tampon and has a nylon string attached to one slightly tapered end to facilitate removal from the vagina. Some sets supply cones in two different diameters to accommodate the range in vaginal diameter. To overcome potential problems with infection control, cones should be single user. Cones can be purchased over the counter in the UK. They are supplied with instructions but ideally the patient should receive instruction from a specialist physiotherapist.

Selecting the appropriate cone   The lightest cone is inserted into the vagina while in the semisquatting or half-lying position, or standing with one foot up on a chair. The cone is inserted with the pointed end and string downwards and must be placed far enough into the vagina to lie just above the level of the pelvic floor. The patient then stands and walks around. If the cone can be retained for 1 minute, the patient progresses on to the next cone, which is slightly heavier, and so on until a cone slips out in under 1 minute. The heaviest cone that can be retained for 1 minute is used for exercise.

Treatment sessions   It is usually suggested that twice a day the patient inserts a cone and walks around for up to 15 minutes. If the cone slips down it is pushed back up. Once the cone can be retained for 15 minutes without slipping, progress is made to the next cone. Over time, coughing, stairs and other activities of daily living may be introduced as a progression. Furthermore, Bø (2002) suggests teaching a patient to resist traction applied to the cone string while standing. A course of at least 1 month is recommended.

A Cochrane review (Herbison et al 2002) of research using cones concluded that there is some evidence that cones are better than no active treatment in the treatment of stress incontinence, but noted that there was a considerable dropout of patients in some of the studies examined, for example that of Cammu & Van Nylen (1998). Research has shown that some older women dislike putting 'things into their vagina' (Prashar et al 2000). Bø (1995, 2002) has also questioned their use from an exercise science perspective. She suggests that retention for as long as 15–20 minutes might cause decreased blood supply, decreased oxygen consumption, muscle fatigue and pain, and recruit other muscles than the PFM. Furthermore when standing, the vagina is not a vertical tube and has soft stretchy walls, Hahn et al (1996) showed a transverse lie of the cone in some women, which would obviously aid containment. However, cone usage unmasks incorrect attempts at contracting the PFM such as valsalva, as the cone is pushed out.

If cone therapy is used, the following should be noted:

- It is often the case that greater weight can be retained in the morning than the evening.
- If the width between the medial edges of the levator ani muscles is very wide, congenitally or as a result of trauma at deliveries, retention may be impossible.
- If the innervation to part of the pelvic floor has been permanently damaged the potential for improvement may be very small.
- Vaginal secretions vary through the menstrual cycle and will be greatest in mid-cycle. Moisture will be increased by sexual intercourse, spermicides or lubricant jelly. Cone retention may thus be adversely effected.
- A full rectum may make retention easier.
- Traction on the cord can be used to give an additional challenge to the PFM.

The Educator See page 358.

ELECTRICAL STIMULATION

The research evidence for using electrical stimulation for patients with urinary dysfunction is limited and it is generally unpopular with patients. For an authoritative review of its use see Fall & Lindstrom (1991). It can be used for two purposes. One is to produce muscle contraction and this can be used to attempt to assist patients who seem unable to produce a VPFMC or have very weak PFM, particularly if they have urodynamic stress incontinence. Once a patient is able voluntarily to contract the PFM reliably then intensive active exercise is probably the best treatment. The other use of electrical stimulation is to utilise the sensory stimulation it causes to inhibit detrusor overactivity and nomalise reflex activity, so this is useful for some patients who experience urgency and urge incontinence (see also Laycock & Vodusek 2002).

Interferential therapy

Interferential therapy (IT) which employed medium-frequency currents in the region of either 4000 Hz (4 kHz) or 2000 Hz (2 kHz) was used extensively therapeutically in the treatment of urinary incontinence in the 1980s in the UK. In a survey of English physiotherapists, Mantle & Versi (1989) found that 77% of the respondents put IT as either their first or second choice of modality for the treatment of stress incontinence, and they considered it to be 63% effective. However, with the increasing use of biofeedback it has become less popular, and some experts have cast doubt on the specificity of the spread of the current even using a vaginal electrode.

Low-frequency muscle stimulation

There are two main types of equipment used to apply electrical stimulation in the treatment of urinary incontinence: computerised clinic-based machines and small battery-operated devices for home use. It is usual to use a vaginal electrode and commonly this is the Periform (see p. 373), provided that it is comfortable for the patient. It is supplied with an indicator, which, if attached, can be used to confirm whether or not a PFM contraction is being obtained by the electrical stimulation. There are narrower vaginal electrodes if these are needed; alternatively flat adhesive electrodes can be used externally.

Computerised clinic-based electrical stimulation equipment

Some equipment can be used for both EMG and electrical stimulation either separately or in combination. The patient should be comfortably positioned and well supported in half-lying such that both patient and physiotherapist can see the screen. The equipment allows for seemingly infinite permutations, but for stimulating PFM contractions it is usual to use a $250\,\mu s$ pulse duration and a frequency of 35–40 Hz. The duty cycle is chosen with great care. In that stimulation is often used for very weak muscles or where the patient is unable to produce a VPFMC, it is wise to select rest periods of double the stimulation period, and a stimulation period which matches, in seconds, the ability of the patient to hold a contraction – if this is possible. The patient is encouraged to join in and, with equipment with EMG facilities, they can compare their efforts to those of the stimulation. Where a patient cannot contract, a starting duty cycle of 2 seconds on and 4 off would be appropriate, for 5 minutes in the first instance and with the patient trying to join in. Intensity needs to be such that a good contraction is produced. Progress will match the patient's ability to hold contractions, need less rest and tolerate longer treatment sessions up to 30 minutes.

It is sometimes claimed that stimulation of this kind *strengthens* muscles. Stimulation for several hours a day is required to strengthen muscles significantly. Complex clinic-based equipment is less well suited to treating urgency and urge incontinence because the patient is best served with daily sessions of 20–30 minutes.

Battery-operated electrical stimulation devices for clinic-based or home electrical stimulation

Ideally these are sturdy and simple to operate, and have facilities for setting the pulse width, frequency and duty cycle to those most appropriate for each patient; it is helpful if the machine records how often and for how long the device is used as a check on compliance. These are particularly well suited to treating urgency and urge incontinence, enabling the patient to be treated daily cost effectively. A vaginal electrode is used. The patient with urgency symptoms must be very carefully instructed, receive an instruction sheet and have a telephone contact number should difficulties arise. A pulse width of about $500\,\mu s$, a frequency of 5–10 Hz and the maximum tolerable intensity are used. Daily treatment sessions start at about 5 minutes but quickly rise to 20–30 minutes if all is well.

Electrical stimulation of the PFM can also be carried out using a battery-operated device in the clinic or at home, or both locations, using the appropriate settings given in the previous section. See also page 367 concerning loaning and maintenance of loaned equipment.

BLADDER RETRAINING

Bladder retraining or drill was first described by Jeffcoate & Francis (1966) and was called 'bladder discipline'. It was used in the management of frequency, urgency without leakage and urge incontinence (*bladder overactivity*) (Frewen 1979, Jarvis & Millar 1980, Jeffcoate & Francis, 1966) and then was extended to the treatment of genuine (*urodynamic*) stress incontinence (Fantl et al 1991, Wyman et al 1998). Originally some patients were admitted to hospital to assist adherence to the strict regimen. The objective is to help patients who are 'ruled by their bladders' and 'tied to the toilet'.

The main aims are to:

- correct faulty habits
- control urgency
- prolong periods between voids
- reduce incontinence episodes
- reduce the daily number of voids and increase voided volumes
- build up the patient's confidence.

To achieve this the patient must be mentally intact, motivated and able to go to the toilet independently. It may be used in combination with pharmacotherapy. The patient needs to understand clearly her problem, the normal mechanisms of continence and how bladder retraining is intended to help her. She is asked to fill in a frequency/volume chart including 'accidents', and what and how much is drunk. The chart is then studied by the patient and physiotherapist or continence advisor. Goals are set and a programme agreed which includes drinking sufficient fluid.

Deferment techniques are taught such as:

- repeated maximal pelvic floor contractions at times when urgency is felt
- perineal pressure (e.g. sitting on a rolled towel or arm of a chair)
- standing on tip toes
- distraction – such as companionship, games, television or music.

After an agreed period, patients are again required to keep a frequency/volume chart including what and how much is drunk. The patient is supervised and monitored frequently by the physiotherapist or continence advisor who offers praise where praise is due, gives advice on progression and helps to maintain motivation till goals are met.

More recently Wyman et al (1998) reported that PFM exercises and biofeedback were as effective as bladder retraining for patients with urodynamic stress incontinence, bladder overactivity or mixed symptoms.

TIMED AND PROMPTED VOIDING

Where patients are unable to toilet independently or are confused, or both, timed voiding may be helpful to avoid 'accidents'. The patient's need for the toilet is observed and charted over several days, a routine of toileting times is then set – ideally this is individualised. Commonly in residential and nursing homes this is set at 2-hourly intervals and the patient is taken to the toilet or sat on a commode whether or not they express a desire to void. Where the patient can go to the toilet independently, a prompt to void with some guidance may be sufficient.

The concept of timed voiding is also useful for patients who have lost sensation of bladder fullness, and for those women whose life is so pressured and intense that they 'forget' or fail to take the opportunity to void until it is really too late. Furthermore, employers who try to place restrictions on when or how often employees are allowed to go to the toilet should be challenged. People need to realise that anyone will 'have an accident' if they 'wait' long enough.

FUNCTIONAL ACTIVITY

In assessing the patient referred with incontinence, it is important for the physiotherapist to determine to what extent poor balance, joint stiffness or lack of strength and endurance in muscles other than the pelvic floor may be actually contributing to the incontinence or aggravating it. Consideration should also be given as to how far general lack of fitness is responsible for weakness of the pelvic floor musculature. An example of joint stiffness as a contributory factor to incontinence would be osteoarthritic knees, which make standing up from sitting a very painful, 'breathholding' struggle, resulting in leakage either because the raised intra-abdominal pressure provokes detrusor contractions or because it overwhelms the urethral closure mechanisms. In addition (or alternatively), such a disability could result in the woman taking so long to reach the toilet that accidents occur. In such a case, one solution would be specific treatment to relieve pain, mobilise joints and strengthen the leg muscles, whereas another would be to change the environment (Muir Gray 1986).

Another possibility is that the inactivity and social withdrawal caused by the incontinence leads to generalised muscular weakness including the perineal muscles. The pelvic floor musculature is active in its urethral closure role and its supportive role to a variable extent round the clock, the degree of muscle activity being related to what the woman is doing. A gradient of activity might be represented by lying, sitting, standing, walking, bending and lifting. Such activities as talking, laughing and shouting interact with these. The amount of work done by the pelvic floor in a day is governed by what a woman does. Reduced activity, if she is sitting at home a great deal, will reduce the daily work of the pelvic floor and lead in time to many muscles (including the PFM) becoming less strong. Gordon & Logue (1985), writing of postpartum women, reported that any form of muscular exercise improved perineal muscle function. They went on to comment that pure perineal exercises were not extensively practised either because women were not convinced of the benefit or because they found them tedious, and that perhaps more emphasis should be placed on exercise that women find interesting and fulfilling.

Functional activities should be part of an integrated treatment programme. Activities that are known to cause leakage should be excluded at the start of such a programme; and being able once again to achieve them without leakage could be used as an objective test of improvement. Bø et al (1989) used this approach, which also included group general exercise sessions. The physiotherapist is the only professional who is able to assess the patient in this holistic way and decide, first, whether specific exercises or more general exercises are required, and if so, to plan and implement the right programme for the individual.

DEVICES

Small intravaginal and intraurethral devices have been produced. Some promote continence by supporting the bladder neck and others are designed to stop urine loss by blocking the urethra. The reader is referred to Anders (2002).

MANAGEMENT OF PERSISTENT URINARY INCONTINENCE

Where, despite exhaustive and repeated assessment and the best of team care, a patient is still left with some degree of incontinence of urine or faeces, efforts should be directed towards management. The continence advisor can give invaluable help to all concerned in finding the best care solutions for each individual case which will maintain dignity and allow social integration, while reducing the workload and keeping down costs. The physiotherapist may be able to contribute toward these goals with treatment that produces just a little more strength or range of movement. This may enable a patient to become independent by coping with manoeuvres such as ISC or pad changing for themselves, or make it possible for the patient, in spite of all the problems, to get out and about and enjoy life. Incontinence, immobility, social deprivation and depression are a lethal cocktail.

References

Abrams P, Blaivas J G, Stanton S, Andersen J T 1988 Standardization of terminology of lower urinary tract function. Neurourology and Urodynamics 7:403–426.

Abrams P, Cardozo L, Fall M et al 2002a Standardisation of terminology of lower urinary tract function: Report from the Standardisation Sub-committee of the ICS. Neurourology and Urodynamics 21:167–178.

Abrams P, Cardozo L, Khoury A et al (eds) 2002b Incontinence, 2nd edn. Health Publications/Plymbridge Distributors, Plymouth, p 117

ACA (Association for Continence Advice) 2003 Examination and assessment of the female pelvic floor: notes on good practice. ACA, London.

Addison R 2002 7.12 Urinalysis. In: Laycock J, Haslam J (eds) Therapeutic management of incontinence and pelvic pain. Springer, London, p 54–63.

Anders K 2002 Non medical management of incontinence. Ch 17 in: MacLean A B, Cardozo L (eds) Incontinence in women. RCOG Press, London, p 225–248.

Artibani W, Andersen J T, Gajewski J et al 2002 Imaging and other investigations. Ch 8c in: Abrams P, Cardozo L, Khoury A et al (eds) Incontinence. Health Publications/Plymbridge Distributors, Plymouth, p 423–477.

Berghmans L, Hendricks L, Bo K et al 1998 Conservative treatment of stress urinary incontinence in women; a systematic review of randomised clinical trials. British Journal of Urology 82:181–191.

Bidmead J, Mantle J, Cardozo L et al 2002 Home electrical stimulation in addition to conventional pelvic floor exercises: a useful adjunct or expensive distraction? Neurourology and Urodynamics 21(4):372–373.

Black N A, Downs S H 1996 The effectiveness of surgery for stress incontinence in women: a systematic review. British Journal of Urology 78:497–510.

Bø K 1990 Pelvic floor muscle exercise for treatment of female SUI. Methodological studies and clinical results. Acta Obstetrica et Gynecologica Scandinavica 70(7–8):637–639.

Bø K 1995 Vaginal weight cones: theoretical framework, effect on pelvic floor strength and female stress urinary incontinence. Acta Obstetrica et Gynecologic Scandinavica 74(2):87–92.

Bø K 2002 Physiotherapy techniques. Ch 19 in: MacLean A, Cardozo L. (eds) Incontinence in women. RCOG Press, London, p 256–271.

Bø K, Larsen S, Oseid S et al 1988 Knowledge about the ability to correct pelvic floor exercises in women with stress urinary incontinence. Neurourology and Urodynamics 69:261–262

Bø K, Hagen R, Jorgenson J et al 1989 The effect of two different pelvic floor muscle exercise programs in treatment of urinary stress incontinence in women. Neurourology and Urodynamics 8(4):355.

Brown J S, Vittingoff E, Wyman J F et al 2000 Urinary incontinence: does it increase the risk for falls and fractures? A study of Osteoporotic Fractures Research Group. Journal of the American Geriatrics Society 48(7):721–725.

Bump R C, Hurt W G, Fantl J A 1991 Assessment of Kegel pelvic muscle exercise performance after brief verbal instruction. American Journal of Obstetrics and Gynecology 165:322–329.

Cammu H , Van Nylen M 1998 Pelvic floor exercises versus vaginal weight cones in genuine stress incontinence. European Journal of Obstetrics, Gynecology and Reproductive Biology 77(1):89–93.

Chandra M, Saharia R, Shi Q, Hill V 2002 Giggle incontinence in children: a manifestation of detrusor instability. Journal of Urology 169(5):2184–2187.

Continence Foundation 2000 Making the case for investment in an integrated continence service. Continence Foundation, London.

CSP (Chartered Society of Physiotherapy) 1996 Information paper no. PA19. Pelvic floor and vaginal assessment. CSP, London.

CSP (Chartered Society of Physiotherapy) 1998 Information paper no. PA19B. Association of Chartered Physiotherapists in Women's Health guidelines for tutors teaching pelvic floor and vaginal assessment. CSP, London.

DoH (Department of Health) 2000 Good practice in continence services. DoH, London.

DoH (Department of Health) 2001 Reference guide to consent for examination or treatment. DoH, London.

Donovan J & committee 2002 Symptom and quality of life assessment. In: Abrams P, Cardozo L, Khoury A et al (eds) Incontinence. Health Publications/Plymbridge Distributors, Plymouth, p 269–316.

Eardley I, Nagendran K, Lecky B 1991 The neurophysiology of the striated urethral sphincter in multiple sclerosis. British Journal of Urology 67:81–88.

Fall M, Lindstrom S 1991 Electrical stimulation. A physiologic approach to the treatment of urinary incontinence. Urologic Clinics of North America 18(2):393–407.

Fantl J A, Wyman J F, Mclish D K et al 1991 Efficacy of bladder training in elderly women with urinary incontinence. Journal of the American Medical Association 265:609–613.

Fowler C, Vodusek D 2001 Nerve conduction studies. Ch 23 in: Cardozo L, Staskin D (eds) Textbook of female urology and urogynaecology. Isis Medical Media, London, p 251–262.

Fowler C, Benson J, Craggs M et al 2002 Clinical neurophysiology. Ch 8B in: Abrams P, Khoury A, Wein A (eds) Incontinence. Plymbridge Distributors, p 389–424.

Frewen W K 1979 Role of bladder training in the treatment of the unstable bladder in the female. Urologic Clinics of North America 6:273–277.

Garnett S, Abrams P 2002 The role of urodynamics. Ch 6 in: MacLean A B, Cardozo L (eds) Incontinence in women. RCOG Press, London, 61–75.

Glazener C M, Evans J H 2003 Desmopressin for nocturnal enuresis in children (Cochrane review). In: The Cochrane Library, Issue 1. Update Software, Oxford.

Gordon H, Logue M 1985 Perineal muscle function after childbirth. Lancet ii:123–125.

Grimley A, Milson L, Molander U et al 1993 The influence of urinary incontinence on quality of life of elderly women. Age and Aging 22:88–89.

Hahn I, Milsom I, Ohlsson B L et al 1996 Comparitive assessment of pelvic floor function using vaginal cones, vaginal palpation and vaginal pressure measurements. Gynecologic and Obstetric Investigation 41(4):269–274.

Hampel C, Weinhold D, Benkin N et al 1997 Definition of overactive bladder and epidemiology of urinary incontinence. Urology 59(suppl 64):4–14.

Hannestad Y S, Rortvelt G, Daltveit A K et al 2003 Are smoking and other lifestyle factors associated with female urinary incontinence? The Norwegian EPINCONT Study. International Journal of Obstetrics and Gynecology 110:247–254.

Harvey M, Versi E 2001 Pad tests. Ch 16 in: Cardozo L, Staskin D (eds) Textbook of female urology and urogynaecology. Isis Medical Media, London, p 175–182.

Haslam J 2002 Biofeedback for assessment and re-education of the pelvic floor musculature. Ch 10 in: Laycock J, Haslam J (eds) Therapeutic management of incontinence and pelvic pain. Springer, London, p 75–80.

Haylen B T, Ashby D, Sutherst J R et al 1989 Maximum and average urine flow rates in normal male and female populations – the Liverpool nomograms. British Journal of Urology 64:30–38.

Haylen B T, Parys B T, Anyaegbunam W I et al 1990 Urine flow rates in male and female urodynamic patients compared with the Liverpool nomograms. British Journal of Urology 65:483–487.

Haylen B T, Law M G, Fraser M I et al 1999 Urine flow rates and residual urine volumes in urogynaecology patients. International Urogynecologic Journal 6:378–383.

Hay-Smith E J, Bø K, Berghmans L C 2001 Pelvic floor muscle training for female urinary incontinence (Cochrane review). In: The Cochrane Library, Issue 1. Update Software, Oxford.

Herbison P, Plevnik S, Mantle J 2002 Weighted vaginal cones for urinary incontinence (Cochrane review). In: The Cochrane Library, Issue 1. Update Software, Oxford.

Herschorn S 2001 Videourodynamics. Ch 24 in: Cardozo L, Staskin D (eds) Textbook of female urology and urogynaecology. Isis Medical Media, London, p 263–274.

Hilton P 1988 Urinary incontinence during sexual intercourse; a common but rarely volunteered symptom. British Journal of Obstetrics and Gynaecology 95:377–381.

Hilton P 2001 Obstetric fistulae and Surgical fistulae. Chs 56 and 55 in: Cardozo L, Staskin D (eds) Textbook of female urology and urogynaecology, Isis Medical Media, London, p 711–772.

Hilton P 2002 Urogenital fistulae. Ch 13 in: MacLean A B, Cardozo L (eds) Incontinence in women. RCOG Press, London, p 163–181.

Hu T W 1990 Impact of urinary incontinence on health-care costs. Journal of the American Geriatrics Society 39(3):292–295.

Hughes P N, Abrams P 2001 Cystometry. Ch 18 in: Cardozo L, Staskin D (eds) Textbook of female urology and urogynaecology. Isis Medical Media, London, p 197–204.

Jarvis G J, Millar D R 1980 Controlled trial of bladder drill for detrusor instability. British Medical Journal 281:1322–1323.

Jeffcoate T N A, Francis W J A 1966 Urgency incontinence in the female. American Journal of Obstetrics and Gynecology 94:604–619.

Jeyaseelan S M, Oldham J A, Roe B H 1997 The use of perineal pad testing to assess urinary incontinence. Reviews in Clinical Gerontology 7:83–92.

Jeyaseelan S M, Haslam J, Winstanley J et al 2001 Digital vaginal assessment: an inter-tester reliability study. Physiotherapy 87(5):243–250.

Jones R, Comerford M, Sapsford R 2002 Pelvic floor stability and trunk coactivation. In: Laycock J, Haslam J (eds) Therapeutic management of incontinence and pelvic pain, Ch. 8. Springer, London, p 66–70.

Jorgensen L, Lose G, Andersen J T 1987 One hour pad weighing tests for objective assessment of female urinary incontinence. Obstetrics and Gynecology 69:39–42.

Kegel A 1948 The non-surgical treatment of genital relaxation. Annals of Western Medical Surgery 2:213–216.

Kelleher C J, Cardozo L, Khullar V 1997 A new questionnaire to assess quality of life of urinary incontinent women. British Journal of Obstetrics and Gynaecology 104:1374–1379.

Khullar V 2001 Ultrasonography. Ch 27 in: Cardozo L, Staskin D (eds) Textbook of female urology and urogynaecology. Isis Medical Media, London, p 299–312.

Khullar V 2002 The role of imaging. Ch 7 in: MacLean A B, Cardozo L (eds) Incontinence in women. RCOG Press, London, p 76–90.

Kiff E S, Barnes P R H, Swash M 1984 Evidence of pudendal neuropathy in patients with perineal descent and chronic constipation. Gut 25:1279–1282.

Kjolhede P, Ryden G 1994 prognostic factors and long term results of the Burch colposuspension. Acta Obstetrica et Gynecologica Scandinavica 73:642–647.

Laycock J, Chiarelli P 1989 Pelvic floor assessment and re-education. Proceedings of the International Continence Society (99):206–207.

Laycock J, Jerwood D 2001 Pelvic floor assessment: the PERFECT scheme. Physiotherapy 87(12):631–642.

Laycock J, Vodusek D 2002 Electrical stimulation. Ch 12 in: Laycock J, Haslam J (eds) Therapeutic management of incontinence and pelvic pain. Springer, London, p 85–88.

Lose G 2001 Urethral pressure measurement. Ch 20 in: Cardozo L, Staskin D (eds) Textbook of female urology and urogynaecology. Isis Medical Media, London, p 215–226.

McGrother C W, Shaw C, Perry S I et al 2001 Epidemiology (Europe). Ch 3 in: Cardozo L, Staskin D (eds) Textbook of

female urology and urogynaecology. Isis Medical Media, London.

Mahony D T, Laferte R O, Blaise J D 1977 Integral storage and voiding reflexes. Urology 9:95–106.

Mantle J, Versi E 1989 Physiotherapy for stress incontinence: a national survey. British Medical Journal 302:753–755.

Miller J, Ashton-Miller J, Delancey J O L 1998a Quantification of cough-related urine loss using the paper towel test. Obstetrics and Gynecology 91(5 Pt 1):705–709.

Miller J, Ashton-Miller J, DeLancey J O L 1998b A pelvic muscle pre-contraction can reduce cough related urine loss in selected women with mild SUI. Journal of the American Geriatrics Society 46:870–874.

Moore K H, Richmond D H, Sutherst J R et al 1991 Crouching over the toilet seat: prevalence among British gynaecological outpatients and its effect upon micturition. British Journal of Obstetrics and Gynaecology 98:569–571.

Muir Gray J A 1986 Incontinence in the community. Ch 7 in: Mandelstam D (ed) Incontinence and its management, 2nd edn. Croom Helm, London, p 135–146.

NICE (National Institute for Clinical Excellence) 2003 Appraisal consultation document: tension free vaginal tape for stress incontinence. www.nice.org.uk.

Peattie A M, Plevnik S, Stanton S 1989 Distal urethral conductance (DUEC): a screening test for incontinent females. Paper presented to the Blair Bell Research Society, 25 April. RCOG, London.

Prashar S, Simons A, Bryant C et al 2000 Attitudes to vaginal/urethral touching and device placement in women with urinary incontinence. International Urogynecologic Journal 11:4–8.

RCOG (Royal College of Obstetricians & Gynaecologists) 2002 Gynaecological examinations: guidelines for specialist practice. RCOG Press, London.

RCP (Royal College of Physicians) 1995 Incontinence causes, management and provision of services 1995, report of a working party. RCP London.

Sapsford R 2001 The pelvic floor. A clinical model for function and rehabilitation. Physiotherapy 87(12):620–630.

Schafer W, Abrams P, Liao L et al 2002 Report on good urodynamic practice. Neurourology and Urodynamics 21(3):261–274.

Shah J, Vakalopoulos J 2002 Urological complications of gynaecological disorders. Ch 14 in: MacLean A B, Cardozo L (eds) Incontinence in women. RCOG Press, London, p 182–198.

Shepherd A 1990 The conservative treatment of genuine stress incontinence. Ch 13 in: Drife J O, Hilton P, Stanton S L (eds) Micturition. Springer Verlag, London, p 209–224.

Snooks S J, Swash M, Setchell M et al 1984 Injury to innervation of pelvic floor sphincter musculature in childbirth. Lancet ii:546–550.

Stanton S L 1986 Gynaecological aspects. Ch 3 in: Mandelstam D (ed). Incontinence and its management. Croom Helm, London, p 55–75.

Sultan A H 2002 Third degree tear repairs. Ch 29 in: MacLean A B, Cardozo L (eds) Incontinence in women. RCOG Press, London, p 379–390.

Swash M 1985 Anorectal incontinence: electrophysiological tests. British Journal of Surgery 72(suppl):S14–S20.

Thomas T M, Plymat K R, Blannin J et al 1980 Prevalence of urinary incontinence. British Medical Journal 281:1243–1245.

Thomas T M, Egan M, Walgrove A et al 1984 The prevalence of faecal and double incontinence. Community Medicine 6:216–220.

Thow M 1990/1 Compliance with a programme of pelvic floor exercise. Journal of the Association of Chartered Physiotherapists in Obstetrics and Gynaecology 68:10–12.

Versi E 1990 Relevance of urethral pressure profilometry to date. Ch 6 in: Drife J O, Hilton P, Stanton S L (eds) Micturition. Springer Verlag, London, p 81–110.

Versi E, Cardozo L, Anand D 1988 The use of pad tests in the investigation of female urinary incontinence. British Journal of Obstetrics and Gynaecology 8:270–273.

Versi E, Orrego G, Hardy E et al 1996 Evaluation of the home pad test in the investigation of female urinary incontinence. British Journal of Obstetrics and Gynaecology 103(7):720.

Vodusek D, Fowler C 2001 Electromyography. Ch 22 in: Cardozo L, Staskin D (eds) Textbook of female urology and urogynaecology. Isis Medical Media, London, p 239–253.

Wall L L 1999 Birth trauma and the pelvic floor: lessons from the developing world. Journal of Women's Health 8(2):149–155.

Wall L L, Davidson T G 1992 The role of muscular re-education by physical therapy in the treatment of genuine stress urinary incontinence. Obstetrical and Gynecological Survey 47(5):322–331.

Warzak W J 1993 Psychological implications of nocturnal enuresis. Clinical Pediatrics (Phila) Spec No:38–40.

Weatherall M 1999 Biofeedback or pelvic floor exercises for female genuine stress incontinence: a meta-analysis of trial identified in a systematic review. British Journal of Urology International 83(9):1015–1016.

Wilson P D, al Samarrai T, Deakin M et al 1987 An objective assessment of physiotherapy for female genuine stress incontinence. British Journal of Obstetrics and Gynaecology 94:575–582.

Wilson P D, Bo K, Hay-Smith J et al 2002 Conservative treatment in women. Ch 12 in: Abrams P, Cardozo L, Khoury A et al (eds) Incontinence. Health Publications/ Plymbridge Distributors, Plymouth, p 573–624.

Wyman J F, Harkins S W, Fantl J A 1990 Psychological impact of urinary incontinence in the community-dwelling population. Journal of the American Geriatrics Society 38(3):282–285.

Wyman J F, Fantl J A, McClish D K et al 1998 Comparitive efficacy of behavioural interventions in the management of female urinary incontinence. American Journal of Obstetrics and Gynecology 179:999–1007.

Further reading

Abrams A, Wein A 1998 The overactive bladder. Pharmacia Upjohn, Milton Keynes.

Cardozo L, Staskin D (eds) 2002 Textbook of female urology and urogynecology. Isis Medical Media, London.

Laycock J, Haslam J (eds) 2002 Therapeutic management of incontinence and pelvic pain. Springer, London.

MacLean A B, Cardozo L (eds) 2002 Incontinence in women. RCOG Press, London.

Sapsford R, Bullock-Saxton J, Markwell S (eds) 1998 Women's health. W B Saunders, London.

Useful addresses

Association of Chartered Physiotherapists in Women's Health
c/o Chartered Society of Physiotherapy, 14 Bedford Row, London WC1R 4ED
Website: www.womensphysio.com

Association for Continence Advice
Astra House, Arklow Road, New Cross, London SE14 6EB
Email info@aca.uk.com
Website: www.aca.uk.com

Chartered Society of Physiotherapy
14 Bedford Row, London WC1R 4ED
Website: www.csp.org.uk

Continence Foundation
307 Hatton Square, 16 Baldwins Gardens, London EC1N 7RJ
Email continence.foundation@dial.pipex.com
Website: www.continence-foundation.org.uk

Enuresis Resource and Information Centre (ERIC)

34 Old School House, Britannia Rd, Kingswood, Bristol BS15 8DB
Email eneuresisompuserve.com
Website: www.eric.org.uk

InconTact
Email edu@incontact.demon.co.uk
Website: www.incontact.org

International Continence Society
ICS Office, Southmead Hospital, Bristol BS10 SNB
Email vicky@icsoffice.org
Website: www.icsoffice.org

NEEN Healthcare
Old Pharmacy Yard, Church Street, East Dereham, Norfolk NR19 1DJ
Tel 0362 698966; Fax 0362 698967
Email info@neenhealth.com
Website: www.neenhealth.com

Chapter **12**

Bowel and anorectal function and dysfunction

Jeanette Haslam and Jill Mantle

CHAPTER CONTENTS

Introduction 383
Normal bowel function 384
Bowel and anorectal dysfunction 388

Physiotherapy assessment of faecal incontinence
    and bowel dysfunction 402
Treatment for bowel and anorectal dysfunction 410

INTRODUCTION

It is encouraging that there is evidence of increasing professional interest in the neglected field of bowel and anorectal function and dysfunction (DoH 2000, 2001, Potter 2002). Up until now, despite the devastating effects of bowel and anorectal dysfunction, whether it be faecal incontinence due to failures in faecal storage or difficulties in emptying, the service for sufferers has been obscure and fragmented or even non-existent in some localities. In addition, physicians have not appreciated how common these dysfunctions are and sufferers have been understandably reluctant to admit to such problems (Johanson & Lafferty 1996). Further difficulties stem from widespread misconceptions as to what is normal (e.g. frequency of defaecation), and from the inappropriate use of laxatives without prior proper assessment. The field has not appealed to many researchers so the evidence base is weak and, as yet, there is no international standardisation of terminology of lower gastrointestinal tract function and dysfunction comparable with that for lower urinary tract function. Gradually terminology is being refined and some of the most useful definitions are included within the text of this chapter.

It is beyond the scope of this book to cover bowel and anorectal dysfunctions in childhood; however a helpful review is found in Norton et al (2002a).

PREVENTION

As ever, prevention is better than cure and, in this field, it begins with an appreciation of the wide range in normal function between individuals and even in the same individual over time. The traditional view that 'the bowels should be opened once a day' is not the case for many people, and many ordinary aspects of day-to-day living can affect an individual's normal habit (e.g. a change in the level of activity, a change in location, spicy foods, the menstrual cycle, the workplace). The education of parents would enable good childhood habits to be established and this aspect of a child's life to be facilitated and unobtrusively monitored without overemphasis. However, at any age, regular meals, a healthy diet, an unhurried environment that enables a person to obey a 'call to stool' and the availability of a private place to defaecate, which allows the person to adopt an individually suitable defaecation position, are all important.

The possibility of the side-effects of medication, resulting in bowel dysfunction, should always be considered by the prescriber. Where there is a possibility of problems arising, the patient should be warned and encouraged to report the fact if the effects become unacceptable. Some drugs are constipating (e.g. anticholinergics, opiates, iron supplements, non-steroidal anti-inflammatory drugs (NSAIDs)) and other medications cause diarrhoea (e.g. antibiotics). There is much health education needed in this area and health professionals would assist in this by routinely 'giving permission' to raise the matter by including appropriate questions in history taking. Bowel and anorectal dysfunction may occur in association with many pathologies such as stroke, Parkinson's disease and inflammatory bowel disease; but, in the absence of serious pathology, even quite minor and temporary reductions in mobility, or dexterity or both may adversely affect functional aspects of independent toileting, causing preventable problems.

NORMAL BOWEL FUNCTION

The anatomy of the lower digestive tract is described in Chapter 1. Food takes from 1 to 3 days to pass through the gut. It is propelled through by peristalsis and on the way digestion takes place; nutrients are absorbed into the bloodstream chiefly in the small intestines. Continence then depends on safe storage of the waste material in the colon and rectum, and appropriate voiding at a chosen time and place.

In a study of 838 men and 1059 women it was determined that a regular 24-hour cycle of defaecation was present in only 40% of men and 33% of women, with 7% of men and 4% of women having a regular two to three times daily bowel habit (Heaton et al 1992). Of more concern was the 1% of women who defaecated once a week or less. Women of childbearing age had a stool type shifted towards constipation in comparison with older women (Fig. 12.1). Normal (types 3 and 4) stool types that were least likely to induce symptoms were reported by only 56% of women and 61% of men. The study concluded that so-called 'normal' bowel function is present in less than half the population, with young women being the most adversely affected (Heaton et al 1992).

THE BRISTOL STOOL FORM SCALE

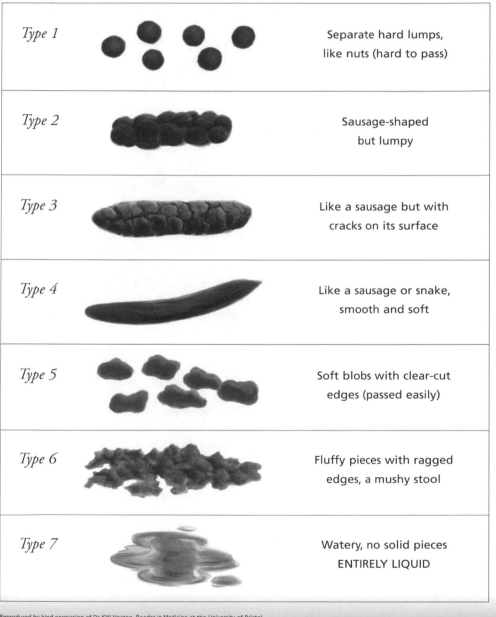

Type 1		Separate hard lumps, like nuts (hard to pass)
Type 2		Sausage-shaped but lumpy
Type 3		Like a sausage but with cracks on its surface
Type 4		Like a sausage or snake, smooth and soft
Type 5		Soft blobs with clear-cut edges (passed easily)
Type 6		Fluffy pieces with ragged edges, a mushy stool
Type 7		Watery, no solid pieces ENTIRELY LIQUID

Reproduced by kind permission of Dr KW Heaton, Reader in Medicine at the University of Bristol.
Produced by Norgine Limited, manufacturer of Movicol®

Figure 12.1   Bristol stool chart. (Reproduced by kind permission of Dr K W Heaton, Reader in Medicine at the University of Bristol; © 2000 Norgine Ltd.)

STORAGE

Residual material, the consistency of soup, is delivered to the colon where water is absorbed and the remainder formed into faeces. To a large extent the consistency of the final stools depends on how long the faecal material remains in the colon having water removed from it; that is, the longer material is in the colon, the dryer and harder is the stool. Finally the faeces are propelled into the rectum by periodic strong mass gut movements, ready for evacuation. These mass movements are triggered by the gastrocolic reflex, which is itself stimulated by eating and activity. Anal continence is maintained so long as the closure pressure at the anus is greater than that being produced by the periodic mass movements of the gut through the colon to the rectum. The initial sensation of the presence of stool in the rectum can be produced by as little as 11–68 mL and the maximal sensation at 250–510 mL. In those with normal compliance and sensation, rectal pressure begins to increase at about 300 mL.

The following factors contribute to the maintenance of anorectal continence:

- The resting pressure of internal anal sphincter (IAS) contributes 70–85% (Frenckner & Euler 1975; Lestar et al 1989) to the total resting pressure at the anus. The actual pressure exerted by the IAS varies with changes in position but the IAS is incapable of hermetically sealing the canal even at its maximum; the shortfall is made up by blood-filled cushions embedded within the canal wall (Lestar et al 1992). The distension of the rectum, caused by waves of rectal filling, elicits the rectoanal inhibitory reflex (RAIR) resulting in relaxation of the IAS. The upper portion of the IAS releases three or four times an hour to allow 'sampling' to take place. By this means a person with normal sensory discrimination in the rectum and anal canal will be able to tell whether there is flatus pressure that can be released without fear of soiling or whether there is liquid or solid material needing a toilet. This sampling mechanism is dependent on the RAIR being intact.
- The remainder of the resting closure pressure is contributed by the striated external anal sphincter (EAS). In addition the EAS reacts by reflex and increases its contribution in response to sudden rectal distension or rises in intra-abdominal pressure, or both, for example on standing or coughing. In addition the EAS can be contracted voluntarily to give added closure pressure when needed, for example in response to a 'call to stool' at an inconvenient time or place. This added pressure can be as much as twice the total resting pressure but can be maintained for only a relatively short time.
- The anorectal angle (Fig. 12.2), supported by the puborectalis muscle, produces a flap valve. The anorectal angle is normally between 60 and 105° but becomes less efficient if it is greater than this. Faecal material in the rectum may increase the angle.
- The vascular anal cushions.
- An intact nerve supply, both autonomic and somatic, sensory and motor.
- The cohesive contact of the moist rectal walls.
- The consistency of stool (i.e. soft yet formed but not liquid).

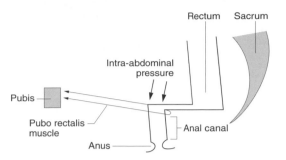

Figure 12.2 Diagrammatic representation of the anorectal flap valve.

- Normal activity of the colon, which is affected by diet, activity and absence of infection.
- The individual is cognitively intact, sufficiently mobile and able to go to the toilet independently.

DEFAECATION

The act of emptying the rectum is called defaecation or 'opening the bowels'. The normal frequency of defaecation varies substantially between individuals from three times a day to three times a week for 94% of the population (Drossman et al 1982). It has also been shown that women defaecate less often and less regularly than men (Heaton et al 1992). For most people the colon is quiet at night but the activity of getting up in the morning and having breakfast stimulates mass peristaltic movements propelling material, which may be solid, liquid or flatus, into the rectum. This may be accompanied by quite urgent sensations that the individual recognises as a 'call to stool'. The presence of material in the rectum causes the upper portion of the IAS to relax allowing 'sampling' to take place. If evacuation is inconvenient or impractical, defaecation can be deferred by repeated strong voluntary squeezes of the external anal sphincter, which has the effect of reversing peristalsis, returning faecal material to the rectum and colon, and facilitating a resumption of contraction of the IAS. The rectum and colon then relax and the sensation of needing to empty wears off. Defaecation can be delayed, but normally there will be reminders as the colon and rectum contract periodically. It must be appreciated that the longer material stays in the colon and rectum the more water is removed and the harder the stools become.

Once the decision to defaecate is taken, an acceptable site is found and clothing arranged; a sitting or squatting position is usually intuitively adopted, which widens the anorectal angle. Expert opinion recommends the position shown in Figure 12.3. The knees should be apart and higher than the hip joints; this may require the feet to be on a support such as a stool, telephone directories or upturned washing bowl. The trunk should be flexed forward at the hips supported on the forearms, *and with the neutral spinal curves maintained*. Where possible the heels should be raised. Physiotherapists will immediately appreciate the possible negative effect on defaecation of providing patients with raised toilet seats! Those providing raised toilet seats must assess this crucial aspect and where necessary seek solutions to avoid possible iatrogenic difficulties in evacuation.

Figure 12.3 Optimal defaecation position.

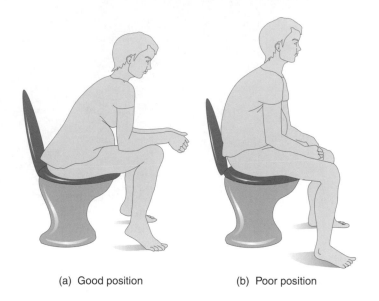

(a) Good position (b) Poor position

Where raised support for the feet is required, there is the obvious danger of the person falling over it when leaving the toilet.

If the call to stool has been urgent and considerable pressure generated by the mass movements of the gut, the IAS will have relaxed. Once the individual is in position, the pelvic floor musculature relaxes such that the floor descends 1–2 cm to the plane of the ischial tuberosities. This further increases the anorectal angle and the anal canal widens and shortens to become a funnel. If all is favourable, the EAS and puborectalis muscles will then release. Either evacuation will then occur without further effort as a result of peristalsis or it will be necessary for the person to produce a rise in intra-abdominal pressure (i.e. 'strain'). Sometimes a short rise in pressure 'to get things started' is all that is needed and peristalsis then takes over; at other times sustained, intense and repeated straining is required, particularly when the stool is hard and dry.

The raised intra-abdominal pressure utilised to assist defaecation is achieved by a complex coordination of trunk muscles, sometimes called 'brace and bulge' (Chiarelli & Markwell 1992); this combines breath holding, descent of the diaphragm, lateral widening of the waist with bulging of the lower abdomen, descent of the pelvic floor, and isometric activity in the pubo-, ilio- and ischiococcygeus muscles to give support to the rectum.

A full description of the importance of coordination between the abdominals, the pelvic floor musculature, diaphragm and multifidus can be found in Sapsford (2001) (see also p. 414).

Once emptying is complete, a closure reflex restores the involved structures to their storage mode and position.

BOWEL AND ANORECTAL DYSFUNCTION

Dysfunctions of the bowel, rectum or anus generally fall into two main groupings: one in difficulty in evacuating faecal material, the other in an inability to store flatus and/or faecal material reliably prior to evacuation at socially acceptable times and places. In a few conditions (e.g. irritable bowel syndrome (IBS)), the patient may alternate between the two states. Patients tend to call the first state constipation, and the second state, variously: farting, diarrhoea, 'messing' or soiling themselves.

SOME USEFUL DEFINITIONS

- *Anal incontinence* is the term used to describe the involuntary loss of flatus, liquid or solid per anus that is a social or hygienic problem.
- *Anismus* is the term used to describe incoordinate activity of anal sphincters and the levator ani muscles such that they fail to relax when defaecation is attempted.
- *Constipation* was generally defined as defaecating twice or less a week and was usually subjective because it relied on self-reporting. However, it became evident that the public frequently use the term to describe the need to strain to evacuate stool. The most recent definition (the Rome 11 criteria) has the support of an international consensus (Thompson et al 1999) and relies on self-reporting of more specific bowel-related symptoms. Functional (non-pathological) constipation is defined as including two or more of the following symptoms for at least 12 weeks in the last 12 months (not necessarily consecutive):
  - straining in >1/4 defaecations
  - lumpy or hard stools in >1/4 defaecations
  - sensation of incomplete evacuation in >1/4 evacuations
  - sensation of anorectal obstruction/blockade in >1/4 defaecations
  - manual manoeuvres to facilitate >1/4 defaecations
  - <3 defaecations per week.

NB Loose stools are not present, and there are insufficient criteria for IBS.

- *Descending perineum syndrome* is the term used to describe abnormal descent and bulging of the perineum associated with defaecation.
- *Dyschezia* is the term used to describe difficulty with rectal evacuation resulting from a long period of voluntary suppression of the urge to defaecate, and a distended rectum.
- *Faecal incontinence* is the term used to describe the involuntary loss of liquid or solid per anus.
- *Megacolon* is an abnormal massive dilation of the colon that may be congenital, toxic or acquired.
- *Megarectum* is an abnormal dilation of the rectum.
- *Paradoxical puborectalis contraction* is a problem of the puborectalis muscle failing to relax to allow defaecation.
- *Paradoxical anal sphincter contraction* is a problem of the anal sphincter failing to relax to allow defaecation.
- *Passive soiling* describes losing stool or liquid per anus without feeling the urge to defaecate.
- *Pelvic floor dyssynergia* describes uncoordinated pelvic floor muscle activity.

- *Proctalgia fugax* is the name given to sudden severe pain affecting the rectum lasting anything from minutes to hours. Attacks may occur days or month apart. The pain is probably caused by muscle spasm and there appears to be no structural disease.

PREVALENCE

Prevalence of constipation

As there has been a wide range of differences in the definition of constipation, it is difficult to define absolutely the prevalence of the condition. However, Thompson et al (1999) stated that constipation is persistent, difficult, infrequent or incomplete defecation, occurring in up to 20% of the population. They also stated that it is more common in women than men and increases with age. This was also shown in a large study of Australian women by Chiarelli et al (2000), who found a prevalence rate of 14.1% in women aged 18–23 years, 26.6% in women aged 45–50 years and 27% in women aged 70–75 years.

Prevalence of anal or faecal incontinence

The prevalence of anal or faecal incontinence is equally difficult to quantify because of the reluctance of sufferers to admit (Khullar et al 1998) to the problem or to report it to a doctor or researcher. There is also the wide variation in frequency and severity of episodes. The picture is further clouded by the fact that much of the research into prevalence has been conducted using samples of persons over the age of 60. Norton et al (2002a), in an analysis for the 2nd International Consultation on Incontinence, considered the available evidence to be level 2 and summarised the prevalence of anal continence thus: it increases with age but is present in all age groups and both genders, varying from 1.5% in children to 50% in nursing home residents.

In a USA community-based study (Roberts et al 1999), using a randomised sample of 762 women aged 50 or more, faecal incontinence was reported by 13.2% of those in their 50s and 20.7% of those of 80 or more. Severity and frequency of faecal incontinence is rarely mentioned in the literature, but in a study by Talley et al (1992) of 328 men and women aged 65–93 living at home, faecal incontinence more than once a week was reported by 3.7%. In addition Roberts et al (1999) found that, of those women with faecal incontinence, 59.6% also experienced urinary incontinence.

FACTORS CONTRIBUTING TO DIFFICULTIES IN DEFAECATION

Abnormal defaecation techniques

If a person has an uncoordinated defaecation pattern, there is a failure of anal relaxation with lowered levator ani while retaining sufficient rectal support; as a result, defecation will be difficult and will cause the person to strain.

There are a variety of types of uncoordinated defaecation pattern. For example, it is thought that intensive abdominal training, or expiratory effort (e.g. in a singer or wind instrument player), may lead to a rigid abdominal wall and to an abnormal pattern of uncoordinated defecation. This may result in a barrier to the diaphragm being able to descend against the abdominal contents to bulge the lower abdominal wall forwards. In addition, any inhibition about sitting on toilet seats can contribute to faulty defaecation postures. Sapsford et al (1996) showed that, during a correct simulated defaecatory pattern, the bulging of the lower abdomen and bracing of the lateral abdominals decreased the activity of the external anal sphincter; this will therefore assist defaecation. At rest the anus should be approximately two centimetres above the ischial tuberosities; this can be noted during the physical assessment of the patient. During defaecation the anus will descend to the level of the ischial tuberosities; however, if there is excessive perineal descent during defaecation, the rectum descends, the anus does not fully open and as a result the person is more likely to have to strain at stool to empty fully, contributing evermore to the likelihood of prolapsed organs. This descending perineum syndrome can also contribute to pudendal nerve stretching and eventual faecal incontinence (see p. 399).

Many women report that they use perineal pressure (perineal splinting) to effect bowel emptying. Gosselink & Schouten (2002) stated that pressure on the perineum stimulates the perineorectal reflex resulting in an increased rectal tone. This effect can be harnessed in those who are having problems with defaecation, although it was shown in the same study that the majority of those with obstructed defaecation ($n = 32$) had a significantly lower perineorectal reflex than controls ($n = 17$).

Women with a rectocoele often use digital posterior vaginal wall pressure to give support and assist rectal emptying, and others with severe constipation assist emptying by extracting stool with their fingers per anus.

(For further details regarding the correct defaecation technique see p. 413.)

Abuse

It is difficult to assess fully the frequency of abuse in the general population as it is often unreported and only few pursue their abusers to the courts. Women often suffer long-term effects of their abuse, which can be triggered into their conscious when attending for bladder or bowel dysfunction therapy. It is thought that an abnormal learned response may occur after sexual assault or abuse (Leroi et al 1995). This may show itself as anismus, paradoxical puborectalis contraction and pelvic floor dyssynergia on attempted defaecation as the pelvic floor muscles fail to release, although the initial examination may appear normal (Bruce & Sletten 2002). It is therefore essential to take a comprehensive history of the patient's condition and important to establish with every patient that they are giving full informed consent before performing any physical examination in the vaginal or anorectal area. However, many patients may not initially relate their previous abuse and therefore it is essential that an examination should be discontinued if there are any signs of mental or physical discomfort during any assessment. Expert opinion considers that if a person has suffered any sexual abuse then it is inappropriate for a physiotherapist to carry out any invasive examination or treatment. Women's health physiotherapists must be aware of the possibility of abuse and know to whom to refer the patient if there is any apparent need. They should not attempt to carry out any psychosexual counselling themselves unless they have had the appropriate specialist training.

Eating disorders

Many patients with eating disorders complain of constipation, often considering it their most incapacitating symptom (Mehler 1997). Anorectal abnormalities have been shown in patients with anorexia nervosa complaining of constipation (Chiarioni et al 2000). It was thought that the delayed colonic transit time was probably due to their abnormal eating habits. Chun et al (1997) showed that once anorexic patients consumed food and had a balanced weight gain or weight maintenance diet for at least 3 weeks, colonic transit returned to normal in the majority of patients.

Dykes et al (2001) showed that, in a group of 28 consecutive patients referred for biofeedback treatment for constipation, 60% had evidence of current affective disorder and 66% previous affective disorder; with 33% reporting a distorted attitude to food. The authors suggested that any patients presenting to surgical departments with chronic intractable constipation should be referred for a psychological assessment.

Binge eaters have also been studied and it was shown that obesity was associated with more frequent constipation, diarrhoea, straining and flatus whether or not the subjects reported binge eating (Crowell et al 1994).

Laxative abuse/overuse/dependence is also common in those with eating disorders suffering with constipation (Bruce & Sletten 2002). This group of patients, with a current eating disorder or history of a former eating disorder, or both, have often had a previous inpatient psychiatric episode of care and very low bodyweight.

Food and drink

Insufficient fluid intake has been suggested as a possible contributory cause to constipation. In one study, eight young men had, in randomised order, 1 week of 2500 mL of beverages per day, a week with less than 500 mL per day with a 1-week washout in between; the week of fluid deprivation (<500 mL) decreased stool frequency and weight (Klauser et al 1990). In older adults a low fluid intake has been associated with constipation (Robson et al 2000). It has also been shown by Brown et al (1990) that coffee (both caffeinated and decaffeinated) affects gut motility in some normal people; hot water had no effect.

Low calorie intake rather than low fibre consumption has been shown to be related to constipation in the elderly (Towers et al 1994). Muller-Lissner (1988) evaluated 20 papers on the effect of wheat bran on large bowel function. He found that bran increased the stool weight and decreased the transit time in healthy controls and in those with IBS, diverticula and constipation. However, those with constipation had lower stool output and slower transit regardless of whether they had taken bran and responded less well to bran treatment than controls. In the elderly it has been shown that a higher intake of bran was associated with greater faecal loading and no decrease in constipation symptoms (Donald et al 1985).

Anti et al (1998) looked at the effects of a high-fibre diet and fluid supplementation in patients with functional constipation with an age range of 18–50 years ($n = 117$). They found that a daily fibre intake of 25 g could increase stool frequency in those with chronic functional constipation; this could be significantly improved by a fluid intake of 1.5–2 litres per day.

It would therefore appear that different types and ages of patients could react differently to an increase in dietary fibre. The women's health physiotherapist should always treat patients individually when giving any advice regarding fluid and food intake. More specialised advice should be obtained from the dietician.

Ignoring the call to stool/workplace constipation

Polite society still considers it inappropriate to discuss bowel activity in general conversation. Therefore members of the general population have little or no awareness as to what may be considered normal bowel activity and even less understanding of how they can potentially harm themselves. If individuals continuously ignore the call to stool and delay defaecation over long periods of time they are inadvertently making constipation more likely. Physical activity levels have further decreased with the use of advancing technology, and many people are computer based using technology such as teleconferencing; a lack of physical activity is known to cause constipation.

Shift working can further affect the normal 'body clock' and normal habits become more difficult to retain. This can affect the nursing profession, the emergency services and all those who work alternate day and night shifts, from factory workers to air travel personnel. Many people can associate with this problem having suffered from 'holiday constipation' when change in time zones and dietary habits affect bowel activity.

Another possible workplace problem can be that of a lack of sufficient pleasant toilet facilities. Small cubicles that may be difficult for pregnant women or large people, irregular cleaning, poor ventilation, and lack of toilet paper, soap and towels all contribute to people putting off emptying their bowels during the working day. This can also apply to schoolchildren. Those people working 'on the move' such as district nurses, community midwives and salesmen are also at the mercy of whatever facilities are available. It has been shown that, in women attending a gynaecology clinic, 85% crouch over (rather than sit on) public toilet seats and 37% even crouch over the toilet seat in a friend's bathroom (Moore et al 1992); this is hardly conducive to bowel emptying when away from home.

There have also been changes in eating habits in recent years: long hours, fast foods, irregular eating, high levels of caffeine intake and highly processed foods – these can all compound the problem.

Irritable bowel syndrome

Irritable bowel syndrome (IBS) affects 10% of people, with a female predominance (Talley & Spiller 2002), and is the commonest functional gastrointestinal disorder. People with IBS can be divided into those who present with spastic constipation having abdominal pain related to bowel spasm, and those with painless diarrhoea complaining of stool frequency without abdominal pain. Most patients seem to report functional abdominal pain, which can be just as severe and disabling as organic pain (Moriarty 1999). The pain of IBS is most commonly felt in either the right or left iliac fossa or right hypochondrium, whereas pain of functional origin tends to be diffuse and may be anywhere in the abdomen or even outside it. Clinically patients report abdominal distension, pain relief with bowel movements, loose, frequent bowel movements or constipation, passage of mucus, excessive flatus, small volumes of pencil-like or 'rabbit' stools and urgency. Blood in the stools is *not* a symptom of IBS and should always be further investigated. Other symptoms can be in the form of back pain, dysmenorrhoea, dyspareunia, dysphagia, nausea and vomiting or the bladder symptoms of frequency, urgency, hesitancy, nocturia or incomplete emptying. This, accompanied by headache, poor sleep, tiredness, pruritus and halitosis, can lead to very unhappy patients. The syndrome is multifactorial in its causation. Silk (1997) considers the possible causes to include disordered motility, disordered sensation in the intestines, central nervous system involvement in the form of stress, anxiety or depression, gastrointestinal infection, antibiotics and diet. Visceral hypersensitivity is claimed by Talley & Spiller (2002) as being the key feature in most patients.

Treatment has to be appropriate to the presenting symptoms. This may include anxiety management for those with psychological disorders and drug therapy in the form of antispasmodic medication and antidiarrhoeal agents if appropriate. Some people require a combination of a laxative and an antidiarrhoeal drug with an antispasmodic drug or anxiolytic drug, or both (Moriarty 1999). Talley & Spiller (2002) further suggest that cognitive behavioural treatment, psychotherapy and hypnosis can be helpful in providing long-lasting benefit in some patients; also tricyclic antidepressants in low doses seem to be effective. Dietary manipulation has also been found to be helpful. In those with symptoms and having a low-fibre diet, an increase in fibre can be helpful, although the converse may be useful in those with symptoms and an existing high-fibre diet. General food intolerance is also reported by 75% of patients with IBS in that they complain of pain after eating. Intolerance to specific foods is also often reported (especially wheat and dairy products) but their role in the pathogenesis of the condition is debatable (Moriarty 1999).

Some people can suffer with IBS as a chronic relapsing disorder in which there is no apparent cure; however, 70% of cases of IBS are virtually symptom free 5 years after presentation (Moriarty 1999). There has also been discussion over whether there is a common aetiology between IBS and the irritable bladder (now known as the overactive bladder). Monga et al (1997) found that there is an irritable bladder associated with the IBS and supports the concept that IBS is part of a generalised smooth muscle disorder.

The women's health physiotherapist should always closely question any patients presenting with bladder or bowel dysfunction regarding their bowel activity, particularly if there have been any recent changes in this activity.

Megacolon and megarectum

Idiopathic megacolon and megarectum may be congenital or acquired. In megacolon the dilated segment shows normal phasic contractility but decreased colonic tone (von der Ohe et al 1994). Those with megarectum have increased rectal compliance with a maximal tolerable volume

(Hémond et al 1995). This is not believed to be a problem of sensation but rather one of the viscoelastic properties of the rectal wall. There may also be an absence or decrease of RAIR.

Menstruation

There have been several studies to investigate the often-reported increase of bowel symptoms premenstrually. Kane et al (1998) studied women with ulcerative colitis ($n = 49$), Crohn's disease ($n = 49$) and IBS ($n = 46$) and 90 healthy community controls. Premenstrual symptoms were reported by 93% of the total of women (most often in those with Crohn's disease). All disease groups had a more cyclical pattern to their bowel habits (diarrhoea, abdominal pain and constipation) than the controls. Moore et al (1998) concluded, in their systematic review, that one-third of otherwise asymptomatic women may experience gastrointestinal symptoms at the time of menstruation; whilst 50% of women with IBS report a perimenstrual increase in symptoms.

Gender has also been investigated, as more women are likely to suffer with IBS than men. Menstrual cycle symptoms were investigated and reported by Lee et al (2001). In this study of 700 people, three groups, all with IBS, were compared: 54 postmenopausal women, 61 premenopausal women and 54 age-matched men. Menstrual-cycle-related worsening of symptoms was reported by 40% of the women, but as there were few differences between pre- and postmenopausal women it was determined that the gender differences were unlikely to be attributable to the menstrual cycle.

Neurological conditions

Constipation can arise in many different neurological conditions. These include Parkinson's disease, multiple sclerosis and spinal cord injury. Any alteration to the normal somatic or autonomic control of the colorectal tract is going to have some effect on normal bowel activity. This can be an additional burden to those already suffering with a neurological condition and can cause them an increasing sense of helplessness. The women's health physiotherapist should have a holistic approach to treatment to optimise healthy function.

Pain associated with anal fissure

An anal fissure is a split or tear in the lining of the lowest part of the anal canal and may be caused by severe constipation or childbirth. Even though the fissure may be comparatively short in length (often less than 5 mm) it can be extremely painful and make life miserable. Each time the person attempts to open their bowels the fissure is stretched provoking acute pain and therefore causing great anxiety each time the person feels the call to stool. If the fissure heals itself it is said to have been an acute fissure; however, if the fissure becomes permanent it is said to be a chronic fissure, sometimes with the formation of a slightly swollen skin tag at the outer margin of the fissure.

Treatment of the chronic fissure is often by the use of glycerol trinitrate (GTN) cream, applied to the lower anal canal and anal margin to facilitate relaxation of the internal sphincter. However, sometimes the pain and bleeding returns after the treatment is discontinued. Calcium channel blockers have also been tried, applied topically or orally; Botox has been suggested although it is not in common use.

Surgery has been used with the aim of reducing anal canal pressure. The anal stretch has been widely used for over 170 years although surgeons are ever more concerned about any resulting sphincter damage that may result in anal incontinence; this may become more significant with advancing age. Sphincterotomy is also sometimes performed but again there is the attendant risk of ensuing anal incontinence. Postnatal fissures do not present as having high anal pressures and should therefore not have surgical intervention (Corby et al 1997).

Pregnancy and postpartum

Constipation and a feeling of bloating are common complaints of pregnancy. It has been reported as being present in 42% of multiparous women and 26% of primiparous women (Marshall et al 1998). This is due mainly to decreasing colonic peristalsis owing to the effect of progesterone on the smooth muscle of the gut. It has also been suggested that there is an increase in water absorption due to increased levels of aldosterone and angiotensin (Hytten 1990). In early pregnancy excessive nausea and vomiting are common and may result in a decrease of fluids passing through the digestive tract. As the pregnancy progresses the decrease in physical activity can affect colonic activity, as can the prescription of iron supplements. Diet may be adversely affected by food cravings in pregnancy and care must be taken to ensure that there is a healthy balanced diet with adequate dietary fibre. Dietary fibre supplementation has been studied by Anderson & Whichelow (1985). After 2 weeks' baseline observation, the two intervention groups were asked to take 10 g of dietary fibre supplement (corn-based biscuit or wheat bran) daily; the third group had no intervention. After 2 weeks of the intervention the number of bowel movements were increased with softer stool consistency in both intervention groups; there were no changes in the non-intervention group.

As the pregnancy develops the enlarging uterus and pelvic floor remodelling may also be contributory factors to defaecatory straining (Brubaker 1996). After delivery the common practice of giving codeine-based analgesia may exacerbate any existing problems with constipation. Pregnant women should be given relevant advice concerning a healthy diet during pregnancy. They should also be taught appropriate defaecation techniques and pelvic floor muscle exercise; this should then be reinforced postnatally.

Prolapse

A rectocoele is a herniation of the anterior rectal wall and the posterior vaginal wall into the vagina. This tear in the rectovaginal septum most commonly occurs above the attachment to the perineal body (Richardson 1993). According to its severity it may protrude through the vaginal introitus and may be associated with anterior vaginal wall defects or enterocoele, or both. Constipation and straining at stool has been thought to be a contributory factor to the formation of a rectocoele (Siproudis et al 1993).

Pelvic denervation, causing thinning of the septum posthysterectomy, is thought to contribute to the formation of rectocoeles. It is believed that a vaginal hysterectomy may put a woman at greater risk owing to the trauma of the transvaginal approach (Lawler & Fleshman 2002). Postmenopausal women may also have general tissue laxity that can contribute to the rectocoele.

Prolonged straining (bearing down/pushing) at childbirth – particularly in those women of certain collagen types – is also an implicating factor for rectocoele; this may also be in addition to constipation and straining at the stool during pregnancy. Spence-Jones et al (1994) have also shown that constipation in addition to obstetric history appears to be an important factor in the pathogenesis of uterovaginal prolapse.

Another possible factor to the formation of a rectocoele is in those patients with a paradoxical sphincter contraction who have resultant higher rectal pressures. A rectocoele can be relatively asymptomatic and not all such prolapses require surgery. However, many women need to give manual pressure on the posterior vaginal wall or on the perineum in order to effect rectal emptying.

Posterior colporrhaphy (see p. 315) corrects the rectovaginal wall defect in 76% of women. Where this is not the case it may even contribute to bowel and sexual dysfunction (Kahn & Stanton 1997). It is therefore appropriate for a women's health physiotherapist to see and advise all women having such surgery regarding pelvic floor muscle exercise and appropriate defaecation techniques.

Psychiatric disorders

It has been found that 27% of patients with major depression report the onset or worsening of constipation with the onset of the depression (Garvey et al 1990). Even higher rates have been found in other studies (Bruce & Sletten 2002). It must be remembered that anticholinergic medication to treat the depression can slow the transit time in the gut and exacerbate any pre-existing constipation. It may therefore be advisable to have selective seretonin reuptake inhibitors (SSRI) prescribed for depression if appropriate, as they do not affect bowel activity.

Anxiety disorders are also prevalent in those with constipation. These include defaecation rituals, bowel obsessions, obsessive–compulsive disorder, panic disorders and generalised anxiety disorder (Bruce & Sletten 2002). They may result in severe restrictions on food, prolonged time on the toilet, avoidance of social situations and a refusal to leave home until the bowels are opened; this can impose severe restrictions on everyday life.

The elderly

With increasing age there may be a decrease in mental function and mobility and an increase in anxiety and confusion. This, together with frailty and a decreased ability to chew food adequately, can lead to a change in dietary habits. A study of elderly ambulatory outpatients showed that those who ate fewer meals and had a lower calorie intake were more likely to suffer with constipation. Calorie intake seemed of greater importance than the consumption of dietary fibre (Towers et al 1994).

Dementia may result in a lack of heeding the urge to defaecate and constipation is one of the ways in which psychiatric illness can sometimes manifest itself. Physical illness such as diabetes may result in constipation owing to an autonomic neuropathy resulting in a slowed colonic transit time (Camilleri 1996).

The risk factors for constipation in the elderly are multifactorial according to Harari (2002); they include polypharmacy, anticholinergic drugs, opiate analgesia, iron supplements, calcium channel antagonists, NSAIDs, immobility, institutionalization, Parkinson's disease, diabetes mellitus, low fluid intake, low dietary fibre intake, dementia, depression and other psychological problems, spinal cord disease or injury, hypothyroidism, uraemia, hypokalaemia and hypercalcaemia. All of these factors should be considered in any elderly person presenting with constipation. It has been reported that it is the primary reason for hospitalisation in 27% of geriatric patients over the course of a year (Read et al 1985).

A further problem may be that of faecal impaction, also known as faecal loading or rectal loading; it is the severe stasis of hard or soft stool in the colon or rectum, or both (Potter 2002). The causes of the condition are unclear but it frequently becomes a problem in elderly patients in rehabilitation and continuing care wards (Barrett 2002). Faecal impaction with overflow incontinence is high in nursing homes; impaction with overflow is often found to be the underlying problem.

Dehydration occurs with long distance air travel; alcohol consumption compounds the problem. As previously stated, constipation has been associated with a low fluid intake in older adults (Robson et al 2000).

CONSEQUENCES OF CONSTIPATION

The failure to recognise or take action on the call to stool can result in other physiological problems. Many authors have reported problems with constipation; these include Koch et al (1997) reporting prolonged and excessive straining, also a need to use digital help to defecate. Camilleri & Szarka (2002) reported that constipation can lead to a feeling of incomplete emptying, abdominal cramping and pain, bloating, perineal pain and nausea. Further symptoms mentioned by Pemberton (2002) include anal pain, perineal descent causing additional problems with emptying, needing to use finger pressure on the perineum or posterior vaginal wall to empty the bowels and rectal prolapse. Constipation and faecal incontinence have also been implicated as contributors to urinary urge incontinence (Ouslander & Schnelle 1995). It is believed that the full rectum exerts pressure on the bladder, which can then trigger sensory urgency, urinary frequency and urge incontinence.

Other symptoms mentioned by constipated patients may include discomfort and pain in emptying the bowels, headache, skin problems and general malaise. It is also known that over a long period of time hard stools can irritate the bowel walls causing them to produce more fluid and mucus that can bypass the hard stool and then leak out. Also haemorrhoids are often associated with constipation and straining.

Constipation associated with delay in the call to stool, discomfort, pain and straining, once established, can severely affect quality of life.

Furthermore Leroi et al (1999) found that 28% of women investigated for urinary incontinence also have anal incontinence with an association with constipation.

Psychological problems

These can also result from constipation. It has been long been known that stress affects bowel function (Drossman et al 1982) and that depression and eating disorders can also be related to constipation. It has been shown that the general well-being of people with constipation is lower than that of the general population (Glia & Lindberg 1997). Therefore stress in the workplace can be part of the downward spiral from an occasional problem to one of chronic constipation and all the other possible problems associated with it. The vicious circle of bad food habits and bad toileting habits may lead to increased anxiety. It may result in a misguided person refraining from eating and drinking on the day of an important meeting owing to fear of needing the toilet, which will only make matters worse. Asbury & White (2001) state that increasing stress can cause many other symptoms. These include:

- *physical symptoms* of muscle tension, palpitations, a churning stomach and fatigue
- *emotional symptoms* of irritability, worry and less enthusiasm for life
- *cognitive symptoms* of poor concentration, indecisiveness and memory changes
- *behavioural symptoms* of agitation, lethargy and poor sleep.

FACTORS CONTRIBUTING TO ANAL INCONTINENCE

Any lack of control of flatus or stool, however temporary or minor, is very unnerving and stressful. At its least severe, there may be loss of flatus in company with the risk of telltale sounds and smell; at its most devastating there is uncontrolled complete emptying of the bowel with little or no warning and in an inappropriate place. The chief adverse factors to continence are those that may contribute to the likelihood of the anal sphincters being overwhelmed (e.g. age, anal sphincter damage, liquid stool). However, the picture is sometimes complicated by the patient's ability to adapt and find ways of compensating for deficits in specific physiological mechanisms by using other biological and behavioural means to maintain continence.

Age

Research shows that resting anal closure pressure and maximum squeeze pressure decline with age and there is an age-dependent increase (particularly in women) in the pressure needed to produce an initial sensation of rectal filling and to trigger the RAIR (Akervall et al 1990). There is also an age-related increase in perineal descent at rest, which would increase the anorectal angle, and a slowed pudendal nerve conduction rate (Jameson et al 1994). This means that the elderly will be more at risk of incontinence of flatus and stool regardless of other factors.

Anal sphincter dysfunction

There is clear evidence that physical disruption of the integrity of either or both of the anal sphincters or the immediate adjacent tissues may jeopardise continence (Kalantar et al 2002). This may occur as a result of childbirth, perianal surgery (e.g. for an anal fissure, fistula or haemorrhoids), forced unwanted anal intercourse or accidental injury. Damage to the external sphincter tends to present as urgency or urge incontinence because the control once the IAS has relaxed is impaired. Damage to the IAS presents as incontinence of flatus or passive soiling (even the passing of solid stool), often following defaecation or on activity, because closure of the IAS for the next storage phase is compromised. Anal sphincter dysfunction may also result from nerve damage or cumulative stretching.

Childbirth   At vaginal delivery, physical damage may occur to the external or internal anal sphincter, or both, as a result of a perineal tear or an episiotomy which extends from vagina to the anus. If the sphincter is involved in any way, the lesion should be classified as a 'third degree tear'. Sultan (1999) has recommended three subdivisions of third degree tears and these have been incorporated into the Royal College of Obstetricians and Gynaecologists guideline no. 29 (RCOG 2001). However, it is now known that occult disruption of one or other sphincter may occur without visible damage, and this is thought to be due to shearing of tissue during labour. Sphincter injuries are more common in primipara, and other associated risk factors include a large baby, forceps delivery, prolonged second stage and occipitoposterior presentation (Sultan et al 1994). Specialist training is required for obstetricians and midwives with respect to examination to detect sphincter disruption, and postpartum repair should be undertaken by an expert in an operating theatre where the light is good (MacLean & Cardozo 2002). Endoanal ultrasound has proved invaluable in detecting and assessing anal sphincter disruption (see p. 409).

Surgery   There has been considerable concern regarding possible iatrogenic damage to the sphincters that can occur as a result of anal surgery (Nelson 1999), for example anal stretch, sphincterotomy or haemorrhoidectomy. Kelly et al (1998) reported a substantial decrease in maximum squeeze pressure following hysterectomy in those who also had multiple vaginal deliveries. Deterioration in bowel function posthysterectomy was also shown by van Dam et al (1997). Of the women in the study ($n = 531$), 59% indicated normal defaecation prior to the hysterectomy; after surgery 31% reported severe deterioration and 11% mentioned a moderate change. The most common symptom of which women complained was severe straining.

Accidents   Damage can also result from accidents (e.g. road traffic accidents), and from abusive or unwanted (rape) penetrative sexual activity. In the latter case, a small study ($n = 7$) by Engel et al (1995) showed that all had IAS damage and three had additional EAS disruption.

Trauma   Trauma to the nerve supply to the anal sphincters or the perineum, or both, as a result of tears, episiotomy or traction on the pudendal nerve during childbirth, may reduce anal sphincter function in the short or long term. Jameson et al (1994) showed that increased parity correlates with decreased squeeze pressure.

Habitual chronic straining at the stool

This may permanently stretch the perineal connective and muscle tissue resulting in descending perineal syndrome. This stretching may damage the nerve supply to the sphincters or the pelvic floor muscles, or both; straining predisposes to haemorrhoids, which may reduce the efficiency of the sealing capability of the closure mechanism, and can even result in rectal prolapse. The stretched perineum cannot give the normal support to the rectum and anus and the lower position of the perineum allows an increase in the anorectal angle. An association between excessive perineal descent and hysterectomy has been reported (Karasick & Spettell 1997). All these possibilities are able to compromise continence.

Liquid stool

Diarrhoea is the term used to describe very frequent bowel evacuation or the passage of very loose watery, poorly formed stools, or both. However, research suggests (Talley et al 1994) that patients use the term variously so it should be interpreted very cautiously. Liquid stool is associated with faecal incontinence (Kalantar et al 2002). The commonest cause is an infection, viral or bacterial, which is usually contracted from infected food or water. The use of laxatives, which stimulate the activity of the gut, can result in material being propelled so quickly through the intestines that there is insufficient time for absorption of water or for stool formation. A number of drugs cause diarrhoea in some people as a side-effect (e.g. some drugs for gastric and duodenal ulcers, hypertension, antibiotics and iron preparations). Women's health physiotherapists should refer to the British National Formulary if concerned.

Patients with certain subtypes of IBS (see p. 393) experience diarrhoea as a result of abnormal contractions of the intestinal musculature and heightened sensitivity to stretching or distension. The cause is as yet unknown and there is no detectable structural disease. The condition is exacerbated by stress and anxiety, and may follow intestinal infection. Sufferers of any condition which results in inflammation and ulceration of segments of the intestinal tract (e.g. Crohn's disease, ulcerative colitis, tumours or radiation enteritis) may experience episodes of diarrhoea.

Patients with faecal impaction (see p. 398) may well present with leakage of stool and apparent diarrhoea but in fact it is due to the impacted material in the rectum stimulating the RAIR, which allows the softer more liquid material from higher up the intestinal tract to leak round and past the impacted material in the rectum, and out through the anus.

Functional faecal incontinence

This term covers all faecal incontinence resulting from failure to reach an appropriate place to defaecate in time, in the absence of any of the factors discussed above. Leaders at children's camps sometimes find children who have 'messed' themselves because they were afraid to go out to the toilets in the dark or could not open the door, etc. Accident and emergency health professionals would do well to consider this aspect of care for patients waiting for hours for diagnoses and treatment for even quite simple traumas like Colles fracture or sprained ankle.

The women's health physiotherapist must ensure that the faecal incontinence is not arising from an inability to achieve toilet transfers, from a lack of adequate mobility and balance, that patients are able to manage their own clothing, especially underclothing, and have adequate manual dexterity to be able to cleanse themselves. The environmental factors to be taken into consideration include: toilet and bed heights, toilet location, clear and unambiguous gender signposting, lighting and flooring, accessibility and adequate manoeuvring space, the bed and the bedding, clothing and footwear, medication and fluids taken, eyesight and hearing, orientation and any help available if needed.

Occupational therapists are members of the multiprofessional team concerned with the functional care of patients; they are experts on matters of functional incontinence. It may be appropriate to refer a patient to occupational therapy for a functional home assessment; this may then result in the provision of appropriate toileting aids, appliances and clothing adaptations.

PHYSIOTHERAPY ASSESSMENT OF FAECAL INCONTINENCE AND BOWEL DYSFUNCTION

HISTORY

When a patient is referred with any symptoms of faecal incontinence or other bowel dysfunction the history taking is an essential requirement prior to any physical examination or treatment. It is crucial that the assessor builds up a good rapport with patients in order to gain their confidence so they are able to relate what may be most distressing symptoms. It is therefore important to establish with patients a mutually understood vocabulary such that there is no misunderstanding regarding the information imparted. Patients may or may not have had investigations prior to the referral; it is therefore essential that the women's health physiotherapist can recognise anything that could be a symptom of more serious underlying pathology. If patients disclose that they have any rectal bleeding, blood or mucus in their stool, rectal pain or a recent change of bowel habit, looser stools or more frequent defaecation, they should be referred back to the appropriate medical person; whether the GP or referring consultant.

There are certain advantages to having a routine questionnaire in that it can be logical in approach and ensure that nothing is forgotten. Reilly et al (2000) found in an American study that a self-administered questionnaire had a greater sensitivity than a standard physician interview. It is thought that people may find it easier to write down responses and are less embarrassed by answering questions on paper. The success of any such self-completed questionnaire will also depend on the literacy level of the patients and the clarity of the questions.

It is useful to send a bowel habit diary to patients prior to them attending for treatment to determine their bowel activity over an average week. There needs to be simple, clear instructions on any such form. An example is shown in Figure 12.4.

It is often helpful to use diagrams and pictures with patients to ensure that they have fully understood what is being told to them regarding bowel function and to determine such matters as their stool type (see Fig. 12.1).

Name: .... **Date of birth:** ....

Please complete the form and bring it with you to your appointment on ....

	Time of bowel movement/s	Consistency: e.g. pellets, soft, hard, pencil thin, diarrhoea etc.	Did you reach the toilet in time? Yes/no	Did you soil your underwear/ pad? Yes/no	Any blood or mucus? Yes/no	Other comments
Monday						
Tuesday						
Wednesday						
Thursday						
Friday						
Saturday						
Sunday						

Figure 12.4 Bowel habit diary.

The initial assessment should ascertain what patients perceive the problem to be, how long they have had the problem for, whether there seemed to be any predisposing event, if the symptoms have changed over time and if they have any of the following symptoms:

- Do they ever pass blood or see blood or mucus in their stools?
- Do they ever have pain before or during opening their bowels?
- How often do they open their bowels and have there been any recent changes?
- What is the stool consistency (use the Bristol stool chart, Fig. 12.1)?
- Have they any symptoms of faecal urgency and for how long are they able to defer?
- Are they having any faecal loss, is it liquid or solid and are they aware of it happening; how often is it happening and how much is lost?
- In what circumstances do they experience the loss?

- Can they control flatus and can they discriminate between flatus, solid and liquid?
- Do they ever have difficulty emptying their bowels; do they strain, use perineal pressure, vaginal pressure or need to empty their bowels manually?
- Do they wear any pads or appliances and how much help are they?
- Do they have/have they had haemorrhoids?
- Do they ever feel a heaviness or anything protruding from the anus or vagina?
- Do they ever strain to empty their bowels?
- In what position do they empty their bowels?
- Do they feel that they completely empty?
- Do they ever experience any abdominal bloating?
- Do they use a lot of toilet paper to cleanse the anal area?
- Do they ever have any skin soreness or other skin problems in the anal region?

General information will need to be gained regarding their height and weight, occupation, usual physical activities that they wish to pursue and family attitudes to the problem. An obstetric history (including birthweights, length of second stage, interventions and perineal trauma), gynaecological history (complaints and treatment), urinary symptomology (see Ch. 11) and surgical history should all be pursued. The medication history (past and present) is of particular importance, especially any use of laxatives, antimotility drugs or any medication that can have either a loosening or drying effect on the stools. It is also useful to ascertain what their normal diet is. The best way to discover this is to provide patients with a simple food diary to show their daily food intake (Fig. 12.5). Questioning regarding past medical history should also include any history of depression and the medication taken and any previous referrals for bowel problems, treatment and outcomes.

As it has been shown that both caffeine (Brown et al 1990) and nicotine (Scott et al 1992) can affect the motility of the gut, patients should also be asked about their smoking and fluid intake history. Quality of life is often affected by bowel dysfunction; it is therefore important to ascertain how much their bowel problem is affecting their everyday life and relationships. The Faecal Incontinence Quality of Life Scale (FIQLS) has been developed, tested and psychometrically evaluated for the assessment of patients with anal incontinence (Rockwood et al 2000).

As bowel problems can occur as a consequence of physical and sexual abuse, the examiner must be acutely aware as to the sensitivities of asking any questions about such matters. A general question such as 'has anybody ever done anything to your body that you were unhappy with?' may be sufficient for them to relate details of abuse that they have previously felt unable to relate. Examiners must take great care not to tender any advice that they are unqualified to offer. However, a listening ear and knowing the appropriate person to whom to make a referral is often all that is needed. Knowledge of any sexual abuse is important owing to the invasive nature of anorectal assessment. Informed consent is essential

FOOD DIARY

Name: ....   Hospital number: ....

Please complete during a normal week all that you eat and drink over a period of 7 days. Note the times of the food and drink and indicate any bowel problems that you experienced on that day

	Breakfast	Lunch	Evening meal	Fluids (type and volume)	Other snacks	Bowel problems on the day
Monday						
Tuesday						
Wednesday						
Thursday						
Friday						
Saturday						
Sunday						

Figure 12.5   Food diary.

before any such examination and sexual abuse can be considered a contraindication to penetrative examination or treatment. Even if there is no history of sexual or physical abuse the patient may have other sexual dysfunction.

The severity of the faecal incontinence may be assessed by the use of a rating scale such as that proposed and validated by Vaizey et al (1999), and a constipation scoring system as proposed by Agachan et al (1996) can be used to assist diagnosis of constipation.

PHYSICAL EXAMINATION

Any physical examination of a person with bowel dysfunction should commence with observation of the patient's gait and posture. Inspection of the lower back may reveal evidence of spina bifida occulta, which could be associated with a congenital neurological defect. After the history taking, informed consent must be gained prior to any physical examination. All infection control protocols in operation in the clinic must be adhered to throughout the examination and treatment.

It is advisable to adhere to the standards for intimate examinations that were proposed by the General Medical Council Standards Committee (2001). These include:

- Explain why an examination is necessary and give an opportunity for the patient to ask questions.
- Explain what the examination will involve in language that the patient will understand.
- Obtain permission prior to the examination, record this and be prepared to discontinue the examination if asked to do so.
- Keep discussion relevant and avoid unnecessary personal comments.
- Offer a chaperone or invite patients (in advance) to have a friend or relative present if they wish. If a chaperone is declined the discussion and its outcome should be recorded.
- Give the patient privacy to undress and dress, with appropriate drapes to maintain dignity.
- Do not assist in removing clothing unless requested to do so.

An abdominal examination should be undertaken with the patient in supine lying to detect any surgical incisions and the presence of any abnormal masses including a full bladder. It should be determined that the patient has not got any latex allergy before proceeding with any examination wearing latex gloves. If there is a latex allergy, appropriate non-latex gloves should be worn.

A neurological assessment will include testing the S4 dermatome by testing the perianal region, asking patients if they can feel both sides equally. The S3 dermatome is checked by sensory testing of the upper two-thirds of the inner surface of the thigh and S2 by checking of the lateral surface of the buttock, lateral thigh, posterior calf and plantar heel. If there is any suspicion of any neurological involvement it is also necessary to check the appropriate myotomes:

- hip flexors (L2–L3)
- adductors (L2–L4)
- peronei/tibialis anterior (L4–L5, S1)
- gluteus medius and minimus (L4–L5, S1)
- gluteus maximus (L5, S1–S3)
- gastrocnemius and soleus (S1–S2)
- toe abductors (S3).

An anorectal examination usually takes place with the patient in left side lying. However, it must be remembered that a person may feel embarrassed when having an anorectal examination and this may provoke spasm of the anal sphincters and glutei (Jones & Irving 1999). Patients should have a clean or disposable sheet provided to lie on, with a clean/disposable sheet to cover them. They should have had the full procedure described to them and be talked through each step as it takes place. The physiotherapist should cease the examination if there are any verbal or body language signs of discomfort or unhappiness with it. The basis of the anorectal examination is shown in Table 12.1.

After the anorectal examination is completed the patient should be covered, and the examiner removes her gloves away from the patient and disposes of them in an appropriate yellow clinical waste bag. The patient should be given privacy to dress whilst the examiner records her findings. After the examination, the findings should be discussed with the patient and a treatment plan determined.

Table 12.1 Anorectal examination of the patient with bowel problems

Examination	Procedure
Visual assessment of the perianal skin	• Observe any signs of gaping, soiling, excoriation, haemorrhoids, skin tags, fissure, congenital abnormalities, redness, rashes or sores
Perineal examination	• Note any signs of scars from an episiotomy or tears, also the length of the perineum
	• Observe any movement of the perineum and anus on bearing down, also when instructed to contract the anal sphincter
Posterior vaginal wall	• Observe any signs of prolapse on rest or strain
Ischial tuberosities	• Consider the relationship of the ischial tuberosities to the anus at rest and at strain
Anorectal examination	
Introduction	• Apply gentle pressure with a gloved, well-lubricated finger on the posterior anal verge, insert the finger in an anterocephalic direction whilst the patient is breathing out, and then curl the end digit of the finger over the puborectalis
	• Note any presence of stools and their consistency
Puborectalis	• Puborectalis can be palpated to determine if there is altered sensation
	• Ask the patient to contract the puborectalis, note the response, the muscle movement (in an anterior direction) and grade the muscle using the modified Oxford scoring scale (see p 357)
	• Ask the patient to bear down and confirm (or otherwise) that the puborectalis relaxes
Anal sphincter	• Withdraw the finger so that the index finger pad can palpate the anal sphincter to detect any scar tissue or other abnormalities
	• Grade the anal sphincter activity when asked to contract the sphincter
Determine an exercise programme as appropriate	• Whilst palpating, determine the hold time, the type and number of contractions that are appropriate for the patient to be practising several times each day
If there are suspicions of rectal prolapse	• Examine the patient in an upright position

INVESTIGATIONS

Anorectal manometry

'Anorectal manometry' subsumes the possibility of conducting the following diagnostic tests which are useful in the assessment of patient complaining of constipation or faecal incontinence or both, that is: (1 resting anal canal pressure, (2) anal canal squeeze pressure – both peal and duration, (3) the RAIR using a balloon to distend the rectum, (4) ana canal pressure in response to coughs, (5) anal canal pressure in response to attempts to defaecate, (6) simulated defaecation in response to balloon distension, (7) compliance of rectum in response to balloon distension and (8) sensory thresholds in response to balloon distention (Azpiros et a 2002). It is carried out using an anal probe to which an inflatable balloon can be fitted.

The actual measurement of anal pressure is dependent on the equipment that is being used. The resting pressure in the anal canal is mainly (70–80%) due to activity in the IAS; this pressure can be doubled by an active EAS contraction. Therefore if the resting pressure is not doubled on active contraction it suggests that there is an EAS problem. In clinical practice a patient may have symptoms of urgency, an inability to get to the toilet in time and also, possible difficulty with expulsion of the faeces owing to a general lack of pelvic floor muscle (PFM) support during defaecation. The assessor must be aware that various artefacts can influence anal manometry, including squeezing of the gluteal muscles.

The RAIR is concerned with the IAS relaxing in response to rectal distension via the enteric system within the rectal wall. This reflex is essential for the sampling mechanism and for normal defaecation to take place. The testing of the RAIR is by a balloon being inflated in the rectum, usually to 20 mL or greater whilst the anal sphincter pressure is being monitored. Initially there is a brief contraction of the EAS but this is then followed by a prolonged relaxation of the IAS.

Rectal sensation can be assessed by a balloon being placed in the rectum and it being inflated with air at a rate of approximately 25 mL/s. It is noted when patients first feel a sensation, when they feel a call to stool and when this becomes a feeling of severe urgency. The normal volumes are considered to be approximately 40 mL of air at first sensation, 80 mL at feeling of need to defaecate and 120 mL for severe urgency. This test is considered to be subjective and will provide only a rough idea of sensitivity. Very low volumes detected suggest hypersensitivity and high volumes undetected suggest some sensory impairment.

Colonic transit studies

Radiological transit studies can be a useful tool in the evaluation of severely constipated patients. They can be carried out by the ingestion of radio-opaque different-shaped and different-sized markers on different days, followed by abdominal X-rays on several days afterwards to track the markers' progression. The studies cannot be carried out if a woman is pregnant or if there is bowel obstruction. A full description of the method can be found in Metcalf (1995).

It has been reported that the rectal tone after a meal is absent or blunted in patients having obstructed defecation with prolonged transit times (Gosselink & Schouten 2001a).

Concentric needle EMG

Electromyography detects electrical activity in a muscle. A concentric needle can determine the amount of activity in about 20 motor units in the vicinity of its tip in the EAS and puborectalis during an active contraction, at rest and on bearing down (when the sphincters and puborectalis should relax).

Defaecating proctogram

The defaecating proctogram is concerned with the fluoroscopic evaluation of rectal emptying. The barium paste is introduced rectally and the evacuation observed during radiography. It can be used to assess the anorectal angle, descent of the pelvic floor and prolapse (including rectocoeles). A full description of evacuation proctography can be found in Bartram & Halligan (2002).

Endoanal ultrasonography (EAUS)

EAUS enables clinicians to visualise and detect accurately defects of both the IAS and EAS. It is a simple procedure using an anal probe that patients generally find acceptable. The 360° rotating ultrasound transducer is placed in the anal canal and is used to gain an image of the subepithelium and both the IAS and EAS. It can detect any damage to the sphincters so that an accurate diagnosis and treatment may be carried out. As experience accumulates it is giving valuable assistance in the selection of patients, particularly postpartum, who may benefit from prompt sphincter repair, either sphincteroplasty (i.e. overlapping of the two ends) or apposition of the two sides. Sadly results of surgery are rarely perfect, many patients have residual symptoms and some may develop new evacuation disorders (Malouf et al 2000a). Further details of transrectal ultrasound imaging of the pelvic floor can be found in Khullar (2002).

Magnetic resonance imaging (MRI)

MRI provides high-resolution images in multiple planes and may be used to evaluate the pelvic floor. However, it is expensive, limited to static studies and mainly considered a research tool. A study by Malouf et al (2000b) compared the use of MRI and anal endosonography in patients with faecal incontinence. They determined that the methods are equivalent in diagnosing EAS injury but MRI is inferior in diagnosing IAS injury.

Pudendal nerve terminal motor latency (PNTML)

A special device is placed intra-rectally with its tip directed to the pudendal nerve where it travels around the ischial spine on one side or the other. There are two electrodes on the device, one at its tip and one at the level of the anal sphincter. Current is passed through the tip electrode and a measurement taken at the other electrode where it detects activity in the anal sphincter. The test is repeated on both sides. The time that it takes for the pulses to pass down the nerve and make the muscle contract is known as the nerve latency. Less than 2.2 ms is considered normal; longer than 2.2 ms indicates some nerve damage. The test is not carried out during pregnancy or if a cardiac pacemaker is in situ.

Real–time ultrasound

Translabial or transperineal real-time ultrasound is being increasingly used as an assessment and biofeedback tool. It enables the practitioner to observe not only the cranioventral direction of bladder neck movement during PFM contraction, but also the movement of the puborectalis on contraction and bearing down. The probe can also be placed abdominally to detect any associated transversus abdominis contraction. As yet there is little or no research-based evidence on its use in bowel dysfunction, but it looks as though it may be a worthwhile but expensive tool.

Strength duration curves

The assessment of the neural innervation of skeletal muscles by the use of strength duration curves was previously common practice for physiotherapists. In more recent times Monk et al (1998) have investigated and proposed the use of the strength duration curve for assessment of the EAS in conjunction with anal manometry for the investigation of faecal incontinence. Further work has been reported (Mills et al 2002) in which the strength duration curve was compared with other methods of diagnostic anorectal testing (manometry, rectal sensation, EMG, PNTML and endoanal ultrasound). It was shown that the strength duration curve of the EAS significantly correlates with established methods of EAS function and its innervation. Therefore the strength duration curve of the EAS can be a simple measure to show EAS denervation.

TREATMENT FOR BOWEL AND ANORECTAL DYSFUNCTION

DIET

Prior to any therapy it is essential to determine the type (see Fig. 12.1) and frequency of the stool. In the case of infective diarrhoea, rectal bleeding, blood or mucus in the stools or a recent change in bowel habit, medical advice must be immediately sought.

If none of these is present, it may be that appropriate dietary modification is all that is necessary. Appropriate soluble and insoluble fibre should be part of a well-balanced diet including five pieces of fruit or portions of vegetables per day. It is believed that prebiotics, which are non-digestible carbohydrates that stimulate the growth of desirable bacteria in the gut, and probiotics, which are supplements of 'friendly' bacteria, help the colonic bacteria to maintain normal digestion. There is no clear evidence to support their use, but they appear to be without side-effects and work well in some patients. Good food sources of prebiotics are bananas, asparagus, garlic, wheat, tomatoes, onions, chicory and Jerusalem artichokes. Probiotics are usually bought as live bacteria added to foods, drinks and yoghurts (e.g. Actimel, Yakult, Bio yoghurts).

It should always be checked that any patient suffering with any bowel or anorectal dysfunction is consuming appropriate types and volumes of fluids. It is generally recommended that approximately 1.5 litres (3 pints) of fluid a day are appropriate. This may increase according to the patient's level of activity; it is best assessed by looking at the patient's fluid output (ideally about 1.5 litres). Alcohol can affect people's bowels in different ways, therefore a food and drink diary is of some importance in ascertaining any effect.

Caffeine also seems to act as a bowel stimulant, therefore it is sensible to recommend a gradual decrease in caffeine (to avoid caffeine withdrawal symptoms) to anyone with symptoms of frequency, urgency and loose stools. It has also been reported that milk products and artificial sweeteners can make the stools looser, whereas arrowroot biscuits, marshmallow sweets or very ripe bananas can help to make stools firmer in some people (Norton 2002).

BOWEL RETRAINING

A regular habit of bowel emptying is often helpful. This can be retrained by a regular healthy diet and toileting 20–30 minutes after a meal or warm drink, especially breakfast, to utilise the gastrocolic response. If it becomes apparent that the call to stool takes place in a particular part of the day then appropriate planning can be made.

Bowel retraining may be necessary for those suffering with bowel frequency and urgency. St Mark's Hospital advocates a four-stage 'holding on' programme (full details obtainable on the internet at www.bowelcontrol.org.uk) in which patients are given the following instructions:

- Sit on the toilet and hold on for as long as you can. Whatever you can manage double it and double it again aiming for 5 minutes.
- When you have mastered this, try holding on for 10 minutes (something to read may be helpful).
- When able, try to hold on for 5 minutes whilst in the bathroom but not sat on the toilet.
- When able to hold on for 10 minutes away from the toilet, move further away from the bathroom.

However, sitting on the toilet may excite the reflexes associated with bowel emptying and people may find they spend the longest time on achieving stage one.

MEDICATION

It may be that the drugs that a person is taking for other conditions are causing a problem of constipation. These drugs include anticholinergics, diuretics, oral iron supplements, sympathomimetics, antacids, antihypertensives and NSAIDs (Emmanuel 2002). It is therefore always worthwhile to ask the GP to review the medication being taken in those suffering with constipation.

However, it may be necessary for a patient to take some form of medication to assist in manipulating the stool consistency to one that is easier both to contain and to expel, also perhaps to stimulate increased peristalsis. The expenditure on laxatives in the UK was reported as being £43 billion by Petticrew et al (1999). It is therefore of great importance that, when it is necessary, the appropriate laxative is used. However, it was also stated in the same study (Petticrew et al 1999) that the reviewed laxative trials have serious methodological shortcomings.

Constipation

Medication may be necessary as part of the treatment of constipation; it is important that the different types of laxative are understood and how they are effective. They have the possible serious side-effects of hypokalaemia (an insufficient amount of potassium in the bloodstream), and an atonic non-functioning colon (Downie et al 1995). The types of medication can be considered in the groups of those that act as a bulking agent, those that act as a stimulant, osmotic laxatives and faecal softeners.

Bulking agents

These include:

- ispaghula husk – Fybogel, Isogel, Regulan
- methylcellulose – Celevac
- sterculia – Normacol.

These absorb water and increase the bulk and weight of the stool; this water is not absorbed in the intestine. They may take a few days to work and cause flatulence, bloating, or crampy abdominal pain. It is most important that the patient should drink sufficient fluids to avoid intestinal obstruction. Bulking agents should not be used in elderly people with atonic bowels. Natural bran is no longer recommended as it can affect the absorption of minerals such as iron and calcium.

Stimulants

These include:

- senna – Senakot, Manevac
- bisacodyl – Dulcolax
- docusate sodium – Dioctyl, Docusol
- glycerol suppositories
- sodium picosulphate.

These stimulate peristalsis and hence intestinal motility with decreased fluid reabsorption and are used when a more rapid reaction time (8–12 hours) is needed. They should only be used in the short term as long-term use can result in atony of the bowel and electrolyte disturbance with laxative use/constipation/laxative use becoming a vicious circle. They may cause griping abdominal pain.

Osmotic laxatives

These include:

- lactulose
- polyethylene glycol (PEG) – Movicol.

These agents reduce the absorption of water from the bowel; this water retention in the stool softens it, increases its bulk and stimulates peristalsis. Adverse effects can include abdominal pain and flatulence. Osmotics may be used when stimulants and bulking agents have failed. A study by Attar et al (1999) showed that PEG (Movicol) was more effective than lactulose, and better tolerated. There was less flatus reported with a higher mean frequency and less straining at stool in the PEG group.

Faecal softeners   These include:

- arachis oil (**NB** not to be used with anyone with any peanut allergy)
- docusate sodium – Docusate, Docusol, Dioctyl.

These preparations aim to lubricate and soften the stool. They can be given as a retention enema but should be used with caution in case of any intestinal obstruction.

Faecal incontinence

Faecal incontinence can be influenced by the stool consistency. It may be necessary to take appropriate medication to thicken the stool.

Antimotility drugs   These include:

- loperamide (Imodium)
- codeine phosphate.

These drugs reduce peristalsis and gastrointestinal motility by stimulating the opioid receptors in the bowel. They can have the adverse effect of constipation. Loperamide has the additional advantage of having a direct effect on the anal sphincter causing an increase in anal sphincter pressure (Read et al 1982).

Absorbents   These include agents such as kaolin. They absorb water without increasing stool bulk, making the stool firmer and smaller.

Antispasmodics   These include preparations such as Mebeverine. Bowel motility is decreased by a reduction of the peristalsis taking place. Anticholinergic drugs are often used in the treatment of the painful spasm that can be experienced in IBS.

Topical agents   It has been reported that application of 10% phenylephrine gel to the anus produces a significant rise in the resting anal pressure in healthy human volunteers (Carapeti et al 1999).

Oestrogen replacement therapy   A pilot study of 20 postmenopausal women with demonstrable faecal incontinence showed a possible benefit of oestrogen replacement for this group of women (Donnelly et al 1997).

PHYSIOTHERAPY FOR BOWEL AND ANORECTAL DYSFUNCTION

It is essential to carry out a detailed appropriate assessment of any patient presenting for treatment for bowel and anorectal dysfunction. It is then necessary to give advice as appropriate and to build up a good patient–therapist interaction. The advice should include appropriate advice regarding defaecation technique, exercise and diet (see p. 410).

Defaecation technique

Effective defaecation is that in which patients have sufficient warning, can delay if necessary, get to the toilet easily, sit comfortably and evacuate with minimal effort and without harm to themselves. This involves coordinated activity between the somatic and autonomic nervous systems to cause contraction in smooth muscle and both contraction and relaxation in striated muscle. The aim is to have rectal contraction with sphincter and puborectalis relaxation, whilst maintaining levator tone to provide rectal support. At the same time, respiration and posture can impinge on the effectiveness for full emptying. It has been known for some time that the forward-lean posture can affect the anal aperture and anorectal angle. The abdominal muscles coordinated with the diaphragm create an increase in intra-abdominal pressure to assist in completing the defaecation.

The Australian physiotherapists Chiarelli & Markwell (1992) did much to popularise the technique for good defaecation dynamics involving sitting with forearm support on the knees, feet resting on the floor, the throat closed, and diaphragm moving down together with a lower abdominal 'brace and bulge'. The word brace means to make the waist wide and bulge to let the abdominals bulge anteriorly. The instructions were those of: 'brace, open out and grunt'. The 'pump brace technique' was advocated to retrain those people who strained to empty their bowels; involving bracing and opening out three or four times in succession, always remembering to contract the anal sphincter at the completion of defecation to reactivate the storage reflexes.

Markwell & Sapsford (1995) published the rationale and reasoning for using the technique to maintain the rectal support whilst releasing the anal outlet with sufficient expulsion to be effective. They described it as being necessary to give the patient a full explanation before commencing training, so that the patient then assumes the correct position for retraining:

- sitting on a chair
- feet supported on a footstool of approximately 15 cm with heels raised
- hips flexed to more than 90°
- the weight of the upper trunk supported on the forearms, resting on the abducted thighs
- neutral spinal curves.

The action was then described as:

- lateral bracing with brief 1–2 second holds and sustained 10–20-seconds holds
- anal release facilitated by lower abdominal bulging
- practice of the combination of bracing and bulging.

Markwell & Sapsford (1998) further describe how the forward-lean sitting position results in the anterior shift of the abdominal contents. The lowering diaphragm pushes the abdomen out and lengthens the rectus abdominis with an isometric hold in its outer range such that puborectalis is then able to release and anal shortening and widening result. It is also believed that diaphragmatic breathing with the breath held with the diaphragm low will assist the defaecation pattern (Chiarelli 2002).

In summary, the women's health physiotherapist should be aware of and assess for the following in any patient with the problem of disordered defaecation:

- posture for effective defaecation – forward lean, neutral spine, forearms resting on abducted thighs, knees higher than hips, heels may be raised
- breathing patterns – diaphragmatic
- abdominal activity during a simulated defaecation – brace and bulge
- pelvic floor activity during bearing down – anal relaxation with rectal support
- return to normal sphincter activity after evacuation.

The correct patterns of movement and positioning should then be taught as necessary. Adaptations may need to be considered for the elderly or those with disability.

Anal sphincter exercise

The EAS and puborectalis are both under somatic control and contribute to the faecal continence control mechanism. Appropriate exercise can therefore improve faecal continence status. However, exercise must be associated with appropriate lifestyle changes where necessary. This includes attention to stool consistency, diet and general exercise, and defaecation training to prevent straining at the stool.

It is first necessary to ensure that the appropriate action is taking place; this is best done by an anorectal examination (see p. 406) but if this is not possible the external signs of puckering and inwards drawing of the anus can be used to assess an appropriate sphincter exercise programme.

Initially it may be an advantage to instruct the patient to sit resting back in the chair (for proprioception of the posterior pelvic floor) with knees slightly apart. The instructions are those of squeezing as though to stop passing wind or stool, and lifting the sphincter off the chair, whilst continuing with normal breathing. There may be further activation by giving the instruction to try the same whilst reducing foot pressure on the floor (but *not* attempting to lift the feet completely off the floor). Once the person has localised the anal sphincter muscles they should then be trained in the same way that other pelvic floor muscles are trained (see Ch. 11). This will include strong holds of maximal length, longer contractions of approximately half the maximum hold for endurance and finally fast contractions. There must always be adequate rest periods depending on the muscle grade and ability. As the patient becomes able, the length and number of contractions are increased and the rest periods shortened. Chiarioni et al (1993) showed that a squeeze of at least 20 seconds is necessary to control faecal urgency when there is more liquid stool.

Instructions to the patient for self-checking can include using a mirror for observation, or feeling a lift of the anal sphincter away from an examining finger.

It is generally found that exercising three times a day is both possible and sufficient to achieve muscle improvement. Concentrated effort is necessary initially, but sphincter exercises must then be incorporated into activities of daily living. It is therefore necessary to practise the exercises in functional positions as well as in sitting. Although there has been no research looking at employing 'the knack' for faecal incontinence, it would seem sensible to advise patients to contract their anal sphincter with their entire pelvic floor muscles when doing any activities that increase intra-abdominal pressure.

Biofeedback

Any women's health physiotherapist who is embarking on the use of biofeedback therapy for either faecal incontinence or constipation is advised to seek training in the practical administration of such from a recognised clinician. Although the present evidence is not robust and does not show an overwhelming benefit from biofeedback, there are many patients seen clinically to whom biofeedback can be a great motivator and challenge to effect improvement. The biofeedback may be via an anal pressure probe or EMG surface electrodes, either intra-anally or externally on the anal sphincter.

Constipation

Biofeedback training for constipation may be of help in some patients. If a paradoxical puborectalis contraction is discovered at the initial anorectal assessment, digital proprioceptive biofeedback may be given to increase patient awareness. However, this distorts the anal sphincter and may be embarrassing for the patient.

After the patient has been given full instructions regarding defaecation technique (see p. 413) some clinicians have found it useful to place small (paediatric) surface electrodes around the anal sphincter at approximately 2 o'clock and 10 o'clock. Initially the patient is asked to observe both contraction and relaxation of the sphincter on a monitor. Then the patient whilst sitting on a commode is asked to simulate defaecation (using the correct technique) whilst observing the anal sphincter EMG activity on the monitor. The aim is to regain the ability to relax the anal sphincter appropriately, whilst maintaining activity in the more lateral levator ani to give rectal support. Alternatively a pressure probe may be used, which may detect the increase or decrease in pressure from puborectalis; however, the use of any probe will distort the anal sphincters. In a study of 26 patients, Glia et al (1997) found that biofeedback using either manometry or surface EMG was effective in improving the symptoms and anorectal function caused by a paradoxical puborectalis contraction.

Faecal incontinence

Norton & Kamm (2001a) systematically reviewed 46 studies published in English that used biofeedback to treat adults complaining of faecal incontinence. It was difficult to evaluate the results as the studies had many variables concerning type of biofeedback and exercise. However, they concluded that the results suggest that biofeedback and exercises help the majority of patients with faecal incontinence.

Norton et al (2002b) further investigated four groups of patients reporting faecal incontinence. Group A received standard medical and nursing care advice, group B advice plus instructions on anal sphincter exercises, group C additional hospital-based computer-assisted biofeedback for five sessions, and group D all of the before-mentioned treatments plus the use of a home EMG biofeedback device. All groups had an increase of anal pressure at rest and on squeeze and increased endurance. The important finding of the study was that the patient–therapist interaction together with coping strategies were of the greatest significance. These benefits were maintained 1 year after treatment.

A study using augmented biofeedback for those suffering with obstetric trauma was reported by Fynes et al (1999). In this study 40 women with anal obstetric injury resulting in impaired faecal continence were randomly assigned for 12 weeks to either a 30-minute session of sensory biofeedback using a Peritron perineometer, or a 35-minute session for augmented biofeedback utilising an Incare PRS 9300 system for both visual EMG biofeedback and stimulation at 20 Hz and 50 Hz. Both groups were instructed to practise pelvic floor muscle exercises daily. Significant improvement was found in both groups but the results in the augmented therapy group were superior to those in the sensory biofeedback group.

Massage for constipation

It has been suggested that abdominal wall massage may be a therapeutic effective treatment for those with chronic constipation. It has been suggested that abdominal massage may: encourage peristalsis, release spasm, relieve flatulence, precipitate bowel opening, may be used in retraining bowel function, is safe, non-invasive and can be performed as self-massage or by a carer (Richards 1998). There has been description in the literature of its use with 32 institutionalised adults having severe disability (Emly et al 1998); it was found to be as effective as laxatives within that environment. Richards (1998) further describes abdominal massage being used to good effect in a mixed group of 10 patients (ages 4–63) with a variety of conditions from IBS to multiple sclerosis. Each participant in the study received at least 35 massage treatments over a 7-week period. It was suggested that such treatment reduces the use of laxatives and is therefore both beneficial to the patient's well-being and cost effective.

However Klauser et al (1992) studied nine constipated patients (aged 63–73 years) and seven healthy volunteer subjects (aged 26–28 years) with a 3-week treatment phase (with nine sessions) and a control phase. They found that the healthy volunteers and patients did not differ significantly during the control and massage periods.

The lack of scientific evidence from large studies in the general constipated population means that at present the practitioner cannot necessarily anticipate successful outcomes from abdominal massage. However, it is easily learnt and is both generally safe and non-invasive, provided that the contraindications to abdominal massage, such as cancer of the bowel, any abdominal herniation or recent abdominal surgery or scarring, are all heeded (Richards 1998).

Massage technique

Before any massage takes place the environment must be conducive to relaxation and the patient positioned in a comfortable position.

Emly (1993) describes a five-part technique taking about 15–20 minutes that she used for a 21-year-old cerebral palsy patient, with olive oil as a couplant:

1. stroking from the stomach to the groin to encourage initial relaxation
2. when relaxation is felt, effleurage along the colon starting in the right iliac fossa and then travelling along the ascending, transverse and descending sections of colon
3. following the effleurage strokes by circular kneeding along the line of the colon in the same direction as previously
4. more effleurage as previously
5. side-to-side stroking across the abdominal wall.

Massage should never be a therapy employed in isolation, but rather be part of a general management plan for the underlying constipation. As recent abdominal surgery is a contraindication to massage of the abdomen, appropriate abdominal exercise postsurgery may be utilised. Other massage 'equipment' has also been reported as being used in spinal units, such as a tennis ball being abdominally rolled along the length of the colon for self-massage (Richards 1998).

Neuromuscular stimulation

Electrical stimulation has been used for many years as a method of re-education of muscle by raising cortical awareness, normalising reflex activity and having a direct affect on the muscle stimulated. However, a Cochrane review by Hosker et al (2003) concluded that at present there is insufficient evidence to draw reliable conclusions on the effect of electrical stimulation for the treatment of faecal incontinence. They reported that there is a suggestion that stimulation may have a therapeutic effect but that this is not certain.

If a patient is assessed to have a low voluntary anal squeeze on examination and exercise does not seem to be leading to any improvement, it may be appropriate to consider a course of stimulation by a home treatment unit preferably for daily use or attendance for clinic-based therapy. It is proposed that an anal electrode should be used to ensure that maximal stimulation can take place, but care must be taken as the anal mucosa is often more sensitive than the vaginal mucosa (Laycock 2002). As it is generally the EAS and posterior pelvic floor compartment that is undergoing treatment, it is appropriate to use a frequency of 35–40 Hz with a pulse duration of 250 μs with a non-fatiguing duty cycle (depending on the patient's ability).

Rectal sensitivity training

If there is a problem with reduced sensation to rectal filling, sensitivity training is used to re-educate the contraction of the EAS in response to rectal distension. This can be achieved by using a simple device: a rectal balloon attached to a plastic tube with a three-way tap to enable air to be introduced by a syringe. A condom covers the balloon and proximal tube to ensure good infection control and assist in the removal of the device.

The patient is in side lying whilst the balloon is introduced into the rectum, then air or water is introduced via the syringe until the patient reports the threshold sensation. The air/water is then removed and the patient instructed to contract the anal sphincter strongly as soon as a similar rectal sensation is felt when the air/water is reintroduced. It has been suggested that sympathetic afferent nerves are stimulated by fast distension and parasympathetic afferent fibres stimulated by both slow and fast distension. Therefore clinicians often repeat the infilling at different speeds of introduction of the same volume of air/water with the patient concentrating on contracting the anal sphincter each time a sensation is felt. However, Gosselink & Schouten (2001b) have shown that rectal sensory perception is blunted or absent in the majority of patients with obstructed defaecation. They further suggest that this may be due to deficient parasympathetic nerves; also, as no patients in their study experienced a non-specific sensation in the lower abdomen or pelvis during fast distension, it was also thought that the sympathetic innervation may also be deficient. They therefore concluded that different distension protocols are unnecessary in patients with obstructed defaecation. However, many clinicians still tend to use different filling speeds and progress to this being repeated with the patient in more functional positions (standing, or sitting on a commode). The aim is for the patient to gradually recognise smaller volumes of air/water. These volumes should be recorded at each attendance.

In a study by Chiarioni et al (2002) using sensory retraining, 24 patients with solid stool incontinence at least once a week were treated with three to four sessions of biofeedback. They were taught to squeeze the anal sphincter voluntarily in response to rectal balloon distention. Thirteen patients became continent and four were substantially improved.

If a rectum is 'overactive', similar sensory training can be used with gradually increased volumes being introduced whilst the patient is asked to contract the sphincter and 'hold on'.

There are also systems available whereby an anorectal-measuring device with two pressure chambers may be used with a computer that allows two pressure screens to be used at once. The deeper-lying chamber measures rectal pressure, whilst the other chamber is positioned at the level of maximal pressure of the anal sphincters. A small amount of air is introduced into the anal sphincter pressure chamber to detect any changes in the sphincter pressure. Air can then be introduced into the rectal pressure chamber and changes in sphincter activity noted. There may be a small increase in sphincter pressure (EAS contraction) as the air is first being introduced; this is then followed by a fall in sphincter pressure (i.e. IAS demonstrating RAIR); this should then be followed by a gradual return to baseline sphincter pressure. The patient may need to be retrained by instruction to contract the EAS. The aim of the training is to increase the awareness of the patient to rectal distension and to be able to take appropriate action to avoid any anal incontinence. It is recommended that any women's health physiotherapist embarking on more complicated anorectal therapy should attend a recognised clinician to observe and undergo supervised practice.

Anal plugs

Disposable anal plugs and tampons have been designed to help control intractable faecal incontinence by obstructing the anal canal; they are inserted into the upper part of the anal canal and removed to allow defaecation. The majority of patients (14/20) in a study by Norton & Kamm (2001b) could not tolerate the discomfort caused on an everyday basis despite finding the plugs generally effective. It seems possible however, that such devices are useful on an occasional basis in order to cope with special circumstances (e.g. a social event).

Anal cones

Specially designed cones for anal incontinence are available via the internet. However, there is no research literature to back up their efficacy.

Skin care and body odours

Sore skin in the anal region is a common problem for those suffering from anal incontinence owing to the effects of faeces on the skin in the area. Some people have problems with properly wiping the area and leaving a residue behind; others can have faecal seepage, especially of liquid stool. Immobility and inactivity make the problem worse. Advice will comprise of using soft toilet paper or moist wipes (avoiding any with an alcohol base) or moist cotton wool, always wiping from front to back, and washing after a bowel movement whenever possible (portable bidets are available, or a jug with warm water or plant spray can all be useful), then gently patting dry. Strongly perfumed soaps, bath foams, disinfectants or antiseptics, talcum powder or deodorants should be avoided. It is also desirable to wear cotton underwear and avoid tights (unless crotchless). Synthetic fibre, tight clothing and biological detergents are also best avoided and great care should be taken in rinsing underwear thoroughly after washing. It is also advisable to avoid creams unless specifically advised to use them; the stoma nurse or continence advisor will often be the person to advise on appropriate creams, skin barriers or barrier wipes. If a continence pad is used, it must be changed at the first sign of soiling. If the anal area does become sore it is sensible to have some time each day when air can circulate in the area. If there is skin irritation it is essential that the patient is instructed to resist the urge to scratch.

There are useful suggestions from St Mark's hospital to be found on the internet at the site www.bowelcontrol.org.uk/tips. These include:

- Unpleasant smells in the bathroom or elsewhere can be counteracted by striking a match.
- Some people also find help in reducing flatus and its smell by ingesting charcoal tablets, mint tea, fennel tea, aloe vera capsules or juice, Yakult drink, Acidophilus or indigestion remedies such as Rennies.
- The use of aromatherapy burners, pot-pourri and air fresheners is a matter of personal taste. However some are obtainable specifically to neutralise unpleasant odours.

A SUMMARY OF THE TREATMENT OPTIONS FOR FAECAL INCONTINENCE

Whitehead et al (2001) reported the results of a consensus conference on the treatment options for faecal incontinence. A summary of their consensus statement is as follows:

- Diarrhoea is the commonest aggravating factor and antidiarrhoeal medication may help; faecal impaction is a common cause of diarrhoea in children and the elderly and it responds to a combination of laxatives and habit training in 60% of cases.

- In those who fail medical management or have evidence of sphincter weakness, anorectal manometry and endoanal ultrasound are recommended in helping to differentiate structural defects from neurological injuries.
- Biofeedback is a harmless and inexpensive treatment, which benefits 75% but cures only 50%, and is possibly more beneficial where there is partial denervation.
- External anal sphincter plication (with or without pelvic floor repair) is effective in about 68% of cases where there is known, repairable structural defect.
- Electrically stimulated gracilis transpositions or colostomy should be reserved for those who cannot or do not benefit from other options.
- Other options include implanted nerve stimulators, artificial sphincters and anal plugs.

References

Agachan F, Chen T, Pfeifer J et al 1996 A constipation scoring system to simplify evaluation and management of constipated patients. Diseases of the Colon and Rectum 39:681–685.

Akervall S, Nordgren S, Fasth S et al 1990 The effects of age, gender, and parity on rectoanal functions in adults. Scandinavian Journal of Gastroenterology 25(12):1247–1256.

Anderson A S, Whichelow M J 1985 Constipation during pregnancy: dietary fibre intake and the effect of fibre supplementation. Human Nutrition – Applied Nutrition 39(3):202–207.

Anti M, Pignareto G, Armuzzi A et al 1998 Water supplementation enhances the effect of high fiber diet on stool frequency and laxative consumption in adult patients with functional constipation. Hepatogastroenterology 45(21):727–732.

Asbury N, White H 2001 Don't make me laugh. How to feel better about living with a weak bladder. Northumbria Healthcare NHS Trust Journal:9–62.

Attar A, Lémann M, Ferguson et al 1999 Comparison of a low dose polyethylene glycol electrolyte solution with lactulose for treatment of chronic constipation. Gut 44:226–230.

Azpiros F, Enck P, Whitehead W E 2002 Anorectal functional testing: review of collective experience. American Journal of Gastroenterology 97(2):232–240.

Barrett J 2002 Pathophysiology of constipation and faecal incontinence in older people. In: Potter J, Norton C, Cottenden A (eds) Bowel care in older people. Research and practice. Clinical Effectiveness Unit, Royal College of Physicians, London, p 5–22.

Bartrum C I, Halligan S 2002 Coloproctology and the pelvic floor – imaging. In: Pemberton J, Swash M, Henry M M (eds) The pelvic floor. Its function and disorders. W B Saunders, London, p 186–212.

Brown S R, Cann P A, Read N W 1990 Effect of coffee on distal colon function. Gut 31:450–453.

Brubaker L 1996 Rectocele. Current Opinion in Obstetrics and Gynecology 8:376–379.

Bruce B K, Sletten C D 2002 Psychological aspects of pelvic floor disorders. In: Pemberton J H, Swash M, Henry M M (eds) The pelvic floor. Its function and disorders. W B Saunders, London, p 441–456.

Camilleri M 1996 Gastrointestinal problems in diabetes. Review. Endocrinology and Metabolism Clinics of North America 25:361–378.

Camilleri M, Szarka L A 2002 Constipation. In: Pemberton J H, Swash M, Henry M M (eds) The pelvic floor. Its function and disorders. W B Saunders, London, p 313–329.

Carapeti E A, Kamm M A, Evans B K et al 1999 Topical phenylephrine increases anal sphincter resting pressure. British Journal of Surgery 86:267–270.

Chiarelli P, Markwell S 1992 Let's get things moving. Gore & Osment, Sydney, p 56–60.

Chiarelli P, Brown W, McElduff P 2000 Constipation in Australian women: prevalence and associated factors. International Urogynecology Journal 11:71–78.

Chiarelli P E 2002 Constipation. In: Laycock J, Haslam J (eds) Therapeutic management of incontinence and pelvic pain. Springer, London, p 143–150.

Chiarioni G, Scattolini C, Bonfante F et al 1993 Liquid stool incontinence with severe urgency: anorectal function and effective biofeedback treatment. Gut 34(11):1576–1580.

Chiarioni G, Bassotti G, Monsignori A et al 2000 Anorectal dysfunction in constipated women with anorexia nervosa. Mayo Clinic Proceedings 75(10):1015–1019.

Chiarioni G, Bassotti G, Stanganini S et al 2002 Sensory retraining is the key to biofeedback therapy for formed stool fecal incontinence. American Journal of Gastroenterology 97(1):109–117.

Chun A B, Sokol M S, Kaye W H et al 1997 Colonic and anorectal function in constipated patients with anorexia nervosa. American Journal of Gastroenterology 92(10):1879–1883.

Corby H, Donnelly V S, O'Herlihy C et al 1997 Anal canal pressures are low in women with postpartum anal fissure. British Journal of Surgery 84:86–88.

Crowell M D, Cheskin L J, Musial F 1994 Prevalence of gastrointestinal symptoms in obese and normal weight binge eaters. American Journal of Gastroenterology 89(3):387–391.

DoH (Department of Health) 2000 Good practice in continence services. DoH, London.

DoH (Department of Health) 2001 National service framework for older people. DoH, London.

Donald I P, Smith R G, Cruikshank J G et al 1985 A study of constipation in the elderly living at home. Gerontology 31:112–118.

Donnelly V, O'Connell P R, O'Herlihy C 1997 The influence of oestrogen replacement on faecal incontinence in postmenopausal women. British Journal of Obstetrics and Gynaecology 104:311–315.

Downie G, Mackenzie J, Williams A 1995 Pharmacology and drug management for nurses. Churchill Livingstone, London, p 55–70.

Drossman D A, Sandler R S, McKee D C et al 1982 Bowel patterns among subjects not seeking health care. Using a questionnaire to identify a population with bowel dysfunction. Gastroenterology 83(3):529–534.

Dykes S, Smilgin-Humphreys S, Bass C 2001 Chronic idiopathic constipation: a psychological enquiry. European Journal of Gastroenterology and Hepatology 13(1):39–44.

Emly M 1993 Abdominal massage. Nursing Times 89(3):34–36.

Emly M, Cooper S, Vail A 1998 Colonic motility in profoundly disabled people. Physiotherapy 84(4):178–183.

Emmanuel A 2002 The use and abuse of laxatives in older people. In: Potter J, Norton C, Cottenden A (eds) Bowel care in older people. Research and practice. Royal College of Physicians, London, p 77–88.

Engel A F, Kamm M A, Bartram C I 1995 Unwanted anal penetration as a physical cause of faecal incontinence. European Journal of Gastroenterology and Hepatology 7(1):65–67.

Frenckner B, Euler C V 1975 Influence of pudendal block on the function of the anal sphincters. Gut 16(6):482–489.

Fynes M M, Marshall K, Cassidy M et al 1999 A prospective randomised study comparing the effect of augmented biofeedback with sensory biofeedback alone on fecal incontinence after obstetric trauma. Diseases of the Colon and Rectum 42:753–761.

Garvey M, Noyes R, Yates W 1990 Frequency of constipation in major depression: Relationship to other clinical variables. Psychosomatics 31(2):204–206.

General Medical Council Standards Committee 2001 Online. Available: www.gmc-uk.org/standards/intimate.htm.

Glia A, Lindberg G 1997 Quality of life in patients with different types of functional constipation. Scandinavian Journal of Gastroenterology 32:1083–1089.

Glia A, Gylin M, Gullberg K et al 1997 Biofeedback retraining in patients with functional constipation and paradoxical puborectalis contraction. Diseases of the Colon and Rectum 40:889–895.

Gosselink M J, Schouten W R 2001a The gastrorectal reflex in women with obstructed defecation. International Journal of Colorectal Disease 16(2):112–118.

Gosselink M J, Schouten W R 2001b Rectal sensory perception in females with obstructed defecation. Diseases of the Colon and Rectum 44(9):1337–1344.

Gosselink M J, Schouten W R 2002 The perineorectal reflex in health and obstructed defecation. Diseases of the Colon and Rectum 45(3):37–36.

Harari D 2002 Epidemiology and risk factors for bowel problems in older people. In: Potter J, Norton C, Cottenden A (eds) Bowel care in older people: research and practice. Clinical Effectiveness Unit, Royal College of Physicians, London, p 23–45.

Heaton K W, Radvan J, Cripps H et al 1992 Defecation frequency and timing, and stool form in the general population: a prospective study. Gut 33:818–824.

Hémond M, Bédard G, Bouchard H et al 1995 Step by step anorectal manometry: small balloon tube. In: Smith L E (ed) Practical guide to anorectal testing. Igaku-Shoin, New York, p 136–137.

Hosker G, Norton C, Brazzelli M 2003 Electrical stimulation for faecal incontinence in adults (Cochrane review). In: The Cochrane Library, Issue 2. Update Software, Oxford.

Hytten F 1990 The alimentary system in pregnancy. Midwifery 6:201–204.

Jameson J S, Chia V W, Kamm M A et al 1994 Effects of age and parity on anorectal function. British Journal of Surgery 81(11):1689–1692.

Johanson J F, Lafferty J 1996 Epidemiology of fecal incontinence: the silent affliction. American Journal of Gastroenterology 91(1):33–36.

Jones D J, Irving M H 1999 Investigation of colorectal disorders. In: Jones D J (ed) ABC of colorectal diseases. BMJ Books, London, p 4–7.

Kahn M A, Stanton S L 1997 Posterior colporrhaphy: its effect on bowel and sexual function. British Journal of Obstetrics and Gynaecology 104:82–86.

Kalantar J S, Howell S, Talley N J 2002 Prevalence of faecal incontinence and associated risk factors: an under-diagnosed problem in the Australian community? Medical Journal of Australia 176(2):54–57.

Kane S V, Sable K, Hanauer S B 1998 The menstrual cycle and its effect on inflammatory bowel disease and irritable bowel syndrome: a prevalence study. American Journal of Gastroenterology 93(10):1867–1872.

Karasick S, Spettell C M 1997 The role of parity and hysterectomy on the development of pelvic floor abnormalities revealed by defecography. American Journal of Roentgenology 169(6):1555–1558.

Kelly J L, O'Riordain D S, Jones E et al 1998 The effect of hysterectomy on anorectal physiology. International Journal of Colorectal Disease 13(3):116–118.

Khullar V 2002 The role of imaging. In: MacLean A B, Cardozo L (eds) Incontinence in women. RCOG Press, London, p 76–90.

Khullar V, Damiano R, Tooz-Hobson P et al 1998 Prevalence of faecal incontinence among women with urinary incontinence. British Journal of Obstetrics and Gynaecology 105(11):1233–1234.

Klauser A G, Beck A, Schindlbeck N E et al 1990 Low fluid intake lowers stool output in healthy male volunteers. Gastroenterology 28(11):606–609.

Klauser A G, Flaschentrager J, Gehrke A et al 1992 Abdominal wall massage: effect on colonic function in healthy volunteers and in patients with chronic constipation. Zeitschrift für Gastroenterologie 30(4):247–251.

Koch A, Voderholzer W A, Klauser A G et al 1997 Symptoms in chronic constipation. Diseases of the Colon and Rectum 40(8):902–906.

Lawler L P, Fleshman J W 2002 Solitary rectal ulcer, rectocele, hemorrhoids and pelvic pain. In: Pemberton J H, Swash M, Henry M M (eds) The pelvic floor. Its function and disorders. W B Saunders, London, p 358–384.

Laycock J 2002 Treatment. In: Laycock J, Haslam J (eds) Therapeutic management of incontinence and pelvic pain. Springer, London, p 136–137.

Lee O Y, Mayer E A, Schmulson M et al 2001 Gender-related differences in IBS symptoms. American Journal of Gastroenterology 96(7):2184–2193.

Leroi A M, Berkelmans I, Denis P et al 1995 Anismus as a marker of sexual abuse. Consequences of abuse on anorectal motility. Digestive Disease Science 40:1411–1416.

Leroi A M, Weber J, Menard J F et al 1999 Prevalence of anal incontinence in 409 patients investigated for stress urinary incontinence. Neurourology and Urodynamics 18:579–590.

Lestar B, Penninckx F, Kerremans R 1989 The composition of anal basal pressure. An in vivo and in vitro study in man. International Journal of Colorectal Disease 4(2):118–122.

Lestar B, Penninckx F, Rigauts H et al 1992 The internal anal sphincter can not close the anal canal completely. International Journal of Colorectal Disease 7(30):159–161.

MacLean A B, Cardozo L (eds) 2002 Incontinence in women. Ch 12 Discussion. RCOG Press, London, p 151–160.

Malouf A J, Norton C S, Engel A F et al 2000a Long term results of overlapping anterior anal-sphincter repair for obstetric trauma. Lancet 355(9200):260–265.

Malouf A J, Williams A B, Halligan S et al 2000b Prospective assessment of accuracy of endoanal MR imaging and endosonography in patients with fecal incontinence. American Journal of Roentgenology 175(3):741–745.

Markwell S, Sapsford R 1995 Physiotherapy management of obstructed defaecation. Australian Journal of Physiotherapy 41:29–83.

Markwell S, Sapsford R 1998 Physiotherapy management of pelvic floor dysfunction. In: Sapsford R, Bullock-Saxton J, Markwell S (eds) Women's health, a textbook for physiotherapists. W B Saunders, London, p 383–407.

Marshall K, Thompson K A, Walsh D M et al 1998 Incidence of urinary incontinence and constipation during pregnancy and postpartum: survey of current findings at the Rotunda Lying-in Hospital. British Journal of Obstetrics and Gynaecology 105(4):400–402.

Metcalf A M 1995 Transit time. In: Smith L (ed.) Practical guide to anorectal testing, 2nd edn. Igaku-Shoin, New York, p 17–21.

Mehler P 1997 Constipation: diagnosis and treatment in eating disorders. Eating Disorders 5(1):41–44.

Mills P M, Hosker G L, Kiff E S et al 2002 Strength-duration testing of the external anal sphincter in females with anorectal dysfunction. Diseases of the Colon and Rectum 45(1):83–90.

Monga A K, Marrero J M, Stanton S L et al 1997 Is there an irritable bladder in the irritable bowel syndrome. British Journal of Obstetrics and Gynaecology 104:1409–1412.

Monk D N, Mills P, Jeacock J et al 1998 Combining the strength duration curve of the external anal sphincter with manometry for the assessment of faecal incontinence. British Journal of Surgery 85(10):1389–1393.

Moore J, Barlow D, Jewell D et al 1998 Do gastrointestinal symptoms vary with the menstrual cycle? British Journal of Obstetrics and Gynaecology 105(12):1322–1325.

Moore K H, Richmond D H, Sutherst J R et al 1992 Crouching over the toilet seat; prevalence among British gynaecological outpatients and its effect on micturition. Gynecology 47(3):186–187.

Moriarty K J 1999 The irritable bowel syndrome. In: Jones D J (ed.) ABC of colorectal diseases, 2nd edn. BMJ Books, London, p 21–24.

Muller-Lissner S A 1988 Effect of wheat bran on weight of stool and gastrointestinal transit time: a meta analysis. British Medical Journal (Clinical Research Edition) 296:615–617.

Nelson R L 1999 Meta-analysis of operative techniques for fissure-in-ano. Diseases of the Colon and Rectum 42(11):1428–1431.

Norton C 2002 Faecal incontinence. In: Laycock J, Haslam J (eds) Therapeutic management of incontinence and pelvic pain. Springer, London, p 129–136.

Norton C, Kamm M A 2001a Anal sphincter biofeedback and pelvic floor exercises for faecal incontinence in adults – a systematic review. Alimentary Pharmacological Therapy 15(8):1147–1154.

Norton C, Kamm M A 2001b Anal plug for faecal incontinence. Colorectal Disease 3(5):323–327.

Norton C, Christiansen J, Butler U et al 2002a Faecal incontinence in children. In: Abrams P, Cardozo L, Khoury S, Wein A (eds) Incontinence, 2nd edn. International consultation on incontinence, Health Publication/Plymbridge Distributors, Plymouth, p 1019–1025.

Norton C, Chelvanayagam S, Kamm M 2002b Randomised controlled trial of biofeedback for faecal incontinence. Neurourology and Urodynamics 21(4):295–296.

Ouslander J, Schnelle J 1995 Incontinence in the nursing home. Annals of Internal Medicine 122:438–449.

Pemberton J H 2002 Clinical features of posterior pelvic floor dysfunction. In: Pemberton J H, Swash M, Henry M M (eds)

The pelvic floor. Its function and disorders. W B Saunders, London, p 167–171.

Petticrew M, Watt I, Brand M 1999 What's the 'best buy' for treatment of constipation? Results of a systematic review of the efficacy and comparative efficacy of laxatives in the elderly. British Journal of General Practice 49(442):387–393.

Potter J 2002 Introduction. In: Potter J, Norton C, Cottenden A (eds) Bowel care in older people: research practice. Clinical Effectiveness Unit, Royal College of Physicians, London, p 1–4.

RCOG (Royal College of Obstetricians and Gynaecologists) 2001 Management of third and fourth degree tears following vaginal delivery. RCOG guideline no.29. RCOG Press, London.

Read M, Read N W, Barber D C et al 1982 Effects of loperamide on anal sphincter function in patients complaining of chronic diarrhea with fecal incontinence and urgency. Digestive Disease Science 27(9):807–814.

Read N W, Abouzekry L, Read M G et al 1985 Anorectal function in elderly patients with fecal impaction. Gastroenterology 89:959–966.

Reilly W T, Talley N J, Pemberton J H et al 2000 Validation of a questionnaire to assess faecal incontinence and associated risk factors: Fecal Incontinence Questionnaire. Diseases of the Colon and Rectum 43(2):146–153.

Richards A 1998 Hands on help. Nursing Times 94(32): 69–72.

Richardson A C 1993 The rectovaginal septum revisited: its relationship to rectocele and its importance to rectocele repair. Clinical Obstetrics and Gynecology 36:976–983.

Roberts R O, Jacobsen S J, Reilly W T et al 1999 Prevalence of combined fecal and urinary incontinence: a community-based study. Journal of the American Geriatrics Society 47(7):837–841.

Robson K M, Kiely D K, Lembo T 2000 Development of constipation in nursing home residents. Diseases of the Colon and Rectum 43(7):940–943.

Rockwood T H, Church J M, Fleshman J W et al 2000 Faecal incontinence quality of life scale: quality of life instrument for patients with fecal incontinence. Diseases of the Colon and Rectum 43:9–17.

Sapsford R 2001 The pelvic floor. A clinical model for function and rehabilitation. Physiotherapy 87(12):620–630.

Sapsford R R, Markwell S J, Richardson C A 1996 Abdominal muscles and the anal sphincter, their interaction during defaecation. Proceedings of the Australian Physiotherapy Association Congress, Brisbane, p 103–104.

Scott A M, Kellow J E, Eckersley G M et al 1992 Cigarette smoking and nicotine delay postprandial mouth-cecum transit time. Digestive Disease Science 37(10):1544–1547.

Silk D B A 1997 Understanding the causes of irritable bowel. In: Silk D. Understanding your irritable bowel. IBS research appeal, Central Middlesex Hospital NHS Trust, p 24–29.

Siproudis L, Dautreme S, Ropert A et al 1993 Dyschezia and rectocoele- a marriage of convenience? Physiologic evaluation of the rectocoele in a group of 52 women complaining of difficulty in evacuation. Diseases of the Colon and Rectum 36:1030–1036.

Spence-Jones C, Kamm M A, Henry M M et al 1994 Bowel dysfunction: a pathogenic factor in uterovaginal prolapse and urinary stress incontinence. British Journal of Obstetrics and Gynaecology 101:147–152.

Sultan A H 1999 Editorial. Obstetric perineal injury and anal incontinence. Clinical Risk 5:193–196.

Sultan A H, Kamm M A, Hudson C N et al 1994 Third degree obstetric anal sphincter tears: risk factors and outcome of primary repair. British Medical Journal 308:887–891.

Talley N J, Spiller R 2002 Irritable bowel syndrome: a little understood organic bowel disease? Lancet 17(360):555–564.

Talley N J, O'Keefe E A, Zinsmeister A R et al 1992 Prevalence of gastrointestinal symptoms in the elderly; a population-based study. Gastroenterology 102(3):895–901.

Talley N J, Weaver A I, Zinsmeister A R et al 1994 Self-reported diarrhea: what does it mean? American Journal of Gastroenterology 89(8):1160–1164.

Thompson W G, Longstreth G F, Drossman D A et al 1999 Functional bowel disorders and functional abdominal pain. Gut 45(suppl 11):1143–1147.

Towers A L, Burgio K L, Locher J L et al 1994 Constipation in the elderly: influence of dietary, psychological and physiological factors. Journal of the American Geriatrics Society 42(7):701–706.

Vaizey C J, Carpetri E A, Cahill J A et al 1999 Prospective comparison of faecal incontinence grading systems. Gut 44:77–80.

van Dam J H, Gosselink M J, Drogendijk A C et al 1997 Changes in bowel function after hysterectomy. Diseases of the Colon and Rectum 40(11):1342–1347.

von der Ohe M R, Camilleri M, Carryer P W 1994 A patient with megacolon and intractable constipation: evaluation for impairment of colonic muscle tone. American Journal of Gastroenterology 84:1867–1870.

Whitehead W E, Wald A, Norton N J 2001 Treatment options for fecal incontinence. Diseases of the Colon and Rectum 44(1):131–142, discussion.

Further reading

Books

Norton C, Kamm M 1999 Bowel control: information and practical advice. Beaconsfield Publishers, Beaconsfield.

Pemberton J H, Swash M, Henry M M 2002 The pelvic floor. Its function and disorders. W B Saunders, London.

Pettigrew M, Watt I, Sheldon T 1997 Systematic review of the effectiveness of laxatives in the elderly. Health Technology Assessment 1(13):i–iv, 1–52.

Potter J, Norton C, Cottenden A (eds) 2002 Bowel care in older people: research and practice. Clinical Effectiveness Unit, Royal College of Physicians, London.

Leaflets
ACA (Association for Continence Advice) 2003 ACA continence resource pack for care homes. ACA, London.
Addison R, Davies C, Haslam D et al 2001 Managing constipation in adults and older people. An interim guide for healthcare professionals. Funded by Norgine and produced by Professional Medical Communications.

Kyle G, Oliver H, Prynn P 2003 The procedure for the digital removal of faeces, guidelines 2003. Collaborative venture between NHS, Thames Valley University and Norgine.
Potter J, Norton C, Cottenden A (eds) 2003 Bowel care in older people: concise guide. Clinical Effectiveness Unit, Royal College of Physicians, London.

Useful addresses

British Digestive Foundation
3 St Andrew's Place, London NW1 4LB
Website: www.bdf.org.uk

Continence Foundation
307 Hatton Square, 16 Baldwin Gardens, London EC1N 7RJ
Website: www.continence-foundation.org.uk

IBS Network
Northern General Hospital, Sheffield S5 7AU
Website: www.ibsys.com

National Association for Colitis and Crohn's Disease,
PO Box 205, St Albans, Herts AL1 1AB
Website: www.nacc.org.uk

Royal College of Physicians
11 St Andrews Place, London NW1 4LE
Website: www.rcplondon.ac.uk

Appendix 1

Standardisation of terminology of lower urinary tract function

Report from the standardisation sub-committee of the International Continence Society. Reproduced with permission of the International Continence Society Committee on Standardisation of Terminology. First published in Neurology and Urodynamics 21:167–178 (2002)

Members: Paul Abrams, Linda Cardozo, Magnus Fall, Derek Griffiths, Peter Rosier, Ulf Ulmsten, Philip van Kerrebroeck, Arne Victor, and Alan Wein

This report presents definitions of the symptoms, signs, urodynamic observations and conditions associated with lower urinary tract dysfunction (LUTD) and urodynamic studies (UDS), for use in all patient groups from children to the elderly.

The definitions restate or update those presented in previous International Continence Society Standardisation of Terminology reports (see references) and those shortly to be published on Urethral Function (Lose et al in press) and Nocturia (van Kerrebroeck et al 2002). The published ICS report on the technical aspects of urodynamic equipment (Rowan et al 1987) will be complemented by the new ICS report on urodynamic practice to be published shortly (Schäfer et al 2002). In addition there are four published ICS outcome reports (Fonda et al 1998, Lose et al 1998, Mattiasson et al 1998, Nordling et al 1998).

New or changed definitions are all indicated, however, recommendations concerning technique are not included in the main text of this report.

The definitions have been written to be compatible with the WHO publication ICIDH-2 (International Classification of Functioning, Disability and Health) published in 2001 and ICD10, the International Classification of Diseases. As far as possible, the definitions are descriptive of observations, without implying underlying assumptions that may later prove to be incorrect or incomplete. By following this principle the International Continence Society (ICS) aims to facilitate comparison of results and enable effective communication by investigators who use urodynamic methods. This report restates the ICS principle that symptoms, signs and conditions are separate categories, and adds a category of urodynamic observations. In addition, terminology related to therapies is included (Andersen et al 1992).

When a reference is made to the whole anatomical organ the vesica urinaria, the correct term is the bladder. When the smooth muscle

Correspondence to: International Continence Society Office, Southmead Hospital, Bristol, BS10 5NB, UK
Email: Vicky@icsoffice.org

structure known as the m.detrusor urinae is being discussed, then the correct term is detrusor.

It is suggested that acknowledgement of these standards in written publications be indicated by a footnote to the section 'Methods and Materials' or its equivalent, to read as follows:

'Methods, definitions and units conform to the standards recommended by the International Continence Society, except where specifically noted'.

The report covers the following areas:

LOWER URINARY TRACT SYMPTOMS (LUTS)

Symptoms are the subjective indicator of a disease or change in condition as perceived by the patient, carer or partner and may lead him/her to seek help from health care professionals. **(NEW)**

Symptoms may either be volunteered or described during the patient interview. They are usually qualitative. In general, Lower Urinary Tract Symptoms cannot be used to make a definitive diagnosis. Lower Urinary Tract Symptoms can also indicate pathologies other than lower urinary tract dysfunction, such as urinary infection.

SIGNS SUGGESTIVE OF LOWER URINARY TRACT DYSFUNCTION (LUTD)

Signs are observed by the physician including simple means, to verify symptoms and quantify them. **(NEW)**

For example, a classical sign is the observation of leakage on coughing. Observations from frequency volume charts, pad tests and validated symptom and quality of life questionnaires are examples of other instruments that can be used to verify and quantify symptoms.

URODYNAMIC OBSERVATIONS

Urodynamic observations are observations made during urodynamic studies. **(NEW)**

For example, an involuntary detrusor contraction (detrusor overactivity) is a urodynamic observation. In general, a urodynamic observation may have a number of possible underlying causes and does not represent a definitive diagnosis of a disease or condition and may occur with a variety of symptoms and signs, or in the absence of any symptoms or signs.

CONDITIONS

Conditions are defined by the presence of urodynamic observations associated with characteristic symptoms or signs and/or non-urodynamic evidence of relevant pathological processes. **(NEW)**

TREATMENT

Treatment for lower urinary tract dysfunction: these definitions are from the 7th ICS report on Lower Urinary Tract Rehabilitation Techniques (Andersen et al 1992).

1 LOWER URINARY TRACT SYMPTOMS (LUTS)

Lower urinary tract symptoms are defined from the individual's perspective, who is usually, but not necessarily a patient within the health-care system. Symptoms are either volunteered by, or elicited from, the individual or may be described by the individual's caregiver.

Lower urinary tract symptoms are divided into three groups, storage, voiding, and post micturition symptoms.

1.1 STORAGE SYMPTOMS

Storage symptoms are experienced during the storage phase of the bladder, and include daytime frequency and nocturia. **(NEW)**

- *Increased daytime frequency* is the complaint by the patient who considers that he/she voids too often by day. **(NEW)** This term is equivalent to pollakisuria used in many countries.
- *Nocturia* is the complaint that the individual has to wake at night one or more times to void. **(NEW)**[1]
- *Urgency* is the complaint of a sudden compelling desire to pass urine, which is difficult to defer. **(CHANGED)**
- *Urinary incontinence* is the complaint of any involuntary leakage of urine. **(NEW)**[2]

In each specific circumstance, urinary incontinence should be further described by specifying relevant factors such as type, frequency, severity, precipitating factors, social impact, effect on hygiene and quality of life, the measures used to contain the leakage, and whether or not the individual seeks or desires help because of urinary incontinence.[3]

Urinary leakage may need to be distinguished from sweating or vaginal discharge.

- *Stress urinary incontinence* is the complaint of involuntary leakage on effort or exertion, or on sneezing or coughing. **(CHANGED)**[4]

---

[1] The term night time frequency differs from that for nocturia, as it includes voids that occur after the individual has gone to bed, but before he/she has gone to sleep; and voids which occur in the early morning which prevent the individual from getting back to sleep as he/she wishes. These voids before and after sleep may need to be considered in research studies, for example, in nocturnal polyuria. If this definition were used then an adapted definition of daytime frequency would need to be used with it.

[2] In infants and small children the definition of Urinary Incontinence is not applicable. In scientific communications the definition of incontinence in children would need further explanation.

[3] The original ICS definition of incontinence, 'Urinary incontinence is the involuntary loss of urine that is a social or hygienic problem', relates the complaint to quality of life (QoL) issues. Some QoL instruments have been, and are being, developed in order to assess the impact of both incontinence and other LUTS on QoL.

[4] The committee considers the term 'stress incontinence' to be unsatisfactory in the English language because of its mental connotations. The Swedish, French and Italian expression 'effort incontinence' is preferable, however, words such as 'effort' or 'exertion' still do not capture some of the common precipitating factors for stress incontinence such as coughing or sneezing. For this reason the term is left unchanged.

- *Urge urinary incontinence* is the complaint of involuntary leakage accompanied by or immediately preceded by urgency. **(CHANGED)**[5]
- *Mixed urinary incontinence* is the complaint of involuntary leakage associated with urgency and also with exertion, effort, sneezing or coughing. **(NEW)**
- *Enuresis* means any involuntary loss of urine. **(ORIGINAL)** If it is used to denote incontinence during sleep, it should always be qualified with the adjective 'nocturnal'.
- *Nocturnal enuresis* is the complaint of loss of urine occurring during sleep. **(NEW)**
- *Continuous urinary incontinence* is the complaint of continuous leakage. **(NEW)**
- *Other types of urinary incontinence* may be situational, for example the report of incontinence during sexual intercourse, or giggle incontinence.
- *Bladder sensation* can be defined, during history taking, by five categories.
  - *Normal:* the individual is aware of bladder filling and increasing sensation up to a strong desire to void. **(NEW)**
  - *Increased:* the individual feels an early and persistent desire to void. **(NEW)**
  - *Reduced:* the individual is aware of bladder filling but does not feel a definite desire to void. **(NEW)**
  - *Absent:* the individual reports no sensation of bladder filling or desire to void. **(NEW)**
  - *Non-specific:* the individual reports no specific bladder sensation, but may perceive bladder filling as abdominal fullness, vegetative symptoms, or spasticity. **(NEW)**[6]

1.2 VOIDING SYMPTOMS

Voiding symptoms are experienced during the voiding phase. **(NEW)**

- *Slow stream* is reported by the individual as his or her perception of reduced urine flow, usually compared to previous performance or in comparison to others. **(NEW)**
- *Splitting or spraying* of the urine stream may be reported. **(NEW)**
- *Intermittent stream (Intermittency)* is the term used when the individual describes urine flow, which stops and starts, on one or more occasions, during micturition. **(NEW)**
- *Hesitancy* is the term used when an individual describes difficulty in initiating micturition resulting in a delay in the onset of voiding after the individual is ready to pass urine. **(NEW)**

---

[5] Urge incontinence can present in different symptomatic forms, for example, as frequent small losses between micturitions, or as a catastrophic leak with complete bladder emptying.

[6] These non-specific symptoms are most frequently seen in neurological patients, particularly those with spinal cord trauma and in children and adults with malformations of the spinal cord.

- *Straining* to void describes the muscular effort used to either initiate, maintain or improve the urinary stream. **(NEW)**[7]
- *Terminal dribble* is the term used when an individual describes a prolonged final part of micturition, when the flow has slowed to a trickle/dribble. **(NEW)**

1.3 POST MICTURITION SYMPTOMS

Post micturition symptoms are experienced immediately after micturition. **(NEW)**

- *Feeling of incomplete emptying* is a self-explanatory term for a feeling experienced by the individual after passing urine. **(NEW)**
- *Post micturition dribble* is the term used when an individual describes the involuntary loss of urine immediately after he or she has finished passing urine, usually after leaving the toilet in men, or after rising from the toilet in women. **(NEW)**

1.4 SYMPTOMS ASSOCIATED WITH SEXUAL INTERCOURSE

Dyspareunia, vaginal dryness and incontinence are amongst the symptoms women may describe during or after intercourse. These symptoms should be described as fully as possible. It is helpful to define urine leakage as: during penetration, during intercourse, or at orgasm.

1.5 SYMPTOMS ASSOCIATED WITH PELVIC ORGAN PROLAPSE

The feeling of a lump ('something coming down'), low backache, heaviness, dragging sensation, or the need to digitally replace the prolapse in order to defaecate or micturate, are amongst the symptoms women may describe who have a prolapse.

1.6 GENITAL AND LOWER URINARY TRACT PAIN[8]

Pain, discomfort and pressure are part of a spectrum of abnormal sensations felt by the individual. Pain produces the greatest impact on the patient and may be related to bladder filling or voiding, may be felt after micturition, or be continuous. Pain should also be characterised by type, frequency, duration, precipitating and relieving factors and by location as defined below:

- *Bladder pain* is felt suprapubically or retropubically, usually increases with bladder filling, and may persist after voiding. **(NEW)**
- *Urethral pain* is felt in the urethra and the individual indicates the urethra as the site. **(NEW)**

---

[7] Suprapubic pressure may be used to initiate or maintain urine flow. The Crede[3] manoeuvre is used by some spinal cord injury patients, and girls with detrusor underactivity sometimes press suprapubically to help empty the bladder.

[8] The terms 'strangury', 'bladder spasm', and 'dysuria' are difficult to define and of uncertain meaning and should not be used in relation to lower urinary tract dysfunction, unless a precise meaning is stated. Dysuria literally means 'abnormal urination', and is used correctly in some European countries however, it is often used to describe the stinging/burning sensation characteristic of urinary infection. It is suggested that these descriptive words should not be used in future.

- *Vulval pain* is felt in and around the external genitalia. **(NEW)**
- *Vaginal pain* is felt internally, above the introitus. **(NEW)**
- *Scrotal pain* may or may not be localised, for example to the testis, epididymis, cord structures or scrotal skin. **(NEW)**
- *Perineal pain* is felt: in the female, between the posterior fourchette (posterior lip of the introitus) and the anus, and in the male, between the scrotum and the anus. **(NEW)**
- *Pelvic pain* is less well defined than, for example, bladder, urethral or perineal pain and is less clearly related to the micturition cycle or to bowel function and is not localised to any single pelvic organ. **(NEW)**

1.7 GENITO–URINARY PAIN SYNDROMES AND SYMPTOM SYNDROMES SUGGESTIVE OF LUTD

Syndromes describe constellations, or varying combinations of symptoms, but cannot be used for precise diagnosis. The use of the word syndrome can only be justified if there is at least one other symptom in addition to the symptom used to describe the syndrome. In scientific communications the incidence of individual symptoms within the syndrome should be stated, in addition to the number of individuals with the syndrome.

The syndromes described are functional abnormalities for which a precise cause has not been defined. It is presumed that routine assessment (history taking, physical examination, and other appropriate investigations) has excluded obvious local pathologies, such as those that are infective, neoplastic, metabolic or hormonal in nature.

1.7.1 Genito–urinary pain syndromes

Genito-urinary pain syndromes are all chronic in their nature. Pain is the major complaint but concomitant complaints are of lower urinary tract, bowel, sexual or gynaecological nature.

- *Painful bladder syndrome* is the complaint of suprapubic pain related to bladder filling, accompanied by other symptoms such as increased daytime and night-time frequency, in the absence of proven urinary infection or other obvious pathology. **(NEW)**[9]
- *Urethral pain syndrome* is the occurrence of recurrent episodic urethral pain usually on voiding, with daytime frequency and nocturia, in the absence of proven infection or other obvious pathology. **(NEW)**
- *Vulval pain syndrome* is the occurrence of persistent or recurrent episodic vulval pain, which is either related to the micturition cycle or associated with symptoms suggestive of urinary tract or sexual dysfunction. There is no proven infection or other obvious pathology. **(NEW)**[10]
- *Vaginal pain syndrome* is the occurrence of persistent or recurrent episodic vaginal pain which is associated with symptoms suggestive of urinary tract or sexual dysfunction. There is no proven vaginal infection or other obvious pathology.

---

[9] The ICS believes this to be a preferable term to 'interstitial cystitis'. Interstitial cystitis is a specific diagnosis and requires confirmation by typical cystoscopic and histological features. In the investigation of bladder pain it may be necessary to exclude conditions such as carcinoma in situ and endometriosis.

[10] The ICS suggests that the term vulvodynia (vulva – pain) should not be used, as it leads to confusion between single symptom and a syndrome.

- *Scrotal pain syndrome* is the occurrence of persistent or recurrent episodic scrotal pain which is associated with symptoms suggestive of urinary tract or sexual dysfunction. There is no proven epididimo-orchitis or other obvious pathology.
- *Perineal pain syndrome* is the occurrence of persistent or recurrent episodic perineal pain, which is either related to the micturition cycle or associated with symptoms suggestive of urinary tract or sexual dysfunction. There is no proven infection or other obvious pathology. **(NEW)**[11]
- *Pelvic pain syndrome* is the occurrence of persistent or recurrent episodic pelvic pain associated with symptoms suggestive of lower urinary tract, sexual, bowel or gynaecological dysfunction. There is no proven infection or other obvious pathology. **(NEW)**

1.7.2 Symptom syndromes suggestive of lower urinary tract dysfunction

In clinical practice, empirical diagnoses are often used as the basis for initial management after assessing the individual's lower urinary tract symptoms, physical findings and the results of urinalysis and other indicated investigations.

- *Urgency,* with or without urge incontinence, usually with frequency and nocturia, can be described as the *overactive bladder syndrome, urge syndrome or urgency-frequency syndrome.* **(NEW)**

These symptom combinations are suggestive of urodynamically demonstrable detrusor overactivity, but can be due to other forms of urethrovesical dysfunction. These terms can be used if there is no proven infection or other obvious pathology.

- *Lower urinary tract symptoms suggestive of bladder outlet obstruction* is a term used when a man complains predominately of voiding symptoms in the absence of infection or obvious pathology other than possible causes of outlet obstruction. **(NEW)**[12]

2 SIGNS SUGGESTIVE OF LOWER URINARY TRACT DYSFUNCTION (LUTD)

2.1 MEASURING THE FREQUENCY, SEVERITY AND IMPACT OF LOWER URINARY TRACT SYMPTOMS

Asking the patient to record micturitions and symptoms[13] for a period of days provides invaluable information. The recording of micturition events can be in three main forms:

- *Micturition time chart:* this records only the times of micturitions, day and night, for at least 24 hours. **(NEW)**

---

[11] The ICS suggests that in men, the term prostatodynia (prostate-pain) should not be used as it leads to confusion between a single symptom and a syndrome.
[12] In women voiding symptoms are usually thought to suggest detrusor underactivity rather than bladder outlet obstruction.
[13] Validated questionnaires are useful for recording symptoms, their frequency, severity and bother, and the impact of LUTS on QoL. The instrument used should be specified.

- *Frequency volume chart (FVC):* this records the volumes voided as well as the time of each micturition, day and night, for at least 24 hours. **(CHANGED)**
- *Bladder diary:* this records the times of micturitions and voided volumes, incontinence episodes, pad usage and other information such as fluid intake, the degree of urgency and the degree of incontinence. **(NEW)**[14]

The following measurements can be abstracted from frequency volume charts and bladder diaries:

- *Daytime frequency* is the number of voids recorded during waking hours and includes the last void before sleep and the first void after waking and rising in the morning. **(NEW)**
- *Nocturia* is the number of voids recorded during a night's sleep: each void is preceded and followed by sleep. **(NEW)**
- *24-hour frequency* is the total number of daytime voids and episodes of nocturia during a specified 24-hour period. **(NEW)**
- *24-hour production* is measured by collecting all urine for 24-hours. **(NEW)**

This is usually commenced *after* the first void produced after rising in the morning, and is completed by including the first void on rising the following morning.

- *Polyuria* is defined as the measured production of more than 2.8 litres of urine in 24 hours in adults. It may be useful to look at output over shorter time frames (van Kerrebroeck et al 2002). **(NEW)**[15]
- *Nocturnal urine volume* is defined as the total volume of urine passed between the time the individual goes to bed with the intention of sleeping and the time of waking with the intention of rising. **(NEW)** Therefore, it excludes the last void before going to bed but includes the first void after rising in the morning.
- *Nocturnal polyuria* is present when an increased proportion of the 24-hour output occurs at night (normally during the 8 hours whilst the patient is in bed). **(NEW)** The night time urine output excludes the last void before sleep but includes the first void of the morning.[16]

---

[14] It is useful to ask the individual to make an estimate of liquid intake. This may be done precisely by measuring the volume of each drink or crudely by asking how many drinks are taken in a 24-hour period. If the individual eats significant quantities of water containing foods (vegetables, fruit, salads) then an appreciable effect on urine production will result. The time that diuretic therapy is taken should be marked on a chart or diary.

[15] The causes of polyuria are various and reviewed elsewhere but include habitual excess fluid intake. The figure of 2.8 is based on a 70 kg person voiding >40 ml/kg.

[16] The normal range of nocturnal urine production differs with age and the normal ranges remain to be defined. Therefore, nocturnal polyuria is present when greater than 20% (young adults) to 33% (over 65 years) is produced at night. Hence the precise definition is dependant on age.

- *Maximum voided volume* is the largest volume of urine voided during a single micturition and is determined either from the frequency/volume chart or bladder diary. **(NEW)**

The maximum, mean and minimum voided volumes over the period of recording may be stated.[17]

2.2 PHYSICAL EXAMINATION

Physical examination is essential in the assessment of all patients with lower urinary tract dysfunction. It should include abdominal, pelvic, perineal and a focussed neurological examination. For patients with possible neurogenic lower urinary tract dysfunction, a more extensive neurological examination is needed.

2.2.1 Abdominal

The bladder may be felt by abdominal palpation or by suprapubic percussion. Pressure suprapubically or during bimanual vaginal examination may induce a desire to pass urine.

2.2.2 Perineal/genital inspection

Perineal/genital inspection allows the description of the skin, for example the presence of atrophy or excoriation, any abnormal anatomical features and the observation of incontinence.

- *Urinary incontinence (the sign)* is defined as urine leakage seen during examination: this may be urethral or extraurethral.
- *Stress urinary incontinence* is the observation of involuntary leakage from the urethra, synchronous with exertion/effort, or sneezing or coughing. **(CHANGED)**[18]

Stress Leakage is presumed to be due to raised abdominal pressure.

- *Extra-urethral incontinence* is defined as the observation of urine leakage through channels other than the urethra. **(ORIGINAL)**
- *Uncategorised incontinence* is the observation of involuntary leakage that cannot be classified into one of the above categories on the basis of signs and symptoms. **(NEW)**

2.2.3 Vaginal examination

Vaginal examination allows the description of observed and palpable anatomical abnormalities and the assessment of pelvic floor muscle function, as described in the ICS report on Pelvic Organ Prolapse. The

---

[17] The term 'functional bladder capacity' is no longer recommended as 'voided volume' is a clearer and less confusing term, particular if qualified e.g. 'maximum voided volume'. If the term bladder capacity is used, in any situation, it implies that this has been measured in some way, if only by abdominal ultrasound In adults, voided volumes vary considerably. In children, the 'expected volume' may be calculated from the formula (30 + (age in years $\times$ 30) in ml). Assuming no residual urine this will be equal to the 'expected bladder capacity'.

[18] Coughing may induce a detrusor contraction, hence the sign of stress incontinence is only a reliable indication of urodynamic stress incontinence when leakage occurs synchronously with the first proper cough and stops at the end of that cough.

definitions given are simplified versions of the definitions in that report (Bump et al 1996)

- *Pelvic organ prolapse* is defined as the descent of one or more of: the anterior vaginal wall, the posterior vaginal wall, and the apex of the vagina (cervix/uterus) or vault (cuff) after hysterectomy. Absence of prolapse is defined as stage 0 support; prolapse can be staged from stage I to stage IV. **(NEW)**

Pelvic organ prolapse can occur in association with urinary incontinence and other lower urinary tract dysfunction and may on occasion mask incontinence.

- *Anterior vaginal wall prolapse* is defined as descent of the anterior vagina so that the urethrovesical junction (a point 3 cm proximal to the external urinary meatus) or any anterior point proximal to this is less than 3 cm above the plane of the hymen. **(CHANGED)**
- *Prolapse of the apical segment of the vagina* is defined as any descent of the vaginal cuff scar (after hysterectomy) or cervix, below a point which is 2 cm less than the total vaginal length above the plane of the hymen. **(CHANGED)**
- *Posterior vaginal wall prolapse* is defined as any descent of the posterior vaginal wall so that a midline point on the posterior vaginal wall 3 cm above the level of the hymen or any posterior point proximal to this, is less than 3 cm above the plane of the hymen. **(CHANGED)**

2.2.4 Pelvic floor muscle function

Pelvic floor muscle function can be qualitatively defined by the tone at rest and the strength of a voluntary or reflex contraction as strong, weak or absent or by a validated grading system (e.g. Oxford 1–5). A pelvic muscle contraction may be assessed by visual inspection, by palpation, electromyography or perineometry. Factors to be assessed include strength, duration, displacement, and repeatability.

2.2.5 Rectal examination

Rectal examination allows the description of observed and palpable anatomical abnormalities and is the easiest method of assessing pelvic floor muscle function in children and men. In addition, rectal examination is essential in children with urinary incontinence to rule out faecal inpaction.

- *Pelvic floor muscle function* can be qualitatively defined, during rectal examination, by the tone at rest and the strength of a voluntary contraction, as strong, weak or absent. **(NEW)**

2.3 PAD TESTING

Pad testing may be used to quantify the amount of urine lost during incontinence episodes, and methods range from a short provocative test to a 24-hour pad test.

3 URODYNAMIC OBSERVATIONS AND CONDITIONS

3.1 URODYNAMIC TECHNIQUES

There are two principal methods of urodynamic investigation:

- *Conventional urodynamic studies* normally take place in the urodynamic laboratory and usually involve artificial bladder filling. **(NEW)**

- *Artificial bladder filling* is defined as filling the bladder, via a catheter, with a specified liquid at a specified rate. **(NEW)**
- *Ambulatory urodynamic studies* are defined as a functional test of the lower urinary tract, utilising natural filling, and reproducing the subject's every day activities.[19]
  - *natural filling* means that the bladder is filled by the production of urine rather than by an artificial medium.

Both filling cystometry and pressure flow studies of voiding require the following measurements:

- *Intravesical pressure* is the pressure within the bladder. **(ORIGINAL)**
- *Abdominal pressure* is taken to be the pressure surrounding the bladder. In current practice it is estimated from rectal, vaginal or, less commonly from extraperitoneal pressure or a bowel stoma. The simultaneous measurement of abdominal pressure is essential for the interpretation of the intravesical pressure trace. **(ORIGINAL)**
- *Detrusor pressure* is that component of intravesical pressure that is created by forces in the bladder wall (passive and active). It is estimated by subtracting abdominal pressure from intravesical pressure. **(ORIGINAL)**

3.2 FILLING CYSTOMETRY

The word 'cystometry' is commonly used to describe the urodynamic investigation of the filling phase of the micturition cycle. To eliminate confusion the following definitions are proposed:

- *Filling cystometry* is the method by which the pressure/volume relationship of the bladder is measured during bladder filling. **(ORIGINAL)**

The filling phase starts when filling commences and ends when the patient and urodynamicist decide that 'permission to void' has been given.[20]

Bladder and urethral function, during filling, need to be defined separately.

The rate at which the bladder is filled is divided into:

- *Physiological filling rate* is defined as a filling rate less than the predicted maximum – predicted maximum body weight in kg divided by 4, expressed as ml/min (17) **(CHANGED)**
- *Non-physiological filling rate* is defined as a filling rate greater than the predicted maximum filling rate – predicted maximum body weight in kg divided by 4, expressed as ml/min (Klevmark 1999). **(CHANGED)**

---

[19] The term Ambulatory Urodynamics is used to indicate that monitoring usually takes place outside the urodynamic laboratory, rather than the subject's mobility using natural filling.

[20] The ICS no longer wishes to divide filling rates into slow, medium and fast. In practice almost all investigations are performed using medium filling rates which have a wide range. It maybe more important during investigations to consider whether or not the filling rate used during conventional urodynamic studies can be considered physiological.

Bladder storage function should be described according to bladder sensation, detrusor activity, bladder compliance and bladder capacity.[21]

3.2.1 Bladder sensation during filling cystometry

- *Normal bladder sensation* can be judged by three defined points noted during filling cystometry and evaluated in relation to the bladder volume at that moment and in relation to the patient's symptomatic complaints.
  - *First sensation of bladder filling* is the feeling the patient has during filling cystometry, when he/she first becomes aware of the bladder filling. **(NEW)**
  - *First desire to void* is defined as the feeling, during filling cystometry, that would lead the patient to pass urine at the next convenient moment, but voiding can be delayed if necessary. **(CHANGED)**
  - *Strong desire to void* this is defined, during filling cystometry, as a persistent desire to void without the fear of leakage. **(ORIGINAL)**
  - *Increased bladder sensation* is defined, during filling cystometry, as an early first sensation of bladder filling (or an early desire to void) and/or an early strong desire to void, which occurs at low bladder volume and which persists. **(NEW)**[22]
- *Reduced bladder sensation* is defined, during filling cystometry, as diminished sensation throughout bladder filling. **(NEW)**
- *Absent bladder sensation* means that, during filling cystometry, the individual has no bladder sensation. **(NEW)**
- *Non-specific bladder sensations,* during filling cystometry, may make the individual aware of bladder filling, for example, abdominal fullness or vegetative symptoms. **(NEW)**
- *Bladder pain,* during filling cystometry, is a self explanatory term and is an abnormal finding. **(NEW)**
- *Urgency*, during filling cystometry, is a sudden compelling desire to void. **(NEW)**[23]
- *The vesical/urethral sensory threshold,* is defined as the least current which consistently produces a sensation perceived by the subject during stimulation at the site under investigation (Andersen et al 1992). **(ORIGINAL)**

3.2.2 Detrusor function during filling cystometry

In everyday life the individual attempts to inhibit detrusor activity until he or she is in a position to void. Therefore, when the aims of the filling study have been achieved, and when the patient has a desire to void, normally the 'permission to void' is given (see Filling Cystometry). That moment is indicated on the urodynamic trace and all detrusor activity before this 'permission' is defined as 'involuntary detrusor activity'.

---

[21] Whilst bladder sensation is assessed during filling cystometry the assumption that it is sensation from the bladder alone, without urethral or pelvic components may be false.
[22] The assessment of the subject's bladder sensation is subjective and it is not, for example, possible to quantify 'low bladder volume' in the definition of 'increased bladder sensation'.
[23] The ICS no longer recommends the terms 'motor urgency' and 'sensory urgency'. These terms are often misused and have little intuitive meaning. Furthermore, it may be simplistic to relate urgency just to the presence or absence of detrusor overactivity when there is usually a concomitant fall in urethral pressure.

- *Normal detrusor function:* allows bladder filling with little or no change in pressure. No involuntary phasic contractions occur despite provocation. **(ORIGINAL)**
- *Detrusor overactivity* is a urodynamic observation characterised by involuntary detrusor contractions during the filling phase which may be spontaneous or provoked. **(CHANGED)**[24]

There are certain patterns of detrusor overactivity:

- *Phase detrusor overactivity* is defined by a characteristic wave form, and may or may not lead to urinary incontinence. **(NEW)**[25]
- *Terminal detrusor overactivity* is defined as a single involuntary detrusor contraction occurring at cystometric capacity, which cannot be suppressed, and results in incontinence usually resulting in bladder emptying (voiding). **(NEW)**[26]
- *Detrusor overactivity incontinence* is incontinence due to an involuntary detrusor contraction. **(NEW)**

In a patient with normal sensation urgency is likely to be experienced just before the leakage episode.[27]

Detrusor overactivity may also be qualified, when possible, according to cause; for example:

- *Neurogenic detrusor overactivity* when there is a relevant neurological condition.

    This term replaces the term 'detrusor hyperreflexia'. **(NEW)**

- *Idiopathic detrusor overactivity* when there is no defined cause. **(NEW)**

This term replaces 'detrusor instability'.[28]

In clinical and research practice, the extent of neurological examination/investigation varies. It is likely that the proportion of neurogenic: idiopathic detrusor overactivity will increase if a more complete neurological assessment is carried out.

Other patterns of detrusor overactivity are seen, for example, the combination of phasic and terminal detrusor overactivity, and the sustained

---

[24] There is no lower limit for the amplitude of an involuntary detrusor contraction but confident interpretation of low pressure waves (amplitude smaller than $5\,cm\,H_2O$) depends on 'high quality' urodynamic technique. The phrase 'which the patient cannot completely suppress' has been deleted from the old definition.

[25] Phasic detrusor contractions are not always accompanied by any sensation, or may be interpreted as a first sensation of bladder filling, or as a normal desire to void.

[26] 'Terminal detrusor overactivity' is a new ICS term: it is typically associated with reduced bladder sensation, for example in the elderly stroke patient when urgency may be felt as the voiding contraction occurs. However, in complete spinal cord injury patients there may be no sensation whatsoever.

[27] ICS recommends that the terms 'motor urge incontinence' and 'reflex incontinence', should no longer be used as they have no intuitive meaning and are often misused.

[28] The terms 'detrusor instability' and 'detrusor hyperreflexia' were both used as generic terms, in the English speaking world and Scandinavia, prior to the first ICS report in 1976. As a compromise they were allocated to idiopathic and neurogenic overactivity respectively. As there is no real logic or intuitive meaning to the terms, the ICS believes they should be abandoned.

high pressure detrusor contractions seen in spinal cord injury patient when attempted voiding occurs against a dyssynergic sphincter.

- *Provocative manoeuvres* are defined as techniques used during urodynamics in an effort to provoke detrusor overactivity, for example, rapid filling, use of cooled or acid medium, postural changes and hand washing. **(NEW)**

3.2.3 Bladder compliance during filling cystometry

- *Bladder compliance* describes the relationship between change in bladder volume and change in detrusor pressure. **(CHANGED)**[29]

Compliance is calculated by dividing the volume change (ΔV) by the change in detrusor pressure (Δpdet) during that change in bladder volume ($C = V. \Delta p$det). It is expressed in mL/cm H_2O.

A variety of means of calculating bladder compliance has been described. The ICS recommends that two standard points should be used for compliance calculations: the investigator may wish to define additional points. The standards points are:

1. *the detrusor pressure at the start of bladder filling and the corresponding bladder volume (usually zero), and*
2. *the detrusor pressure (and corresponding bladder volume) at cystometric capacity or immediately before the start of any detrusor contraction that causes significant leakage (and therefore causes the bladder volume to decrease, affecting compliance calculation). Both points are measured excluding any detrusor contraction.*

3.2.4 Bladder capacity: during filling cystometry

- *Cystometric capacity* is the bladder volume at the end of the filling cystometrogram, when 'permission to void' is usually given. The end point should be specified, for example, if filling is stopped when the patient has a normal desire to void. The cystometric capacity is the volume voided together with any residual urine. **(CHANGED)**[30]
- *Maximum cystometric capacity,* in patients with normal sensation, is the volume at which the patient feels he/she can no longer delay micturition (has a strong desire to void). **(ORIGINAL)**
- *Maximum anaesthetic bladder capacity* is the volume to which the bladder can be filled under deep general or spinal anaesthetic and should be qualified according to the type of anaesthesia used, the speed

---

[29] The observation of reduced bladder compliance during conventional filling cystometry is often related to relatively fast bladder filling: the incidence of reduced compliance is markedly lower if the bladder is filled at physiological rates, as in ambulatory urodynamics.

[30] In certain types of dysfunction, the cystometric capacity cannot be defined in the same terms. In the absence of sensation the cystometric capacity is the volume at which the clinician decides to terminate filling. The reason (s) for terminating filling should be defined, e.g. high detrusor filling pressure, large infused volume or pain. If there is uncontrollable voiding, it is the volume at which this begins. In the presence of sphincter incompetence the cystometric capacity may be significantly increased by occlusion of the urethra e.g. by Foley catheter.

of filling, the length of time of filling, and the pressure at which the bladder is filled. **(CHANGED)**

3.2.5 Urethral function during filling cystometry

The urethral closure mechanism during storage may be competent or incompetent.

- *Normal urethral closure mechanism* maintains a positive urethral closure pressure during bladder filling even in the presence of increased abdominal pressure, although it may be overcome by detrusor overactivity. **(CHANGED)**
- *Incompetent urethral closure mechanism* is defined as one which allows **leakage of urine in the absence of a detrusor contraction. (ORIGINAL)**
- *Urethral relaxation incontinence* is defined as leakage due to urethral relaxation in the absence of raised abdominal pressure or detrusor overactivity. **(NEW)**[31]
- *Urodynamic stress incontinence* is noted during filling cystometry, and is defined as the involuntary leakage of urine during increased abdominal pressure, in the absence of a detrusor contraction. **(CHANGED)**

Urodynamic stress incontinence is now the preferred term to 'genuine stress incontinence'.[32]

3.2.6 Assessment of urethral function during filling cystometry

- *Urethral pressure measurement*
  - *Urethral pressure* is defined as the fluid pressure needed to just open a closed urethra. **(ORIGINAL)**
  - *The urethral pressure profile* is a graph indicating the intraluminal pressure along the length of the urethra. **(ORIGINAL)**
  - *The urethral closure pressure profile* is given by the subtraction of intravesical pressure from urethral pressure. **(ORIGINAL)**
  - *Maximum urethral pressure* is the maximum pressure of the measured profile. **(ORIGINAL)**
  - *Maximum urethral closure pressure (MUCP)* is the maximum difference between the urethral pressure and the intravesical pressure. **(ORIGINAL)**
  - *Functional profile length* is the length of the urethra along which the urethral pressure exceeds intravesical pressure in women.
  - *Pressure 'transmission' ratio* is the increment in urethral pressure on stress as a percentage of the simultaneously recorded increment in intravesical pressure.

---

[31] Fluctuations in urethral pressure have been defined as the 'unstable urethra'. However, the significance of the fluctuations and the term itself lack clarity and the term is not recommended by the ICS. If symptoms are seen in association with a decrease in urethral pressure a full description should be given.

[32] In patients with stress incontinence, there is a spectrum of urethral characteristics ranging from a highly mobile urethra with good intrinsic function to an immobile urethra with poor intrinsic function. Any delineation into categories such as 'urethral hypermobility' and 'intrinsic sphincter deficiency' may be simplistic and arbitrary, and requires further research.

- *Abdominal leak point pressure* is the intravesical pressure at which urine leakage occurs due to increased abdominal pressure in the absence of a detrusor contraction. **(NEW)**[33]
- *Detrusor leak point pressure* is defined as the lowest detrusor pressure at which urine leakage occurs in the absence of either a detrusor contraction or increased abdominal pressure. **(NEW)**[34]

3.3 PRESSURE FLOW STUDIES

Voiding is described in terms of detrusor and urethral function and assessed by measuring urine flow rate and voiding pressures.

- *Pressure flow studies* of voiding are the method by which the relationship between pressure in the bladder and urine flow rate is measured during bladder emptying. **(ORIGINAL)**

The voiding phase starts when 'permission to void' is given or when uncontrollable voiding begins, and ends when the patient considers voiding has finished.

3.3.1 Measurement of urine flow

Urine flow is defined either as continuous, that is with out interruption, or as **intermittent**, when an individual states that the flow stops and starts during a single visit to the bathroom in order to void. The continuous flow curve is defined as a **smooth** arc shaped curve or **fluctuating** when there are multiple peaks during a period of continuous urine flow.[35]

- *Flow rate* is defined as the volume of fluid expelled via the urethra per unit time. It is expressed in mL/s. **(ORIGINAL)**
- *Voided volume* is the total volume expelled via the urethra. **(ORIGINAL)**
- *Maximum flow rate* is the maximum measured value of the flow rate after correction for artefacts. **(CHANGED)**
- *Voiding time* is total duration of micturition, i.e. includes interruptions. When voiding is completed with out interruption, voiding time is equal to flow time. **(ORIGINAL)**
- *Flow time* is the time over which measurable flow actually occurs. **(ORIGINAL)**
- *Average flow rate* is voided volume divided by flow time. The average flow should be interpreted with caution if flow is interrupted or there is a terminal dribble. **(CHANGED)**

---

[33] The leak pressure point should be qualified according to the site of pressure measurement (rectal, vaginal or intravesical) and the method by which pressure is generated (cough or valsalva). Leak point pressures may be calculated in three ways from the three different baseline values which are in common use: zero (the true zero of intravesical pressure), the value of p_{ves} measured at zero bladder volume, or the value of p_{ves} immediately before the cough or valsalva (usually at 200 or 300 ml bladder capacity). The baseline used and the baseline pressure, should be specified.

[34] Detrusor leak point pressure has been used most frequently to predict upper tract problems in neurological patients with reduced bladder compliance. ICS has defined it 'in the absence of a detrusor contraction' although others will measure DLPP during involuntary detrusor contractions.

[35] The precise shape of the flow curve is decided by detrusor contractility, the presence of any abdominal straining and by the bladder outlet. (11)

- *Time to maximum flow* is the elapsed time from onset of flow to maximum flow. **(ORIGINAL)**

3.3.2 Pressure measurements during pressure flow studies (PFS)

The following measurements are applicable to each of the pressure curves: intravesical, abdominal and detrusor pressure.

- *Premicturition pressure* is the pressure recorded immediately before the initial isovolumetric contraction. **(ORIGINAL)**
- *Opening pressure* is the pressure recorded at the onset of urine flow (consider time delay). **(ORIGINAL)**
- *Opening time* is the elapsed time from initial rise in detrusor pressure to onset of flow. **(ORIGINAL)**

This is the initial isovolumetric contraction period of micturition. Flow measurement delay should be taken into account when measuring opening time.

- *Maximum pressure* is the maximum value of the measured pressure. **(ORIGINAL)**
- *Pressure at maximum flow* is the lowest pressure recorded at maximum measured flow rate. **(ORIGINAL)**
- *Closing pressure* is the pressure measured at the end of measured flow. **(ORIGINAL)**
- *Minimum voiding pressure* is the minimum pressure during measurable flow. This is not necessarily equal to either the opening or closing pressures.
- *Flow delay* is the time delay between a change in bladder pressure and the corresponding change in measured flow rate.

3.3.3 Detrusor function during voiding

- *Normal detrusor function:*

Normal voiding is achieved by a voluntarily initiated continuous detrusor contraction that leads to complete bladder emptying within a normal time span, and in the absence of obstruction. For a given detrusor contraction, the magnitude of the recorded pressure rise will depend on the degree of outlet resistance. **(ORIGINAL)**

- *Abnormal detrusor activity* can be subdivided:
  o *Detrusor underactivity* is defined as a contraction of reduced strength and/or duration, resulting in prolonged bladder emptying and/or a failure to achieve complete bladder emptying within a normal time span. **(ORIGINAL)**
  o *Acontractile detrusor* is one that cannot be demonstrated to contract during urodynamic studies. **(ORIGINAL)**[36]
  o *Post void residual (PVR)* is defined as the volume of urine left in the bladder at the end of micturition. **(ORIGINAL)**[37]

---

[36] A normal detrusor contraction will be recorded as: a high pressure if there is high outlet resistance, normal pressure if there is normal outlet resistance: or low pressure if urethral resistance is low.

[37] If after repeated free flowmetry no residual urine is demonstrated, then the finding of a residual urine during urodynamic studies should be considered an artifact, due to the circumstances of the test.

3.3.4 Urethral function during voiding

During voiding, urethral function may be:

Normal urethra function is defined as a urethra that opens, and is continuously relaxed to allow the bladder to be emptied at a normal pressure (CHANGED)

Abnormal urethra function may be due to either obstruction to urethra overactivity, or a urethra that cannot open due to anatomic abnormality such as an enlarged prostate or a urethral stricture.

- **Bladder outlet obstruction** is the generic term for obstruction during voiding and is characterised by increased detrusor pressure and reduced urine flow rate. It is usually diagnosed by studying the synchronous values of flowrate and detrusor pressure. (CHANGED)[38]
- *Dysfunctional voiding* is defined as an intermittent and/or fluctuating flow rate due to involuntary intermittent contractions of the periurethral striated muscle during voiding, in neurologically normal individuals. (CHANGED)[39]
- *Detrusor sphincter dyssynergia* is defined as a detrusor contraction concurrent with an involuntary contraction of the urethral and/or periurethral striated muscle. Occasionally flow may be prevented altogether. (ORIGINAL)[40]
- *Non-relaxing urethral sphincter obstruction* usually occurs in individuals with a neurological lesion and is characterised by a non-relaxing, obstructing urethra resulting in reduced urine flow. (NEW)[41]

4 CONDITIONS

- *Acute retention of urine* is defined as a painful, palpable or percussable bladder, when the patient is unable to pass any urine. (NEW)[42]

---

[38] Bladder outlet obstruction has been defined for men but as yet, not adequately in women and children.

[39] Although dysfunctional voiding is not a very specific term it is preferred to terms such as 'non-neurogenic neurogenic bladder'. Other terms such as 'idiopathic detrusor sphincter dyssynergia', or 'sphincter overactivity voiding dysfunction', may be preferable. However, the term dysfunctional voiding is very well established. The condition occurs most frequently in children. Whilst it is felt that pelvic floor contractions are responsible, it is possible that the intra-urethral striated muscle may be important.

[40] Detrusor sphincter dyssynergia typically occurs in patients with a supra-sacral lesion, for example after high spinal cord injury and is uncommon in lesions of the lower cord. Although the intraurethral and periurethral striated muscles are usually held responsible, the smooth muscle of the bladder neck or urethra may also be responsible.

[41] Non-relaxing sphincter obstruction is found in sacral and infra-sacral lesions such as meningomyelocoele, and after radical pelvic surgery. In addition there is often urodynamic stress incontinence during bladder filling. This term replaces 'isolated distal sphincter obstruction'.

[42] Although acute retention is usually thought of as painful, in certain circumstances pain may not be a presenting feature, for example when due to prolapsed intervertebral disc, post partum, or after regional anaesthesia such as an epidural anaesthetic. The retention volume should be significantly greater than the expected normal bladder capacity. In patients after surgery, due to bandaging of the lower abdomen or abdominal wall pain, it may be difficult to detect a painful, palpable or percussable bladder.

- *Chronic retention of urine* is defined as a non-painful bladder, which remains palpable or percussable after the patient has passed urine. Such patients may be incontinent. **(NEW)**[43]
- *Benign prostatic obstruction* is a form of *bladder outlet obstruction;* and may be diagnosed when the cause of outlet obstruction is known to be benign prostatic enlargement, due to histologic benign prostatic hyperplasia. **(NEW)**
- *Benign prostatic hyperplasia* is a term used (and reserved for) the typical histological pattern which defines the disease. **(NEW)**
- *Benign prostatic enlargement* is defined as prostatic enlargement due to histologic benign prostatic hyperplasia. The term 'prostatic enlargement' should be used in the absence of prostatic histology. **(NEW)**

5 TREATMENT

The following definitions were published in the 7th ICS report on Lower Urinary Tract Rehabilitation Techniques (3) and remain in their original form.

5.1 LOWER URINARY TRACT REHABILITATION

Lower urinary tract rehabilitation is defined as non-surgical, non-pharmacological treatment for lower urinary tract function and includes:

- *Pelvic floor training* defined as repetitive selective voluntary contraction and relaxation of specific pelvic floor muscles.
- *Biofeedback* is the technique by which information about a normally unconscious physiological process is presented to the patient and/or the therapist as a visual, auditory or tactile signal.
- *Behavioural modification* is defined as the analysis and alteration of the relationship between the patient's symptoms and his or her environment for the treatment of maladaptive voiding patterns.

This may be achieved by modification of the behaviour and/or environment of the patient.

5.2 ELECTRICAL STIMULATION

Electrical stimulation is the application of electrical current to stimulate the pelvic viscera or their nerve supply.

The aim of electrical stimulation may be to directly induce a therapeutic response or to modulate lower urinary tract, bowel or sexual dysfunction.

5.3 CATHETERISATION

Catheterisation is a technique for bladder emptying employing a catheter to drain the bladder or a urinary reservoir.

---

[43] The ICS no longer recommends the term 'overflow incontinence'. This term is considered confusing and lacking a convincing definition. If used, a precise definition and any associated pathophysiology, such as reduced urethral function, or detrusor overactivity/low bladder compliance, should be stated. The term chronic retention, excludes transient voiding difficulty, for example after surgery for stress incontinence, and implies a significant residual urine; a minimum figure of 300 mL has been previously mentioned.

5.3.1 Intermittent (in/out) catheterisation

Intermittent (in/out) catheterisation is defined as drainage or aspiration of the bladder or a urinary reservoir with subsequent removal of the catheter.

The following types of intermittent catheterisation are defined:

- *Intermittent self-catheterisation* is performed by the patient himself/herself
- *Intermittent catheterisation* is performed by an attendant (e.g. doctor, nurse or relative)
- *Clean intermittent catheterisation*: use of a clean technique. This implies ordinary washing techniques and use of disposable or cleansed reusable catheters.
- *Aseptic intermittent catheterisation:* use of a sterile technique. This implies genital disinfection and the use of sterile catheters and instruments/gloves.

5.3.2 Indwelling catheterisation

Indwelling catheterisation: an indwelling catheter remains in the bladder, urinary reservoir or urinary conduit for a period of time longer than one emptying.

5.4 BLADDER REFLEX TRIGGERING

Bladder reflex triggering comprises various manoeuvres performed by the patient or the therapist in order to elicit reflex detrusor contraction by exteroceptive stimuli.

The most commonly used manoeuvres are; suprapubic tapping, thigh scratching and anal/rectal manipulation.

5.5 BLADDER EXPRESSION

Bladder expression comprises various manoeuvres aimed at increasing intravesical pressure in order to facilitate bladder emptying.

The most commonly used manoeuvres are abdominal straining, Valsalva's manoeuvre and Credé manoeuvre.

ACKNOWLEDGEMENTS

The authors of this report are very grateful to Vicky Rees, Administrator of the ICS, for her typing and editing of numerous drafts of this document.

ADDENDUM

Formation of the ICS terminology committee

The terminology committee was announced at the ICS meeting in Denver 1999 and expressions of interest were invited from those who wished to be active members of the committee and they were asked to comment in detail on the preliminary draft (the discussion paper published in Neurourology and Urodynamics). The nine authors replied with a detailed critique by 1st April 2000 and constitute the committee: **Paul Abrams, Linda Cardozo, Magnus Fall, Derek Griffiths, Peter Rosier, Ulf Ulmsten, Philip van Kerrebroeck, Arne Victor, and Alan Wein**.

We thank other individuals who later offered their written comments: **Jens Thorup Andersen, Walter Artibani, Jerry Blaivas, Linda Brubaker, Rick Bump, Emmanuel Chartier-Kastler, Grace Dorey, Clare Fowler, Kelm Hjalmas, Gordon Hosker, Vik Khullar, Guus Kramer, Gunnar Lose, Joseph Macaluso, Anders Mattiasson, Richard Millard, Rien**

Nijman, Arwin Ridder, Werner Schäfer, David Vodusek, and Jean Jacques Wyndaele.

A ½ day workshop was held at the ICS Annual Meeting in Tampere (August 2000) and a two-day meeting in London, January 2001, which produced draft 5 of the report which was then placed on the ICS website (www.icsoffice.org). Discussions on draft 6 took place at the ICS meeting in Korea September 2001, draft 7 then remained on the ICS website until final submission to journals in November 2001.

References

Abrams P (Chair), Blaivas J G, Stanton S, Andersen J T. 1988. ICS standardisation of terminology of lower urinary tract function. Neurourol Urodyn 7:403–426.

Abrams P, Blaivas J G, Stanton S L, Andersen J. 1992. ICS 6th report on the standardisation of terminology of lower urinary tract function. Neurourol Urodyn 11:593–603.

Andersen J T, Blaivas J G, Cardozo L, Thüroff J. 1992. ICS 7th report on the standardisation of terminology of lower urinary tract function: lower urinary tract rehabilitation techniques. Neurourol Urodyn 11:593–603.

Bump R C, Mattiasson A, Bo K, Brubaker L P, DeLancey J O L, Klarskov P, Shull B L, Smith A R B. 1996. The standardisation of terminology of female pelvic organ prolapse and pelvic floor dysfunction. Am J Obstet Gynecol 175:10–11.

Fonda D, Resnick N M, Colling J, Burgio K, Ouslander J G, Norton C, Ekelund P, Versi E, Mattiasson A. 1998. Outcome measures for research of lower urinary tract dysfunction in frail and older people. Neurourol Urodyn 17:273–281.

Griffiths D, Höfner K, van Mastrigt R, Rollema H J, Spangberg A, Gleason D. 1997. ICS report on the standardisation of terminology of lower urinary tract function: pressure-flow studies of voiding, urethral resistance and urethral obstruction. Neurourol Urodyn 16:1–18.

International Classification of Functioning, Disability and Health. ICIDH-2 website http://www.who.int/icidh.

Klevmark B. 1999. Natural pressure: volume curves and conventional cystometry. Scand J Urol Nephrol Suppl 201:1–4.

Lose G, Fanti J A, Victor A, Walter S, Wells T L, Wyman J, Mattiasson A. 1998. Outcome measures for research in adult women with symptoms of lower urinary tract dysfunction. Neurourol Urodyn 17:255–262.

Lose G, Griffiths D, Hosker G, Kulseng-Hanssen S, Perucchini D, Schäfer W, Thind P, Versi E. Standardisation of urethral pressure measurement: report from the standardisation sub-committee of the International Continence Society. Neurourol Urodyn (In press).

Mattiasson A, Djurhuus J C, Fonda D, Lose G, Nordling J, Stöhrer M. 1998. Standardisation of outcome studies in patients with lower urinary dysfunction: a report on general principles from the standardisation committee of the International Continence Society. Neurourol Urodyn 17:249–253.

Nordling J, Abrams P, Ameda K, Andersen J T, Donovan J, Griffiths D, Kobayashi S, Koyanagi T, Schäfer W, Yalla S, Mattiasson A. 1998. Outcome measures for research in treatment of adult males with symptoms of lower urinary tract dysfunction. Neurourol Urodyn 17:263–271.

Stöhrer M, Goepel M, Kondo A, Kramer G, Madersbacher H, Millard R, Rossier A, Wyndaele J J. 1999. ICS report on the standardisation of terminology in neurogenic lower urinary tract dysfunction. Neurourol Urodyn 18:139–158.

Schäfer W, Sterling A M, Liao L, Spangberg A, Pesce F, Zinner N R, van Kerrebroeck P, Abrams P, Mattiasson A. 2002. Good urodynamic practice: report from the standardisation sub-committee of the International Continence Society. Neurourol Urodyn (In press).*

van Waalwijk van Doorn E, Anders K, Khullar V, Kulseng-Hansen S, Pesce F, Robertson A, Rosario D, Schäfer W. 2000. Standardisation of ambulatory urodynamic monitoring: report of the standardisation sub-committee of the International Continence Soceity for ambulatory urodynamic studies. Neurourol Urodyn 19:113–125.

van Kerrebroeck P, Abrams P, Chaikin D, Donovan J, Fonda D, Jackson S, Jennum P, Johnson T, Lose G, Mattiasson A, Robertson G, Weiss J. 2002. ICS standardisation report on nocturia: report from the standardisation sub-committee of the International Continence Society. Neurourol Urodyn 21:193–199.

wan D, James E D, Kramer A E J L, Sterling A M, Suhel P F. 1987. ICS report on urodynamic equipment: technical aspects. J Med Eng Technol 11(2):57–64.

*Now published as: Schäfer W, Abrams P, Liao L, Mattiason A, Pesce F, Spangberg A, Sterling A, Zinner N, van Kerrebroeck P 2002 Good urodynamic practices: uroflow-metry, filling cystometry and pressure-flow studies. Neurourol Urodyn 21:261–274.

Appendix 2

Standardisation of terminology of lower urinary tract function

Reproduced with permission of the International Continence Society Committee on Standardisation of Terminology. First published in Scandinavian Journal of Urology and Nephrology, Supplementum 114, 1988

Members: Paul Abrams, Jerry G. Blaivas, Stuart L. Stanton and Jens T. Andersen (Chairman)

1 INTRODUCTION

The International Continence Society established a committee for the standardisation of terminology of lower urinary tract function in 1973. Five of the six reports (1,2,3,4,5) from this committee, approved by the Society, have been published. The fifth report on 'Quantification of urine loss' was an internal I.C.S. document but appears, in part, in this document.

These reports are revised, extended and collated in this monograph. The standards are recommended to facilitate comparison of results by investigators who use urodynamic methods. These standards are recommended not only for urodynamic investigations carried out on humans but also during animal studies. When using urodynamic studies in animals the type of any anaesthesia used should be stated. It is suggested that acknowledgement of these standards in written publications be indicated by a footnote to the section 'Methods and Materials' or its equivalent, to read as follows:

'Methods, definitions and units conform to the standards recommended by the International Continence Society, except where specifically noted'.

Urodynamic Studies involve the assessment of the function and dysfunction of the urinary tract by any appropriate method. Aspects of urinary tract morphology, physiology, biochemistry and hydrodynamics affect urine transport and storage. Other methods of investigation such as the radiographic visualisation of the lower urinary tract is a useful adjunct to conventional urodynamics.

This monograph concerns the urodynamics of the lower urinary tract.

2 CLINICAL ASSESSMENT

The clinical assessment of patients with lower urinary tract dysfunction should consist of a detailed history, a frequency/volume chart and a physical examination: In urinary incontinence, leakage should be demonstrated objectively.

2.1 HISTORY

The general history should include questions relevant to neurological and congential abnormalities as well as information on previous urinary infections and relevant surgery. Information must be obtained on medication with known or possible effects on the lower urinary tract. The general history should also include assessment of menstrual, sexual and bowel function, and obstetric history.

The urinary history must consist of symptoms related to both the storage and the evacuation functions of the lower urinary tract.

2.2 FREQUENCY/VOLUME CHART

The frequency/volume chart is a specific urodynamic investigation recording fluid intake and urine output per 24 hour period. The chart gives objective information on the number of voidings, the distribution of voidings between daytime and nighttime and each voided volume. The chart can also be used to record episodes of urgency and leakage and the number of incontinence pads used. The frequency/volume chart is very useful in the assessment of voiding disorders, and in the follow-up of treatment.

2.3 PHYSICAL EXAMINATION

Besides a general urological and, when appropriate, gynaecological examination, the physical examination should include the assessment of perineal sensation, the perineal reflexes supplied by the sacral segments S2–S4, and anal sphincter tone and control.

3 PROCEDURES RELATED TO THE EVALUATION OF URINE STORAGE

3.1 CYSTOMETRY

Cystometry is the method by which the pressure/volume relationship of the bladder is measured. All systems are zeroed at atmospheric pressure. For external transducers the reference point is the level of the superior edge of the symphysis pubis. For catheter mounted transducers the reference point is the transducer itself.

Cystometry is used to assess detrusor activity, sensation, capacity and compliance.

Before starting to fill the bladder the residual urine may be measured. However, the removal of a large volume of residual urine may alter detrusor function especially in neuropathic disorders. Certain cystometric parameters may be significantly altered by the speed of bladder filling (see 6.1.1.4).

During cystometry it is taken for granted that the patient is awake, unanaesthetised and neither sedated nor taking drugs that affect bladder function. Any variations should be specified.

Specify

(a) Access (transurethral or percutaneous).
(b) Fluid medium (liquid or gas).
(c) Temperature of fluid (state in degrees Celsius).
(d) Position of patient (e.g. supine, sitting or standing).
(e) Filling may be by diuresis or catheter. Filling by catheter may be continuous or incremental; the precise filling rate should be stated.

 When the incremental method is used the volume increment should be stated. For general discussion, the following terms for the range of filling rate may be used:
   (i) up to 10 ml per minute is slow fill cystometry ('physiological' filling).
   (ii) 10–100 ml per minute is medium fill cystometry.
   (iii) over 100 ml per minute is rapid fill cystometry.

Technique

(a) Fluid-filled catheter – specify number of catheters, single or multiple lumens, type of catheter (manufacturer), size of catheter.
(b) Catheter tip transducer – list specifications.
(c) Other catheters – list specifications.
(d) Measuring equipment.

Definitions

Intravesical pressure is the pressure within the bladder.

 Abdominal pressure is taken to be the pressure surrounding the bladder. In current practice it is estimated from rectal or, less commonly, extraperitoneal pressure.

 Detrusor pressure is that component of intravesical pressure that is created by forces in the bladder wall (passive and active). It is estimated by subtracting abdominal pressure from intravesical pressure. The simultaneous measurement of abdominal pressure is essential for the interpretation of the intravesical pressure trace. However, artifacts on the detrusor pressure trace may be produced by intrinsic rectal contractions.

 Bladder sensation. Sensation is difficult to evaluate because of its subjective nature. It is usually assessed by questioning the patient in relation to the fullness of the bladder during cystometry.

 Commonly used descriptive terms include:

First desire to void
Normal desire to void (this is defined as the feeling that leads the patient to pass urine at the next convenient moment, but voiding can be delayed if necessary).
Strong desire to void (this is defined as a persistent desire to void without the fear of leakage).
Urgency (this is defined as a strong desire to void accompanied by fear of leakage or fear of pain).

Pain (the site and character of which should be specified). Pain during bladder filling or micturition is abnormal.

The use of objective or semi-objective tests for sensory function, such as electrical threshold studies (sensory testing), is discussed in detail in 5.5.

The term 'Capacity' must be qualified.

Maximum cystometric capacity, in patients with normal sensation, is the volume at which the patient feels he/she can no longer delay micturition. In the absence of sensation the maximum cystometric capacity cannot be defined in the same terms and is the volume at which the clinician decides to terminate filling. In the presence of sphincter incompetence the maximum cystometric capacity may be significantly increased by occlusion of the urethra e.g. by Foley catheter.

The *functional bladder capacity*, or voided volume is more relevant and is assessed from a frequency/volume chart (urinary diary).

The *maximum (anaesthetic) bladder capacity* is the volume measured after filling during a deep general or spinal/epidural anaesthetic, specifying fluid temperature, filling pressure and filling time.

Compliance indicates the change in volume for a change in pressure. Compliance is calculated by dividing the volume change (ΔV) by the change in detrusor pressure (Δpdet) during that change in bladder volume ($C = \Delta V/\Delta p$det). Compliance is expressed as mls per cm H_2O (see 6.1.1.4).

3.2 URETHRAL PRESSURE MEASUREMENT

It should be noted that the urethral pressure and the urethral closure pressure are idealized concepts which represent the ability of the urethra to prevent leakage (see 6.1.5). In current urodynamic practice the urethral pressure is measured by a number of different techniques which do not always yield consistant values. Not only do the values differ with the method of measurement but there is often lack of consistency for a single method. For example the effect of catheter rotation when urethral pressure is measured by a catheter mounted transducer.

Intraluminal urethral pressure may be measured:

(a) At rest, with the bladder at any given volume.
(b) During coughing or straining.
(c) During the process of voiding (see 4.4).

Measurements may be made at one point in the urethra over a period of time, or at several points along the urethra consecutively forming a *urethral pressure profile* (U.P.P.).

Storage phase

Two types of U.P.P. may be measured:

(a) Resting urethral pressure profile – with the bladder and subject at rest.
(b) Stress urethral pressure profile – with a defined applied stress (e.g. cough, strain, valsalva).

In the storage phase the *urethral pressure profile* denotes the intraluminal pressure along the length of the urethra. All systems are zeroed at atmospheric pressure. For external transducers the reference point is the superior edge of the symphysis pubis. For catheter mounted transducers the reference point is the transducer itself. Intravesical pressure should be measured to exclude a simultaneous detrusor contraction. The subtraction of intravesical pressure from urethral pressure produces the *urethral closure pressure profile*.

The simultaneous recording of both intravesical and intra-urethral pressures are essential during stress urethral profilometry.

Specify

(a) Infusion medium (liquid or gas).
(b) Rate of infusion.
(c) Stationary, continuous or intermittent withdrawal.
(d) Rate of withdrawal.
(e) Bladder volume.
(f) Position of patient (supine, sitting or standing).

Technique

(a) Open catheter – specify type (manufacturer), size, number, position and orientation of side or end hole.
(b) Catheter mounted transducers – specify manufacturer, number of transducers, spacing of transducers along the catheter, orientation with respect to one another; transducer design e.g. transducer face depressed or flush with catheter surface; catheter diameter and material. The orientation of the transducer(s) in the urethra should be stated.
(c) Other catheters, e.g. membrane, fibreoptic – specify type (manufacturer), size and number of channels as for microtransducer catheter.
(d) Measurement technique: For stress profiles the particular stress employed should be stated e.g. cough or valsalva.
(e) Recording apparatus: Describe type of recording apparatus. The frequency response of the total system should be stated. The frequency response of the catheter in the perfusion method can be assessed by blocking the eyeholes and recording the consequent rate of change of pressure.

Definitions

Fig. A2.1: Referring to profiles measured in storage phase.

Maximum urethral pressure is the maximum pressure of the measured profile.

Maximum urethral closure pressure is the maximum difference between the urethral pressure and the intravesical pressure.

Functional profile length is the length of the urethra along which the urethral pressure exceeds intravesical pressure.

Functional profile length (on stress) is the length over which the urethral pressure exceeds the intravesical pressure on stress.

Pressure 'transmission' ratio is the increment in urethral pressure on stress as a percentage of the simultaneously recorded increment in intravesical pressure. For stress profiles obtained during coughing, pressure transmission ratios can be obtained at any point along the urethra. If single values

Figure A2.1   Diagram of a female urethral pressure profile (static) with I.C.S. recommended nomenclature.

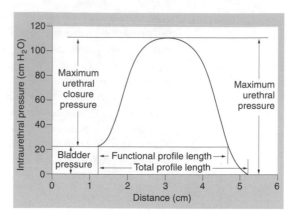

are given the position in the urethra should be stated. If several pressure transmission ratios are defined at different points along the urethra a pressure 'transmission' profile is obtained. During 'cough profiles' the amplitude of the cough should be stated if possible.

Note: the term 'transmission' is in common usage and cannot be changed. However transmission implies a completely passive process. Such an assumption is not yet justified by scientific evidence. A role for muscular activity cannot be excluded.

Total profile length is not generally regarded as a useful parameter.

The information gained from urethral pressure measurements in the storage phase is of limited value in the assessment of voiding disorders.

3.3 QUANTIFICATION OF URINE LOSS

Subjective grading of incontinence may not indicate reliably the degree of abnormality. However it is important to relate the management of the individual patients to their complaints and personal circumstances, as well as to objective measurements.

In order to assess and compare the results of the treatment of different types of incontinence in different centres, a simple standard test can be used to measure urine loss objectively in any subject. In order to obtain a representative result, especially in subjects with variable or intermittent urinary incontinence, the test should occupy as long a period as possible; yet it must be practical. The circumstances should approximate to those of everyday life, yet be similar for all subjects to allow meaningful comparison. On the basis of pilot studies performed in various centres, an internal report of the I.C.S. (5th) recommended a test occupying a one-hour period during which a series of standard activities was carried out. This test *can* be extended by further one hour periods if the result of the first one hour test was not considered representative by either the patient or the investigator. Alternatively the test can be repeated having filled the bladder to a defined volume.

The total amount of urine lost during the test period is determined by weighing a collecting device such as a nappy, absorbent pad or condom appliance. A nappy or pad should be worn inside waterproof underpants or should have a waterproof backing. Care should be taken to use a collecting device of adequate capacity.

Immediately before the test begins the collecting device is weighed to the nearest gram.

Typical test schedule

(a) Test is started without the patient voiding.
(b) Preweighed collecting device is put on and first one hour test period begins.
(c) Subject drinks 500 ml sodium free liquid within a short period (max. 15 min), then sits or rests.
(d) Half hour period: subject walks, including stair climbing equivalent to one flight up and down.
(e) During the remaining period the subject performs the following activities:
    (i)   standing up from sitting, 10 times
    (ii) coughing vigorously, 10 times
    (iii) running on the spot for 1 minute
    (iv) bending to pick up small object from floor, 5 times
    (v)   wash hands in running water for 1 minute
(f) At the end of the one hour test the collecting device is removed and weighed.
(g) If the test is regarded as representative the subject voids and the volume is recorded.
(h) Otherwise the test is repeated preferably without voiding.

If the collecting device becomes saturated or filled during the test it should be removed and weighed, and replaced by a fresh device. The total weight of urine lost during the test period is taken to be equal to the gain in weight of the collecting device(s). In interpreting the results of the test it should be born in mind that a weight gain of up to 1 gram may be due to weighing errors, sweating or vaginal discharge.

The activity programme may be modified according to the subject's physical ability. If substantial variations from the usual test schedule occur, this should be recorded so that the same schedule can be used on subsequent occasions.

In principle the subject should not void during the test period. If the patient experiences urgency, then he/she should be persuaded to postpone voiding and to perform as many of the activities in section (e) as possible in order to detect leakage. Before voiding the collection device is removed for weighing. If inevitable voiding cannot be postponed then the test is terminated. The voided volume and the duration of the test should be recorded. For subjects not completing the full test the results may require separate analysis, or the test may be repeated after rehydration.

The test result is given as grams urine lost in the one hour test period in which the greatest urine loss is recorded.

Additional procedures

Additional procedures intended to give information of diagnostic value are permissible provided they do not interfere with the basic test. For example, additional changes and weighing of the collecting device can give information about the timing of urine loss. The absorbent nappy may be an electronic recording nappy so that the timing is recorded directly.

Presentation of results

Specify

(a) collecting device
(b) physical condition of subject (ambulant, chair-bound, bedridden)
(c) relevant medical condition of subject
(d) relevant drug treatments
(e) test schedule.

In some situations the timing of the test (e.g. in relation to the menstrual cycle) may be relevant.

Findings

Record weight of urine lost during the test (in the case of repeated tests greatest weight in any stated period). A loss of less than one gram is within experimental error and the patients should be regarded as essentially dry. Urine loss should be measured and recorded in grams.

Statistics

When performing statistical analysis of urine loss in a group of subjects, non-parametric statistics should be employed, since the values are not normally distributed.

4 PROCEDURES RELATED TO THE EVALUATION OF MICTURITION

4.1 MEASUREMENT OF URINARY FLOW

Urinary flow may be described in terms of *rate* and *pattern* and may be *continuous* or *intermittent*. *Flow rate* is defined as the volume of fluid expelled via the urethra per unit time. It is expressed in ml/s.

Specify

(a) Voided volume.
(b) Patient environment and position (supine, sitting or standing).
(c) Filling:
    (i) by diuresis (spontaneous or forced: specify regimen),
    (ii) by catheter (transurethral or suprapubic).
(d) Type of fluid.

Technique

(a) Measuring equipment.
(b) Solitary procedure or combined with other measurements.

Definitions

(a) Continuous flow (Fig. A2.2)
Voided volume is the total volume expelled via the urethra.
   Maximum flow rate is the maximum measured value of the flow rate.
   Average flow rate is voided volume divided by flow time. The calculation of average flow rate is only meaningful if flow is continuous and without terminal dribbling.
   Flow time is the time over which measurable flow actually occurs.
   Time to maximum flow is the elapsed time from onset of flow to maximum flow.
   The flow pattern must be described when flow time and average flow rate are measured.

(b) Intermittent flow (Fig. A2.3)
The same parameters used to characterise continuous flow may be applicable if care is exercised in patients with intermittent flow. In measuring flow time the time intervals between flow episodes are disregarded.

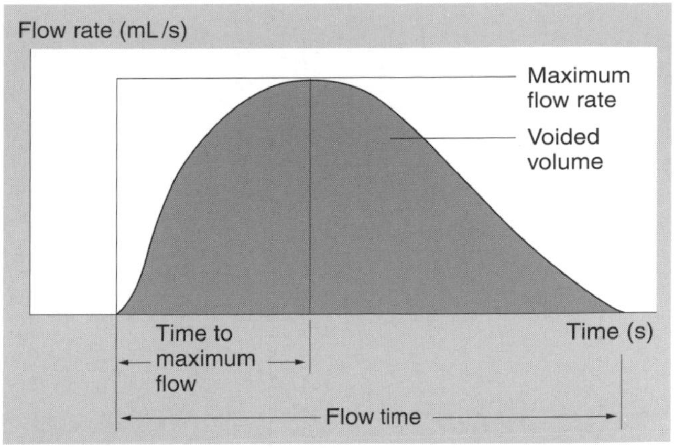

Figure A2.2   Diagram of a continuous urine flow recording with I.C.S. recommended nomenclature.

Figure A2.3   Diagram of an interrupted urine flow recording with I.C.S. recommended nomenclature.

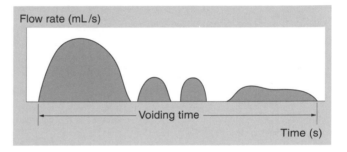

Voiding time is total duration of micturition, i.e. includes interruptions. When voiding is completed without interruption, voiding time is equal to flow time.

4.2 BLADDER PRESSURE MEASUREMENTS DURING MICTURITION

The specifications of patient position, access for pressure measurement, catheter type and measuring equipment are as for cystometry (see 3.1).

Definitions (Fig. A2.4)

Opening time is the elapsed time from initial rise in detrusor pressure to onset of flow. This is the initial isovolumetric contraction period of micturition. Time lags should be taken into account. In most urodynamic systems a time lag occurs equal to the time taken for the urine to pass from the point of pressure measurement to the uroflow transducer.

The following parameters are applicable to measurements of each of the pressure curves: intravesical, abdominal and detrusor pressure.

Premicturition pressure is the pressure recorded immediately before the initial isovolumetric contraction.

Opening pressure is the pressure recorded at the onset of measured flow.

Maximum pressure is the maximum value of the measured pressure.

Pressure at maximum flow is the pressure reorded at maximum measured flow rate.

Contraction pressure at maximum flow is the difference between pressure at maximum flow and premicturition pressure.

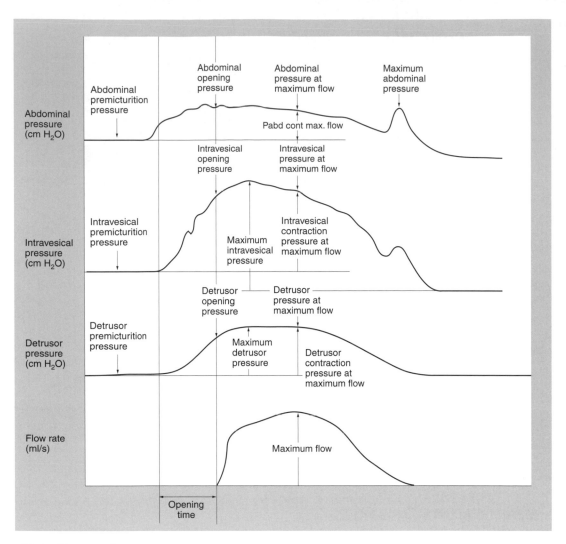

Figure A2.4 Diagram of a pressure-flow recording of micturition with I.C.S. recommended nomenclature.

Postmicturition events (e.g. after contraction) are not well understood and so cannot be defined as yet.

4.3 PRESSURE FLOW RELATIONSHIPS

In the early days of urodynamics the flow rate and voiding pressure were related as a 'urethral resistance factor'. The concept of a resistance factor originates from rigid tube hydrodynamics. The urethra does not generally behave as a rigid tube as it is an irregular and distensible conduit whose walls and surroundings have active and passive elements and hence, influence the flow through it. Therefore a resistance factor cannot provide a valid comparison between patients.

There are many ways of displaying the relationships between flow and pressure during micturition, an example is suggested in the I.C.S. 3rd Report (4) (Fig. A2.5). As yet available data do not permit a standard presentation of pressure/flow parameters.

Figure A2.5 Diagram
illustrating the presentation of
pressure flow data on individual
patients in three groups of 3
patients: obstructed, equivocal
and unobstructed.

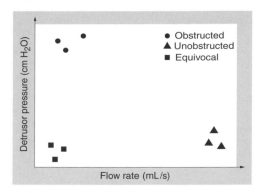

When data from a group of patients are presented, pressure-flow relationships may be shown on a graph as illustrated in Fig. A2.5. This form of presentation allows lines of demarcation to be drawn on the graph to separate the results according to the problem being studied. The points shown in Fig. A2.5 are purely illustrative to indicate how the data might fall into groups. The group of equivocal results might include either an unrepresentative micturition in an obstructed or an unobstructed patient, or underactive detrusor function with or without obstruction. This is the group which invalidates the use of 'urethral resistance factors'.

4.4 URETHRAL PRESSURE MEASUREMENTS DURING VOIDING (V.U.P.P.)

The V.U.P.P. is used to determine the pressure and site of urethral obstruction.

Pressure is recorded in the urethra during voiding. The technique is similar to that used in the U.P.P. measured during storage (the resting and stress profiles (see 3.2)).

Specify: as for U.P.P. during storage (see 3.2).

Accurate interpretation of the V.U.P.P. depends on the simultaneous measurement of intravesical pressure and the measurement of pressure at a precisely localised point in the urethra. Localisation may be achieved by radio opaque marker on the catheter which allows the pressure measurements to be related to a visualised point in the urethra.

This technique is not fully developed and a number of technical as well as clinical problems need to be solved before the V.U.P.P. is widely used.

RESIDUAL URINE

Residual urine is defined as the volume of fluid remaining in the bladder immediately following the completion of micturition. The measurement of residual urine forms an integral part of the study of micturition. However voiding in unfamiliar surroundings may lead to unrepresentative results, as may voiding on command with a partially filled or overfilled bladder. Residual urine is commonly estimated by the following methods:

(a) Catheter or cystoscope (transurethral, supra-pubic).
(b) Radiography (excretion urography, micturition cystography).
(c) Ultrasonics.
(d) Radioisotopes (clearance, gamma camera).

When estimating residual urine the measurement of voided volume and the time interval between voiding and residual urine estimation should be recorded: this is particularly important if the patient is in a diuretic phase. In the condition of vesicoureteric reflux, urine may re-enter the bladder after micturition and may falsely be interpreted as residual urine. The presence of urine in bladder diverticula following micturition present special problems of interpretation, since a diverticulum may be regarded either as part of the bladder cavity or as outside the functioning bladder.

The various methods of measurement each have limitations as to their applicability and accuracy in the various conditions associated with residual urine. Therefore it is necessary to choose a method appropriate to the clinical problems. The absence of residual urine is usually an observation of clinical value, but does not exclude infravesical obstruction or bladder dysfunction. An isolated finding of residual urine requires confirmation before being considered significant.

5 PROCEDURES RELATED TO NEUROPHYSIOLOGICAL EVALUATION OF THE URINARY TRACT DURING FILLING AND VOIDING

5.1 ELECTROMYOGRAPHY

Electromyography (EMG) is the study of electrical potentials generated by the depolarisation of muscle. The following refers to striated muscle EMG. The functional unit in EMG is the motor unit. This is comprised of a single motor neurone and the muscle fibres it innervates. A motor unit action potential is the recorded depolarisation of muscle fibres which results from activation of a single anterior horn cell. Muscle action potentials may be detected either by needle electrodes, or by surface electrodes.

Needle electrodes are placed directly into the muscle mass and permit visualisation of the individual motor unit action potentials.

Surface electrodes are applied to an epithelial surface as close to the muscle under study as possible. Surface electrodes detect the action potentials from groups of adjacent motor units underlying the recording surface.

EMG potentials may be displayed on an oscilloscope screen or played through audio amplifiers. A permanent record of EMG potentials can only be made using a chart recorder with a high frequency response (in the range of 10 kHz).

EMG should be interpreted in the light of the patients symptoms, physical findings and urological and urodynamic investigations.

General information

(a) EMG (solitary procedure, part of urodynamic or other electrophysiological investigation).

Specify

(b) Patient position (supine, standing, sitting or other).
(c) Electrode placement:
   (i) Sampling site (intrinsic striated muscle of the urethra, periurethral striated muscle, bulbocavernosus muscle, external anal sphincter, pubococcygeus or other). State whether sites are single or multiple, unilateral or bilateral. Also state number of samples per site.

(ii) Recording electrode: define the precise anatomical location of the electrode. For needle electrodes, include site of needle entry, angle of entry and needle depth. For vaginal or urethral surface electrodes state method of determining position of electrode.

(iii) Reference electrode position.

Note: ensure that there is no electrical interference with any other machines, e.g. X-ray apparatus.

Technical information

(a) Electrodes.

Specify

    (i) Needle electrodes
- design (concentric, bipolar, monopolar, single fibre, other)
- dimensions (length, diameter, recording area).
- electrode material (e.g. platinum).

    (ii) Surface electrodes.
- type (skin, plug, catheter, other)
- size and shape
- electrode material
- mode of fixation to recording surface
- conducting medium (e.g. saline, jelly)

(b) Amplifier (make and specifications).

(c) Signal processing (data: raw, averaged, integrated or other).

(d) Display equipment (make and specifications to include method of calibration, time base, full scale deflection in microvolts and polarity).

    (i) oscilloscope

    (ii) chart recorder

    (iii) loudspeaker

    (iv) other

(e) Storage (make and specifications).

    (i) paper

    (ii) magnetic tape recorder

    (iii) microprocessor

    (iv) other

(f) Hard copy production (make and specifications).

    (i) chart recorder

    (ii) photographic/video reproduction of oscilloscope screen

    (iii) other.

EMG Findings

(a) Individual motor unit action potentials – Normal motor unit potentials have a characteristic configuration, amplitude and duration. Abnormalities of the motor unit may include an increase in the amplitude, duration and complexity of waveform (polyphasicity) of the potentials. A polyphasic potential is defined as one having more than 5 deflections. The EMG findings of fibrillations, positive sharp waves and bizarre high frequency potentials are thought to be abnormal.

(b) Recruitment patterns – In normal subjects there is a gradual increase in 'pelvic floor' and 'sphincter' EMG activity during bladder filling. At the onset of micturition there is complete absence of activity. Any sphincter EMG activity during voiding is abnormal unless the patient is attempting to inhibit micturition. The finding of increased sphincter EMG activity, during voiding, accompanied by characteristic simultaneous detrusor pressure and flow changes is described by the term, detrusor-sphincter-dyssynergia. In this condition a detrusor contraction occurs concurrently with an inappropriate contraction of the urethral and or periurethral striated muscle.

5.2 NERVE CONDUCTION STUDIES

Nerve conduction studies involve stimulation of a peripheral nerve, and recording the time taken for a response to occur in muscle, innervated by the nerve under study. The time taken from stimulation of the nerve to the response in the muscle is called the 'latency'. Motor latency is the time taken by the fastest motor fibres in the nerve to conduct impulses to the muscle and depends on conduction distance and the conduction velocity of the fastest fibres.

General information

(Also applicable to reflex latencies and evoked potentials – see below.)

Specify

(a) Type of investigation.
  (i)   nerve conduction study (e.g. pudendal nerve)
  (ii) reflex latency determination (e.g. bulbocavernosus)
  (iii) spinal evoked potential
  (iv) cortical evoked potential
  (v)   other
(b) Is the study a solitary procedure or part of urodynamic or neurophysiological investigations?
(c) Patient position and environmental temperature, noise level and illumination.
(d) Electrode placement: Define electrode placement in precise anatomical terms. The exact interelectrode distance is required for nerve conduction velocity calculations.
  (i)   Stimulation site (penis, clitoris, urethra, bladder neck, bladder or other).
  (ii) Recording sites (external anal sphincter, periurethral striated muscle, bulbocavernosus muscle, spinal cord, cerebral cortex or other).
         When recording spinal evoked responses, the sites of the recording electrodes should be specified according to the bony landmarks (e.g. L4). In cortical evoked responses the sites of the recording electrodes should be specified as in the International 10–20 system (6). The sampling techniques should be specified (single or multiple, unilateral or bilateral, ipsilateral or contralateral or other).
  (iii) Reference electrode position.
  (iv) Grounding electrode site: ideally this should be between the stimulation and recording sites to reduce stimulus artefact.

Technical information

(Also applicable to reflex latencies and evoked potential – see below.)

Specify (a) Electrodes (make and specifications). Describe *separately* stimulus and recording electrodes as below
  (i) design (e.g. needle, plate, ring, and configuration of anode and cathode where applicable)
  (ii) dimensions
  (iii) electrode material (e.g. platinum)
  (iv) contact medium
(b) Stimulator (make and specifications)
  (i) stimulus parameters (pulse width, frequency, pattern, current density, electrode impedance in Kohms. Also define in terms of threshold e.g. in case of supramaximal stimulation)
(c) Amplifier (make and specifications)
  (i) sensitivity (mV–μV)
  (ii) filters – low pass (Hz) or high pass (kHz)
  (iii) sampling time (ms)
(d) Averager (make and specifications)
  (i) number of stimuli sampled
(e) Display equipment (make and specifications to include method of calibration, time base, full scale deflection in microvolts and polarity)
  (i) oscilloscope
(f) Storage (make and specifications)
  (i) paper
  (ii) magnetic tape recorder
  (iii) microprocessor
  (iv) other
(g) Hard copy production (make and specification)
  (i) chart recorder
  (ii) photographic/video reproduction of oscilloscope screen
  (iii) XY recorder
  (iv) other.

Description of nerve conduction studies

Recordings are made from muscle and the latency of response of the muscle is measured. The latency is taken as the time to onset, of the earliest response.

(a) To ensure that response time can be precisely measured, the gain should be increased to give a clearly defined takeoff point. (Gain setting at least $100\,\mu V/div$ and using a short time base e.g. $1–2\,ms/div$).

(b) Additional information may be obtained from nerve conduction studies, if, when using surface electrodes to record a compound muscle action potential, the amplitude is measured. The gain setting must be reduced so that the whole response is displayed and a longer time base is recommended (e.g. $1\,mV/div$ and $5\,ms/div$). Since the amplitude is proportional to the number of motor unit potentials within the vicinity of the recording electrodes, a reduction in amplitude indicates loss of motor units and therefore denervation. (Note: A prolongation of latency is not necessarily indicative of denervation).

5.3 REFLEX LATENCIES

Reflex latencies require stimulation of sensory fields and recordings from the muscle which contracts reflexly in response to the stimulation. Such responses are a test of reflex arcs which are comprised of both afferent and efferent limbs and a synaptic region within the central nervous system. The reflex latency expresses the nerve conduction velocity in both limbs of the arc and the integrity of the central nervous system at the level of the synapse(s). Increased reflex latency may occur as a result of slowed afferent or efferent nerve conduction or due to central nervous system conduction delays.

GENERAL INFORMATION and TECHNICAL INFORMATION. The same technical and general details apply as discussed above under nerve conduction studies (see 5.2).

Description of reflex latency measurements

Recordings are made from muscle and the latency of response of the muscle is measured. The latency is taken as the time to onset, of the earliest response.

To ensure that response time can be precisely measured, the gain should be increased to give a clearly defined take-off point. (Gain setting at least $100\,\mu V/div$ and using a short time base e.g. 1–2 ms/div).

5.4 EVOKED RESPONSES

Evoked responses are potential changes in central nervous system neurones resulting from distant stimulation usually electrical. They are recorded using averaging techniques. Evoked responses may be used to test the integrity of peripheral, spinal and central nervous pathways. As with nerve conduction studies, the conduction time (latency) may be measured. In addition, information may be gained from the amplitude and configuration of these responses.

GENERAL INFORMATION and TECHNICAL INFORMATION. See above under nerve conduction studies (see 5.2).

Description of evoked responses

Describe the presence or absence of stimulus evoked responses and their configuration.

Specify

(a) Single or multiphasic response.
(b) Onset of response: defined as the start of the first reproducible potential. Since the onset of the response may be difficult to ascertain precisely, the criteria used should be stated.
(c) Latency to onset: defined as the time (ms) from the onset of stimulus to the onset of response. The central conduction time relates to cortical evoked potentials and is defined as the difference between the latencies of the cortical and the spinal evoked potentials. This parameter may be used to test the integrity of the corticospinal neuraxis.
(d) Latencies to peaks of positive and negative deflections in multiphasic responses (Fig. A2.6). P denotes positive deflections, N denotes negative deflections. In multiphasic responses, the peaks are numbered

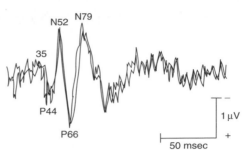

Figure A2.6 Multiphasic evoked response recorded from the cerebral cortex after stimulation of the dorsal aspect of the penis. The recording shows the conventional labelling of negative (N) and positive (P) deflections with the latency of each deflection from the point of stimulation in milliseconds.

consecutively (e.g. P1, N1, P2, N2 ...) or according to the latencies to peaks in milliseconds (e.g. P44, N52, P66 ...).

(e) The amplitude of the responses is measured in μV.

5.5 SENSORY TESTING

Limited information, of a subjective nature, may be obtained during cystometry by recording such parameters as the first desire to micturate, urgency or pain. However, sensory function in the lower urinary tract, can be assessed by semi-objective tests by the measurement of urethral and/or vesical sensory thresholds to a standard applied stimulus such as a known electrical current.

General information

Specify

(a) Patients position (supine, sitting, standing, other).
(b) Bladder volume at time of testing.
(c) Site of applied stimulus (intravesical, intraurethral).
(d) Number of times the stimulus was applied and the response recorded. Define the sensation recorded, e.g. the first sensation or the sensation of pulsing.
(e) Type of applied stimulus
    (i) electrical current: it is usual to use a constant current stimulator in urethral sensory measurement
       – state electrode characteristics and placement as in section on EMG
       – state electrode contact area and distance between electrodes if applicable
       – state impedance characteristics of the system
       – state type of conductive medium used for electrode/epithelial contact. *Note: topical anaesthetic agents should not be used.*
       – stimulator make and specifications.
       – stimulation parameters (pulse width, frequency, pattern, duration, current density).
    (ii) other – e.g. mechanical, chemical.

Definition of sensory thresholds

The vesical/urethral sensory threshold is defined as the least current which consistently produces a sensation perceived by the subject during stimulation at the site under investigation. However, the absolute values will vary in relation to the site of the stimulus, the characteristics of the equipment and the stimulation parameters. Normal values should be established for each system.

6 A CLASSIFICATION OF URINARY TRACT DYSFUNCTION

The lower urinary tract is composed of the *bladder* and *urethra*. They form a functional unit and their interaction cannot be ignored. Each has two functions, the bladder to store and void, the urethra to control and convey. When a reference is made to the hydrodynamic function or to the whole anatomical unit as a storage organ – the vesica urinaria – the correct term is the *bladder*. When the smooth muscle structure known as the m.detrusor urinae is being discussed then the correct term is *detrusor*. For simplicity the bladder/detrusor and the urethra will be considered separately so that a classification based on a combination of functional anomalies can be reached. Sensation cannot be precisely evaluated but must be assessed. This classification depends on the results of various objective urodynamic investigations. A complete urodynamic assessment is not necessary in all patients. However, studies of the filling and voiding phases are essential for each patient. As the bladder and urethra may behave differently during the storage and micturition phases of bladder function it is most useful to examine bladder and urethral activity separately in each phase.

Terms used should be objective, definable and ideally should be applicable to the whole range of abnormality. When authors disagree with the classification presented below, or use terms which have not been defined here, their meaning should be made clear.

Assuming the absence of inflammation, infection and neoplasm, *Lower urinary tract dysfunction* may be caused by:

(a) Disturbance of the pertinent nervous or psychological control system.
(b) Disorders of muscle function.
(c) Structural abnormalities.

Urodynamic diagnoses based on this classification should correlate with the patients symptoms and signs. For example the presence of an unstable contraction in an asymptomatic continent patient does not warrant a diagnosis of detrusor overactivity during storage.

6.1 THE STORAGE PHASE

6.1.1 Bladder function during storage

This may be described according to:

(a) Detrusor activity (6.1.1.1).
(b) Bladder sensation (6.1.1.2).
(c) Bladder capacity (6.1.1.3).
(d) Compliance (6.1.1.4).

6.1.1.1 Detrusor activity

In this context detrusor activity is interpreted from the measurement of detrusor pressure (pdet).
Detrusor activity may be:

(a) Normal.
(b) Overactive.

Normal detrusor function   During the filling phase the bladder volume increases without a significant rise in pressure (accommodation). No involuntary contractions occur despite provocation.

A normal detrusor so defined may be described as 'stable'.

Figure **A2.7** Diagrams of filling cystometry to illustrate: (a) Typical phasic unstable detrusor contraction. (b) The gradual increase of detrusor pressure with filling characteristic of reduced bladder compliance.

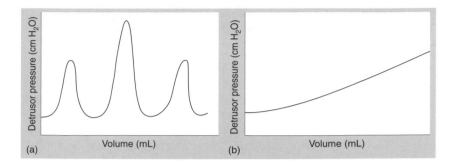

Overactive detrusor function Overactive detrusor function is characterised by involuntary detrusor contractions during the filling phase, which may be spontaneous or provoked and which the patient cannot completely suppress. Involuntary detrusor contractions may be provoked by rapid filling, alterations of posture, coughing, walking, jumping and other triggering procedures. Various terms have been used to describe these features and they are defined as follows.

The *unstable detrusor* is one that is shown objectively to contract, spontaneously or on provocation, during the filling phase while the patient is attempting to inhibit micturition. Unstable detrusor contractions may be asymptomatic or may be interpreted as a normal desire to void. The presence of these contractions does not necessarily imply a neurological disorder. Unstable contractions are usually phasic in type (Fig. A2.7A). A gradual increase in detrusor pressure without subsequent decrease is best regarded as a change of compliance (Fig. A2.7B).

Detrusor hyperreflexia is defined as overactivity due to disturbance of the nervous control mechanisms. The term detrusor hyperreflexia should only be used when there is objective evidence of a relevant neurological disorder. The use of conceptual and undefined terms such as hypertonic, systolic, uninhibited, spastic and automatic should be avoided.

6.1.1.2 Bladder sensation

Bladder sensation during filling can be classified in qualitative terms (see 3.1) and by objective measurement (see 5.5). Sensation can be classified broadly as follows:

(a) Normal.
(b) Increased (hypersensitive).
(c) Reduced (hyposensitive).
(d) Absent.

6.1.1.3 Bladder capacity

See 3.1.

6.1.1.4 Compliance

Compliance is defined as: $\Delta V / \Delta p$ (see 3.1).
Compliance may change during the cystometric examination and is variably dependent upon a number of factors including:

(a) Rate of filling.
(b) The part of the cystometrogram curve used for compliance calculation.

(c) The volume interval over which compliance is calculated.
(d) The geometry (shape) of the bladder.
(e) The thickness of the bladder wall.
(f) The mechanical properties of the bladder wall.
(g) The contractile/relaxant properties of the detrusor.

During normal bladder filling little or no pressure change occurs and this is termed 'normal compliance'. However at the present time there is insufficient data to define normal, high and low compliance.

When reporting compliance, specify:

(a) The rate of bladder filling.
(b) The bladder volume at which compliance is calculated.
(c) The volume increment over which compliance is calculated.
(d) The part of the cystometrogram curve used for the calculation of compliance.

6.1.2 Urethral function during storage

The urethral closure mechanism during storage may be:

(a) normal
(b) incompetent.

(a) The *Normal urethral closure mechanism* maintains a positive urethral closure pressure during filling even in the presence of increased abdominal pressure. Immediately prior to micturition the normal closure pressure decreases to allow flow.

(b) *Incompetent Urethral Closure Mechanism* An incompetent urethral closure mechanism is defined as one which allows leakage of urine in the absence of a detrusor contraction. Leakage may occur whenever intravesical pressure exceeds intraurethral pressure (Genuine stress incontinence) or when there is an involuntary fall in urethral pressure. Terms such as 'the unstable urethra' await further data and precise definition.

6.1.3 Urinary incontinence

Urinary incontinence is involuntary loss of urine which is objectively demonstrable and a social or hygienic problem. Loss of urine through channels other than the urethra is extraurethral incontinence.

Urinary incontinence denotes:

(a) A symptom
(b) A sign
(c) A condition.

The symptom indicates the patients statement of involuntary urine loss.
The sign is the objective demonstration of urine loss.
The condition is the urodynamic demonstration of urine loss.

Symptoms   *Urge incontinence* is the involuntary loss of urine associated with a strong desire to void (urgency). *Urgency* may be associated with two types of dysfunction:

(a) Overactive detrusor function *(motor urgency).*
(b) Hypersensitivity *(sensory urgency).*

Stress incontinence: the symptom indicates the patient's statement of involuntary loss of urine during physical exertion.

'Unconscious' incontinence. Incontinence may occur in the absence of urge and without conscious recognition of the urinary loss.

Enuresis means any involuntary loss of urine. If it is used to denote incontinence during sleep, it should always be qualified with the adjective 'nocturnal'.

Post-micturition dribble and *Continuous leakage* denotes other symptomatic forms of incontinence.

Signs

The sign stress-incontinence denotes the observation of loss of urine from the urethra synchronous with physical exertion (e.g. coughing). Incontinence may also be observed without physical exercise. Post-micturition dribble and continuous leakage denotes other signs of incontinence. Symptoms and signs alone may not disclose the cause of urinary incontinence. Accurate diagnosis often requires urodynamic investigation in addition to careful history and physical examination.

Conditions

Genuine stress incontinence is the involuntary loss of urine occurring when, in the absence of a detrusor contraction, the intravesical pressure exceeds the maximum urethral pressure.

Reflex incontinence is loss of urine due to detrusor hyperreflexia and/or involuntary urethral relaxation in the absence of the sensation usually associated with the desire to micturate. This condition is only seen in patients with neuropathic bladder/urethral disorders.

Overflow incontinence is any involuntary loss of urine associated with over-distension of the bladder.

6.2 THE VOIDING PHASE

6.2.1 The detrusor during voiding

During micturition the detrusor may be:

(a) acontractile
(b) underactive
(c) normal.

(a) *The acontractile detrusor* is one that cannot be demonstrated to contract during urodynamic studies. *Detrusor areflexia* is defined as acontractility due to an abnormality of nervous control and denotes the complete absence of centrally coordinated contraction. In detrusor areflexia due to a lesion of the conus medullaris or sacral nerve outflow, the detrusor should be described as *decentralised* – not denervated, since the peripheral neurones remain. In such bladders pressure fluctuations of low amplitude, sometimes known as 'autonomous' waves, may occasionally occur. The use of terms such as atonic, hypotonic, autonomic and flaccid should be avoided.

(b) *Detrusor underactivity.* This term should be reserved as an expression describing detrusor activity during micturition. Detrusor underactivity is defined as a detrusor contraction of inadequate magnitude and/or duration to effect bladder emptying with a normal time span. Patients may have underactivity during micturition and detrusor overactivity during filling.

(c) *Normal detrusor contractility.* Normal voiding is achieved by a voluntarily initiated detrusor contraction that is sustained and can usually be suppressed voluntarily. A normal detrusor contraction will effect comlete bladder emptying in the absence of obstruction. For a given detrusor contraction, the magnitude of the recorded pressure rise will depend on the degree of outlet resistance.

6.2.2 Urethral function during micturition

During voiding urethral function may be:

(a) normal
(b) obstructive
  – overactivity
  – mechanical.

(a) *The normal urethra* opens to allow the bladder to be emptied.
(b) *Obstruction due to urethral overactivity:* this occurs when the urethral closure mechanism contracts against a detrusor contraction or fails to open at attempted micturition. Synchronous detrusor and urethral contraction is *detrusor/urethral dyssynergia.* This diagnosis should be qualified by stating the location and type of the urethral muscles (striated or smooth) which are involved. Despite the confusion surrounding 'sphincter' terminology the use of certain terms is so widespread that they are retained and defined here. The term *detrusor/external sphincter dyssynergia or detrusor-sphincter-dyssynergia (D.S.D.)* describes a detrusor contraction concurrent with an involuntary contraction of the urethral and/or periurethral striated muscle. In the adult, detrusor sphincter dyssynergia is a feature of neurological voiding disorders. In the absence of neurological features the validity of this diagnosis should be questioned. The term *detrusor/bladder neck dyssynergia* is used to denote a detrusor contraction concurrent with an objectively demonstrated failure of bladder neck opening. No parallel term has been elaborated for possible detrusor/distal urethral (smooth muscle) dyssynergia.

Overactivity of the striated urethral sphincter may occur in the absence of detrusor contraction, and may prevent voiding. This is not detrusor/sphincter dyssynergia.

Overactivity of the urethral sphincter may occur during voiding in the absence of neurological disease and is termed *dysfunctional voiding.* The use of terms such as 'non-neurogenic' or 'occult neuropathic' should be avoided.

Mechanical obstruction: is most commonly anatomical e.g. urethral stricture.

Using the characteristics of detrusor and urethral function during storage and micturition an accurate definition of lower urinary tract behaviour in each patient becomes possible.

7 UNITS OF MEASUREMENT

In the urodynamic literature pressure is measured in cm H_2O and *not* in millimeters of mercury. When Laplace's law is used to calculate tension

Table A2.1

Quantity	Acceptable unit	Symbol
Volume	Millilitre	ml
Time	Second	s
Flow rate	Millilitres/second	$ml\ s^{-1}$
Pressure	Centimetres of water[1]	$cm\ H_2O$
Length	Metres or submultiples	m, cm, mm
Velocity	Metres/second or submultiples	$m\ s^{-1}, cm\ s^{-1}$
Temperature	Degrees Celsius	°C

[1]The SI unit is the pascal (Pa), but it is only practical at present to calibrate our instruments in cm H_2O. One centimetre of water pressure is approximately equal to 100 pascals (1 cm H_2O = 98.07 PA = 0.098 kPa).

in the bladder wall, it is often found that pressure is then measured in $dyne\ cm^{-2}$. This lack of uniformity in the systems used leads to confusion when other parameters, which are a function of pressure, are computed, for instance, 'compliance', contraction force, velocity etc. From these few examples it is evident that standardisation is essential for meaningful communication. Many journals now require that the results be given in SI Units. This section is designed to give guidance in the application of the SI system to urodynamics and defines the units involved. The principal units to be used are listed below (Table A2.1).

SYMBOLS

It is often helpful to use symbols in a communication. The system in Table A2.2 has been devised to standardise a code of symbols for use in

Table A2.2   List of symbols

Basic symbols		Urological qualifiers		Value	
Pressure	p	Bladder	ves	Maximum	max
Volume	V	Urethra	ura	Minimum	min
Flow rate	Q	Ureter	ure	Average	ave
Velocity	v	Detrusor	det	Isovolumetric	isv
Time	t	Abdomen	abd	Isotonic	ist
Temperature	T	External stream	ext	Isobaric	isb
Length	l			Isometric	ism
Area	A				
Diameter	d				
Force	F				
Energy	E				
Power	P				
Compliance	C				
Work	W				
Energy per unit volume	e				

Examples: pdet,max = maximum detrusor pressure; e.ext = kinetic energy per unit volume in the external stream.

urodynamics. The rationale of the system is to have a basic symbol representing the physical quantity with qualifying subscripts. The list of basic symbols largely conforms to international usage. The qualifying subscripts relate the basic symbols to commonly used urodynamic parameters.

References

1. Abrams P, Blaivas JG, Stanton SL, Andersen JT, Fowler CJ, Gerstenberg T, Murray K. Sixth report on the standardisation of terminology of lower urinary tract function. Procedures related to neurophysiological investigations: Electromyography, nerve conduction studies, reflex latencies, evoked potentials and sensory testing. World J Urol 1986; 4: 2–5. Scand J Urol Nephrol 1986; 20: 161–164.

2. Bates P, Bradley WE, Glen E, Melchior H, Rowan D, Sterling A, Hald T. First report on the standardisation of terminology of lower urinary tract function. Urinary incontinence. Procedures related to the evaluation of urine storage: Cystometry, urethral closure pressure profile, units of measurement. Br J Urol 1976; 48: 39–42. Eur Urol 1976; 2: 274–276. Scand J Urol Nephrol 1976; 11: 193–196. Urol Int 1976; 32: 81–87.

3. Bates P, Glen E, Griffiths D, Melchior H, Rowan D, Sterling A, Zinner NR, Hald T. Second report on the standardisation of terminology of lower urinary tract function. Procedures related to the evaluation of micturition: Flow rate, pressure measurement, symbols. Acta Urol Jpn 1977; 27: 1563–1566. Br J Urol 1977; 49: 207–210. Eur Urol 1977; 3: 168–170. Scand J Urol Nephrol 1977; 11: 197–199.

4. Bates P, Bradley WE, Glen E, Griffiths D, Melchior H, Rowan D, Sterling A, Hald T. Third report on the standardisation of terminology of lower urinary tract function. Procedures related to the evaluation of micturition: Pressure flow relationships, residual urine. Br J Urol 1980; 52: 348–350. Eur Urol 1980; 6: 170–171. Acta Urol Jpn 1980; 27: 1566–1568. Scand J Urol Nephrol 1980; 12: 191–193.

5. Bates P, Bradley WE, Glen E, Melchior H, Rowan D, Sterling A, Sundin T, Thomas D, Torrens M, Turner-Warwick R, Zinner NR, Hald T. Fourth report on the standardisation of terminology of lower urinary tract function. Terminology related to neuromuscular dysfunction of lower urinary tract. Br J Urol 1981; 52: 333–335. Urology 1981; 17: 618–620. Scand J Urol Nephrol 1981; 15: 169–171. Acta Urol Jpn 1981; 27: 1568–1571.

6. Jasper HH. Report to the committee on the methods of clinical examination in electroencephalography. Electroencephalography in Clinical Neurophysiology, 1958; 10: 370–75.

Index

A

Abdomen
  examination 406, 435
  gynaecological surgery 310, 325, 327
  massage 182, 183 (fig.), 417
  muscles *see* abdominal muscles
  pain *see* abdominal pain
  shape change during labour 58
Abdominal hysterectomy *see* hysterectomy, abdominal
Abdominal muscles 11–12, 12 (fig.)
  defaecation 388, 414
    'brace and bulge' 414
  during labour 54–5
  exercise 152, 213, 214, 227, 325
    home 219
  gynaecological surgery 325, 327
  postnatal 205
  postnatal status 206–7
  see also individual muscles
Abdominal pain 291–2, 291 (fig.)
  in labour 62 (fig.), 160, 182, 183 (fig.)
  irritable bowel syndrome (IBS) 393
  pregnancy 160
  see also intra-abdominal pressure
Abdominal pressure 437, 451
Abdominal retraction 227
Abscess(es)
  Bartholin's glands 273
  breast, postnatal 243
Abuse
  associated with incontinence 334
  bowel dysfunction 391, 404
  violence in pregnancy 98
Accidents, anal incontinence 400
Acquired immune deficiency syndrome (AIDS) 276–7

see also human immunodeficiency virus (HIV)
Active Birth Movement 105
Acupuncture, pain relief in labour 189
Acyclovir 46
Addictive drugs, pregnancy 125
Adrenaline (epinephrine), labour and 63–4
Age
  anal incontinence and 399
  first time mothers 109
  menopause 249
  sexuality 301–2
AIDS 276–7
  see also human immunodeficiency virus (HIV)
Alcohol
  bowel dysfunction 410
  effect on continence 368
  pregnancy 122–3
Alpha fetoprotein (AFP) level 100
Amenorrhoea 27, 288–9
  exercise effect 103
  pregnancy sign 33
  secondary 288–9
American College of Obstetricians and Gynecologists (ACOG 2002) 75
Amniocentesis 101
Amnion 30
  artificial rupture 79, 198
  rupture (breaking of waters) 55–6
Amniotic fluid 30
  loss, sign of labour 55–6
  screening during pregnancy 101
Amniotic sac *see* amnion
Amniotomy, labour induction 79, 198
Anaemia in pregnancy 43
  dilution anaemia 36

Anal canal 22, 23 (fig.)
Anal columns 22
Anal cones, faecal incontinence 419–20
Anal continence 386
Anal fissure
  defaecation pain 395–6
  postnatal 396
Anal incontinence
  causative factors 399–402
    accidents 400
    age 399
    anal sphincter dysfunction 399–400
    childbirth 400
    functional faecal incontinence 401–2
    liquid stool 401
    straining 401
    surgery 400
    trauma 400
  definition 389
  prevalence 390
  see also faecal incontinence
Anal plugs, faecal incontinence 419–20
Anal sphincter
  dysfunction 399–400
  exercise 415–16
  external 23, 386, 387, 388
  internal 22, 386, 387, 388
  paradoxical contraction 389
Andropause syndrome 253
Anismus 389
Anococcygeal body 22
Anorectal angle 386
  defaecation 387
Anorectal dysfunction 383–425
  associated pathologies 384
  definitions 384–90
  prevalence 390
  prevention 384

Anorectal dysfunction (*contd*)
  skin care 420
  treatment 410–21
    bowel retraining 411
    diet 410–11
    medication 411–20
    physiotherapy 413–20
  see also individual disorders
Anorectal examination 406–7, 407
    (table)
Anorectal flap 387 (fig.)
Anorectal function 384–8
  abnormal *see* anorectal dysfunction
  continence maintenance 386
Anorectal manometry 408
Anorectal region 22–3
Anorexia nervosa
  defaecation difficulties 392
  menstruation effect 27
Anorgasmia 295
Antenatal care 93–140
  aims 94
  care team 96–7
  early pregnancy 104
  emotional distress 109
  fatigue 109
  lifestyle 109–10
  neuromuscular control teaching
      111–13
    breathing 112–13
    contrast method 112
    touch and massage 112
    visualisation and imagery 112
  NICE guidelines 98
  options 95–7
  preconceptual care 102–4
  relaxation 109–10, 112 (fig.)
  routine care 97–100
    booking visit 97–8
  screening 100–2
    acceptability 101–2
  stress 109–10
  working during 110
  see also antenatal classes; midwives
Antenatal classes 104–19, xxii
  6-week course 128–9
  class reunion 130–1
  crash courses 127
  criteria 105
  'early bird' classes 105–6, 126
  education in back pain 143
  environment 127–8
  exercise in water 37
  history xvii–xviii
  planning 126–38
  self-help strategies 131
  see also parenthood classes
Antepartum haemorrhage (APH) 43–4

Antimotility drugs 413
Antispasmodics 413
Anus 390–1
Anxiety
  defaecation difficulties 397
  fathers 132–3
  irritable bowel syndrome (ISB) 394
  pain during labour 60, 184
  postnatal 233
Apgar score 71–2, 72 (table)
Aponeurosis 11
Arcus tendineus fascia of the pelvis
    (ATFP) 8
Areola 12
  pigmentation changes 38
Aromatherapy, pain relief in labour 190
Artificial rupture of membrane (ARM)
    79, 198
Association for Continence Advice
    (ACA), guidelines for intimate
    examinations 355
Association of Chartered
    Physiotherapists in Obstetrics
    and Gynaecology (ACPOG)
    xviii–xix
Atrophic vaginitis 251–2

B

Babies
  bathing, posture advice 219
  feeding
    after caesarean section 238
    multiple births 239–40
    posture advice 217–18
    see also breastfeeding
  loss of 199–200
  macrosomic, diabetes and 45
  massage 220–1
  pre-term 200
  suckling
    difficulty 12
    uterine contraction and 59, 79,
      84, 197
'Baby blues' 234
Backache *see* back pain
Back care, pregnancy 106, 106 (fig.),
    107 (fig.)
  gynaecological surgery 325, 327
Back pain 227–8, 291–2, 291 (fig.)
  coping strategies 155 (fig.)
  epidural anaesthesia and 195–6, 228
  low (lumbar) *see* low back pain
  postnatal 207, 242
  postural 154
  pregnancy 142–9
    assessment 147–9

back-care principles 143–6
    examination 148–9
    factors influencing 142–3
    management 146–7
    prevention 143–6
    previous pregnancies 147–8
    treatment 149–55
  see also posture
Bacterial infections 272, 274
Bartholin's glands 10
  abscess 273
  cyst 277, 278
    marsupialisation 320
Baths/bathing
  baby, posture advice 219
  warm 185
    first stage of labour 70
    perineal dysfunction/pain 223
Bearing down urge 54–5, 175
Bed mobility, gynaecological surgery
    324–5
Bed wetting *see* nocturnal enuresis
Behavioural modification, lower
    urinary tract dysfunction 445
Bicornuate uterus 15
Bilateral salpingo-oophorectomy 311
  endometriosis 283
Billings ovulation method 29
Biofeedback
  constipation 416
  faecal incontinence 416–17
  lower urinary tract dysfunction 445
  PFM assessment 357–60, 372–5
    manometry 372–3
Birth canal, formation 55, 65
Birthing pool 70–1, 190
Birth partner
  massage 181
  role 166
Birth plans 197–8
Birth weight, effects on labour 66
Bishop score 33, 53, 54 (table)
Bisphosphonates, osteoporosis
    treatment 263
Bladder 19–20
  capacity 440–1, 452, 467
  compliance volume 337, 440, 452,
    467–8
  cystometry *see* cystometry
  displacement 284
  dysfunction *see* urinary
    incontinence
  expression 446
  filling 336, 437–8
    neurophysiological evaluation
      460–5
    non-physiological filling rate
      437–8

physiological filling rate 437
imaging 360–1
pain, definition 432
position 341
pregnancy 41
pressure 336–7
    closure 337
    factors contributing 337
    measurement 361–2
    measurements during
        micturition 457–8
puerperium 85
reflex triggering 446
retraining 377
sensation 430, 438, 451, 467
urine storage 336–7, 339–41, 466–8
    detrusor function 466–8
    urethral function 468
voiding (emptying) see micturition
wall, stretch receptors 339
Bladder diary 352–4, 353 (fig.), 434
Bladder outlet obstruction 444
Bladder pain syndrome, definition 432
Blastocyst 29
Bleeding
    breakthrough 290
    dysfunctional uterine bleeding
        (DUB) 291
    during labour 43–4
    postmenopausal 249
    see also haemorrhage
Blood group, antenatal tests 100
Blood, in stools 394
Blood pressure
    labour, effect on 64
    measurement
        labour 70
        pregnancy 98
    pregnancy
        effects on 37
        pregnancy-induced
            hypertension 48–9
Blood supply
    anorectal region 23
    breasts 13
    urethra 21
Blood tests, antenatal 99–100
Blood volume, increase in pregnancy
    36
Body image
    cancer and 303
    postnatal 205, 220, 234
Body mass index (BMI) 97, 119
Booking visit 97–8
Bowel dysfunction 383–425
    assessment 402–10
        history 402–5
        investigations 408–10

physical examination 405–7
associated pathologies 384
definitions 384–90
drug induced 384
patients at risk 335
prevalence 390
prevention 384
skin care 420
treatment 410–21
    bowel retraining 411
    diet 410–11
    medication 411–20
    physiotherapy 413–20
    see also individual disorders
Bowel function 383–425
    abnormal see bowel dysfunction
    anatomy 22–23
    defaecation see defaecation
    normal 384–8
    storage 386–7
Bowel habits
    diary 402–3, 403 (fig.)
    questionnaires 402–4
Brachial plexus pain, pregnancy 156
Brachytherapy 314
Braxton Hicks contractions 36, 56
    breathing 173
    see also uterine contractions
Breakthrough bleeding 290
Breast(s) 12–13, 13 (fig.)
    antenatal care 133–4, 134
    awareness 270
    blood supply 13
    growth 12
    increase in size 134
    menopause 13
    milk production 12, 85–6
        see also breastfeeding
    postnatal 207
    pregnancy effects 38
    problems, postnatal 231–2, 243
Breast abscess 243
Breast cancer
    HRT and 255, 260
    pregnancy 44
Breast engorgement 231–2
Breastfeeding 86, 208–10
    antenatal care 133–4
    antenatal classes 129
    older mothers 134
    posture advice 134–5, 217–18, 217
        (fig.), 232
    problems 209, 231–2
    suckling difficulty 12
    weight loss assistance 119
    WHO recommendations 133–4
Breathing 170–7
    labour 172

alteration during 171
contractions and 172–6
first stage 173–4
pushing 176–7
second stage 176–7
teaching techniques 172
transition stage 174–5
neuromuscular control 112–13
Breech position 44, 74–5, 199
    types 75
Bristol stool chart 385 (fig.)
British Council for Cervical Cytology,
    classification of smear results
    271
British National Formulary (BNF) 124
Bulbospongiosus muscle 10
Bulking agents, bowel dysfunction 412
Burning vulva syndrome see
    vulvodynia

C

Caesarean section 81–4, 199
    classical 82
    ectopic pregnancy and 84
    elective 197
        breech presentation 75
        indications 81–2
        procedure 83
    emergency, indications 82
    epidural anaesthesia 193, 196
    increasing rates xxi
    multiple births 125
    Pfannenstiel (bikini line) 82, 83
    postnatal care 237–9
        exercises 238
        feeding 238
        massage 238
        physiotherapist's role 237–9
        posture 238
        wound healing 238
    postoperative complications
        83–4
Caffeine
    bowel dysfunction 404, 411
    incontinence 368
    pregnancy 120, 122
Calcitonin, osteoporosis treatment 263
Calcitriol, osteoporosis treatment 264
Calcium
    osteoporosis 258
    pregnancy 120
Calcium channel blockers, anal fissure
    396
Calorie intake
    defaecation difficulties 392
    pregnancy 114, 119

Cancer
  benign tumours 277
  body image 303
  breast 44, 255, 260
  cervical 279–80
  endometrium 280
  malignant tumours 277
  ovary 280–1
  sexuality after 303
  vulva 277–8
Candida albicans 272
Capacitation 15
Carbon dioxide, in labour 171
Carcinoma
  endometrium 280
  fallopian tubes 280
Cardiac decompensation, labour 45
Cardiac disease 44–5
Cardinal (transverse cervical)
    ligaments 18
Cardiotocograph (CTG) 70
Cardiovascular disease (CVD)
  incidence 255
  postmenopause 254, 255
  pregnancy 44–5
  protection 255
Cardiovascular system
  demands during maternal exercise
    114
  labour effects 64, 170–1
  pregnancy effects 36–7
Carpal tunnel syndrome
  postnatal 243
  pregnancy 155–6
Catecholamines, labour and 64
Catheter, cystometry 361–2
Catheterisation, lower urinary tract
    dysfunction 445–6
Cauphyllum 190
Centers for Disease Control and
    Prevention and the American
    College of Sports Medicine
    (CDC-ACSM) 42
Cephalic presentation 54
Cephalopelvic disproportion (CPD)
    77, 198
Cervical dystocia 77, 198
Cervical ligaments, transverse 18
Cervicitis 274–5
Cervix 16
  benign tumour 278–9
  cytology 270–1
  dilation during labour 33, 54,
    55 (fig.)
    assessment 58–9
    pain 60
  disorders 274–5
  erosion 274

malignancy 279–80
pregnancy effects 16, 33
suspensory ligaments 18 (fig.)
'Changing childbirth' xxi–xxii
Chest infection, postoperative 328
Chignon 81
Childbirth *see* labour
Chlamydia trachomatis 274–5
Chloasma (mask of pregnancy) 38
Chondromalacia patellae, pregnancy
    159
Chorion 29
Chorionic villus sampling (CVS) 29,
    100, 101
Circulatory system
  disorders in pregnancy 157–9
    haemorrhoids 158
    muscle cramps 158–9
    thrombosis/thromboembolism
      159
    varicose veins 157
    vulval varicose veins 157–8
  exercises during pregnancy 108–9
  gynaecological surgery 324
  reproductive tract 17
Climacteric 249–68
  adverse effects 251
  age of occurrence 249
  hormone changes 250, 253
  hot flushes 251
  neurological symptoms 253
  organ atrophy 250, 251–2
  physical symptoms 251–2
  sexuality 253–4, 301–2
  skin changes 252
  terminology 250 (fig.)
  urinary disorders 252
  vaginal changes 250
    soreness 251–2
  see also menopause
Clomifene, preconceptual care 103
Coccydynia 142, 153–4, 228–9
  physiotherapeutic measures 228
Coccygeus (ischiococcygeus) 7
Cognitive performance, oestrogen 253
Collagenous tissue
  breakdown during pregnancy 42,
    143, 147
  uterus 35
Colon, defaecation 387
Colonic transit studies 408
Colporrhaphy 314
  anterior 314–15
  posterior 315–16
  risks/complications 315–16
  sacral 316
Colposcopy 320
Colposuspension 317–18

Combined oral contraceptive (COC),
    endometriosis 282
Compressor urethrae 21
Concentric needle electromyography
    409
Constipation 384, 389
  biofeedback therapy 416
  consequences 398–9
  diastasis recti abdominis 225
  elderly 398
  irritable bowel syndrome (IBS) 39.
  massage 417–18
  optimal defaecation position 388,
    388 (fig.)
  postnatal 225
  pregnancy 396
  prevalence 390
  psychological problems 399
  treatment 411–13
  workplace 393
Consultant obstetric units, antenatal
    care 96
Consultants, antenatal care 96
Continence 333
  advice 368
  neurological control 339–41, 340
    (fig.)
  problems *see* incontinence
Continence Foundation xx–xxi
  guidelines for continence care xx
Contraception, postnatal advice 210
Contractions *see* uterine contractions
Cooley's anaemia, pregnancy 49
Coronary artery disease, HRT 255
Corpus luteum 14
  hormone production 29
Cot death 201
Coulevaire uterus 77
Cramp, exercises for during pregnancy
    108–9
Cystitis 344
  honeymoon 347
Cystocoele 284, 285, 285 (fig.)
  micturition difficulties 348
  surgical treatment 314
Cystometry 361–2, 450–2
  definitions 451–2
  disadvantages 362
  filling 437–42
    bladder capacity 440–1
    bladder compliance 440
    bladder sensation 438
    detrusor function 438–40
    urethral function 441–2
  specify 451
  technique 451
Cystoscopy 364
Cystourethrocoele 285

ystourethroscopy 364
ysts 277–83
    Bartholin's glands 277, 278, 320
    ovary 280
    physiotherapy 283
    vagina 278

D

Decidua 15
Deep vein thrombosis (DVT)
    postnatal 230–1
    postoperation complications 328
Defaecating proctogram 409
Defaecation 387–8
    difficulties
        elderly 397–8
        factors contributing 390–8
        see also constipation
    ignoring call 393
    optimal position 388, 388 (fig.)
    technique 413–15
        abnormal 390–1
    workplace constipation 393
    see also faecal incontinence
Dehydration 39
    during labour 65
Dementia
    defaecation difficulties 398
    oestrogen 253
Depression, defaecation difficulties
    397
Dermatology see skin
Descent of foetal head 34 (fig.)
Descending perineum syndrome 225,
    389
Detrusor 19
    function 466–7
        filling cystometry 438–40
        micturition 443, 469–70
        overactivity see urinary
            incontinence
    pressure 437, 451
    sphincter dyssynergia 444
Diabetes mellitus
    pregnancy and 45
    pregnancy-related (gestational)
        41, 46
Diaphragm
    displacement during pregnancy
        38
    in labour 54–5
Diaries
    bladder diary 352–4, 353 (fig.)
    bowel habit diary 402–3,
        403 (fig.)
    food diary 405 (fig.)

Diarrhoea
    irritable bowel syndrome (IBS) 393
    treatment 420–1
Diastasis recti abdominis 43, 206, 206
        (fig.), 242
    assessment 226–7
    constipation 225
    exercises 227
    re-education 227
Dick-Read, Grantly Dr xviii
Diet
    incontinence management 347
    irritable bowel management 394
    pregnancy 119–26
        foods to avoid 121–3
        nutrients 120–1
Dilatation and curettage (D&C) 320
Dilution anaemia (physiological
        anaemia of pregnancy) 36
Discharge advice, gynaecological
        surgery 329–30
Displacement
    anterior compartment 285
    middle compartment 286–7
    physiotherapy 287
    posterior compartment 287
    types 285 (fig.)
    see also genital prolapse
Doula, support during labour 70
'Dowager's hump' 256
Down's syndrome, screening for 100,
        101
Drinking, recommendations during
        labour 64–5
Drug-induced diarrhoea 401
Drugs of abuse, pregnancy 125
Dysaesthetic vulvodynia 298–9
Dyschezia 389
Dysfunctional uterine bleeding (DUB)
        291
Dysmenorrhoea 289
Dyspareunia 240–1, 296–8
    treatment 298
    types 296
Dysuria 343

E

'Early bird' antenatal classes 105–6,
        126
Eating disorders, defaecation
        difficulties 391
Eating, recommendations during
        labour 64–5
Eclampsia 48–9
Ectopic pregnancy 15, 45
    following caesarean section 84

Edinburgh postnatal depression scale
        132
Education, preparation for labour 167
Educator 358–9, 359 (fig.)
Egg (ovum) 14
Elderly
    constipation 398
    defaecation difficulties 397–8
    faecal incontinence 390
    sexuality 302
Electrical stimulation, lower urinary
        tract dysfunction 445
Electromyography (EMG) 373–5
    computerised 373–4
    concentric needle 409
    incontinence 363–4
    motor conduction tests 364
    muscle activity 8–9
    PFM assessment 358, 359
    single fibre density 363
    urinary tract 460–2
    vaginal cones 374–5
        considerations 375
        selection of appropriate 374
        treatment sessions 374–5
Electrophysiological tests,
        incontinence 363–4
Embryo 30
Emotional distress 74
    antenatal period 109
    pain, effect on 62
    postnatal 233–4
    see also maternal distress
Emotional vulnerability, postnatal
        209–10
Endoanal ultrasonography (EAUS) 409
Endocrine system, pregnancy effects
        32–3
    see also hormones
Endometriosis 281–3
    aetiology 282
    fertility 283
    investigations 282
    prevalence 281
    symptoms 281
    treatment 282–3
Endometritis 275
Endometrium 15
    ablation 320
    carcinoma 280
Endopelvic fascia 5, 6, 8
Energy expenditure, in pregnancy 39
Enterocoele 286
Entonox 190–1
Enuresis 342, 430
Environmental factors, faecal
        incontinence 402
Enzymes, prelabour role 53

Epidural anaesthesia 185, 192–6
  advantages 192–3
  back pain 195–6, 228
  caesarean section 193, 196
  complications 193–5
  foetal effects 195
  haematoma 195
  maternal position and 67
  pre-booked 165
  technique 193
Episiotomy 65–6, 78, 80, 199
  anal incontinence 400
  position 80 (fig.)
Erectile dysfunction (ED) 253
Ergometrine 196
Estimated date of delivery (EDD) 30
Exercise
  caesarean section and 238
  foot, DVT prevention 231
  gentle, during labour 70
  postnatal 210–11
    community classes 220
    educational principles 214–16
    home exercises 219–20
    return to sport 220
  preconceptual 102
  during pregnancy 36, 103, 113–19,
      132
    benefits 118
    contraindications 116, 116
        (table)
    foetal risks 115–16
    guidelines 116–18
    low back pain 150
    physiological effects 114–15
    pre-term labour 115–16
    signs for medical review 117
    walking 42
    water based 36, 37, 118–19
External anal sphincter (EAS) 23
  defaecation 387, 388
  resting pressure 386
External cephalic version (ECV) 44
Extremely low birth weight infants
    (ELBW) 31

F

Faecal impaction 398, 401
Faecal incontinence 8, 224–5, 242, 389
  assessment 402–10
    history 402–5
    investigations 408–10
    physical examination 405–7
  biofeedback therapy 416–17
  elderly 390
  functional 401–2

liquid stool 401
passive soiling 389
prevalence 390
skin care 420
treatment 413, 415, 416–7, 418
see also anal incontinence; anorectal
    dysfunction; bowel
    dysfunction
The Faecal Incontinence Quality of
    Life Scale (FIQLS) 404
Faecal softeners 413
Fallopian tubes 15
  carcinoma 280
  ectopic pregnancy 15, 45
  infections 275
  surgery 313, 316
False labour 36
Faradism 364
Fathers 132–3
Fatigue
  postnatal 232–3
  pregnancy 109, 161
Fat, increase during pregnancy 39
Female anatomy 1–25
Ferguson's reflex 71, 194
Fertility
  endometriosis 283
  problems see infertility
Fibre 39, 410
  defaecation difficulties 392–3
  pregnancy requirement 121
Fibroareolar lateral ligaments 20
Fibroids 45–6, 278–9
  pregnancy 160
Fibromyoma 278
'Fight or flight' response 63–4, 110
Fish oils, pregnancy 120
Fluid
  input/output during labour 70
  intake 410
    defaecation difficulties 392
  retention, pregnancy 37
Fluoride, osteoporosis treatment 264
Fluoroscopic evaluation, rectal
    emptying 409
Foetal adrenal hormones, labour
    induction 57
Foetal alcohol syndrome (FAS) 123
Foetal distress
  labour complications 73–4
  maternal exercising 115
  prolonged labour 59
Foetal growth 29–31
  fundal height 34 (fig.), 98–9
  maternal exercising, effect on 115
  patterns 31 (table)
Foetal heart 36
  monitoring 70, 73, 99

Foetal hypoglycaemia, maternal
    exercising 114
Foetal hypoxia 73–4
Foetal malformations, maternal
    temperature and 115
Foetal movements 99
  cessation 99
Foetal positions, labour 53–4
Foetal thorax, compression 64
Foetus 30
  descent of head 34 (fig.), 63
  development see foetal growth
  drug sensitivity 30
    pethidine effects 191–2
  HIV transmission 46–7
  intrauterine death 46
  labour effects 63–5
  macrosomic 45
  maternal exercise effects 115–16
  maternal hyperventilation 171
  positioning 53–4
    breech see breech position
    head, engaged 34–5
    unstable/transverse lie 49–50
  premature delivery 31
  sex detection 101
  TENS effect 187–8
  see also entries beginning foetal
Folic acid 102
Food diary 405 (fig.)
Foot exercise, DVT prevention 231
Forceps delivery 199
  incontinence risk 224
  labour interventions 80–1
  unassisted vaginal birth vs. 211–12
Fracture 256–7
  risk reduction 259–60
Frequency volume chart (FVC) 352–4,
    353 (fig.), 434
Fundal height
  antenatal care 98–9
  gestational age vs. 34 (fig.)
Fungal infections 272, 274

G

Gardnerella vaginalis 274
Gartner's ducts, infection 273
Gastric reflex, pregnancy 39
Gastrocolic reflex 386
Gastrointestinal system
  labour effects 64–5
  pregnancy 39
General Medical Council Standards
    Committee 406
General practitioner (GP), antenatal
    care 96

enetic counselling, preconceptual care 102
enital assessment 435
enital herpes, pregnancy 46
Genital muscles, external 6
Genital organs, external 10, 11 (fig.)
Genital prolapse 283–7
  anterior compartment 285
  HRT 284
  hysterectomy 284
  middle compartment 286
  physiotherapy 287
  posterior compartment 286
  surgery see gynaecological surgery
Genital tract, infection susceptibility 17
Genitourinary dysfunction/pain 224–6, 431–3
Gestational diabetes mellitus 41, 46
Giggle incontinence 347
Gilliam's ventrosuspension 316
'Glazer' protocol 299
Glycerol trinitrate (GTN) cream, anal fissure 395
Gonorrhoea 273, 274
Gravitational oedema, puerperium 88
Gravity (centre of), pregnancy effects 42–3
Gynaecological conditions 269–308
  backache/abdominal pain 291–2, 291 (fig.)
  common disorders 271–5
  cysts and new growths 277–83
  emotional/psychological implications 302–3
  infections 271–7
    physiotherapy 276
  physical check-up 270–1
  physiotherapist attitudes 269
  physiotherapy 276
  screening 269
  surgery for see gynaecological surgery
Gynaecological health 269–71
Gynaecological surgery 309–32
  bed mobility 324–5
  circulatory system 324
  excision 309–13
  physiotherapy 322–8
    abdominal muscle exercise 325, 327
    mobilisation 327–8
    pelvic floor muscle exercise 325, 326–7
  postoperative issues 326–8
    complications 328
    discharge advice 329
    leaving hospital 328
    lifelong advice 330

posture and backcare 325, 327
preoperative issues 322–6
  assessment 322–3
  instruction/preparation 323–6
  patient discussion 326
  treatment 326
psychological aspects 321–2
radiotherapy 314
repair 314–16
respiratory system 323–4
rest 328
stress incontinence 317–20
terminology 320
wind pain 326

H

Haemoglobin monitoring, antenatal care 99
Haemoglobinopathies
  pregnancy 49
  testing in antenatal care 100
Haemorrhage
  antepartum 43–4
  labour complications 77, 196
  postpartum 87
Haemorrhoids
  anal incontinence 401
  ice therapy 231
  postnatal 231
  pregnancy 158
Hair loss, postnatal 243
Hammock hypothesis 6 (fig.), 8
Hartmann's solution 193
The Health Committee (Maternity Services 1992), water births 190
Health professionals, labour preparation 165
Health visitor, role xix
Health Visitors' Association (HVA) xix
Heartburn, pregnancy 39, 161–2
Heart, pregnancy and 36–7
HELLP syndrome 48
Herpes genitalis 273
Herpes simplex virus, pregnancy 46
Hilum 18–19
HIV see human immunodeficiency virus (HIV)
Homan's signs 230
Home births 95–6
  UK rates 95
Homeopathy, pain relief in labour 190
'Honeymoon cystitis' 347
Hormone replacement therapy (HRT) 13, 251
  administration 261–2
  benefits 255

diseases associated 260
implant 261–2
long-term risks 254
nasal spray 262
oral 261
osteoporosis treatment 260–2
progestogen administration 262
prolapse 284
skin 252
topical (vaginal) 262
transdermal 262
Hormones
  joint laxity effects 41–2
  measurement during pregnancy 100
  menopause
    changes 250–3
    replacement see hormone replacement therapy (HRT)
  menstruation control 27, 28 (fig.), 29
  preconceptual treatments 103
  pregnancy 32–3
    pain role 143
  see also individual hormones
Hot flushes 251
HRT see hormone replacement therapy (HRT)
Human chorionic gonadotrophin (HCG) 29
  morning sickness, role 30
Human immunodeficiency virus (HIV) 276–7
  pregnancy 46–7, 99
  transmission 276
Human papilloma virus (HPV) 273
Hyperemesis gravidarum 39
Hyperglycaemia, maternal 45
Hypertension, pregnancy-induced 48–9
Hyperventilation 171, 171 (table), 173
Hypnosis, pain relief in labour 189
Hypogastric nerve 20
Hypogastric plexus, autonomic 22
Hypoglycaemia, maternal exercising 114
Hypomenorrhoea 288
Hypotension, pregnancy 37
Hysterectomy 309–13, 320
  abdominal 310–12
    postoperative condition 311
    procedure 310–11
    risks/complications 312
  endometriosis 283
  indications 309–10
  menopause 251

Hysterectomy (*contd*)
  number performed 310
  ovarian failure 251
  prolapse following 284
  route 310
  subtotal 311
  vaginal 312–13
    LAVH 312–13
    postoperative condition 312
    procedure 312
    risks/complications 312
    Wertheim's 311
Hysteroscopy 320

I

Ice therapy
  haemorrhoids 231
  perineal dysfunction/pain 222–3
Iliac arteries 17
Iliococcygeus 5–6, 7, 8
Imaging, incontinence assessment 364
Incontinence 334
  definitions 334, 435
  diet 347
  double 334
  extra-urethral 435
  faecal *see* faecal incontinence
  functional activity 378–9
  imaging 364
  prevention 335
  urinary *see* urinary incontinence
Infants *see* babies
Infection(s) 271–7
  anal incontinence 401
  bacterial 272, 274
  differential diagnosis, importance 299
  fallopian tubes 275
  fungal 272, 274
  Gartner's ducts, 273
  genital tract, susceptibility 17
  organisms 272–3, 274
  parasitic 273
  physiotherapy 276
  postoperation complications 328
  puerperal 88
  urinary *see* urinary infections
  uterine 275
  viral 273
  vulval 271–3
  see also specific infections
Infertility 103–4, 293
  caesarean section, after 83
  primary 293
  secondary 293
  in vitro fertilisation (IVF) 103

Injuries, pregnancy and exercise 42
Insomnia, pregnancy 161
Intercostal arteries 13
Interferential therapy (IT), incontinence treatment 375
Internal anal sphincter (IAS) 22
  defaecation 387, 388
  resting pressure 386
International Consultation on Incontinence Questionnaire (ICIQ) 360
International Continence Society (ICS), terminology 342, 344
  lower urinary tract function (1988) 449–72
  lower urinary tract function (2002) 427–47
International Society for the Study of Vulvar Disease (SSVD), classification 272
Intra-abdominal pressure 337, 361, 386, 388
  see also bearing down, straining
Intracytoplasmic sperm injection (ICSI) 103
Intrauterine death 46
Intrauterine growth retardation (IUGR) 47, 98–9
  foetal AIDS 46
Intravesical pressure 437, 451
In vitro fertilisation (IVF) 103
Iron, pregnancy 120
Irritable bowel syndrome (IBS) 393–4
Ischiocavernosus muscle 10
Ischiococcygeus (coccygeus) 7
Isthmus 57

J

Joint laxity in pregnancy 4, 41–2, 150

K

Kidneys 18–19
Kielland forceps 81
Kneeling, puerperium posture 217

L

Labial lacerations 78, 199
Labour 53–91
  'after-pains' 229–30
  anal incontinence 400
  anteversion 58
  bear down urge 54–5, 175
  bleeding during 43–4

complications 73–9
  breech birth *see* breech position
  cephalopelvic disproportion 7?
  contracted pelvis 77
  failure to progress 73
  foetal distress 73–4
  haemorrhage 77, 196
  incoordinate uterine activity 76–7
  knotted cord 76
  malposition 75–6
  malpresentation 74
  maternal distress 74
  multiple births 78
  perineal trauma 78–9
  placental abruption 44, 77
  placenta praevia 44
  prolapsed cord 76
  retained placenta 79
  see also specific complications
coping strategies 184
drive angle 58, 58 (fig.)
duration 66
dyspareunia 297
false 36
fear/embarrassment 175
first stage 54
  active 58
  breathing 170–4
  coping strategies 129
  latent 58
  management 70–1
  pain 54, 60–1
  position 66–7, 179 (fig.)
  variations 198–9
foetal head, descent of 34 (fig.), 63
foetal physiology, effect on 63–5
foetal position 53–4
history xix–xx
home births 95–6
interventions 79–84, 198
  after effects 236–40
  amniotomy 79, 198
  caesarean section *see* caesarean section
  episiotomy *see* episiotomy
  forceps *see* forceps delivery
  oxytocin 79
  prostaglandins 79
  vacuum extraction (ventouse delivery) 81, 199, 211–12
management (normal labour) 68–73
  recording progress 68, 70
massage *see* massage
maternal physiology, effect on 63–5
maternal position during 66–8
  see also posture, labour

mechanics 63
pain 59–63, 187
    anxiety 60, 184
    causes 60–3
    control *see* pain relief
    coping strategies 63
    zone change 62 (fig.), 183 (fig.)
physical/physiological changes 53–6
    pelvic floor 65–6
    perineum 65–6
    positioning in labour 66–8, 177–81, 178 (fig.), 179 (fig.), 180 (fig.)
prelabour 36, 53–4
preparation for 126–38, 165–203
    birth plans 197–8
    breathing *see* breathing
    education 167
    relaxation *see* relaxation
    'tool kit' of coping skills 166–7
pre-term 31, 200
    maternal exercising and 115–16
process of normal 56–68
prolonged 66
    defaecation difficulties 397
    pushing 176
rest after 86–7
second stage 54–5
    assistance 80–1
    breathing 176–7
    contractions 59
    descent 59
    management 71–2
    maternal positioning 71
    pain 61
    perineal 59
    position 67
    positioning 180 (fig.)
    variations 199
signs of 55–6, 129
third stage 55
    labour preparation 196–7
    management 72–3, 196–7
    position 68
    variations 199
transition stage, breathing 174–5
trial of 77
uterine retraction 15
variations 198–9
warm bath and 70, 185
water births 95
Lactation 12, 85–6
    puerperium 85–6
    see also breastfeeding
Lactiferous ducts 12
Lactiferous sinus 12

Laparoscopic assisted vaginal hysterectomy (LAVH) 312–13
Laparoscopic colposuspension 318
Laparoscopy 320
Laparotomy 320
Laplace's law 470–1
Large loop excision of the transformation zone (LLETZ) 313
Laxatives 401, 411
    abuse 392
    constipation 412
    osmotic 412
Legal cases, PMT 290
Let-down reflex 86, 209
Levator ani muscles 5–6
    muscle fibres 8–9
    sub division 8
Libido loss 235–6
Lidocaine 78
Lifelong advice, gynaecological surgery 320
Lifestyle
    antenatal period 109–10
    changes, parenthood 132
Lifting, pregnancy 146
    gynaecological surgery 329
Ligament(s)
    postnatal damage 206–7
    reproductive tract 17–18, 18 (fig.)
    see also individual ligaments
Linea alba 227
Listeria, pregnancy 121
Liver (dietary), pregnancy 122
Lochia 85
Low back pain 228
    pregnancy 149–50
        exercise programme 150
        TENS and 149
        treatment 149–50
Lower urinary tract
    abnormal function *see* lower urinary tract dysfunction
    normal function 336–42
    terminology
        International Continence Society (1988) 449–72
        International Continence Society (2002) 427–47
    urine storage evaluation 450–6
Lower urinary tract dysfunction 342–3
    classification 466–70
        storage phase 466–9
        voiding phase 469–70
    clinical assessment 450
        frequency/volume charts 450
        history 450
        physical disease 450

genitourinary pain and syndromes 432–3
signs 428, 434–6
    measuring frequency and severity 434–5
    pad testing 436
    physical examination 435–6
    symptoms 433
treatment 445–6
    behavioural modification 445
    biofeedback 445
    bladder expression 446
    bladder reflex triggering 446
    catheterisation 445–6
    electrical stimulation 445
    pelvic floor muscle training 445
see also urinary incontinence
Lower urinary tract symptoms 428, 429–33
    associated with pelvic organ prolapse 431
    associated with sexual intercourse 431
    pain 431–2
    post micturition 431
    storage 429–30
    voiding symptoms 430–1
Lumbar lordosis 4, 42, 142
Lying down
    postnatal posture 214–15, 216–17
    pregnancy 143–4
Lymphatic system, reproductive tract 17

M

Mackenrodt's ligaments 18
Macrosomic babies, diabetes and 45
Magnetic resonance imaging (MRI), bowel dysfunction 409
Male sexual dysfunction 253–4
Manchester repair 316
Manometry 372–3
Marsupialisation of Bartholin's cyst 320
Mask of pregnancy (chloasma) 38
Massage
    baby 220–1
    caesarean section 238
    constipation 417–18
    history xvii
    ice cube 223
    during labour 180–4
        abdomen 182, 183 (fig.)
        back 181–2, 181 (fig.), 182 (fig.)
        legs 182
        perineal 182–4

Mastitis, postnatal 243
Maternal alkalosis 64
Maternal apnoea 171
Maternal dehydration 39
Maternal distress
  labour 74, 184–5
  related thoughts, pain increase
    62
Maternal fatality 93–4
  pre-eclamptic toxaemia 49
  UK rate 94
Maternal hyperglycaemia 45
Maternal hyperventilation 36
Maternal serum screening 100
'Maternity blues' 234
Maternity leave 233
McGill pain questionnaire 60, 61
  pain scores 62 (table)
Medications during pregnancy
    124–5
Megacolon 389, 394–5
Megarectum 389, 394–5
Menarche 288
Mendelson's syndrome 64
Menopause
  associated disease 254
    breast cancer 255
    cardiovascular 255
    osteoporosis see osteoporosis
    stroke 255
  breast 13
  defined 249
  dyspareunia 297
  HRT see hormone replacement
    therapy (HRT)
  non-HRT drug therapy 263–4
  premature 293–4
  see also climacteric
Menorrhagia 288, 291
Menstrual cycle 27–9, 28 (fig.)
  cognitive ability 290
  defaecation difficulties 395
  disorders 287–91
  hormone effects 28 (fig.)
  physiological changes 15
  premenstrual tension (PMT) 290
    legal cases 290
Meralgia paraesthetica, pregnancy
    156–7
Methoxyflurane (Penthrane) 190
Micturition 336, 337–9
  cycle 336, 336 (fig.), 434
    urodynamic investigation 437–42
    see also cystometry
  detrusor function 443, 469–70
  difficulties 348–9
  evaluation procedures 456–60
    bladder pressure 457–8

neurophysiological 460–5
  pressure flow relationships
    458–9, 458 (fig.), 459 (fig.)
  urethral pressure 459
  urinary flow 456–7, 457 (fig.)
flow rate 338, 338 (fig.)
  stopping 339
frequency 160, 342, 345, 429
frequency/volume chart (bladder
    diary) 352–4, 353 (fig.)
  collection 352
  results 354
hesitancy 343
increased daytime frequency 342–3
during labour 70
lower urinary tract symptoms 431
neurological control 341
normal desire 343
pelvic floor 338–9
position 338
privacy 338
residual urine 459–60
stream 343
timed/prompted 377–8
urethral function 443, 470
urgency 343
  treatment 368
Midwives
  antenatal care 96
  home births 95–6
  independent 97
  pain management 185
  postnatal care 208
  puerperium care 87
  role xix
  shortage xxi
  TENS 189
Midwives and Health Visitors
    (Midwives' Amendment) Rule
    1986 189
Milk ejection reflex 86, 208
Miscarriage 200
  caesarean section, after 83
Mitchell, Laura xviii
Mitchell method of physiological
    relaxation 109, 111–12, 168, xviii
Monilial infection, differential
    diagnosis 299
Montgomery's tubercles 12, 38
Morning sickness 39, 162
  excessive 39
  human chorionic gonadotrophin
    role 30
Morula 29
Mucoid show 55, 57
Multiple pregnancy 47, 125
  labour complications 78
  postnatal complications 239–40

Multiple sclerosis, pregnancy 44
Muscle(s)
  increased load on during
    pregnancy 43
  postnatal condition 206–7
  strengthening in pregnancy 145–6
  see also individual muscles
Muscle cramps, pregnancy 158
Muscle fibres
  levator ani muscles 8–9
  type I 9
  type II 9, 10 (table)
  uterus 35–6
Musculoskeletal system
  assessment 147–9
  bad posture 217–19
  pain 156
  pregnancy effects 41
  trauma during maternal exercise 114
Myomectomy 313
Myometrium 15

N

Naegele's rule 30
Nappy changing, posture advice
    218–19, 218 (fig.)
National Childbirth Trust (NCT) 105
National Institute for Clinical
    Excellence (NICE), guidelines
    for antenatal care 98
National Health Service (NHS), role in
    antenatal care 95
Nausea in pregnancy 39, 162
  HCG role 30
Neisseria gonorrhoeae 274
Neonatal herpes 46
Neonates see babies
Nerve compression syndromes,
    pregnancy 155–7
Nerve supply
  anorectal region 23
  pelvis 17
Nervous system
  labour pain 60–1, 61 (fig.)
  pregnancy effects 40
Neural tube defects (NTDs), screening
    100
Neurogenic detrusor overactivity 439
Neurological complications
  defaecation difficulties 395
  epidural anaesthesia 195
Neurological control
  continence 339–41, 340 (fig.)
  voiding 341
Neuromuscular control, teaching
    111–13

euromuscular stimulation, anorectal
    dysfunction 418
europhysiological evaluation,
    urinary tract 460–5
Neuropraxia 224
Neville Barnes' forceps 81
Nicotine, bowel dysfunction 404
Nightmares, pregnancy 161
Night sweats 251
Nipple 12
    inverted 12
    sore and cracked 232
    stimulation, uterine contraction
        and 59
Nitrous oxide, labour 190–1
Nocturia 342, 429
    pregnancy 162
Nocturnal enuresis 342, 346–7, 430
    diet 347
    management 347
Nocturnal polyuria 434
Nocturnal urine volume, definition
    434
Non-steroidal anti-inflammatory drugs
    (NSAIDs), endometriosis 282
Nutrients, pregnancy 120–1

O

Obesity, pregnancy 39
Oblique muscles 11
Obstetric care, antenatal 96–7
Obstetric history, bowel dysfunction
    404
Obstetric physiotherapist, role
    xix–xx
Obturator internus 7
Occipitoposterior position (OP) 75–6,
    198–9
Occupational therapists, faecal
    incontinence 402
Oedema
    gravitational 88
    postnatal 207, 230
    pregnancy 43
        measurement 98
Oestrogens 14, 30
    bone metabolism 256
    breasts 38
    cognitive performance 253
    deficiency 254
    effects in pregnancy 4, 33
    fluid retention 37
    in labour 57
    replacement 261
        cardiovascular disease and
            255

faecal incontinence 413
    see also hormone replacement
        therapy (HRT)
Oligohydramnios 30, 47
Oligomenorrhoea 288, 289
Omega-3 fatty acids, pregnancy
    120
Oophorectomy 313
Orgasm, dysfunction 295
Osmotic laxatives 412
Osteoporosis 256–64
    calcium 258
    development 256
    diagnosis 258
    exercise 259–60
    fractures 256–7
        risk reduction 259
    oestrogen and 256
    pharmacological management
        260–4
        HRT and 254, 260–2
            see also hormone replacement
                therapy (HRT)
        non-HRT drug therapy 263–4
    pregnancy-associated 154–5
    prevention 257–8
    risk factors 257 (box)
    treatment 259–60
    vitamin D 258
Ovarian cystectomy 313
Ovaries 14
    cancer 280–1
    cysts 280
        removal 313
    follicles 14
    premature failure 293–4
Ovum (egg) 14
Oxygen, increased demand
    labour 64
    pregnancy 37
Oxytocic injection 72–3
Oxytocin
    labour interventions 72–3, 79
    labour role 56, 57
    rise during labour 56

P

Pad test 354–5, 436
Pain
    control see pain relief
    definition 59–60
    labour see labour
Pain relief
    labour 63, 129, 184–96
        acupuncture 189
        Entonox 190–1

epidural anaesthesia see
        epidural anaesthesia
    homeopathy/aromotherapy
        190
    hypnosis 189
    pethidine 191–2
    TENS see TENS
    water 190
    postnatal 209
        advice 213
Paper towel test 355
Paracetamol, pregnancy 124
Paradoxical anal sphincter contraction
    389
Parasitic infections 273
Parathyroid hormone (PTH),
    osteoporosis treatment 263–4
Parenthood classes 126–38, xx
    lifestyle changes 132
    support network 130
    transition 131–2
    see also antenatal classes
Partogram 68, 69 (fig.), 70
Peak bone mass (PBM) 256
Peanuts, pregnancy 122
Pediculosis pubis 273
Pelvic denervation 397
Pelvic diaphragm see levator ani
    muscles
Pelvic floor 5–10, 9 (fig.)
    dyssynergia 389
    exercises see pelvic floor muscle
        exercises
    labour and 55, 65–6
    ligaments 5
    muscles see pelvic floor muscles
        (PFM)
    neuropathy due to prolonged
        labour 59
Pelvic floor muscle exercises 108,
    108 (fig.)
    antenatal 108
    home 219
    importance 335, 347
    lower urinary tract dysfunction 445
    misconceptions 349
    perineal dysfunction/pain 222
    postnatal 212, 213
        physiotherapist's role 211
    practice sessions 371
        progression 371–2
    stress incontinence 241
    teaching 368–72
        contractions 370
        instructions 369–70
        language 369
        starting position 369
        visualisation 369

Pelvic floor muscles (PFM) 5–10, 11
   assessment
      biofeedback 357–60, 372–5
      computerised manometric
         359–60
      electromyography (EMG) 358–9
   confirmation of contraction 357, 370
   damage 207
   electrical stimulation 375–6
   examination 355–7
      chaperone 356
      consent 356
      guidelines 355
      procedure 356–7
   exercise see pelvic floor muscle
      exercises
   function 6
      definition 436
   gynaecological surgery 325, 326–7
   micturition 338–9
   neurological control 341
   strength grading 357
   stress incontinence 225, 241
   voluntary contraction (VPFMC)
      344–5, 346
   weakness 346
   see also specific muscles
Pelvic girdle
   pain, pregnancy 142–9
      assessment 147–9
      examination 148–9
      management 146–7
   pregnancy effects 42
Pelvic inflammatory disease (PID)
   275–6
   cause 274
Pelvic organ prolapse
   definition 436
   lower urinary tract symptoms 431
Pelvic pain
   childbirth during/after 5
   definition 432
   pregnancy 142–9
   syndrome 433
Pelvic radiotherapy 314
Pelvic splanchnic nerves 20, 22
Pelvic tilt 42, 108, 227
'Pelvic trampoline' 5, 8
Pelvis 1–5, 2 (fig.)
   circulation 17
   contracted 77
   diameters 3 (table)
   different types 3 (fig.)
   female vs. male 1
   in labour 3
   muscles 5–10
   nerve supply 17
   see also entries beginning pelvic

Penthrane (methoxyflurane) 190
PERFECT scheme 357
Periform 376
Perimenopause 250
   see also climacteric
Perineal body 10
Perineal membrane 6, 9–10
Perineal pain syndrome 433
Perineometer 358
Perineum 10
   assessment 355–7, 435
      chaperone 356
      consent 356
      guidelines 355
      procedure 356–7
   dysfunction/pain
      ice therapy 222–3
      physiotherapist's role 222
      postnatal 213, 221–4, 240
      treatment 222–4
   labour, effect on 65–6
   massage 78, 182–4
   postnatal 85, 207
   superficial muscles 7
   support during defaecation 391
   tears
      anal incontinence 400
      classification 78
      labour complications 78–9
      support following 213
Peritron 358 (fig.)
Pethidine 191–2
Pfannenstiel incision 82, 310
Phenylephrine gel 413
Physiotherapy 94
   bowel function assessment 402–10
   breastfeeding assistance 208–9
   gynaecological surgery
      postoperative 326–30
      preoperative 322–6
   labour education 167
   labour preparation 166
   postnatal 210–13
      assessment 211–12
      classes 214–21
      exercise 212–13
      exercise advice 214–21
      individual vs. group 212
      posture advice 214–21
      role 210–11
      venue 212
   postnatal check 210
   postnatal depression 235
   pregnancy
      back pain 143
      breastfeeding 134–5
      exercise advice 117–18
      interaction with father 133

   stress reduction 111–12
   relaxation methods 169
   TENS 188, 189
   urinary function assessment 349–5
Phyto-oestrogens, osteoporosis
      treatment 264
Pilates, maternal exercising 119
Pinard stethoscope 99
Piriformis 7
Placenta 29–30
   delivery 55, 59, 72
   passage of substances across 30, 191
   retained 79, 199
Placenta accreta 79
   following caesarean section 83–4
Placental abruption 44
   labour complications 77
Placenta praevia 44, 47–8, 198
   diagnosis 48
   following caesarean section 83–4
Pollakisuria 342–3, 429
Polycystic ovarian syndrome 103, 292
Polyhydramnios 30, 48
Polymenorrhoea 288
Polyp 278
Polyuria, measurement 434
Postcoital dysuria 347
Postmenopausal women 250
   bleeding 249
   problems 254–5
Postnatal care 208–21
   breastfeeding 208–10
   classes see postnatal classes
   following caesarean section 237–9
   physiotherapy 210–11
   postnatal check 209–10
   posture 214–15
   routine 208
Postnatal classes 214–21
   baby massage 220–1
   community exercise classes 220
   educational principles 215
   home exercises 219–20
   relaxation 215
   return to sport 220
   setting up class 214
   teaching ergonomics 216–19
   teaching points 214–15
Postnatal depression (PND) 132, 233,
   235
   baby massage 221
   long term 244
Postnatal period 205–48
   after-effects of instrumental
      intervention 236–40
   care during see postnatal care
   circulatory dysfunction/pain
      230–1

depression *see* postnatal
  depression (PND)
genitourinary dysfunction/pain
  224–6
immediate problems 221–4
long-term complications 240–4
  dyspareunia 240–1
  perineal pain/discomfort 240
  vaginal pain/discomfort 240
multiple births 239–40
musculoskeletal dysfunction/pain
  226–30
psychological symptoms 233–6
puerperium *see* puerperium
sexual problems 235–6
Postpartum headache, epidural
  anaesthesia 195
Posture
  bad, musculoskeletal symptoms
    217–19
  caesarean section 238
  defaecation 387–8, 388 (fig.), 414
  gynaecological surgery 325, 327
  infant feeding 217 (fig.)
  kneeling 217
  labour 177–80
    'all-fours' 67
    birth cushion 178
    birth partner's role 177–8
    first stage 179 (fig.)
    kneel fall 180 (fig.)
    leaning forward 177, 178 (fig.)
    second stage 71, 180 (fig.)
    sitting position 67
    squatting position 67, 178
    supine position 68, 178 (fig.)
    upright position 66
  postnatal 216 (fig.)
    bathing baby 219
    feeding 217–18, 217 (fig.)
    lying 214–15, 216–17
    nappy changing 218–19, 218
      (fig.)
    sitting 214, 216
    standing 214, 216
    teaching points 214–15
  pregnancy 42, 148–9
    back pain prevention 143–6
      lifting 146
      lying 143–4
      rolling 144
      sitting 144–5
      standing and walking
        145–6
  see also back pain
Postvoid residual (PVR) 343
Potter's syndrome 47
Pouch of Douglas 22

Prebiotics 410
Preconceptual care 102–4
Pre-eclamptic toxaemia 48–9
Pregnancy 27–53
  back care 106, 106 (fig.), 107 (fig.)
  comorbidity 44
  complications 43–52
  defaecation difficulties 396
  diaphragm 38
  diet during *see* diet
  discomfort relief 141–64, 157–9
    back and pelvic pain 142–50
    chondromalacia patellae 159
    circulatory disorders 157–9
    coccydynia 153–4
    fatigue 161
    fibroids 160–1
    heartburn 161–2
    incontinence (urinary) 162
    insomnia 161
    morning sickness 162
    nerve compression syndromes
      155–7
    nightmares 161
    osteoporosis 154–5
    postural backache 154
    pruritus 161
    restless leg syndrome 159–60
    sacroiliac joint dysfunction
      150–2
    sciatica 152
    symphysis pubis dysfunction
      153
    urinary disorders 162
    uterine ligament pain 160
    see also individual problems
  early care 104
  ectopic 15, 45
  estimated date of delivery (EDD)
    30
  exercise during *see* exercise
  father's role 132–3
  foetal development 29–31
    see also foetus
  insomnia 161
  mask of (chloasma) 38
  medications during 124–5
  multiple 47, 125
    preterm delivery 125
  myths 300
  physical/physiological changes
    31–43, 35 (fig.)
    breasts 38
    cardiovascular system 36–7
    endocrine system 32–3
    gastrointestinal system 39
    musculoskeletal system 41
    nervous system 40

  reproductive system 33–6
  respiratory system 37–8
  skin 38–9
  urinary system 41
  weight gain 40 (fig.)
  physiological anaemia of 36
  sexuality 300
  smoking 123–4
  unstable/transverse lie 49–50
  see also antenatal care
Pregnancy-associated osteoporosis
  154–5
Pregnancy hypotensive syndrome
  37
Pregnancy test 41
Prelabour 36, 53–4
Premature delivery 31, 200
  maternal exercising and 115–16
Premature ovarian failure (POF)
  293–4
Premenopausal women 250
  sexuality 301
Premenstrual tension (PMT) 290
  legal cases 290
Pressure flow studies 442–4
Private antenatal care 97
Procidentia 286
Proctalgia fugax 389
Progesterone 14
  blood vessels, effect on 36
  effects in pregnancy 32–3
Progestogens, foetal development
  30
Prolactin 85
Prolapse *see* genital prolapse
Prolapsed cord 56, 76
Prostaglandins
  labour interventions 79
  production in labour 57
Pruritus
  pregnancy 161
  vulval 272
Psychiatric disorders, defaecation
  difficulties 397
Psychological aspects, gynaecological
  surgery 321–2
Psychological effects, childbirth 167
Psychological problems, constipation
  399
Psychological symptoms, postnatal
  233–6
Psychosexual problems 294–8
  aetiology 294–5
  see also sexual dysfunction
Pubocervical fascia 18
Pubococcygeus 5–6
  during labour 55
  type ll muscle fibres 10 (table)

Puborectalis muscles 6
    defaecation 388
    during labour 55
    paradoxical contraction 389
Pubovaginalis 6
Puboviceralis 5–6
Pudendal nerve 10
    damage during labour 65
    elderly 399
Pudendal nerve terminal motor
        latency (PNTML) 409
Puerperal infection 88
Puerperal psychosis 234–5
Puerperium 84–8
    'after-pains' 84, 229–30
    complications 87–8
    defaecation difficulties 396
    lactation 85–6
    loss of baby 199–200, 201
    management 86–7
    perineum 85
        dysfunction/pain 221–4
    physical condition 206–7
    psychological state 207
    psychosis 234–5
    sexuality 300–1
    sexual problems 300
    stillbirth 200–1
    uterus 84–5
    vagina 85
Pulmonary embolism, postnatal 87–8,
        231
Pulsed electromagnetic energy
        (PEME), perineal
        dysfunction/pain 224

Q

Quality of life questionnaire,
        incontinence assessment 360

R

Radiotherapy, pelvis 314
Raloxifene, osteoporosis treatment 263
Randell, Minnie xvii
Rectal sensitivity training 418–19
Rectoanal inhibitory reflex (RAIR) 386
    testing 408
Rectocoele 285 (fig.), 287, 396–7
    surgical treatment 315–6
Rectovaginal fistula 225
Rectovaginal septum, tear 396
Rectum 22, 23 (fig.)
    defaecation 387
Reflex latencies, urinary tract 462–3
Relaxation 130, 167–70

antenatal 109–10, 112 (fig.), 219
    benefits 168
    in labour 129
    postnatal 215
    techniques 167–9
        assessment 169
        dissociation and unblocking
            168–9
        imagery 170
        Mitchell method 168
        teaching 169–70
        tense–relax technique 168
        touch relaxation 169
Relaxin 33, 38, 42
Renal disorders, preconceptual care
        102
Reproductive tract 13–18, 14 (fig.)
    circulation and nerve supply 17
    fallopian tubes 15
    ovaries see ovaries
    pregnancy effects 33–6
    suspensory ligaments 17–18, 18
        (fig.)
    uterus (womb) see uterus
    vagina see vagina
Respiratory system
    gynaecological surgery 323–4
    labour, effect on 64, 170–1
    maternal exercising 115
    pregnancy effects 37–8
    see also breathing
Rest
    after labour 86–7
    antenatal 219
Restless leg syndrome, pregnancy
        159–60
Retraction 15
Rhabdosphincter (striated urogenital
        sphincter muscle) 20
Rhesus negative blood group,
        umbilical cord clamping 72
Rheumatoid arthritis, pregnancy 44
Royal College of Midwives (RMC) xvii
Royal College of Obstetricians and
        Gynaecologists (RCOG)
    intimate examinations guidelines
        355
    water birth guidelines 190

S

Sacral colpopexy 316
Sacroiliac joint 1
Sacroiliac joint dysfunction 5, 146–7,
        150–2
    treatment 150–2
        Cyriax 151
        leg pull 151

self-help 151 (fig.), 152 (fig.)
        side lying 152
        TENS 152
Sacroiliac ligaments, ventral (anterior)
        posterior 2 (fig.), 3
Sacrum 3–4
    rotation under loading 4, 4 (fig.)
Safe Motherhood Initiative 95
Salmonella, in pregnancy 121
Salpingectomy 313
Salpingitis 275
Salpingostomy 316
Scabies 273
Sciatica 152
Sclerosis, sacroiliac joints 150
Scrotal pain 432, 433
Seat belts, correct position 106, 107
        (fig.)
Selective oestrogen receptor
        modulators (SERMS),
        osteoporosis treatment 263
Sensory blockade, epidural
        anaesthesia 194
Sexual abuse
    bowel dysfunction 404
    defaecation difficulties 391
Sexual dysfunction 295
    male 253–4
    postnatal 235–6
    see also psychosexual problems
Sexual intercourse
    labour induction 57
    lower urinary tract symptoms
        431
    urinary incontinence and 347–8
Sexuality 300–3
    ageing 301–2
    cancer 303
    climacteric 253–4, 301–2
    pregnancy 300
    premenopause 301
    puerperium 300–1
Sexually transmitted disease (STD)
        273, 274
    pelvic inflammatory disease 275
    testing in antenatal care 99–100
Sexual self rating (SSR) scale,
        premenopause 301
Sickle cell disease (SCD), pregnancy
        49
Sitting
    postnatal care 216
    pregnancy 144–5
    puerperium 214
Skin
    menopause 252–3
    pregnancy 38–9
Small for gestational age (SFGA) 31
Smoking

cessation 124
  menopause and 249
  pregnancy 123–4
oiling, passive 389
onic-aid monitor 99
pecial care baby unit (SCBU) 200
phincterotomy, anal fissure 396
pinal anaesthesia, total 195
tages of labour 54–5
tanding
  postnatal posture 214, 216
  pregnancy 145–6
Staphylococcus 272
Statins, osteoporosis treatment 264
Stillbirth 200–1
Stimulants, bowel dysfunction 412
St Mark's Hospital, four stage
    'holding on' programme 411
Stoma cells 14
Stool(s)
  blood in 394
  Bristol stool chart 385 (fig.)
  liquid 401
Straining
  anal incontinence 401
  prolonged, defaecation difficulties
      397
Strength duration curves 410
Stress
  antenatal period 109–10
  constipation 399
  labour 64
  physiological effects 110–11
  reducing techniques 103
  scale 111 (table)
Stress incontinence 225, 317–18, 430,
    469
  definition 435
  gynaecological surgery 317–20
  postnatal complication 241
  surgical procedures 317–20
  treatment 367
  urodynamic (USI) 345–6
Stretch marks (striae) 39
Stretch receptors
  anorectal region 23
  bladder wall 339
Striated urogenital sphincter muscle
    20
Stroke, HRT and 255
Stroke volume, pregnancy effect 37
Subfertility 103–4, 293
Subtotal hysterectomy 311
Sudden infant death syndrome (SIDS)
    201
  smoking risk 124
Suicide 94
Supervisor of Midwives 95
Supine hypotension 114

Surgery
  anal fissure 396
  anal incontinence 400
  endometriosis 282–3
  see also gynaecological surgery
Suspensory ligaments 17–18, 18 (fig.)
Swimming 118–19, 220
Symphysis pubis 1
  diastasis 242
  dysfunction (SPD) 106–8, 153
  pain 5, 142, 229
Syntocinon 196

T

Tamoxifen, osteoporosis treatment 263
Temperature (body)
  foetal malformations and 115
  labour effects 65
TENS 185–9
  brief intense 186–7
  burst train 186
  considerations 188
  electrode placement 187
  low back pain in pregnancy 149
  meralgia paraesthetica 157
  midwives 189
  modes of stimulation 186–7
  obstetric units 189
  sacral electrodes 188
  sacroiliac joint dysfunction 152
  safety 187–8
  spinal electrodes 188
  trials 185–6
Tension-free vaginal tape (TVT)
    317–18, 319
Term Breech Trial 75
Testosterone
  female implants 261
  male decline 253
Tetracycline, pregnancy 124
Thalassaemia, pregnancy 49
Thalidomide, pregnancy 124
'The knack' 367, 371
Thermoregulation, maternal
    exercising 114
Thighs, discomfort during labour 61
'Third day blues' 234
Thoracic arteries, internal 13
Thoracic region
  lordosis 142
  pain 142, 228
  spine pain 154
Thromboembolism 159
Thrombosis
  deep vein thrombosis (DVT)
    postnatal 230–1
    postoperative 328

pregnancy 159
  puerperium 87–8, 230
Thrush 272
Tibial nerve compression, pregnancy
    157
Tibolone, osteoporosis treatment
    263
Toxoplasmosis, pregnancy 121–2
Transcutaneous electrical nerve
    stimulation *see* TENS
Transformation zone, large loop
    excision 313
Translabial real-time ultrasound
    410
Transperineal real-time ultrasound
    410
Transvaginal sacrospinous fixation
    316
Transverse abdominis contractions,
    position for 108 (fig.)
'Transverse arrest' 76
Transverse cervical ligaments 18
Transverse lie 49–50
Transversus abdominis muscle
    11
Trauma, anal incontinence 400
Triangular ligament *see* perineal
    membrane
Trichlorethylene (Trilene) 190
Trichomonas vaginalis 274
Trigone 19
Trilene (trichlorethylene) 190
Trophoblast 29
Tumour(s) *see* cancer
Tuohy needle 193
TVT *see* tension-free vaginal tape
Twins and Multiple Birth Association
    (TAMBA) 240

U

UK Central Council, TENS
    recommendations 189
Ultrasound
  antenatal screening 101
  bladder 360–1
  foetal heart monitor 70
  perineal dysfunction/pain 223
  real-time 410
Umbilical cord
  clamping 72
  controlled traction 73
  knotted 76
  prolapse 56, 76
Umbilical ligament, median (urachus)
    20
Undeveloped countries, maternal
    deaths 93–4

UNICEF UK Baby Friendly Initiative, ten steps of successful breastfeeding 134
Unstable lie 49–50
Ureter 19
Urethra 17, 20–2
blood supply 21
distal electric conductance 363
dyssynergia 349
function 470
filling cystometry 441–2
micturition 443, 444
storage phase 468
pain 432
Urethral pain syndrome 432
Urethral pressure profile (UPP) 362, 452–4
definitions 453–4
female, ICS recommended nomenclature 454 (fig.)
storage phase 452–3
technique 453
voiding (VUPP) 362, 459
Urethral sphincter 20–1, 21 (fig.)
Urethral syndrome 252
Urethrocoele 285, 285 (fig.)
treatment 314
Urethrovaginal sphincter 21
Urethrovesical angle 20, 338
Urge incontinence 345, 377, 430
see also urinary dysfunction and urinary incontinence, detrusor overactivity
Urinalysis 352
Urinary dysfunction 342–82
causes 365 (table)
incontinence see urinary incontinence
lower urinary tract see lower urinary tract dysfunction
menopause 252
preconceptual care 103
pregnancy 162
understanding 364
urgency 226, 343–5, 429–30
Urinary function 333–42
continence 333
problems 334
factors in normal 341–2
micturition see micturition
understanding 364
Urinary incontinence 20, 224, 225, 343–82, 429, 430, 468–9
assessment
bladder ultrasound 360–1
cystometry 361–2
distal urethral electric conductance 363

electrophysiological tests 363–4
form 350–1 (fig.)
imaging 364
physiotherapy 349–61
questionnaires 360
urethral pressure profilometry 362
urinalysis 352
urinary flow 456–7, 457 (fig.)
urodynamic/radiological/EMG 361–4
uroflowmetry 362–3
VAS 360
definition 435
detrusor overactivity 343–5, 346
idiopathic 344
neurogenic 344
terminology 344–5
VPFMC 344–5
exercises to prevent 108
extra-urethral 343
factors leading to 335
frequency 342, 429
functional 348
giggle incontinence 347
history 351–2
caution 352
infection 361
mixed 345
treatment 368
nocturnal enuresis 342, 346–7
pad test 354–5
paper towel test 355
patients at risk 335
perineal/vaginal assessment 355–6
persistant 379
pregnancy 41, 162
prevalence 334
prevention 335
recent developments 335
sexual activity-associated 347–8
stress see stress incontinence
treatment 364–79
additional techniques 367–8
attendance 372
bladder retraining 377
continence-promoting advice 368
devices 379
electrical stimulation 375–6
home 367, 376
persistent problems 379
principles 367
sociological problems 366
types 343–8
see also lower urinary tract dysfunction
Urinary infections 17, 20, 361

Urinary leaking 430
Urinary output, pregnancy 41
Urinary retention 349
acute 444
chronic 445
epidural anaesthesia 194
postnatal 225–6
Urinary tract 18–22
bladder see bladder
infection 361
kidney 18–19
lower see lower urinary tract
neurophysiological evaluation 460–5
electromyograph (EMG) 460–2
evoke responses 464–5
nerve conduction studies 462–3, 464–3
reflex latencies 464
sensory testing 465
pregnancy effects 41
urether 19
urethra see urethra
Urinary urgency 398, 429, 433
postnatal 226
Urine
analysis during pregnancy 98
average flow rate (AUFR) 338
increased output after labour 85
loss, quantification 454–6
maximul urine flow rate (MUFR) 338
pressure flow studies 442–3
residual 459–60
storage 337, 339
storage evaluation 450–6
cystometry 450–2
quantification of urine loss 454–6
urethral pressure measurement 452–4
voiding see micturition
Urodynamic conditions 444–5
see also lower urinary tract dysfunction
Urodynamic stress incontinence (USI) 345–6
Urodynamic studies 428, 436–44
ambulatory 437
conventional 436–7
filling cystometry 361, 437–42
pressure flow studies 362, 442–4
symbols 471–2
units of measurement 470–1
Uroflowmetry 362–3
Urogenital diaphragm see perineal membrane
Uterine contractions
Braxton Hicks 36

breathing 172–7
first stage of labour 54
hypertonic 198
hypotonic 198
labour sign 56
oxytocin effect 56, 57, 84, 197
Uterine ligament, pain, pregnancy 160
Uterine muscles 17
Uterine prolapse 286–7, 286 (fig.)
surgical repair 316
Uterine tissue, in puerperium 84–5
Uterosacral ligaments 5, 18
Uterus 15–16
anteflexed 283
anteverted 283
benign tumour 278–9
collagenous tissue 35
congenital malformations 15–16
didelphys 15–16
fibroids 45–6
growth during pregnancy 33–6, 34 (fig.)
infections 275
malignant tumour 280
muscle fibres 16 (fig.), 35–6
puerperium 84–5
removal see hysterectomy
retroflexed 284
retroverted 284
see also entries beginning uterine

V

Vacuum extraction (ventouse delivery) 199
labour interventions 81
unassisted vaginal birth vs. 211–12
Vagina 16–17
atrophy 250, 251–2
cysts 278
disorders 273–4
menopause 250
soreness 251
prolapse 436
in puerperium 85
tearing during labour 65
see also entries beginning vaginal
Vaginal assessment 355–7, 391, 435–6
chaperone 356
consent 356

during labour 58–9
guidelines 355
labour 68
procedure 356–7
stress incontinence 241
transition stage 174–5
vaginal cones 374
Vaginal discharge 273–4
family planning method 27, 29
menstruation cycle, changes during 27, 29
Vaginal haematoma 221
labour complications 78
Vaginal hysterectomy see hysterectomy
Vaginal pain/discomfort 240
definitions 432, 433
Vaginal pain syndrome 433
Vaginal vault prolapse – surgical repair 316
Vaginal wall, repair 314
Vaginismus 295–6
primary 295
secondary 296
Vaginitis 273
Valsalva manoeuvre 64
Varicose veins
postnatal 230
pregnancy 37, 157
vulval 157–8
Vascular plexus 21
Vena cava 17
Venereal Disease Research Laboratory (VDRL) 100
Venous thromboembolism (VTE), HRT 260
Ventouse delivery see vacuum extraction (ventouse delivery)
Very low birth weight infants (VLBW) 31
Vesicovaginal fistula 88, 94
Violence, in pregnancy 98
Viral infections 273
Visual analogue scale (VAS), incontinence assessment 360
Visualisation and imagery, neuromuscular control 112
Vitamin D, osteoporosis 258
Vocalisation, in labour 174–5, 176
Voiding, prompted, timed 377
Voiding difficulties 348
Voiding dysfunction 444

postoperative complications 328
symptoms 430–1
see also micturition
Vomiting in pregnancy 39
HCG role 30
hyperemesis gravidarum 39
Vulva
cancer 277–8
disorders 272
infections 271–3
pain 432, 433
surgery 313
varicose veins 157–8
Vulval pain syndrome 433
Vulvar vestibulitis 299
Vulvectomy 313
Vulvitis 271–2
Vulvodynia 298–9
Vulvovaginitis 271

W

Walking
postnatal exercise 219
pregnancy 145–6
Water births 95, 190
safety 190
Water retention, pregnancy 40, 43
'Waters,' breaking of 55–6
Weight gain in pregnancy 39, 40 (fig.), 119–26
labour duration, effect on 66
measurement during 98
normal 119
Wertheim's hysterectomy 311
Womb see uterus
Workplace, defaecation difficulties 393
World Health Organization (WHO), breastfeeding recommendations 133–4
Wound healing, caesarean section 238
Wound infection, postoperation complications 328
Wrigley's forceps 81

Y

Yoga, maternal exercising 119